Nursing Care Plans and Documentation

Nursing Diagnoses and Collaborative Problems

NursingCarePlans andDocumentation

Nursing Diagnoses and Collaborative Problems

Lynda Juall Carpenito, R.N., M.S.N.

Nursing Consultant, Mickleton, New Jersey

With 30 Contributors

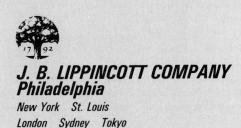

J. B. LIPPINCOTT COMPANY
Philadelphia
New York   St. Louis
London   Sydney   Tokyo

Acquisitions Editor: Donna Hilton, R.N., B.S.N.
Coordinating Editorial Assistant: Barbara Nelson Cullen
Project Editor: Tom Gibbons
Indexer: Ellen Murray
Art Director: Ellen C. Dawson
Interior Designer: Ellen C. Dawson
Cover Designer: Louis Fuiano
Production Manager: Helen Ewan
Production Coordinator: Pamela Milcos
Compositor: Tapsco, Inc.
Printer/Binder: Courier Westford, Inc.

3 5 6 4

Library of Congress Cataloging-in-Publication Data

Carpenito, Lynda Juall.
    Nursing care plans and documentation: nursing diagnosis and collaborative prob-
lems/Lynda Juall Carpenito with 30 contributors.
        p.   cm.
    Includes bibliographical references.
    Includes index.
    ISBN 0-397-54681-5
    1. Nursing care plans.   2. Nursing assessment.   3. Diagnosis.
I. Title.
    [DNLM: 1. Nursing Diagnosis.   2. Patient Care Planning.   WY 100
C294n]
RT49.C38   1991
610.73—dc20
DNLM/DLC
for Library of Congress   90-6362
                                                                                  CIP

Any procedure or practice described in this book should be applied by the health-care practitioner under appropriate supervision in accordance with professional standards of care used with regard to the unique circumstances that apply in each practice situation. Care has been taken to confirm the accuracy of information presented and to describe generally accepted practices. However, the authors, editors, and publisher cannot accept any responsibility for errors or omissions or for any consequences from application of the information in this book and make no warranty, express or implied, with respect to the contents of the book.

Every effort has been made to ensure drug selections and dosages are in accordance with current recommendations and practice. Because of ongoing research, changes in government regulations and the constant flow of information on drug therapy, reactions and interactions, the reader is cautioned to check the package insert for each drug for indications, dosages, warnings and precautions, particularly if the drug is new or infrequently used.

To Pati, my sister

Your lessons to the children you teach
go beyond the book

You offer strength to those in need

You will not be silenced by power

We have feared together, cried together
and rejoiced together

Blood has made us sisters, trust has
made us friends

Contributors

Caroline McAlpine Alterman, R.N., M.S.N.
Clinical Nurse Specialist, Shepherd Spinal Center, Atlanta, Georgia
(Spinal Cord Injury)

Lynn M. Bobel, R.N., C., M.S.N.
Clinical Nurse Specialist, Nursing Manager, Huron Valley Hospital, Milford, Michigan
(Total Parenteral Nutrition, Peptic Ulcer Disease, Enteral Nutrition)

Sharon Varga Buckingham, B.S.N.
Nursing Education Coordinator, Huron Valley Hospital, Milford, Michigan
(Hypertension, Chronic Obstructive Pulmonary Disease, Gastroenteritis)

Nancy Denton, R.N.
Admission Manager Surgical ISCU, Harper Hospital, Detroit, Michigan
(Hysterectomy)

Sandy K. DeSalvo, R.N., C.C.R.N.
Clinical Nurse III, Renal Dialysis Unit, St. Vincent Infirmary, Little Rock, Arkansas
(Hemodialysis, External Arteriovenous Shunting)

Mary Ann Ducharme, R.N., M.S.N.
Case Manager, Harper Hospital, Detroit, Michigan
(Hemodynamic Monitoring, Peritoneal Dialysis)

Rita Dundon, R.N., M.S.N., C.S.
Oncology Clinical Nurse Specialist, Harper Hospital, Detroit, Michigan
(Cancer [Initial Diagnosis], Chemotherapy, Radiation Therapy, End-Stage Cancer, Long-Term Venous Access Devices)

Doris Fleming, R.N., C., M.S.N.
Clinical Nurse Specialist—Diabetes, Harper Hospital, Detroit, Michigan
(Diabetes Mellitus)

Jill Grodecki, R.N., M.S.N.
Clinical Nurse Specialist, Harper Hospital, Detroit, Michigan
(Leukemia)

Deborah Guziatek-Karwan, R.N., B.S.N.
Assistant Patient Care Coordinator, Harper Hospital, Detroit, Michigan
(Prostatectomy)

Sandra A. Halquist, R.N., B.S.N.
Assistant Patient Care Coordinator, Harper Hospital, Detroit, Michigan
(Radical Vulvectomy)

Evelyn Howard, R.N.
Head Nurse Renal Dialysis Unit, St. Vincent Infirmary, Little Rock, Arkansas
(Acute Renal Failure, Chronic Renal Failure)

Debra Lynn-McHale, R.N., M.S.N., C.C.R.N.
Clinical Nurse Specialist/Critical Care, Thomas Jefferson Hospital, Philadelphia, Pennsylvania
(Percutaneous Transluminal Coronary Angioplasty, Coronary Artery Bypass Grafting)

JoAnn Maklebust, R.N., M.S.N., C.S.
Case Manager, Harper Hospital, Detroit, Michigan
(Colostomy, Ileostomy, Urostomy, Pressure Ulcers, Inflammatory Bowel Disease, Neurogenic Bladder)

Silvia S. Maxwell, R.N.
Clinical Nurse, Harper Hospital, Detroit, Michigan
(Casts)

Linda C. Mondoux, R.N., M.S., C.S.
Clinical Specialist, Botsford Hospital, Farmington, Michigan
(Fractured Hip and Femur, Pneumonia, Osteoporosis, Hypothyroidism)

Patricia Mosko, C.R.N.P.
Adult Nurse Practitioner, Temple University Hospital, Philadelphia, Pennsylvania
(Inflammatory Joint Disease [Rheumatoid Arthritis, Infectious Arthritis], Systemic Lupus Erythematosus, Anticoagulant Therapy, Corticosteroid Therapy)

Victoria Navarro, R.N., M.S.A.
Assistant Director of Nursing, Wilmer Ophthalmological Institute, The Johns Hopkins Hospital, Baltimore, Maryland
(Penetrating Keratoplasty [Corneal Transplant])

Beth Ormandy, R.N.
Clinical Nurse, Harper Hospital, Detroit, Michigan
(Casts)

Rhonda Rhea Panfilli, R.N., M.S.N.
Clinical Nurse Specialist, Harper Hospital, Detroit, Michigan
(Obesity)

Jeanne S. Parzuchowski, R.N., M.S.
Case Manager, Harper Hospital, Detroit, Michigan
(Tracheostomy, Radical Neck Dissection, Laryngectomy)

Lee-Anne M. Placzek, R.N., B.S.N.
Administrative Manager, Harper Hospital, Detroit, Michigan
(Cesium Implant)

Margaret P. Price, R.N., M.S.
Nursing Director Critical Care Unit, Huron Valley Hospital, Milford, Michigan
(Cranial Surgery, Laminectomy)

Hattie L. Robinson, R.N.
Assistant Administrative Manager, Harper Hospital, Detroit, Michigan
(Casts)

Pamela S. Schremp, R.N., M.S.N.
Clinical Nurse Specialist, Lorain Community Hospital, Lorain, Ohio
(Glaucoma, Cataract Extraction, Enucleation, Ophthalmic Surgery)

Mary Sieggreen, R.N., M.S.N., C.S.
Clinical Nurse Specialist Vascular, Harper Hospital, Detroit, Michigan
(Carotid Endarterectomy, Amputation, Abdominal Aortic Aneurysm Resection, Arterial Bypass Grafting in the Lower Extremity, Arteriography, Deep Venous Thrombosis, Venous Stasis Ulcers, Peripheral Arterial Disease [Atherosclerosis], Raynaud's Syndrome, Percutaneous Transluminal Coronary Angioplasty)

Carolyn Sipes, R.N., M.S.N.
Clinical Nurse Specialist, Program Coordinator, Immunodeficient Clinic, Children's Hospital, Columbus, Ohio
(Acquired Immunodeficiency Syndrome)

Frances Tolley, R.N., B.S.N.
Head Nurse, Wilmer Ophthalmological Institute, The Johns Hopkins Hospital, Baltimore, Maryland
(Penetrating Keratoplasty [Corneal Transplant])

Susan A. Walthall, R.N., M.S.N.
Clinical Nurse Specialist, Harper Hospital, Detroit, Michigan
(Cardiac Catheterization, Pacemaker Insertion)

Peter Wozniak, R.N.
Clinical Director, Harper Hospital, Detroit, Michigan
(Casts)

Preface

*Nursing is primarily assisting individuals (sick or well) with those activities con-
tributing to health, or its recovery (or to a peaceful death) that they perform unaided
when they have the necessary strength, will or knowledge; nursing also helps individuals carry out prescribed therapy and to be independent of assistance as soon
as possible (Henderson, 1960)*

Historically, nurses have represented the core of the health care delivery system (acute, long term,
and community agencies), but their image continues to be one of individuals whose actions are
dependent on physician supervision. However, as Diers (1981) wrote, "Nursing is exceedingly
complicated work since it involves technical skill, a great deal of formal knowledge, communication
ability, use of self, timing, emotional investment and any number of other qualities." What it also
involves—and what is hidden from the public—is the complex process of thinking that leads from
the knowledge to the skill, from the perception to the action, from the decision to the touch, from
the observation to the diagnosis. Yet it is this process of nursing care, which is at the center of
nursing's work, that is so little described.

One way for this process of nursing work to be made visible is for every nurse to describe,
discuss and publicize the plan of nursing care. Physicians regularly and openly explain the measures
they plan to the public, especially clients and families. However, nurses often fail to consistently
explain their plan of care. This book provides both a framework for nurses to provide quality
nursing care and guidelines for them to document and communicate that care.

The focus of this book is independent nursing care—the management of client situations
that the nurse can treat legally and independently. It will assist students in transferring their
theoretical knowledge to clinical practice; it can help experienced nurses to provide quality care
in a variety of clinical situations. The care plans presented in this book can also be used to
formulate standards of care in a health care agency. The author recommends that committees of
staff nurses review the care plans that directly relate to their units. During the review, the staff
nurses can evaluate whether the plan represents the care that is regularly provided to the clients
in their population. Revisions (additions or deletions) can be made to create the agency-specific
standard. In this way, the standard of care will reflect actual practice, as is necessary both legally
and professionally.

The Bifocal Clinical Practice Model underpins this book and serves to organize the nursing
care plans in Unit II. Chapter 1 describes and discusses the Bifocal Clinical Practice Model, which
differentiates nursing diagnoses from other problems that nurses treat. In this chapter, nursing
diagnoses and collaborative problems are explained and differentiated. The relationship of the type
of diagnosis to outcome criteria and nursing interventions is also emphasized.

Effective and appropriate documentation of nursing care is outlined in Chapter 2. Legal
issues, standards, and regulatory agencies and their effect on nursing documentation are discussed.
The chapter explains a documentation system from admission to discharge. Sample forms are used
to emphasize efficient, professional charting.

Chapter 3 explores the issues and human responses associated with illness and hospitalization.
Coping strategies of the client and family are described. The chapter emphasizes the importance
of assisting the client and family with end-of-life discussions whenever possible, before a crisis
occurs.

Chapter 4 focuses on the surgical experience and the related nursing care to discuss the
human response to the experience. Preoperative assessment and preparation are described for
preadmitted surgical clients. The nursing responsibilities in the postanesthesia recovery room are
described, and the related documentation forms are included. This chapter also outlines the in-

tegration of the nursing process in caring for same-day surgery clients; again, the corresponding forms that will help the nurse do this are included.

Unit II presents care plans that represent a compilation of the complex work of nursing in caring for individuals (and their families) experiencing medical disorders or surgical interventions or undergoing a diagnostic or therapeutic procedure. It uses the nursing process to present the type of nursing care that is expected to be necessary for persons experiencing similar situations. The plans provide the nurse with a framework for providing initial, or essential, care. This is the nursing care known to be provided when a certain clinical situation is present—for example, preoperative teaching for persons awaiting surgery or the management of fatigue in individuals with arthritis. As the nurse intervenes and continues to assess, additional diagnoses, goals, and interventions can be added to the initial plan. Even though the type of care that is warranted for persons in certain clinical situations is predictable, the nurse must still assess the individual for unexpected responses.

The book concludes with three Appendices. Appendix I presents a generic care plan for hospitalized clients, along with guidelines for its use in a health care agency; Appendix II is a generic care plan for general surgery clients, focusing on both pre- and postoperative care; and Appendix III shows a generic care plan for a client experiencing outpatient (same-day) surgery.

The intent of this book is to assist the nurse to identify the responsible care that nurses are accountable to provide. By using the Bifocal Clinical Practice Model, it clearly defines the scope of independent practice. The author invites comments and suggestions from readers. Correspondence can be directed to the publisher or to the author's address: 66 East Rattling Run Road, Mickleton, NJ 08056.

References

Diers, D. (1981). Why write? Why publish? *Image, 13;*1–7
Henderson, V., & Nite, G. (1960). *Principles and practice of nursing* (5th ed.), New York: Macmillan, p. 14

Acknowledgments

This project was more difficult than I anticipated. Thank you, Nancy Mullins, for your encouragement in the early developmental work. I am also grateful for the continued support from other J.B. Lippincott personnel, including Ellen Campbell, Barbara Nelson Cullen, and Diana Intenzo. The copy editing by Kevin Law was tenacious and thorough. A special note to Donna Hilton, who joined this project midstream as my editor; thank you for your professional challenges and support.

My family was asked once again to live through the pain of developing a new book. My son Olen continues to provide me with reminders of what is important: love, health, and trust. My husband Richard continues to nurture me through the difficult times. Together we *are* because of each other.

Contents

UNIT II
CLINICAL NURSING CARE PLANS

Section 1
Medical Disorders

Section 2
Surgical Procedures

Section 3
Diagnostic and Therapeutic Procedures

UNIT 1

Introduction to Care Planning

The path to universal recognition of nursing as a profession has been tumultuous. When any occupational group seeks to claim professional status, the following requisites are universally demanded:

- [ ] An extensive university education
- [ ] A unique body of knowledge
- [ ] An orientation of service to others
- [ ] A professional society
- [ ] Autonomy and self-regulation (Styles, 1982)

The classification activities of the North American Nursing Diagnosis Association (NANDA) have been instrumental in defining nursing's unique body of knowledge. This unified system of terminology

- [ ] Provides consistent language (oral and written)
- [ ] Stimulates nurses to acquire new knowledge
- [ ] Establishes a system for automation, reimbursement
- [ ] Provides an educational framework
- [ ] Allows efficient information retrieval for research and quality assurance
- [ ] Provides a consistent structure for literature presentation of nursing knowledge
- [ ] Clarifies nursing as an art and a science for its members and society
- [ ] Establishes standards to which nurses are held accountable

Table 1-1 provides a list of NANDA-approved nursing diagnoses.

Clearly, nursing diagnosis has positively influenced the nursing profession. However, integration of nursing diagnosis into nursing practice has proven problematic. Although references to nursing diagnosis in the literature have increased one hundredfold since the first meeting in 1973 of the National Group for the Classification of Nursing Diagnosis (which later became NANDA), nurses have not seen efficient and representative applications. For example, nurses have been directed to use nursing diagnoses exclusively to describe their clinical focus. However, nurses who strongly support nursing diagnosis often become frustrated when they try to attach a nursing diagnosis label to every facet of nursing practice. Some of the dilemmas that result from the attempt to label as nursing diagnoses all situations in which nurses intervene are as follows:

1. *Using nursing diagnoses without validation.* When the nursing diagnostic categories are the only labels or diagnostic statements that can be used by the nurse, the nurse is encouraged to "change the data to fit the label,"

for example, using the Altered Nutrition category for all NPO patients. Potential for Injury frequently serves as a "waste basket" diagnosis, because all potentially injurious situations (e.g., bleeding) can be captured within a Potential for Injury diagnosis.

2. *Renaming medical diagnoses.* Clinical nurses know that an important component of their practice is monitoring for the onset and status of physiological complications and initiating both nurse-prescribed and physician-prescribed interventions. Morbidity and mortality are reduced and prevented because of nursing's expert management.

    If nursing diagnoses would describe all situations in which nurses intervene, then clearly a vast number must be developed to describe the situations identified on the International Code of Diseases (ICD-9). Table 1-2 represents examples of misuse of nursing diagnoses and the renaming of medical diagnoses. Examination of the substitution of nursing diagnosis terminology for medical diagnoses or pathophysiology in Table 1-2 gives rise to several questions:
    - [ ] Should nursing diagnoses describe all situations in which nurses intervene?
    - [ ] If a situation is not called a nursing diagnosis, is it then less important or scientific?
    - [ ] How will it serve the profession to rename as nursing diagnoses the pathophysiological situations that nurses co-treat with physicians?
    - [ ] Will using the examples in Table 1-2 improve communication and clarify nursing?

3. *Omitting problem situations in documentation.* If a documentation system requires the use of nursing diagnosis exclusively, and if the nurse does not choose to "change the data to fit a category" or "to rename pathophysiology," then the nurse has no terminology to describe a critical component of nursing practice. Failure to describe these situations can seriously jeopardize nursing's effort to justify and affirm the need for professional nurses in all health care settings (Carpenito, 1983).

THE DIMENSIONS OF NURSING

In the 20th century, nursing has been challenged to differentiate itself from medicine for legislative and educational purposes. Into the 1970s, nursing education in many schools continued to focus on medical diagnoses rather than nursing problems. At the same time, various theoretical or conceptual frameworks were developed to organize nursing knowledge and practice, such as Roy's Adaptation Model, Johnson's Behavioral System Model, Orem's Self-care Model, Roger's Life Process Theory, and Newman's Health Systems Model.

Frameworks or theories of nursing should help to distinguish nursing within the broad field of health care. The Bifocal Clinical Practice Model serves to distinguish nursing from other health care disciplines.

THE BIFOCAL CLINICAL PRACTICE MODEL

Nursing's theoretical knowledge derives from the natural, physical, and behavioral sciences, the humanities, and nursing research. Nurses can use various theories in practice, including family systems, loss, growth and development, crisis intervention, and general systems theories.

TABLE 1-1. *Nursing Diagnostic Categories Grouped Under Functional Health Patterns**

1. HEALTH PERCEPTION-HEALTH MANAGEMENT
   Growth and Development, Alt.
   Health Maintenance, Alt.
   Health Seeking Behaviors
   Noncompliance
   High Risk for Injury
      High Risk for Suffocation
      High Risk for Poisoning
      High Risk for Trauma
2. NUTRITIONAL-METABOLIC
   Body Temperature, High Risk for Alt.
      Hypothermia
      Hyperthermia
      Thermoregulation, Ineffective
   †Breastfeeding, Effective
   Breastfeeding, Ineffective
   Fluid Volume Deficit
   Fluid Volume Excess
   Infection, High Risk for
   ‡Infection Transmission, High Risk for
   Nutrition, Alt: Less Than Body Requirements
      Swallowing, Impaired
   Nutrition, Alt: More Than Body Requirements
   Nutrition, Alt: Potential for More Than Body Requirements
   †Protection, Alt.
      Tissue Integrity, Imp.
         Oral Mucous Membrane, Alt.
         Skin Integrity, Imp.
3. ELIMINATION
   ‡Bowel Elimination, Alt.
      Constipation
      Colonic Constipation
      Perceived Constipation
      Diarrhea
      Bowel Incontinence
   Urinary Elimination, Alt. Patterns of
      Urinary Retention
      Total Incontinence
      Functional Incontinence
      Reflex Incontinence

   Urge Incontinence
   Stress Incontinence
   ‡Maturational Enuresis
4. ACTIVITY-EXERCISE
   Activity Intolerance
   Cardiac Output, Decreased
   Disuse Syndrome, High Risk for
   Diversional Activity Deficit
   Home Maintenance Management, Imp.
   Mobility, Imp. Physical
   ‡Respiratory Function, High Risk for Alt.
      Ineffective Airway Clearance
      Ineffective Breathing Patterns
      Imp. Gas Exchange
   ‡Self-Care Deficit Syndrome
      Bathing/Hygiene Self-Care Deficit
      Dressing/Grooming Self-Care Deficit
      Feeding Self-Care Deficit
      Instrumental Self-Care Deficit
      Toileting Self-Care Deficit
   Tissue Perfusion, Alt: (Specify) (Cerebral, Cardiopulmonary, Renal, Gastrointestinal, Peripheral)
5. SLEEP-REST
   Sleep Pattern Disturbance
6. COGNITIVE-PERCEPTUAL
   ‡Comfort, Alt.
      Pain
      Chronic Pain
   Decisional Conflict
   Dysreflexia
   Knowledge Deficit: (Specify)
   High Risk for Aspiration
   Sensory-Perceptual Alteration: (Specify) (Visual, Auditory, Kinesthetic, Gustatory, Tactile, Olfactory)
   Thought Processes, Alt.
   Unilateral Neglect

7. SELF-PERCEPTION
   Anxiety
   Fatigue
   Fear
   Hopelessness
   Powerlessness
   ‡Self-Concept Disturbance
      Body Image Disturbance
      Personal Identity Disturbance
      Self-Esteem Disturbance
         Chronic Low Self-Esteem
         Situational Low Self-Esteem
8. ROLE-RELATIONSHIP
   ‡Communication, Imp.
      Communication, Imp. Verbal
   Family Processes, Alt.
   ‡Grieving
      Grieving, Anticipatory
      Grieving, Dysfunctional
   Parenting, Alt.
   Parental Role Conflict
   Role Performance, Alt.
   Social Interactions, Imp.
   Social Isolation
9. SEXUALITY-REPRODUCTIVE
   Sexual Dysfunction
   Sexuality Patterns, Alt.
10. COPING-STRESS TOLERANCE
    Adjustment, Imp.
    Coping, Ineffective Individual
       Defensive Coping
       Ineffective Denial
    Coping, Disabling, Ineffective Family
    Coping, Compromised, Ineffective Family
    Coping: Potential for Growth, Family
    Post-Trauma Response
       Rape Trauma Syndrome
    Self-Harm, High Risk for
    Violence, High Risk for
11. VALUE-BELIEF
    Spiritual Distress

alt., altered; *imp.*, impaired

* The Functional Health Patterns were identified in Gordon M: Nursing Diagnosis: Process and Application. New York, McGraw-Hill, 1982, with minor changes by the author.

† These categories were accepted by the North American Nursing Diagnosis Association in 1990.

‡ These diagnostic categories are not currently on the NANDA list but have been included for clarity and usefulness.

TABLE 1-2. *Renaming Medical Diagnoses With Nursing Diagnosis Terminology*

Medical Diagnosis	Nursing Diagnosis
Myocardial Infarction	Decreased Cardiac Output
Shock	
Adult Respiratory Distress	Impaired Gas Exchange
Chronic Obstructive Lung	
Disease	
Asthma	
Alzheimer's Disease	Altered Cerebral Tissue
Increased Intracranial	Perfusion
Pressure	
Retinal Detachment	Sensory–Perceptual Alterations:
	Visual
Thermal Burns	Impaired Tissue Integrity
Incisions, Lacerations	Impaired Skin Integrity
Hemorrhage	Fluid Volume Deficit
Congestive Heart Failure	Fluid Volume Excess

The difference between nursing and the other health care disciplines with which it interfaces lies in nursing's depth and breadth of focus. Other disciplines are restricted to a narrower focus than nursing is. Certainly, the nutritionist has more expertise in the field of nutrition, and the pharmacist in the field of therapeutic pharmacology, than any nurse. Every nurse, however, brings a knowledge of nutrition and pharmacology to client interactions. The depth of this knowledge is sufficient for many client situations; when it is insufficient, then consultation is required. No other discipline has this varied knowledge, thus explaining why attempts to substitute other disciplines for nursing have proved costly and ultimately unsuccessful.

The Bifocal Clinical Practice Model represents the situations that influence persons, groups, and communities, as well as the classification of these responses from a nursing perspective. The situations are organized into five broad categories: pathophysiological, treatment-related, personal, environmental, and maturational. Nursing students should be taught the situations that are regularly encountered in practice. Without an understanding of such situations, the nurse will be unable to diagnose responses and intervene appropriately. Figure 1-1 illustrates examples of each category.

Clinically, these situations are important to nurses. Thus, as nursing diagnoses evolved, nurses sought to substitute nursing terminology for these situations, for example, Impaired Tissue Integrity for burns and Potential for Injury for dialysis. Nurses do not prescribe for and treat these situations, e.g., dialysis and burns. Rather, they prescribe for and treat the *responses* to these situations.

The practice focus for clinical nursing is at the response level, not at the situation level. For example, a client who has sustained burns may exhibit a wide variety of responses to the burns and the treatments. Some may be predicted, such as Potential for Infection; others may not be, such as fear of losing a job. In the past, nurses focused on the nursing interventions associated with treating burns rather than on those associated with the client's responses. This resulted in nurses being described as "doers" rather than "knowers," as technicians rather than scientists.

What this approach to nursing obscured was the fact that embedded in each intervention lay scientific rationales for what was prescribed and why. Although applying a single term—burns—appears attractive from a documentation efficiency standpoint, relying on a single term to describe the entire span of nursing focus has proved to be not conducive to nursing autonomy. A better solution is to establish standards of documentation that are efficient and relevant (Burke and Murphy, 1988). See Chapter 2 for a discussion of documenting nursing care.

Nursing Diagnoses and Collaborative Problems

The Bifocal Clinical Practice Model describes the two foci of clinical nursing: nursing diagnoses and collaborative problems.

A nursing diagnosis is a clinical judgment about individual, family, or community responses to actual or potential health problems/life processes. Nursing diagnosis provides the basis for selection of nursing interventions to achieve outcomes for which the nurse is accountable (NANDA, 1990). *Collaborative problems are certain physiological complications that nurses monitor, to detect their onset or changes in status.* Nurses manage collaborative problems by utilizing both physician-prescribed and nursing-prescribed interventions to minimize the complications of the events (Carpenito, 1990). Figure 1-2 diagrams the Bifocal Clinical Practice Model.

The nurse makes independent decisions for both collaborative problems and nursing diagnoses. The difference is that in nursing diagnoses, nursing prescribes the definitive treatment to achieve the desired outcome, but in collaborative problems, prescription for definitive treatment comes from both nursing and medicine. Some physiological complications (such as Potential for Infection and Impaired Skin Integrity) are nursing diagnoses, for nurses can order the definitive treatment. In a collaborative problem, the nurse primarily monitors for the onset and change in status of physiological complications, to prevent morbidity and mortality. These physiological complications usually are related to disease, trauma, treatments, medications, or diagnostic studies. Thus, collaborative problems can be labeled Potential Complication: (Specify), for example,

Pathophysiological
Myocardial infarction
Borderline personality
Burns

Treatment-related
Anticoagulants
Dialysis
Arteriogram

Personal
Dying
Divorce
Relocation

Environmental
Overcrowded school
No handrails on stairs
Rodents

Maturational
Peer pressure
Parenthood
Aging

Figure 1-1. Examples of pathophysiological, treatment-related, personal, environmental, and maturational situations.

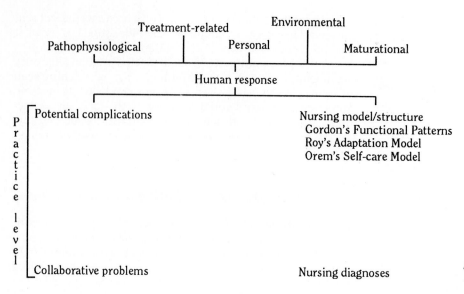

Figure 1-2. Bifocal clinical nursing model. (© 1985, Lynda Juall Carpenito)

Potential Complication: Hemorrhage or Potential Complication: Renal Failure.

Monitoring is not the sole nursing intervention for collaborative problems, however. For example, in addition to monitoring a client with increased intracranial pressure, the nurse also restricts certain activities, maintains head elevation, implements the medical regimen, and continually addresses the client's psychosocial and educational needs.

Below are some collaborative problems that commonly apply to certain situations:

Situation	Collaborative Problem
Myocardial infarction	Potential complication (PC): Dysrhythmias
Craniotomy	PC: Increased intracranial pressure
Hemodialysis	PC: Fluid/electrolyte imbalance
Surgery	PC: Hemorrhage
Cardiac catheterization	PC: Allergic reaction

If the situation calls for the nurse to monitor for a cluster or group of physiological complications, the collaborative problems may be documented as

PC: Cardiac

or

PC post-op   Urinary retention
Hemorrhage
Hypovolemia
Hypoxia
Thrombophlebitis
Renal insufficiency
Paralytic ileus
Evisceration

Table 1-3 provides a list of common collaborative problems.

All physiological complications are not collaborative problems, however. Nurses themselves can prevent some physiological complications, such as infections from external sources (for example, wounds and catheters), contractures, in-

continence, and pressure ulcers. Thus, such complications fall into the category of nursing diagnosis.

Nursing Interventions

Carpenito (1987) stated that the relationship of diagnosis to interventions is a critical element in defining nursing diagnoses. Many definitions of nursing diagnoses focus on the relationship of selected interventions to the diagnoses. A certain type of intervention appears to distinguish a nursing diagnosis from a medical diagnosis or other problems that nurses treat. According to Bulechek and McCloskey (1985), a nursing intervention is "an autonomous action based on scientific rationale that is executed to benefit the client in a predicted way related to the nursing diagnosis and goal." Nursing interventions can be categorized into two types: independent and delegated (Maryland, 1986). Independent interventions are nurse prescribed; delegated interventions are physician prescribed. However, both types of interventions require independent nursing judgment. By law, the nurse must determine whether it is appropriate to initiate an action, regardless of whether it is independent or delegated (Carpenito, 1989).

The type of intervention distinguishes a nursing diagnosis from a collaborative problem and also differentiates between actual, potential, and possible nursing diagnoses. Table 1-4 outlines definitions of each type and the corresponding intervention focus. For example, for a nursing diagnosis of Impaired Tissue Integrity related to immobility as manifested by a 2-cm epidermal lesion on the client's left heel, the nurse would order interventions to monitor the lesion and to eliminate it. In another client with a surgical wound, the nurse would focus on prevention of infection and promotion of healing. Potential for Infection would better describe the situation than Impaired Tissue Integrity. Impaired Tissue Integrity should not be used to describe wounds or burns that require nursing and medical treatment. Instead, the nurse should identify the response to the burn or wound that the nurse can prevent or reduce (i.e., Impaired Physical Mobility, Potential for Infection, Potential for Disuse Syndrome). Nursing diagnoses are not more important than collaborative problems, and collaborative problems are not more important than nursing diagnoses. Priorities are determined by the client's situation, not by whether it is a nursing diagnosis or a collaborative problem.

A *diagnostic cluster* represents those nursing diagnoses and collaborative problems that have a high likelihood of occurring in a client population. The nurse validates their presence in the individual client. Figure 1-3 represents the diagnostic cluster for a client after abdominal surgery. (For more information on differentiating between nursing diagnoses and collaborative problems, refer to Carpenito, 1989, Chapter 2.)

TABLE 1-3.   Collaborative Problems*

Potential Complication: Gastrointestinal–Hepatic
PC: Paralytic Ileus/Small Bowel Obstruction
PC: Hepatorenal Syndrome
PC: Hyperbilirubinemia
PC: Evisceration
PC: Hepatosplenomegaly
PC: Curling's Ulcer
PC: Ascites
PC: Gastrointestinal Bleeding

Potential Complication: Metabolic/Immune
PC: Hypoglycemia
PC: Hyperglycemia
PC: Negative Nitrogen Balance
PC: Electrolyte Imbalances
PC: Thyroid Dysfunction
PC: Hypothermia (severe)
PC: Hyperthermia (severe)
PC: Sepsis
PC: Acidosis/Alkalosis
PC: Diabetes
PC: Anasarca
PC: Hypo/Hyperthyroidism
PC: Allergic Reaction
PC: Donor Tissue Rejection
PC: Adrenal Insufficiency

Potential Complication: Neurologic/Sensory
PC: Increased Intracranial Pressure
PC: Stroke
PC: Seizures
PC: Spinal Cord Compression
PC: Autonomic Dysreflexia
PC: Birth Injuries
PC: Hydrocephalus
PC: Microcephalus
PC: Meningitis
PC: Cranial Nerve Impairment
PC: Paresis/Paresthesia/Paralysis
PC: Peripheral Nerve Impairment
PC: Increased Intraocular Pressure
PC: Corneal Ulceration
PC: Neuropathies

Potential Complication: Cardiovascular
PC: Dysrhythmias
PC: Congestive Heart Failure
PC: Cardiogenic Shock
PC: Thromboemboli/Deep Vein Thrombosis
PC: Hypovolemic Shock
PC: Peripheral Vascular Insufficiency
PC: Hypertension
PC: Congenital Heart Disease
PC: Thrombocytopenia
PC: Polycythemia
PC: Anemia
PC: Compartmental Syndrome
PC: Disseminated Intravascular Coagulation
PC: Endocarditis
PC: Sickling Crisis
PC: Embolism (air, fat)
PC: Spinal Shock
PC: Ischemic Ulcers

Potential Complication: Respiratory
PC: Atelectasis/Pneumonia
PC: Asthma
PC: Chronic Obstructive Pulmonary Disease (COPD)
PC: Pulmonary Embolism
PC: Pleural Effusion
PC: Tracheal Necrosis
PC: Ventilator Dependency
PC: Pneumothorax
PC: Laryngeal Edema
PC: Pneumothorax

Potential Complication: Renal/Urinary
PC: Acute Urinary Retention
PC: Renal Failure
PC: Bladder Perforation

Potential Complication: Reproductive
PC: Fetal Compromise
PC: Uterine Atony
PC: Pregnancy-Induced Hypertension
PC: Eclampsia
PC: Hydramnios
PC: Hypermenorrhea
PC: Polymenorrhea
PC: Syphilis

Potential Complication: Muscular/Skeletal
PC: Stress fractures
PC: Osteoporosis
PC: Joint Dislocation

* The most frequently encountered collaborative problems are represented on this list.

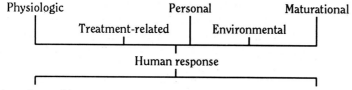

Abdominal surgery (post-op)

Physiologic   Personal   Maturational
  └── Treatment-related ── Environmental ──┘
              Human response

Collaborative problems   Nursing diagnoses

Potential complications:

Hemorrhage
Hypovolemia/shock
Urinary retention
Peritonitis
Urinary retention
Thrombophlebitis
Paralytic ileus
Evisceration
Dehiscence
Infection

Potential Altered Respiratory Function related to immobility
    secondary to postanesthesia state and pain
Potential for Infection related to increased susceptibility
    to bacteria secondary to wound
Altered Comfort related to surgical interruption of
    body structures, flatus, and immobility
Potential Altered Nutrition: Less than Body Requirements
    related to increased protein/vitamin requirements for
    wound healing and decreased intake secondary to pain,
    nausea, vomiting, and diet restrictions
Potential Colonic Constipation related to decreased
    peristalsis secondary to immobility, effects of anesthesia,
    and narcotics
Activity Intolerance related to pain and weakness secondary
    to anesthesia, tissue hypoxia, and insufficient
    fluids/nutrients
Potential Altered Health Maintenance related to insufficient
    knowledge of care of operative site, restrictions (diet,
    activity), medications, signs and symptoms of
    complications, follow-up care

Figure 1-3. Diagnostic cluster for client recovering from abdominal surgery.

Outcome Criteria

In a nursing care plan, outcome criteria are "statements describing a measurable behavior of client/family which denote a favorable status (changed or maintained) after nursing care has been delivered" (Alfaro, 1989). They help determine the success or appropriateness of the nursing care plan. If a favorable status cannot be achieved by the nursing care plan, and the diagnosis is correct, the nurse must change the goal or change the plan. If neither of these options is indicated, the nurse then confers with the physician for delegated orders.

Nursing diagnoses should *not* represent situations that require physician orders for treatment. Otherwise, how can nurses assume accountability for diagnosis and treatment? For example, consider a client with a nursing diagnosis:

Potential Altered Cerebral Tissue Perfusion related to effects of recent head injury

TABLE 1-4.   Differentiation Among Types of Diagnoses

Diagnostic Statement	Corresponding Client Outcome or Nursing Goals	Focus of Intervention
Actual Diagnosis		
Three-part statement including nursing diagnostic label, etiology, and signs/symptoms	Change in patient behavior moving toward resolution of the diagnosis or improved status	Reduce or eliminate problem
Potential Diagnosis		
Two-part statement including nursing diagnostic label and risk factors	Maintenance of present condition	Reduce risk factors to prevent an actual problem from occurring
Possible Diagnosis		
Two-part statement including nursing diagnostic label and unconfirmed etiology or unconfirmed defining characteristics	Undetermined until problem is validated	Collect additional data to confirm or rule out signs/symptoms or risk factors
Collaborative Problem		
Potential physiological complication	Nursing goals	Determine onset or status of the problem Management of change in status

and these outcome criteria:

> The client will demonstrate continued optimal cerebral pressure as evidenced by
> - Pupils equally reactive to light and accommodation
> - Absence of change in orientation or consciousness

If this client were to exhibit evidence of increased intracranial pressure, would it be appropriate for the nurse to change the goals? What changes in the nursing care plan would the nurse make to stop the cranial pressure from increasing? Actually, neither action is warranted. Rather, the nurse should confer with the physician for delegated orders to treat increased intracranial pressure. When the nurse formulates client goals or outcomes that require delegated medical orders for goal achievement, the situation is not a nursing diagnosis but a collaborative problem. Thus, in this case the client's problem would be described better as a collaborative problem:

> Potential Complication: Increased Intracranial Pressure

and the nursing goal:

> The nurse will manage and minimize increased intracranial pressure episodes

Outcome criteria are not indicated for collaborative problems, because they do not serve as indicators for evaluating nursing care. Nursing goals are used for collaborative problems for they serve to represent the accountability for the situation. For collaborative problems, nurses use monitoring criteria to evaluate the client's status, such as normal range for blood pressure and serum potassium. For nursing diagnoses, nurses use outcome criteria to evaluate the effectiveness of the nursing plan.

For this reason, the care plans presented in Unit II include client goals for nursing diagnoses and nursing goals for collaborative problems.

Summary

The Bifocal Clinical Practice Model provides nurses with a framework to diagnose the unique responses of a client and significant others to various situations. Clear definition of the two dimensions of nursing practice enhances the use, and minimizes the misuse, of nursing diagnoses.

References/Bibliography

Alfaro, R. (1989). *Applying nursing diagnosis and nursing process: A step-by-step guide* (2nd ed.). Philadelphia: J.B. Lippincott.

Bulechek, G., & McCloskey, J. (1985). *Nursing interventions: Treatments for nursing diagnoses.* Philadelphia: J.B. Lippincott.

Burke, L., & Murphy, J. (1988). *Charting by exception.* Philadelphia: W.B. Saunders.

Carpenito, L.J. (1989). *Nursing diagnosis: Application to clinical practice* (3rd ed.). Philadelphia: J.B. Lippincott.

Carpenito, L.J. (1987). Nursing interventions as indicators for differentiating diagnoses. *MINDA News, 3*(2), 2–3.

Maryland Nurse Practice Act, July 1986, p. 4.

NANDA nursing diagnosis definition (1990). *Nursing Diagnosis,* in press.

Styles, M.M. (1982). *On nursing: Toward a new endowment.* St. Louis: C.V. Mosby.

Historically, nurses have had an uneasy relationship with nursing documentation. Although the *quantity* of nursing documentation certainly has increased over the years, the same cannot necessarily be said about the *quality* of the information documented.

Nursing documentation is varied, complex, and time consuming. Studies reflect that nurses spend from 35 to 140 minutes on charting per shift. Logically, the severity of the client's condition should determine charting time; in reality, however, the nurse spends the most time in repetitive, duplicative charting of routine care and observations. As a result, too often specific significant observations or dialogues are not recorded because of time constraints. Moreover, significant information that is recorded may be missed because nurses and doctors do not regularly read nurses' progress notes.

Physicians rely on oral communication with nurses to acquire information about a client's status. Nurses rely on oral communication among the nursing staff to transmit status reports, significant findings, and nursing orders. Interestingly, physicians' orders never would be left to chance with oral communications only. Today's health care environment, with its increasing demands on professional nurses, necessitates the development of a professional and efficient documentation system.

LEGAL ISSUES AND STANDARDS OF PRACTICE

The delivery and documentation of nursing care must meet the standard of the profession. The American Nurses Association (ANA) defines a standard as an "authoritative statement by which the quality of practice, service, and education can be judged" (Flanagan, 1974). A standard is a generally accepted practice that reasonably prudent nurses in similar circumstances would perform. Similar circumstances could include available resources (equipment, number of staff), educational preparation of staff, client census, client acuity, case load, and geographical region (Northrop and Kelly, 1987).

In order for care or charting to be judged, it must be compared to a standard. Standards governing nursing documentation come from many different sources. Knowledge of these standards provides a department of nursing with the authority to determine their philosophy and policies of documentation in accordance with applicable standards.

The ANA's *Standards of Nursing Practice* (1973) directs

Sources of Standards for Nursing Documentation

- Federal statutes (e.g., Medicare, Medicaid)
- State statutes (e.g., Nurse Practice Act, Department of Health)
- American Nurses Association
- Joint Commission on Accreditation of Healthcare Organizations (JCAHO)
- Specialty nursing associations (e.g., American Association of Operating Room Nurses, American Association of Critical Care Nurses)
- Institutional policies and procedures

nurses in documenting the nursing process by mandating the following:

1. The collection of data about the health status of the client/patient is systematic and continuous. The data are accessible, communicated, and recorded.
2. Nursing diagnoses are derived from health status data.
3. The plan of nursing care includes goals derived from the nursing diagnoses.
4. The plan of nursing care includes priorities and the prescribed nursing approaches or measures to achieve the goals derived from the nursing diagnoses.
5. Nursing actions provide for client/patient participation in health promotion, maintenance, and restoration.
6. Nursing actions assist the client/patient to maximize his health capabilities.
7. The client's/patient's progress or lack of progress toward goal achievement is determined by the client/patient and the nurse.
8. The client's/patient's progress or lack of progress toward goal achievement directs reassessment, reordering of priorities, new goal-setting, and revision of the plan of nursing care.

The Joint Commission on Accreditation of Healthcare Organizations (JCAHO) has voluntary standards for nursing documentation. Approximately 33% of hospitals receive recommendations for improvement of nursing documentation after a JCAHO survey visit. Accreditation by JCAHO is required for a hospital to receive Medicare reimbursement. JCAHO states

The nursing process (assessment, planning, intervention, evaluation) shall be documented for each hospitalized patient from admission through discharge. Each patient's nursing needs shall be assessed by a registered nurse at the time of admission or within the period established by nursing department/service policy. These assessment data shall be consistent with the medical plan of care and shall be available to all nursing personnel involved in the care of the patient.

A registered nurse must plan each patient's nursing care whenever possible, and nursing goals should be mutually set with the patient and/or family. Goals shall be based on the nursing assessment and shall be realistic, measurable, and consistent with the therapy prescribed by the responsible medical practitioner. Patient education and patient/family knowledge of self-care shall be given special consideration in the nursing plan. The instructions and counseling given to the patient must be consistent with that of the responsible medical practitioner. The plan of care must be documented and should reflect current standards of nursing practice. The plan shall include nursing measures that will facilitate the medical care prescribed and that will restore, maintain, or promote the patient's well-being. As appropriate, such measures should include physiological, psychosocial, and environmental factors; patient/family education; and patient discharge planning. The scope of the plan shall be determined by the anticipated needs of the patient and shall be revised as the needs of the patient change. Exceptions to the requirement for a care plan shall be defined in writing.

Documentation of nursing care shall be pertinent and concise and shall reflect the patient's needs, problems, capabilities, and limitations. Nursing intervention and patient response must be noted. When a patient is transferred within or discharged from the hospital, a nurse shall note the patient's status in the medical record. As appropriate, patients who are discharged from the hospital requiring nursing care should receive instructions and individualized counseling prior to discharge, and evidence of the instructions and the patient's or family's understanding of these instructions should be noted in the medical record. Such instructions and counseling must be consistent with the responsible medical practitioner's instructions.

The nursing department/service is encouraged to standardize documentation of routine elements of care and repeated monitoring of, for example, personal hygiene, administration of medications, and physiological parameters.

Examination of the JCAHO standards reveals that a department of nursing can select how the standard is to be met. Most hospitals receive an unsatisfactory JCAHO review because they fail to provide evidence that they actually do what they say they do. For example, if a hospital states that indwelling (Foley) catheter care must be charted as provided, JCAHO would expect to find evidence of this charting. However, a hospital could take a different approach by stating that all clients with indwelling catheters will be provided with catheter care each shift and as needed, and that no charting is needed unless this care is *not* provided.

JCAHO does specifically identify selected documentation requirements, such as admission assessment and discharge planning; however, JCAHO does not specify the documentation method, leaving that up to the individual hospitals. The *Code of Federal Regulations* also has directions for documentation that provide for flexibility by hospitals. In summary, hospitals have the authority to define their own documentation requirements as long as these requirements are in compliance with legal, accreditation, and professional standards.

ATTRIBUTES OF NURSING DOCUMENTATION

Historically, nurses have believed that the more information a nurse has charted, the better one's legal defense in any litigation. Today, however, nurses recognize that a comprehensive, streamlined documentation system actually can document more data in less time and space. Nursing documentation must be objective and comprehensive and must accurately reflect the status of the client and what has happened to him. If legally challenged, the nursing records must represent what reasonably prudent nurses chart and must demonstrate compliance with the institution's policy.

Unfortunately, most hospitals and other agencies have not seriously examined what actually is required in documentation. Many nurses have been taught to write as much as possible, operating under the philosophy, "If it wasn't charted, it wasn't done." Does poor charting represent poor care? Inherent in this question are others: What is poor charting? By what standard is it poor?

If a department of nursing does not establish specific policies for charting, then the charting in question can be held to standards from another department of nursing or from expert testimony. Case law does not determine the standards for nursing documentation but instead passes a judgment regarding compliance with a standard.

Nursing documentation has two professional purposes— administrative and clinical. The administrative purposes are as follows:

☐ To define the nursing focus for the client or group
☐ To differentiate the accountability of the nurse from that of other members of the health care team
☐ To provide the criteria for reviewing and evaluating care (quality assurance)
☐ To provide the criteria for patient classification
☐ To provide justification for reimbursement
☐ To provide data for administrative and legal review
☐ To comply with legal, accreditation, and professional standard requirements
☐ To provide data for research and educational purposes

A nursing documentation system has several components. Most components focus primarily on documenting these items:

☐ Assessment
☐ Planning
☐ Implementation
☐ Evaluation

NURSING ADMISSION
DATA BASE

Date _____ Arrival Time _____ Contact Person _____ Phone _____

ADMITTED FROM: ___ Home alone   ___ Home with relative   ___ Long-term care
                ___ Homeless   ___ Home with ___   ___ facility
                ___ ER   ___ (Specify)   ___ Other _____

MODE OF ARRIVAL: ___ Wheelchair   ___ Ambulance   ___ Stretcher

REASON FOR HOSPITALIZATION: _____

_____

LAST HOSPITAL ADMISSION: Date _____ Reason _____

_____

PAST MEDICAL HISTORY: _____

MEDICATION (Prescription/Over-the-Counter)	DOSAGE	LAST DOSE	FREQUENCY

HEALTH MAINTENANCE–PRESCRIPTION PATTERN
USE OF:

Tobacco: ___ None ___ Quit (date) ___ Pipe ___ Cigar ___ <1 pk/day
              ___ 1–2 pks/day ___ >2 pks/day Pks/year history _____

Alcohol: ___ None ___ Type/amount ___ /day ___ /wk ___ /month

Other Drugs: ___ No ___ Yes Type _____ Use _____

Allergies (drugs, food, tape, dyes): _____ Reaction _____

_____

ACTIVITY/EXERCISE PATTERN
SELF-CARE ABILITY:

  0 = Independent   1 = Assistive device   2 = Assistance from others
  3 = Assistance from person and equipment   4 = Dependent/Unable

	0	1	2	3	4
Eating/Drinking					
Bathing					
Dressing/Grooming					
Toileting					
Bed Mobility					
Transferring					
Ambulating					
Stair Climbing					
Shopping					
Cooking					
Home Maintenance					

ASSISTIVE DEVICES: ___ None ___ Crutches ___ Bedside commode ___ Walker
                    ___ Cane ___ Splint/Brace ___ Wheelchair ___ Other ___

CODE: (1) Non-applicable (2) Unable to acquire
       (3) Not a priority at this time (4) Other (specify in notes)

Figure 2-1. Sample admission data base. *(Carpenito LJ: Nursing Diagnosis: Application to Clinical Practice, ed 3. Philadelphia, JB Lippincott, 1989)*

(continued)

NUTRITION/METABOLIC PATTERN

Special Diet/Supplements _____

Previous Dietary Instruction: ____ Yes ____ No

Appetite: ____ Normal ____ Increased ____ Decreased ____ Decreased taste sensation
____ Nausea ____ Vomiting ____ Stomatitis

Weight Fluctuations Last 6 Months: ____ None _____ lbs. Gained/Lost

Swallowing Difficulty (Dysphagia): ____ None ____ Solids ____ Liquids

Dentures: ____ Upper (_ Partial _ Full) ____ Lower (_ Partial _ Full)
With Patient ____ Yes ____ No

History of Skin/Healing Problems: ____ None ____ Abnormal Healing ____ Rash
____ Dryness ____ Excess Perspiration

ELIMINATION PATTERN

Bowel Habits: ____ # BMs/day ____ Date of last BM ____ Within normal limits
____ Constipation ____ Diarrhea ____ Incontinence
____ Ostomy: Type ____ Appliance ____ Self-care ____ Yes ____ No

Bladder Habits: ____ WNL ____ Frequency ____ Dysuria ____ Noctuna ____ Urgency
____ Hematuria ____ Retention

Incontinency: ____ No ____ Yes ____ Total ____ Daytime ____ Nighttime
____ Occasional ____ Difficulty delaying voiding
____ Difficulty reaching toilet

Assistive Devices: ____ Intermittent catheterization
____ Indwelling catheter ____ External catheter
____ Incontinent briefs ____ Penile implant type _____

SLEEP/REST PATTERN

Habits: ____ hrs/night ____ AM nap ____ PM nap
Feel rested after sleep ____ Yes ____ No

Problems: ____ None ____ Early waking ____ Insomnia ____ Nightmares

COGNITIVE–CONCEPTUAL PATTERN

Hearing: ____ WNL ____ Impaired (_ Right _ Left) ____ Deaf (_ Right _ Left)
____ Hearing Aid ____ Tinnitus

Vision: ____ WNL ____ Eyeglasses ____ Contact lens
____ Impaired ____ Right ____ Left
____ Blind ____ Right ____ Left
____ Cataract ____ Right ____ Left
____ Glaucoma
____ Prosthetis ____ Right ____ Left

Vertigo: ____ Yes ____ No

Discomfort/Pain: ____ None ____ Acute ____ Chronic ____ Description _____
_____

Pain Management: _____

COPING STRESS TOLERANCE/SELF-PERCEPTION/SELF-CONCEPT PATTERN

Major concerns regarding hospitalization or illness (financial, self-care): _____
_____

Major loss/change in past year: ____ No ____ Yes _____
_____

CODE: (1) Non-applicable (2) Unable to acquire
(3) Not a priority at this time (4) Other (specify in notes)

Figure 2-1 *(continued)*

SEXUALITY/REPRODUCTIVE PATTERN

LMP: _____

Menstrual Problems: ____ Yes ____ No _____

Last Pap Smear: _____

Monthly Self-Breast/Testicular Exam: ____ Yes ____ No

Sexual Concerns R/T Illness: _____

_____

ROLE-RELATIONSHIP PATTERN

Occupation: _____

Employment Status: ____ Employed ____ Short-term disability
____ Long-term disability ____ Unemployed

Support System: ____ Spouse ____ Neighbors/Friends ____ None
____ Family in same residence ____ Family in separate residence
____ Other _____

Family concerns regarding hospitalization: _____

_____

VALUE-BELIEF PATTERN

Religion: ____ Roman Catholic ____ Protestant ____ Jewish ____ Other

Religious Restrictions: ____ No ____ Yes (Specify) _____

Request Chaplain Visitation at This Time: ____ Yes ____ No

PHYSICAL ASSESSMENT (Objective)

1. **CLINICAL DATA**

   Age _____ Height _____ Weight _____ (Actual/Approximate)

   Temperature _____

   Pulse: ____ Strong ____ Weak ____ Regular ____ Irregular

   Blood Pressure: Right Arm ____ Left Arm ____ Sitting ____ Lying ____

2. **RESPIRATORY/CIRCULATORY**

   Rate _____

   Quality: ____ WNL ____ Shallow ____ Rapid ____ Labored ____ Other _____

   Cough: ____ No ____ Yes/Describe _____

   Auscultation:

   Upper rt lobes ____ WNL ____ Decreased ____ Absent ____ Abnormal sounds ____

   Upper lt lobes ____ WNL ____ Decreased ____ Absent ____ Abnormal sounds ____

   Lower rt lobes ____ WNL ____ Decreased ____ Absent ____ Abnormal sounds ____

   Lower lt lobes ____ WNL ____ Decreased ____ Absent ____ Abnormal sounds ____

   Right Pedal Pulse: ____ Strong ____ Weak ____ Absent

   Left Pedal Pulse: ____ Strong ____ Weak ____ Absent

3. **METABOLIC-INTEGUMENTARY**

   SKIN:

   Color: ____ WNL ____ Pale ____ Cyanotic ____ Ashen ____ Jaundice ____ Other ____

   Temperature: ____ WNL ____ Warm ____ Cool

   Turgor: ____ WNL ____ Poor

   Edema: ____ No ____ Yes/Description/location _____

   Lesions: ____ None ____ Yes/Description/location _____

   Bruises: ____ None ____ Yes/Description/location _____

   Reddened: ____ No ____ Yes/Description/location _____

   Pruritus: ____ No ____ Yes/Description/location _____

   Tubes: Specify _____

   MOUTH:

   Gums: ____ WNL ____ White plaque ____ Lesions ____ Other _____

   Teeth: ____ WNL ____ Other _____

   ABDOMEN:

   Bowel Sounds: ____ Present ____ Absent

Figure 2-1 *(continued)*

4. NEURO/SENSORY
Mental Status: ____ Alert ____ Receptive aphasia ____ Poor historian
____ Oriented ____ Confused ____ Combative ____ Unresponsive
Speech: ____ Normal ____ Slurred ____ Garbled ____ Expressive aphasia
Spoken language_____ Interpreter _____
Pupils: ____ Equal ____ Unequal

Left: • • • • • • • ● ●

Right: • • • • • ● ● ● ●

Reactive to light:
Left: ____ Yes ____ No/Specify _____
Right: ____ Yes ____ No/Specify _____

Eyes: ____ Clear ____ Draining ____ Reddened ____ Other _____

5. MUSCULAR–SKELETAL
Range of Motion: ____ Full ____ Other _____
Balance and Gait: ____ Steady ____ Unsteady
Hand Grasps: ____ Equal ____ Strong ____ Weakness/Paralysis (__ Right __ Left)
Leg Muscles: ____ Equal ____ Strong ____ Weakness/Paralysis (__ Right __ Left)

DISCHARGE PLANNING
Lives: Alone ____ With _____ No known residence _____
Intended Destination Post Discharge: ____ Home ____ Undetermined ____ Other _____
Previous Utilization of Community Resources:
__ Home care/Hospice __ Adult day care __ Church groups __ Other _____
__ Meals on Wheels __ Homemaker/Home health aide __ Community support group
Post-discharge Transportation:
____ Car ____ Ambulance ____ Bus/Taxi
____ Unable to determine at this time
Anticipated Financial Assistance Post-discharge?: ____ No ____ Yes _____
Anticipated Problems with Self-care Post-discharge?: ____ No ____ Yes _____
Assistive Devices Needed Post-discharge?: ____ No ____ Yes _____
Referrals: (record date)
Discharge Coordinator _____ Home Health _____
Social Service _____ V.N.A. _____
Other Comments: _____
_____
_____

SIGNATURE/TITLE _____ DATE _____

Figure 2-1 *(continued)*

Assessment

In assessment—the deliberate collection of data about a client, family, or group—the nurse obtains data by interviewing, observing, and examining. There are two types of assessment: admission screening interview and focus assessment.

ADMISSION SCREENING INTERVIEW

The admission interview has two parts: functional patterns and physical assessment. It focuses on determining the client's present health status and ability to function (see Figure 2-1 for a nursing admission data base). Specific functional pattern assessment categories include the following:

- ☐ Ability to bathe self
- ☐ Presence of confusion
- ☐ Condition of skin
- ☐ Ability to control urination
- ☐ Ability to tolerate activities

The physical examination uses the skills of inspection, auscultation, and palpation to assess areas such as these:

- ☐ Pulses
- ☐ Skin condition
- ☐ Muscle strength
- ☐ Lung fields

After completing and recording the screening assessment, the nurse analyzes the data, asking questions such as the following:

☐ Does the client have a problem that requires nursing interventions (e.g., assistance with ambulation)?

☐ Is the client at risk for developing a problem (e.g., pressure sores)?

☐ Does the client's medical condition put him or her at high risk for complications (e.g., problems associated with increased blood glucose in diabetes mellitus)?

☐ Do the prescribed treatments put the client at high risk for complications (e.g., phlebitis from IV therapy)?

FOCUS ASSESSMENT

Focus assessment involves the acquisition of selected or specific data as determined by the nurse and the client or family, or as directed by the client's condition (Carpenito, 1983). These assessments are continuous. The nurse can perform a focus assessment during the initial interview if the data suggest that additional questions should be asked. For example, on admission most clients would be questioned about eating patterns. A client with chronic obstructive lung disease would also be asked whether dyspnea interferes with eating. This represents a focus assessment, for not every client would be asked whether dyspnea affects food intake.

Certain focus assessments—such as vital signs, bowel and bladder function, and nutritional status—are done every shift for every client. (Appendix I presents a generic care plan for all hospitalized adults that includes these routine focus assessments.) The nurse determines the need for additional focus assessments based on the client's condition. For example, in a postoperative client, the nurse assesses and monitors the surgical wound and IV therapy.

Each care plan in Unit II of this book contains specific focus assessment criteria for each listed nursing diagnosis. These criteria represent specific data that must be assessed to confirm or rule out the diagnosis, or to identify etiologic, contributing, and risk factors. The sample below shows the focus assessment criteria for a patient with multiple sclerosis.

Planning

The clinical purposes of documentation are to direct care and to record the client's status or response. Directions for nursing care originate in both nursing and medicine. Interventions prescribed by physicians are transferred to various forms; e.g., Kardex or treatment and medication administration records. Nurses prescribe both routine interventions and those specific to the client. Routine nursing interventions can be found in nursing care standards. These client-specific interventions are listed on the nursing care plan.

Care plans serve the following purposes:

☐ They represent the priority set of diagnoses (collaborative problems and/or nursing diagnoses) for a client.

☐ They provide a "blueprint" to direct charting.

☐ They communicate to the nursing staff what to teach, what to observe, and what to implement.

☐ They provide outcome criteria for reviewing and evaluating care.

☐ They direct specific interventions for the client, family, and other nursing staff members to implement.

To direct and evaluate nursing care effectively, the care plan should include the following:

☐ Diagnostic statements (collaborative problems or nursing diagnoses)

☐ Outcome criteria or nursing goals

☐ Nursing orders or interventions

☐ Evaluation (status of diagnosis)

DIAGNOSTIC STATEMENTS

Diagnostic statements can be either collaborative problems or nursing diagnoses. Refer to Chapter 1, The Bifocal Clinical Practice Model, for information on these two types of diagnostic statements.

OUTCOME CRITERIA

Outcome criteria, or client goals, are statements describing a measurable behavior of the client or family, denoting a favorable status (changed or maintained) after nursing care has been delivered (Alfaro, 1986). They serve as standards for measuring the care plan's effectiveness. Outcome criteria for nursing diagnoses should represent favorable statuses that can be achieved or maintained through nursing-prescribed (indepen-

---

Potential Self-concept Disturbance related to the effects of prolonged debilitating condition on achieving developmental tasks and life style

Focus Assessment Criteria	Clinical Significance
1. Prior exposure to individuals with multiple sclerosis	1–4. This information enables the caregiver to detect patterns of response due to adaptation. It is helpful to note how the client's support system views the client's self-concept. They can provide insight into factors that may have affected self-concept development and may be sensitive to the subtle effects of recent changes.
2. Ability to express feelings about condition	
3. Ability to share feelings with significant others	
4. Evidence of negative self-concept	
5. Participation in self-care	5, 6. Participation in self-care and adaptation of goals to disability indicate attempts to cope with the changes (Hamburg).
6. Evidence of adapting life style to disabilities	

dent) interventions (Carpenito, 1989). If outcome criteria are not being achieved, the nurse must reevaluate the diagnosis and revise the goal and/or the plan, or collaborate with a physician.

When the nurse collaborates with the physician, the diagnosis is a collaborative problem, not a nursing diagnosis. For example, if a client with a collaborative problem of Potential Complication: Dysrhythmia experiences premature ventricular contractions, the nurse would not change the nursing care plan but instead would initiate physician-prescribed interventions.

Collaborative problems should not have outcome criteria, because they do not serve as indicators for evaluating nursing care. Any outcome criteria written for collaborative problems would need to represent the criteria for evaluating both nursing and medical care. Physiological stability is the overall goal for collaborative problems.

NURSING INTERVENTIONS

In 1987, Carpenito wrote that the relationship of diagnosis to intervention is a critical element in defining nursing diagnosis. Many definitions of nursing diagnosis focus on the relationship of selected interventions to the diagnosis. A certain type of intervention appears to distinguish a nursing diagnosis from a medical diagnosis or other problems that nurses treat. Bulechek and McCloskey (1985) stated that a "nursing intervention is an autonomous action based on scientific rationale that is executed to benefit the client in a predicted way related to the nursing diagnosis and goal."

Nursing interventions can be categorized as either independent or delegated (Maryland, 1984). *Independent interventions* are nurse prescribed; *delegated interventions* are physician prescribed. Both types of interventions require nursing judgment; for either, the nurse is legally bound to determine whether it is appropriate to initiate.

So, the nurse makes independent decisions regarding both collaborative problems and nursing diagnoses. The decisions differ in that for nursing diagnoses, the nurse prescribes the definitive treatment for the situation; for collaborative problems, the nurse primarily monitors the client's condition to detect physiological complications. The nurse confers with a physician or initiates physician protocols to manage the complication. The nurse utilizes physican- and nurse-prescribed interventions to assist the client to return to pre-complication stability.

Care plans should not contain directions for nurses regarding delegated (physician-prescribed) interventions. Instead, physicians' orders are transferred to care and treatment records, Kardexes, and medication administration records. For this reason, the care plans presented in Unit II list only nurse-prescribed (independent) interventions. At the end of the Collaborative Problems section in each care plan, a section titled Related Physician-Prescribed Treatments provides these interventions as additional information.

In the care plans, the interventions listed under nursing diagnoses generally consist of these types, described by Alfaro (1986):

☐ Performing activities for the client or assisting the client with activities
☐ Performing nursing assessments to identify new problems and to determine the status of existing problems

☐ Teaching to help the client gain new knowledge concerning his or her health or the management of a disorder
☐ Counseling the client to make decisions about his or her own health care
☐ Consulting with other health care professionals
☐ Performing specific actions to remove, reduce, or resolve health problems
☐ Assisting the client to perform activities himself or herself
☐ Assisting the client to identify risks or problems and to explore available options

In contrast, the interventions listed under collaborative problems focus primarily on the following:

☐ Monitoring for physiological instability
☐ Consulting with a physician to obtain appropriate interventions
☐ Performing specific actions to manage and reduce the severity of the event

CARE PLANNING SYSTEMS

For years, practicing nurses have held an ambivalent view of care planning. Staff nurses' common oppositions to written care plans include those listed here:

☐ Not enough time to write them
☐ Not necessary except for JCAHO accreditation
☐ Not used after they are written

Supporters of care planning in nursing cite these benefits:

☐ Care plans provide written directions to nursing staff rather than relying on verbal communication.
☐ They help ensure continuity of care for a client.
☐ They direct nurses to intervene in the priority set of problems for this client for this hospitalization.
☐ They provide a means of reviewing or evaluating care.
☐ They demonstrate the complex role of professional nurses to validate their position in health care settings.

Since care plans usually contain only routine interventions (because including more detail is a burden in a manual system), nurses often do not use them. A care plan that is not used is not revised. As a result, the care plan that a nurse reads commonly does not represent the most current plan for the client. In order to update the staff on the care that the client requires, the nurse then uses oral communication. This type of communication makes the delivery of nursing care very inefficient and costly.

An efficient, professional, and useful care planning system is possible. This system utilizes standards of care, client problem lists, and standardized and addendum care plans.

Standards of Care

Standards of care are detailed guidelines that represent the predicted care indicated in a specific situation.

Standards of care should represent the care that nurses are responsible for providing, not an ideal level of care. The nurse cannot hope to address all or even most of the problems that a client may have. Rather, the nurse must select those problems that are the most serious or most important to the client. Ideal standards that are unrealistic only frustrate nurses and hold them legally accountable for care that they cannot provide. Nurses must create realistic standards based on client acuity, length of stay, and available resources.

A care planning system can contain three levels of directions:

☐ Level I—Generic Unit Standards Of Care
☐ Level II—Diagnostic Cluster or Single Diagnosis Standardized Plans
☐ Level III—Addendum Care Plans

Level I Standards of Care predict the generic care that will be needed for all or most individuals or families on the unit. Examples of generic unit standards of care are medical, surgical, oncologic, pediatric, post-partum, operating room, emergency room, mental health unit, rehabilitation unit, and newborn nursery. Figure 2-2 presents a diagnostic cluster for most hospitalized adults. Appendices I and II are Level I standards.

Level II care plans contain a diagnostic cluster or a single nursing diagnosis or collaborative problem. A diagnostic cluster is a set of nursing diagnoses and collaborative problems that have been predicted to be present and of high priority for a given population.

Examples of Level II single-diagnosis standards are Potential Impaired Skin Integrity, Potential for Violence, and PC: Fluid/Electrolyte Imbalances.

Collaborative Problems

Potential Complication: Cardiovascular
Potential Complication: Respiratory

Nursing Diagnoses

Anxiety related to unfamiliar environment, routines, diagnostic tests and treatments, and loss of control

Potential for Injury related to unfamiliar environment and physical/mental limitations secondary to condition, medications, therapies, and diagnostic test

Potential for Infection related to increased microorganisms in environment, the risk of person-to-person transmission, and invasive tests and therapies

Self-care Deficit related to sensory, cognitive, mobility, endurance, or motivation problems

Potential Altered Nutrition: Less Than Body Requirements related to decreased appetite secondary to treatments, fatigue, environment, and changes in usual diet, and increased protein/vitamin requirements for healing

Potential Constipation related to change in fluid/food intake, routine and activity level, effects of medications, and emotional stress

Sleep Pattern Disturbance related to unfamiliar, noisy environment, change in bedtime ritual, emotional stress, and change in circadian rhythm

Potential Spiritual Distress related to separation from religious support system, lack of privacy, or inability to practice spiritual rituals

Altered Family Process related to disruption of routines, change in role responsibilities, and fatigue associated with increase workload and visiting hour requirements

---

Figure 2-2. Generic diagnostic cluster for hospitalized adults.

Because they apply to all clients, the nursing diagnoses or collaborative problems associated with the generic standard of care do not need to be written on an individual client's care plan. Instead, institutional policy can specify that the generic standard will be implemented for all clients. Documentation of the generic standard is discussed later in this chapter.

Although standards of care do not have to be part of the client's record, the record should specify what standards have been selected for the client. The problem list serves this purpose. The problem list represents the priority set of nursing diagnoses and collaborative problems for an individual client. Figure 2-3 presents a sample problem list. Next to each diagnosis, the nurse indicates where the directions for the care can be found—on a standardized form or on the addendum plan. The last column can be used to indicate the progress of the client.

Standardized Care Plans

Standardized care plans are standards of care that become permanent chart records because of additions or deletions. A standard of care that has not been changed does not have to be a permanent chart record, although it is still a legal standard to which the nurse is held accountable. If the standard or standardized care plan is not in the permanent record, the problem list (as a part of the permanent record) will indicate the diagnoses that are to be addressed.

Addendum Care Plans

An addendum care plan represents additional interventions to be provided for the client. These specific interventions can be added to a standardized care plan or may be associated with additional priority nursing diagnoses or collaborative problems not included on the standardized plan.

The initial care of most hospitalized clients can be directed responsibly using standards of care. With subsequent nurse–client interactions, specific data may warrant specific addendum additions to the client's care plan to ensure holistic, empathic nursing care. Figure 2-4 presents a problem list and addendum care plan for a client recovering from gastric surgery. In addition to the diagnostic cluster in the postoperative standard of care, this client has three addendum diagnoses. Potential Impaired Skin Integrity is being managed with interventions from a standard for this diagnosis. Documentation will be completed each shift on the flow record. Impaired Swallowing is being treated with generic interventions and with addendum intervention specifying foods that this client can tolerate. The last diagnosis, Impaired Physical Mobility, involves only addendum interventions prescribed to increase the client's motivation and to promote correct ambulation techniques.

DOCUMENTATION AND EVALUATION

Care plans represent documentation of the nursing care planned for a client. They also reflect the status of the diagnosis: active, resolved, or ruled out. The documentation of care delivered

Nursing Problem List/Care Plan

Nursing Diagnosis/Collaborative Problem	Status	Standard	Addendum	Evaluation of Progress			

Status Code: A = Active   R = Resolved   RO = Ruled-out
Evaluation Code: S = Stable   I = Improved   *W = Worsened   *U = Unchanged   P = Progressing   *NP = Not Progressing

Addendum Care Plan

NSG DX/COLL PROB	CLIENT/NURSING GOALS	DATE/INITIALS	INTERVENTIONS

Initials/Signature			
1.	3.	5.	7.
2.	4.	6.	8.

Figure 2-3.   Nursing problem list and care plan.

and the client's status or response after care are recorded on specific forms, including the following:

☐ Graphic records
☐ Flow records
☐ Progress notes
☐ Teaching records
☐ Discharge planning/summary

Evaluation

The nurse is responsible to evaluate a client's status and progress to outcome achievement daily. Evaluation of the client's status and progress is different for collaborative prob-

lems versus nursing diagnoses. For nursing diagnoses the nurse will:

☐ Assess the client's status
☐ Compare this response to the outcome criteria
☐ Conclude if the client is progressing to outcome achievement

The nurse can record this evaluation on a flow record as

	7–3 PM
Comfort	Report satisfaction relief from measures

or on a progress note as

Nursing Problem List/Care Plan

Nursing Diagnosis/Collaborative Problem	Status	Standard	Addendum	Evaluation of Progress				
1. STANDARD — POST-OP	A 6/8 LJC	✓		6/9 LJC *NP	6/10 JW P			
2. POT. IMPAIRED SKIN INTEGRITY RT IMMOBILITY	A 6/8 LJC			6/9 LJC S	6/10 JW S			
3. Impaired Swallowing RT Unknown etiology aEB choking with liquids	A 6/9 LJC	✓	✓	6/9 LJC P	6/10 JW P			
4. Impaired physical mobility RT fatigue, decreased motivation and uncoordinated movements 2° to Parkinson's	A 6/10 JW		✓	—	6/10 JW *NP			

Status Code: A = Active   R = Resolved   RO = Ruled-out
Evaluation Code: S = Stable   I = Improved   *W = Worsened   *U = Unchanged   P = Progressing   *NP = Not Progressing

Addendum Care Plan

NSG DX/COLL PROB	CLIENT/NURSING GOALS	DATE/INITIALS	INTERVENTIONS
3. Impaired Swallowing	—	6/9 LJC	5. Stay with him during meals
			6. Teach to moisten dry foods
4. Imp. Phys. mobility Mobility	Will walk to Nsg Station with walker by 6/14	6/10 JW	1. Establish distance goal before walking
			2. Talk about something interesting during walking

Initials/Signature			
1. LJC L.J. Carpenito RN	3.	5.	7.
2. JWm J. Woolsey RN	4.	6.	8.

Figure 2-4.   Sample problem list and addendum care plan.

Altered Comfort

Sub. The medication relieved my pain well. It is easier to move and cough.

Eval. Pain controlled, continue plan

Not all nursing diagnoses require a progress note in order to record evaluation. A well-designed flow record can be used.

For collaborative problems the nurse will:

☐ Collect selected data
☐ Compare the data to the established norms
☐ Judge if the data are within an acceptable range

The nurse can record the assessment data for collaborative problems on flow records. Progress notes can be used if the findings are significant, followed by the nursing management of the situation. The last column of Figure 2-3 represents the place where the nurse can document the progress of the client for each diagnosis on the problem list. The frequency of this documentation will be determined by the institution, e.g., q 24h. If a client has not improved or has worsened, an I* or N* is used. In addition, a progress note is required to record the nursing actions undertaken.

Thus the evaluation for nursing diagnoses is focused on progress to achievement of client outcome, whereas the eval-

---

Nursing/Physician Order Flowsheet

Date 6-28-1990

NRSG DX	NURSING/PHYSICIAN ORDER									
	Incisional assess/care	✓ IJC¹⁰	* JM¹⁸	→MS⁴						

* SIGNIFICANT FINDINGS ▼   NURSE INITIAL ►

NRSG DX #	TIME	
	18:00	2cm erythematic area left incisional line. Dr. Tomm notified. J Maklehurst RN

Guidelines:

Upon carrying out an order that has no significant findings, a " → " in the appropriate category box is sufficient to indicate it was done. If the order includes an assessment, the following parameters will be considered a negative assessment and constitute the use of a "*".

"Surgical dressing/Incisional assessment"—Dressing dry and intact. No evidence of redness, increased temperature, or tenderness in surrounding tissue. Sutures/staples/steri-strips intact. Wound edges well-approximated. No drainage present.

Figure 2-5. Charting by exception flow record. *(Burke L, Murphy J. Charting by Exception. New York: John Wiley & Sons, 1988; used with permission)*

uation for collaborative problems is focused on the client's condition compared with established norms.

Graphic Records

Used to record vital signs, weights, 24-hour intake and output totals, and selected assessments, graphic records document the client's status in selected areas. If the assessments are normal, additional charting on the progress notes is unnecessary.

Flow Records

Flow records are used to record repetitive data, e.g., intake and output, treatments, and medication administration. They also can be used to document the client's status or response after nursing interventions. Treatments, assessments, and the nurse's interpretation of the data can be recorded on a flow record, as shown in Figure 2-5. On this sample, the check mark next to "wound assess./care" indicates that wound care was provided and that the wound was assessed to be healing within normal limits. If the wound was not healing properly, the nurse would indicate this with an asterisk (*) and would also write a progress note describing the abnormal findings (see below). The nurse would use the → symbol to indicate that a previous finding was found again (Burke and Murphy, 1988).

Progress Notes

Progress notes, or nursing progress notes, provide the format for recording significant data or events. Progress notes should contain only unusual events or responses, or significant observations or interactions that are inappropriate for a flow record. For example, if the results of a neurovascular assessment were normal, the nurse would record the data on a flow record (pulses, color, capillary filling, sensation); no progress note

would be needed. But if the data were abnormal, the nurse would record it on the flow sheet with an associated explanatory progress note. Figure 2-6 illustrates the use of an asterisk on a flow record to indicate that a related progress note exists.

Historically, the format for progress notes is a narrative. However, exclusively narrative charting produces notes from which information is difficult to retrieve—a reason, perhaps, why very few health care professionals read progress notes.

To allow efficient retrieval of information about the status of a certain problem or situation, progress notes should be organized under the topic being addressed. Both *problem-oriented charting* and *focus charting* serve this purpose. (Figure 2-7 illustrates examples of each format.) Regardless of the charting format used, the nurse sometimes will need to use a narrative notation to record an observation or interaction that does not relate to a nursing diagnosis or a collaborative problem. For such a situation, the note should be identified as an addendum.

If the nursing documentation system used flow records correctly, progress notes would better represent the depth and breadth of professional nursing practice. Too often, however, progress notes present only repetitive, routine interventions and assessments, while the significant dialogue between the nurse and client or family member goes unrecorded.

Teaching Records

All clients have learning needs. The generic client-teaching interventions that apply to all clients—e.g., safety measures, preparation for routine x-ray films and lab studies—should be outlined in the generic standard of care. Documentation of this teaching is unnecessary unless something unusual occurs.

Besides such generic teaching, most clients have other teaching needs. Specific teaching on a standard of care—e.g., ostomy care, wound care, exercises—can be preprinted on a teaching record. Figure 2-8 presents a sample preprinted client teaching record taken from a standard of care for a diabetic client. Teaching records should provide space for the nurse to indicate that the teaching was done and whether or not the desired outcome was achieved.

	8-12-89				
Peripheral pulses	90				
Color	Pink				
Capillary filling	3 sec				
Sensation	*				

8-12-89	c/o Tingling in left foot. Dr. Green notified.
	L.J. Carpenito RN.

Figure 2-6. Example of flow record with a corresponding progress note.

Problem-oriented Charting

DATE	HOUR	NRSG. DX #	NOTES	SIGNATURE OF NURSE
9/23/90	1400	3	Impaired Physical Mobility	
			Sub: states "I feel tired after being out of bed"	
			Obj: Walked 6 feet, OOB in chair 30 mins.	
			Assess: Physically tolerated ambulation of 6 feet. Walked slowly with the aid of one person but was steady.	
			Impl: Explained that fatigue was normal. Told him he did very well. He agreed to increase distance tomorrow.	
			Eval: Care plan revised	*LJ Carpenito RN*

Focus Charting

Date 9/23/90

HOUR	FOCUS	PATIENT CARE NOTES
1400	Imp Phy Mob	Data: Walked 6 feet with 1 person assisting, slowly but steady. OOB in Chair 30 mins. c/o he was tired but agreed to increase distance tomorrow.
		Action: Reinforced that he would be tired, praised him. Care plan revised. *LJ Carpenito RN*

Figure 2-7. Problem-oriented and focus charting.

Client Teaching Record	Diabetes Mellitus		(Stamp)
	Instructed Date/Initial	**Goals Accomplished** Date/Initial	**Comments**
A. Will Correctly Explain:			
1. DIABETES (Pathophysiology)			
a. Causes			
b. Treatment			
c. Relationship of diet, exercise, insulin			
2. INSULIN			
a. Types utilized			
b. Action/time of each			
3. HYPOGLYCEMIA*			
a. Signs and symptoms			
b. Causes/treatment			
• Carry sugar			
• Glucagon			
4. HYPERGLYCEMIA/KETOACIDOSIS*			
a. Signs and symptoms			
b. Treatment			
c. Causes/prevention			
5. DIETARY			
a. Exchange diet			
6. SICK DAYS*			
a. Liquid exchange diet			
b. Insulin requirements			
7. PHONE CONTACT			
a. Call-in-hour			
b. Emergency			
B. Will Demonstrate:			
1. URINE TESTS*			
a. Type			
2. BLOOD MONITORING*			
a. Machine			
b. Visual			
3. RECORD KEEPING			
a. Urine and blood results			
b. Symptoms experienced			
4. INSULIN ADMINISTRATION*			
a. Mixing two types of insulin			
b. Choosing, preparing, and rotating site			
c. Injection			
d. Storage of supplies			

* If outcome not achieved by patient by discharge, initiate a referral.

Initial	Signature	Initial	Signature

Figure 2-8. Sample teaching record. *(Copyright © 1988 by Lynda Juall Carpenito)*

I. Planning (initiate on admission)

Lives alone _____ With _____ No known residence _____
Intended destination after discharge:

  Home _____ Other _____ Undetermined _____

Anticipated caregiver: Self _____ Other _____
Prehospital functioning ability
- Home management: Independent / Assistance needed / Dependent
- Cooking: Independent / Assistance needed / Dependent
- Shopping: Independent / Assistance needed / Dependent
- Self-care: Independent / Assistance needed / Dependent

Anticipated financial assistance post discharge?　No _____　Yes _____

Anticipated problems with self-care post discharge?　No _____　Yes _____

Assistive devices needed post discharge?　No _____　Yes _____
Referrals: (record date)
Discharge coordinator _____　Home health _____

Social service _____　Other _____

II. Discharge Criteria and Instructions

1. Nutrition:

_____ Explain diet to be followed upon discharge.

  Diet _____

          _____

  Restrictions _____

2. Medications:

_____ State correct dose, time, special precautions, and side effects of medications

Name/Dose	Time(s)	Special instructions (in addition to those on container)

3. Activity

_____ State activity restrictions

_____ Demonstrate prescribed exercises

_____ Demonstrate correct use of appliances/assistive devices
☐ Resume normal activity
☐ Sponge bath only　　☐ Tub bath　　☐ Shower

☐ Restricted activity for _____ (length of time)
　☐ No lifting　☐ No climbing stairs　☐ No driving

☐ No sexual activity　☐ Other _____

_____

_____

4. Special instructions

_____ Correctly describe or demonstrate the prescribed treatment

_____ State signs and symptoms that necessitate reporting

Figure 2-9. Discharge planning and summary record.
(continued)

Symptoms to report: _____

_____

_____

Other: _____

_____

_____

_____

_____ Describe follow-up care and available community resources

☐ Appointment with _____ Date _____ Time _____

☐ Patient/Family to make appointment in _____ days/weeks

☐ Referral to _____

☐ Records sent with patient (list) _____

_____

III. Discharge Summary

Discharge criteria met?   Yes _____   No _____

Action taken if discharge criteria not met: _____

_____

_____

_____

Discharged to _____ Date _____ Time _____

Mode of transportation _____

Accompanied by _____

Personal effects/Valuables sent home?   Yes _____   No _____

List _____

Medications sent home from pharmacy?   Yes _____   No _____

Other comments _____

_____

_____

_____

Discharge nurse's signature _____

Figure 2-9 *(continued)*

DISCHARGE PLANNING

Discharge planning is a systematic process of appraisal, preparation, and coordination done to facilitate provision of health care and social services before and after discharge. Discharge planning can be categorized as standard or addendum.

Standard discharge planning includes the teaching deemed necessary based on the client's specific medical or surgical condition. The standard of care usually can address the content to be taught under two nursing diagnoses: Potential Altered Health Maintenance and Potential Impaired Home Maintenance Management. Standard discharge planning is the responsibility of the professional nurse caring for the client or family.

Addendum discharge planning requires coordinated and collaborative action among health care providers within the institution and in the community at large. Multidisciplinary actions may be indicated. This type of discharge planning should be coordinated by a nurse discharge coordinator. The discharge coordinator should be a nurse because most post-hospital care involves nursing care, and because the nurse has the following attributes (Waters, 1980):

☐   Is the expert on the type of care and services required at home

☐   Is the center of hospital and community agency services
☐   Has a strong collaborative relationship with physicians
☐   Can predict what impact the medical diagnosis and nursing diagnoses will have upon client function
☐   Has the most comprehensive knowledge, which can produce the most economically coordinated health care services

Staff nurses usually do not have the time or resources available for addendum discharge planning. However, it is the staff nurse who refers high-risk clients or families to the discharge coordinator.

The goal of discharge planning is to identify the specific needs for maintaining or achieving maximum function after discharge. The discharge needs of clients and families can result in two types of nursing actions:

☐   Teaching the client or family how to manage the situation at home
☐   Referring the client or family to support services (e.g., community nurses, physical therapists, self-help groups) for assistance with management at home.

All unresolved outcome criteria on the problem list require either teaching for self-management or referrals before discharge.

Discharge planning should begin at admission. After the admission assessment, the nurse must analyze the data to identify whether the client or family needs addendum discharge planning and referrals. Figure 2-9 presents questions that can help the nurse identify high-risk clients and families. These questions can be placed either as a section at the end of the admission assessment form or as a section on a combined discharge planning and summary record, as illustrated in Figure 2-9. High-risk clients and families require a referral to the discharge coordinator at admission.

Certain events that may not be predicted on admission also necessitate referral to a discharge coordinator. Some examples follow (Burgess and Raglands, 1983):

☐   Newly diagnosed chronic disease
☐   Prolonged recuperation after illness or surgery
☐   Complex home-care regimens
☐   Terminal illness
☐   Emotional instability

Discharge Summary

JCAHO recommends that a discharge summary represent instructions given, referrals, client status, and the client's understanding of the instructions. The nurse can use progress notes to record this information; however, a more efficient system for recording the discharge summary can be designed. Refer to Figure 2-9 to review a sample discharge planning and summary record. This record could be adapted with specific outcomes related to the medical or surgical condition. For example, a preprinted discharge summary record for a postoperative client could include these items:

☐   The client will correctly describe wound care measures.
☐   The client will state signs and symptoms that must be reported to a health care professional: fever, chills, redness or drainage of wound, increasing pain.

A systematic, efficient discharge planning program can promote continuity of care by identifying a client's discharge needs early. Early identification of discharge needs also may help eliminate unnecessary hospital days and unnecessary readmissions.

Summary

The development of an efficient, professional nursing documentation system is possible within the scope of existing standards of practice. The elimination of repetitive, narrative charting on progress notes can reduce the total time spent in charting and produce a more accurate, useful representation of professional practice and client or family response. A streamlined documentation system that integrates the nursing process from admission to discharge with the designated charting requirements also presents the nurse with an optimum defense in the event of litigation proceedings and legal challenges.

References/Bibliography

Alfaro, R. (1986). *Application of nursing process: A step by step guide.* Philadelphia: J.B. Lippincott.

American Nurses Association. (1973). *Standards of nursing practice.* Kansas City, MO: American Nurses Association.

Bulechek, G.M., & McCloskey, J.C. (1985). *Nursing interventions: Treatments for nursing interventions.* Philadelphia: W.B. Saunders.

Burgess, W., & Raglands, E. (1983). *Community health nursing: Philosophy, process, practice.* Norwalk, CT: Appleton-Century-Crofts.

Burke, L., & Murphy, J. (1988). *Charting by exception.* New York: John Wiley & Sons.

Carpenito, L.J. (1983). *Nursing diagnosis: Application to clinical practice.* Philadelphia: J.B. Lippincott.

Carpenito, L.J. (1987). *Nursing diagnosis: Application to clinical practice* (2nd ed.). Philadelphia: J.B. Lippincott.

Carpenito, L.J. (1989). *Nursing diagnosis: Application to clinical practice* (3rd ed.). Philadelphia: J.B. Lippincott.

Flanagan, L. (1974). *One strong voice.* Kansas City, MO: American Nurses Association.

Joint Commission on Accreditation of Healthcare Organizations (JCAHO). (1984, 1985). *Accreditation manual for hospitals.*

Maryland Nurse Practice Act, July 1986, p. 4.

Northrop, C., & Kelly, M. (1987). *Legal issues in nursing.* St. Louis: C.V. Mosby.

Waters, E. (1980). *How to do patient discharge planning.* Miami: E.J. Waters.

Illness, trauma, hospitalization, diagnostic studies, and treatments can precipitate various client responses. Depending on the situation, the client's individual personality, and other factors, these responses may include the following:

☐ Fear
☐ Anxiety
☐ Anger
☐ Denial
☐ Grief
☐ Apathy
☐ Confusion
☐ Hopelessness
☐ Feelings of powerlessness and loss of control

The nurse, as the primary presence 24 hours a day and as the practitioner of the science and art of nursing, represents the optimal health care provider for an ill client and his or her support persons (family members or significant others).

According to Henderson and Nite (1960), "Nursing is primarily assisting individuals (sick or well) with those activities contributing to health or its recovery (or to a peaceful death) that they perform unaided when they have the necessary strength, will, or knowledge." Nursing also helps clients carry out prescribed therapy and to become independent of assistance as soon as possible (Henderson and Nite, 1960).

STRESS AND ADAPTATION

According to Hoskins (1988), ". . . stress is a state produced by a change in the environment that is perceived as challenging, threatening or damaging to the person's dynamic equilibrium." Lazarus and Folkman (1980) have developed a theory of stress that focuses on the interaction or transaction between the person and the external environment. Lazarus and Monat (1977) describe coping as the psychological and behavioral activities done to master, tolerate, or minimize external or internal demands and conflicts.

Every person has a concept of self that encompasses feelings about self-worth, attractiveness, lovability, and capabilities (Peretz, 1970). Everyone also has implicit or explicit goals. Illness, other disruptions of health, and associated treatments can negatively affect a person's self-concept and ability to achieve goals. These negative effects are losses, which precipitate grieving. The extent of a person's grief response is directly related to the extent of interference in goal-directed activity and the significance of the goal.

COPING STRATEGIES

Adaptive and effective coping strategies produce these results (Visotsky, 1961):

☐ Distress is kept or returned to a manageable level.
☐ Hope is maintained or renewed.
☐ Positive self-esteem is maintained or restored.
☐ Cooperative relationships are maintained.

Cohen and Lazarus (1983) have described five modes of coping:

☐ Information-seeking
☐ Direct action
☐ Inhibition of actions
☐ Intrapsychic processes
☐ Turning to others for support.

Table 3–1 presents examples of these five modes.

Information-Seeking

A person attempting to cope with a disturbing or unfamiliar situation often seeks out knowledge to help in managing the situation. Many nurses assume that a client always needs to know as much information as possible about his or her condition and treatments. In reality, according to Burckhardt (1987), ". . . sometimes little attention is paid to whether the patient is seeking information and, if so, what information is most valuable." Burckhardt goes on to state that some clients may need to be allowed *not* to acquire information. However, if a client's lack of information for self-care is seen as detrimental, the nurse must continue to supervise the client or initiate a referral so that the client can be supervised.

In today's health care delivery system, interaction time between nurses and clients has been reduced as a direct result of reduced lengths of hospital stays. To facilitate the coping strategy of information-seeking despite decreased interaction time, the nurse can provide the client and family with opportunities to acquire information in the following ways:

☐ By creating and distributing printed material
☐ By developing audio or visual programs

☐ By providing information on community groups or commercial products that provide relevant information

☐ By directing them to call the unit with questions

Direct Action

This coping strategy incorporates any change or effort (except cognitive) that a person does to manage a situation. For example, having an ample supply of work- or leisure-related items when traveling by air or waiting for an appointment can help reduce the frustration associated with delays. Initiation of a regular exercise program is another example of direct action.

Inhibition of Action

Commonly, effective coping requires avoiding or limiting certain situations or actions. This strategy sometimes can cause problems, however. A person has to weigh the advantages and disadvantages of each action. In some cases, coping that protects or enhances physical health but compromises self-esteem can have more detrimental effects. For example, a person with Parkinson's disease may be safer using a wheelchair than a walker; however, if embarrassment and loss of control result from wheelchair use, the outcome may be decreased mobility and social isolation.

Sometimes, well-intentioned family members may inhibit the actions of the ill person without evaluating the other losses that co-exist with the loss of these actions. For example, prohibiting an elderly woman from continuing to host Thanksgiving dinner may damage her self-esteem and reduce her per-

ception of her purpose in life. Instead, it may be more constructive to allow her to supervise the meal preparation.

Intrapsychic Processes

The coping strategies involved in intrapsychic processes represent attempts to manage a stressful situation through the cognitive activities of defense mechanisms or stress reduction strategies. Table 3–2 lists examples of these cognitive coping activities.

These coping activities provide the person with much-needed control over the emotions of fear and anxiety. Although some health care professionals view defense mechanisms as pathological (Burckhardt, 1987), in most cases these mechanisms actually are constructive. If, however, the person does not use any other coping strategy (i.e., information-seeking, direct action, or support-seeking), then defense mechanisms may produce unsatisfactory or destructive outcomes. If a person delays dealing with a situation or retreats, this may be seen as maladaptive, when actually it may give the person a reprieve for internal readjustment (White, 1974). The nurse must proceed cautiously when determining how much time a client or family needs for internal readjustment. Reduced lengths of stay often propel nurses into pushing clients faster than their coping abilities can adapt. Again, it may be more constructive to provide clients and families with community resources that they can contact after internal readjustment has been achieved.

Turning to Others

This coping response involves a client's social network and social support. *Social network* is defined as the structural in-

---

TABLE 3-1. *Emotion-Focused Behaviors Versus Problem-Focused Behaviors*

	Description	Advantages/Disadvantages
Emotion-Focused Behaviors		
Intrapsychic processes		
Minimization	Reduces the seriousness of the event or problem	Provides time for appraisal and adjustment
Projection, displacement, suppression of anger	Directs anger to a less threatening person or object	Suppressed anger may increase stress
Anticipatory preparation	Rehearsal of possible consequences of behavior in stressful situations	Provides opportunity to prepare for worst; becomes dysfunctional when it produces unmanageable stress
Attribution	Finds personal meaning in the problem situation, e.g., religious faith	Offers consolation, becomes dysfunctional when self-responsibility is lost
Problem-Focused Behaviors		
Goal-setting	Setting time limitations on behaviors	May increase stress if unrealistic
Information-seeking	Learning all about the problem	Reinforces self-control
Direct action or mastery	Learning new skills	Facilitates self-esteem by providing control
Help-seeking	Sharing feelings with others for support	Provides an emotional release and comfort; if excessive, may alienate others
Inhibition of action	Eliminating an action	May increase stress if action is valued

TABLE 3-2.   Examples of Cognitive Coping Activities

Defense Mechanisms	Stress-Reduction Strategies
Denial	Thought-stopping
Avoidance	Relaxation
Rationalization	Biofeedback
Detachment	

terrelationship of the client's family, friends, neighbors, co-workers, and others who provide support; *social support* is the psychological and tangible aid provided by the social network (Tilden and Weinert, 1987). House (1981) has defined four basic types of social support:

☐ Emotional
☐ Appraisal
☐ Informational
☐ Instrumental

Table 3–3 lists characteristics of these four types.

The nurse assesses and evaluates the client's perception that he or she received enough support and the extent to which the client can return support to others—a quality known as *reciprocity.* Reciprocity is crucial to balanced, healthy relationships. According to Tilden and Weinert (1987), ". . . ill persons, unlike healthy people, who can terminate relationships that fail to satisfy their needs, often are locked into unsatisfactory relationships." In an ill client, impaired ability to reciprocate often leads to feelings of depression, dependency, and low self-esteem. Moreover, caregiver burnout can result from "one-way giving," particularly when caring for a chronically ill client (Tilden and Weinert, 1987). The nurse may be able to help a client identify effective ways of reciprocating. For example, an ill client may not be able to cook but can offer appreciation to the caregiver for meals and communicate enjoyment.

COPING WITH CHRONIC ILLNESS

Chronic illness is the number one health problem in the United States. More than 30 million Americans have chronic disabil-

TABLE 3-3.   Types of Social Support

Type of Support	Effect
Emotional support	Communicates concern, trust, caring, liking, or love
Appraisal support	Communicates respect and affirms self-worth
Informational support	Communicates useful advice and information for problem-solving
Instrumental support	Provides assistance (besides cognitive) or tangible goods, e.g., money or help with chores

ities, and over 15 million have limited ability for independent self-care (Anderson and Bauwens, 1983). In American culture, the ability to be productive is a highly valued trait. Vitality, productivity, and success often are linked; thus, chronic illness assaults a person's core values.

According to Burckhardt (1987), ". . . persons with chronic illness face permanent changes in life style, threats to dignity and self-esteem, disruption of normal life-transitions, and decreasing resources." The nurse must assist an ill client's family in recognizing and agreeing on how chronic illness has affected the family system and individual members. Open dialogue about the influences of the chronic illness may help to preserve family relationships. Failure to acknowledge the effects and changes likely will lead to destruction and dissolution of the family system (Larkin, 1987).

Social supports can buffer stress and reduce adverse health effects (Broadhead, Kaplan, and James, 1983). Unfortunately, chronic illness can negatively influence social supports and networks (Table 3–4).

As discussed earlier, chronic illness presents a unique and often frustrating challenge for clients, support networks, and health care professionals. Numerous care plans, applicable to clients and families experiencing chronic illness, can be found in Unit II of this book.

Responses to the losses associated with the experience of illness and its aftermath can include denial, anger, fear, anxiety, guilt, and sadness.

Denial

In order to cope with a difficult situation, sometimes a person disavows or minimizes the seriousness of the situation and also the feelings connected to the situation. In many cases, denial is a very useful and healthy way to deal with a problematic situation, because it provides the time needed to regain and maintain emotional equilibrium. However, denial can be harmful if it leads to detrimental outcomes, e.g., refusal of appropriate treatment or drug abuse.

Anger

Anger can be and should be an appropriate response to an unacceptable situation. Unfortunately, direct expressions of anger usually are considered inappropriate and commonly evoke feelings of guilt afterward. But a person who habitually suppresses angry feelings cultivates hostility. As a result of the person's inability or unwillingness to express anger, conflicts remain unresolved; unresolved conflicts can lead to depression.

Nurses, like others, typically are uncomfortable with clients' expressions of anger. However, anger may be a productive response for a client in a vulnerable position. A person typically expresses anger to those he or she deems least likely to retaliate or least important; thus, nurses are often the target of the anger of clients or their families (just as nurses may use peers or family as targets for their anger at hospital administration or the "system"). A nurse may deal with an angry client by avoiding him or her. In most persons, this avoidance is commonly seen as a benign response; however, for a nurse, avoidance is a malignant response, because it results in reducing or withholding nursing care.

To deal effectively with an angry client, the nurse must first examine her or his feelings about and responses to angry behavior. Did the nurse witness anger as a child? Was she or he allowed to express anger as a child? Next, the nurse should examine the client's or family's anger, asking herself or himself these questions:

- What could be the source(s) of the anger? Loss of control? Fear? Embarrassment?
- Is this the client's or family's usual response to stress?
- Is the anger serving a useful purpose?

When intervening with an angry client, the nurse may find it productive to give the client a direct message that he or she has a right to be angry (if appropriate), but that screaming, verbal abuse, obscene language, and physical violence are not acceptable. Helping a client express anger without alienation is a difficult but productive strategy. Communicating the message that "if I were in your position or situation, I would be angry too; however, screaming at me will not reduce your anger or contribute to finding satisfying options" validates that the client has a right to feel anger but not to express it in a hurtful manner.

Anxiety

Anxiety is a state in which a person experiences feelings of uneasiness or apprehension and activation of the autonomic nervous system in response to a vague, nonspecific threat. Anxiety differs from fear in that an anxious person cannot identify the threat, whereas a fearful person can. Anxiety can occur without fear; however, fear usually does not occur without anxiety (Carpenito, 1987).

Feelings of uneasiness, dread, and inadequacy accompany anxiety. The response to a threat may range from mild anxiety to panic. The four degrees of anxiety—mild, moderate, severe, and panic—are differentiated in Table 3–5. Mild anxiety has been described as normal anxiety, moderate anxiety as chronic anxiety, and severe anxiety as acute anxiety. Mild anxiety is necessary for a person to function and respond effectively to the environment and events.

END-OF-LIFE DECISIONS

Families and health care providers experience intense stress when faced with decisions regarding either initiation or discontinuation of life support systems or other medical interventions that prolong life (Johnson and Justin, 1988). Additional conflicts arise if the client's wishes are unknown, especially if the family disagrees with the decisions of health care providers or vice versa. For this reason, clients and families should be encouraged to discuss and record their directions to guide possible future clinical decision-making (Johnson and Justin, 1988).

The nurse should instruct a client and family members to provide the following information (Carpenito, 1989):

- Person(s) to contact in an emergency
- Person the client trusts most with personal decisions
- Person(s) who will be consulted for decisions if the client becomes mentally incompetent
- Preference to die at home, in the hospital, or no preference
- Desire to sign a living will
- Decision on organ donation
- Funeral arrangements; burial or cremation
- Circumstances in which information should be withheld from the client, if any

TABLE 3-4. *Effects of Chronic Illness on Social Supports and Social Networks*

Resulting Factors (Contributory/Risk Factors)	Resulting Nursing Diagnoses (Possible, Actual, Potential)
Decreased mobility Loss of control of bodily functions Fatigue Loss of employment Avoidance by others Fluctuations in functioning Anger, depression, self-preoccupation	Self-Care Deficits Social Isolation Impaired Social Interactions Fatigue

Changes in family functioning
    Role reversal
    Financial burden
    Reduction of free time
    Avoidance of social functions
    Reduced reciprocity
	Altered Family Process
	Ineffective Coping (family, individual)

All decisions made should be documented. One copy should be given to the person designated as the decision-maker if the client becomes incompetent or unable to make decisions, and the other copy should be retained in a safe deposit box.

A living will is a document that reflects a person's desires or choices should terminal illness occur. Living wills do not apply to initial treatment decisions, only to situations in which no reasonable possibility of recovery exists. Many states have laws governing living wills; however, all are not necessarily legally binding. Nurses should be familiar with their state's laws regarding living wills. To obtain a copy of your state's living will, write to the Society for the Right to Die, 250 West 57th Street, New York, NY 10107.

NURSING ACCOUNTABILITY

Health care raises conflicts for both clients and health care providers. Often, nurses experience conflict when it is unclear to whom they are accountable. Nursing accountability involves both legal and ethical obligations for the nurse. Legally, nurses are accountable to state regulations known as nurse practice acts. Nurse practice acts vary greatly from state to state; some

specify that nurses address diagnosis and case planning. Unfortunately, nurses sometimes allow their practice to be sanctioned by other members of the health care team even when these practices are within the legal boundaries of the applicable nurse practice act.

Besides legal considerations, most situations also involve ethical implications. According to Carpenito and Duespohl (1985), ethical behavior is "a moral obligation, as opposed to a legal one imposed by the law." Carpenito and Duespohl went on to state

> Whereas the professional nurse is held accountable to the law for providing safe nursing care to the consumer, ethical accountability is a personal responsibility that nurses and all other health professionals must accept. Protecting the rights of the client who has entered the health care system is a responsibility the professional nurse shares with others in the medical professions. As the client's advocate, the professional nurse is obligated to coordinate the health services provided to the client by all members of the health team. Every professional nurse has an ethical obligation to place the client's best interest first.

Many state nurse practice acts state specifically that the nurse is ethically accountable to the health care consumer. The

---

TABLE 3-5.   Types of Anxiety

Mild Anxiety

    Perception and attention heightened; alert
    Able to deal with problem situations
    Can integrate past, present, and future experiences
    Uses learning; can consensually validate; formulates meanings
    Curious, repeats questions
    Sleeplessness

Moderate Anxiety

    Perception somewhat narrowed; selectively inattentive, but can direct attention
    Slightly more difficult to concentrate; learning requires more effort
    Views present experiences in terms of past
    May fail to notice what is happening in a peripheral situation; will have some difficulty in adapting and analyzing
    Voice/pitch changes
    Increased respiratory and heart rates
    Tremors, shakiness

Severe Anxiety

    Perception greatly reduced; focuses on scattered details; cannot attend to more even when instructed to do so
    Learning severely impaired; highly distractable, unable to concentrate
    Views present experiences in terms of past; almost unable to understand current situation
    Functions poorly; communication difficult to understand
    Hyperventilation, tachycardia, headache, dizziness, nausea

Panic

    Perception distorted; focuses on blown-up detail; scattering may be increased
    Learning cannot occur
    Unable to integrate experiences; can focus only on present; unable to see or understand situation; has lapses in recall of thoughts
    Unable to function; usually increased motor activity or unpredictable responses to even minor stimuli; communication not able to be understood
    Vomiting; feelings of impending doom

(Carpenito LJ: *Nursing Diagnosis: Application to Clinical Practice*, ed. 2. Philadelphia: JB Lippincott, 1987, p 121)

American Nurses' Association's code of ethics for nurses has no legal basis, but it has been used to revoke the nursing licenses of nurses who have behaved in direct contradiction to its precepts.

STANDARD OF CARE FOR HOSPITALIZED ADULTS

Hospitalization, illness, trauma, diagnostic studies, and treatments affect clients and their families in various ways. All hospitalized clients share experiences that can be predicted prior to admission, e.g., changes in diet, activity, and environment, and preparation for diagnostic studies. The optimal nursing assessments and interventions for these situations have been determined through research and practice, taking into account length of stay, resource allocation, and other factors. Besides the generic diagnostic cluster and interventions outlined in Appendix I, Generic Care Plan for Hospitalized Adults, each client and family will have additional specific diagnoses, as determined through nursing assessment. The care plans in Unit II cover many of these possible diagnoses.

As discussed in Chapter 2, the nurse should not include generic nursing diagnoses and collaborative problems on individual client problem lists. Rather, they are assumed to be present in all clients and are addressed routinely, then documented on flow records, with progress notes written only if something unusual occurs. For example, most clients experience some sleep problems in the hospital. For optimal rest, each night a client should go through at least three or four uninterrupted sleep cycles of about 90 minutes each. If this does not occur, a progress note identifying this sleep disturbance is indicated; otherwise, no documentation is necessary. If additional specific nursing interventions beyond the generic interventions are indicated, the nurse adds Sleep and Rest Disturbance to this client's problem list and appropriate interventions to the addendum care plan.

ANA Code of Ethics for Nurses

1. The nurse provides services with respect for human dignity and the uniqueness of the client unrestricted by considerations of social or economic status, personal attributes, or the nature of health problems.
2. The nurse safeguards the client's right to privacy by judiciously protecting information of a confidential nature.
3. The nurse acts to safeguard the client and the public when health care and safety are affected by the incompetent, unethical, or illegal practice of any person.
4. The nurse assumes responsibility and accountability for individual nursing judgments and actions.
5. The nurse maintains competence in nursing.
6. The nurse exercises informed judgment and uses individual competence and qualifications as criteria in seeking consultation, accepting responsibilities, and delegating nursing activities to others.
7. The nurse participates in activities that contribute to the ongoing development of the profession's body of knowledge.
8. The nurse participates in the profession's efforts to implement and improve standards of nursing.
9. The nurse participates in the professions' efforts to establish and maintain conditions of employment conducive to high quality nursing care.
10. The nurse participates in the profession's effort to protect the public from misinformation and misrepresentation and to maintain the integrity of nursing.
11. The nurse collaborates with members of the health professions and other citizens in promoting community and national efforts to meet the health needs of the public.

(American Nurses' Association: *The Code for Nurses*, rev. ed. Kansas City, MO: ANA, 1976. Reprinted with permission)

Summary

Illness, trauma, and hospitalization, like other stressors that affect lives and life events, have the potential to leave the involved parties (clients and families or significant others) disorganized and devastated, but they may also provide an opportunity for increased growth and cohesiveness. The nurse can be instrumental in directing clients and families to the path of mutual support and individual autonomy.

References/Bibliography

Anderson, S.V., & Bauwens, E.E. (Eds.). (1983). *Chronic health problems.* St. Louis: C.V. Mosby.

Broadhead, W.E., Kaplan, B.H., & James, S.A. (1983). The epidemiologic evidence for a relationship between social support and health. *American Journal of Epidemiology, 117,* 521–537.

Burckhardt, C.S. (1987). Coping strategies of the chronically ill. *Nursing Clinics of North America, 22*(3), 543–549.

Carpenito, L.J. (1987). *Nursing diagnosis: Application to clinical practice* (2nd ed.). Philadelphia: J.B. Lippincott.

Carpenito, L.J. (1989). *Nursing diagnosis: Application to clinical practice* (3rd ed.). Philadelphia: J.B. Lippincott.

Carpenito, L.J., & Duespohl, T.A. (1985). *A guide to effective clinical instruction* (2nd ed.). Rockville, MD: Aspen Systems Corp.

Cohen, F., & Lazarus, R.S. (1983). Coping and adaptation in health and illness. In D. Mechanic (Ed.). *Handbook of health, health care, and health professions.* New York: Free Press.

Hathaway, D. (1987). Health promotion and disease prevention for hospitalized patient's family. *Nursing Administration Quarterly, 11*(3), 1–7.

Henderson, V., & Nite, G. (1960). *Principles and practice of nursing* (5th ed.). New York: Macmillan.

Hoskins, L. (1988). Stress and adaptation. In L. Brunner & D. Suddarth. *Textbook of medical-surgical nursing* (6th ed.). Philadelphia: J.B. Lippincott.

House, J.S. (1981). *Work stress and social support.* Reading, MA: Addison-Wesley.

Informed consent in hospital liability and risk management. (1981). New York: Practicing Law Institute.

Johnson, R.A., & Justin, R. (1988). Documenting patients' end of life decisions. *Nurse Practitioner, 13*(6), 41.

Larkin, J. (1987). Factors influencing one's ability to adapt to chronic illness. *Nursing Clinics of North America, 22*(3), 535–542.

Lazarus, R.S., & Folkman, S. (1980). Analysis of coping in a middle age community sample. *Journal of Health Behavior, 21*(9), 219–239.

Lazarus, R.S., & Folkman, S. (1984). *Stress, appraisal and coping.* New York: Springer-Verlag.

Lazarus, R.S., & Monat, A. (1977). *Stress and coping: An anthology.* New York: Columbia University Press.

Marsh, F.L. (1986). Refusal of treatment. *Clinics in Geriatric Medicine, 2*(3), 511–520.

Peretz, D. (1970). Reaction to loss. In A.C. Carr & D. Peretz (Eds.). *Loss and grief: Psychological management in medicine.* New York: Columbia University Press.

Salmond, S. (1980). How to assess the nutritional status of acutely ill patients. *American Journal of Nursing, 80*(5), 922.

Springhouse Corp. (1985). *Nurse's legal handbook.* Springhouse, PA: Springhouse Corp.

Taylor, C., Lillis, C., & LaMone, P. (1989). *Fundamentals of nursing.* Philadelphia: J.B. Lippincott.

Tilden, V., & Weinert, C. (1987). Social support and the chronically ill individual. *Nursing Clinics of North America, 22*(3), 613–620.

Visotsky, H. (1961). Coping behavior under extreme stress. *Archives of General Psychiatry, 5,* 27–32.

Weber, J. (1989). Hopelessness. In L.J. Carpenito. *Nursing diagnosis: Application to clinical practice* (3rd ed.). Philadelphia: J.B. Lippincott.

White, R.W. (1974). Strategies of adaptation: An attempt at systematic description. In G.V. Coelho, D.A. Hamburg, & J.E. Adams (Eds.). *Coping and adaption.* New York: Basic Books.

A planned trauma, surgery evokes a range of physiological and psychological responses in a client, based on personal and unique past experiences, coping patterns, strengths, and limitations. Most clients and their families view any surgery, regardless of its complexity, as a major event, and they react with some degree of anxiety and fear.

Perioperative nursing is the term used to describe the nursing responsibilities associated with the preoperative, intraoperative, postanesthesia recovery, and postoperative surgical phases. Throughout the perioperative period, the nurse applies the nursing process to identify the client's positive functioning, altered functioning, and potential for altered functioning. The nursing responsibilities for each phase (Table 4–1) focus on specific actual or potential health problems.

Surgical trauma and anesthesia disrupt all major body system functions, but most clients have the compensatory capability to restore homeostasis. However, certain clients are at greater risk for ineffective compensation for the adverse effects of surgery and anesthesia on cardiac, circulatory, respiratory, and other functions (Table 4–2). Again, the nursing process provides the nurse with a guide for identifying client responses to the surgical experience.

PREOPERATIVE ASSESSMENT

The nursing history and physical assessment of a preoperative client focus on present status and the potential for complications. Because all clients receive a nursing assessment on admission, these criteria can be integrated into the general nursing interview. (See Figure 2-1, Nursing Admission Data Base, page 12.)

In addition to the general data collected on admission, the nurse caring for a client in any phase of the perioperative period completes focus assessments—acquisition of selected or specific data as determined by the nurse and the client or family or as directed by the client's condition. The nurse who assesses a new postoperative client's condition (e.g., vital signs, incision, hydration, comfort) is performing a focus assessment (Carpenito and Duespohl, 1985). Preoperative focus assessments involve evaluating certain factors that can influence the client's risk for intraoperative or postoperative complications:

- [ ] Client's understanding of events
- [ ] Acute or chronic condition
- [ ] Client's previous surgical experience
- [ ] Nutritional status
- [ ] Fluid and electrolyte status
- [ ] Emotional status

Another alternative is a specific preoperative assessment that the nurse completes the evening before surgery or the morning of surgery, in the operating or postanesthesia room. Morbidity and mortality may be reduced with a planned, deliberate preoperative nursing assessment.

Understanding of Events

The surgeon is responsible for explaining the nature of the operation, any alternative options, the expected results, and the possible complications that may occur. The surgeon obtains two consents—one for the procedure and one for anesthesia. The nurse is responsible for determining the client's understanding of the information, then notifying the surgeon if more information is needed for a valid informed consent.

Acute or Chronic Condition

In order to compensate for the effects of surgical trauma and anesthesia, the human body needs optimal respiratory, circulatory, cardiac, renal, hepatic, and hematopoietic function. Any condition that interferes with any of these systems' functions (e.g., diabetes mellitus, congestive heart failure, chronic obstructive pulmonary disease, anemia, cirrhosis, renal failure, lupus erythematosus) compromises recovery. In addition to pre-existing medical conditions, advanced age, obesity, and alcohol abuse also make a client more vulnerable to complications, as outlined in Table 4-3.

Previous Surgical Experience

The nurse must ask the client and family specific questions regarding past surgical experiences. The information obtained is used to promote comfort (physical and psychological) and to prevent serious complications.

To detect a possible predisposition to malignant hyperthermia, the nurse should ask, "Has a doctor or a nurse ever mentioned to you or a family member that you had difficulty with anesthesia—excessive somnolence, vomiting, allergic reaction, or hyperthermia?" and, "Has a family member experienced difficulty with anesthesia?" Malignant hyperthermia—a life-threatening syndrome occurring during surgery, predominantly in apparently healthy children and young adults—is associated with a hereditary predisposition and the use of muscle relaxants and inhalation anesthetics. Incidence is estimated

TABLE 4-1. Focus of Nursing Care in the Perioperative Period

Preoperative Phase

Preoperative assessment
Preoperative teaching
Preparation for transfer to operating room
Psychological support
Support of significant other

Intraoperative Phase

Environmental safety
Asepsis control
Physiological monitoring
Psychological support (preinduction)
Transfer to postanesthesia recovery room (PAR)

Postanesthesia Recovery Phase

Physiological monitoring (cardiac, respiratory, circulatory, renal, neurologic)
Psychological support
Environmental safety
Comfort measures
Stability for transfer to unit

Postoperative Phase

Physiological monitoring
Psychological support
Comfort measures
Support of significant other
Physiological equilibrium (nutrition, fluid, elimination)
Mobilization
Wound healing
Discharge teaching

as 1 in 50,000 surgical clients, with a mortality rate of 30% to 40%.

Nutritional Status

The client's preoperative nutritional status directly influences his or her response to surgical trauma and anesthesia. After any major wound, from either trauma or surgery, the body must build and repair tissue and protect itself from infection. To facilitate these processes, the client must increase protein–carbohydrate intake sufficiently to prevent negative nitrogen balance, hypoalbuminemia, and weight loss. Malnourished states result from inadequate intake, compromised metabolic function, or increased metabolic demands. Healthy clients can tolerate short periods of negative nitrogen balance postoperatively, but clients who are malnourished before surgery are at high risk for infections, sepsis, and evisceration (McConnell, 1987).

Wound healing requires the following nutritional components (Constantian, 1980):

☐ Increased protein–carbohydrate intake sufficient to prevent negative nitrogen balance, hypoalbuminemia, and weight loss
☐ Increased daily intake of vitamins and minerals:
Vitamin A—10,000 to 50,000 IU

Vitamin B—0.5 mg to 1.0 mg/1,000 dietary calories
Vitamin B_2—0.25 mg/1,000 dietary calories
Vitamin B_6—2 mg
Niacin—15 to 20 mg
Vitamin B—400 mg
Vitamin C—75 to 300 mg
Vitamin D—400 mg
Vitamin E—10 to 15 IU
Traces of zinc, magnesium, calcium, and copper
☐ Adequate oxygen supply and the blood volume and ability to transport it

Preoperatively, the nurse should identify those clients who are malnourished and those who are at higher risk for postoperative nutritional compromise. The nurse then can consult with the nutritionist and physician for preoperative treatment to correct nutritional deficits.

Fluid and Electrolyte Status

A client with a fluid and electrolyte imbalance is prone to complications of shock, hypotension, hypoxia, and dysrhythmias both intraoperatively and postoperatively. Fluid volume fluctuations result from decreased fluid intake or abnormal fluid loss, both of which occur in surgical trauma. Table 4-4 lists factors that decrease fluid intake and increase fluid loss.

The nurse can assess a client's daily fluid balance by evaluating the following:

☐ Daily weights
☐ Intake and output
☐ Urine specific gravity (in adults under age 65)
☐ Condition of mucous membranes (in infants and children)

Additional parameters assessed when monitoring fluid and electrolyte status include these:

☐ Central venous pressure
☐ Pulmonary arterial pressure
☐ Serum electrolytes
☐ Hemoglobin and hematocrit
☐ Blood urea nitrogen
☐ Creatinine

Adults with no preexisting fluid and electrolyte problem usually can compensate for the losses associated with surgery. However, clients of advanced age and those with cirrhosis, cancer, chronic pulmonary disease, diabetes mellitus, renal disorders, adrenal or thyroid dysfunction, or cardiovascular disorders, or those on corticosteroid therapy, may be unable to compensate.

Emotional Status

A client's, family's, and significant other's response to anticipated surgery depends on the following:

☐ Past experiences
☐ Usual coping strategies
☐ Significance of the surgery
☐ Support system (quality and availability)

TABLE 4-2. Adverse Consequences of Surgery and Anesthesia and Factors That Interfere With Compensatory Mechanisms

Consequence	Factors That Impair Ability to Compensate	Results
Nothing by mouth	Elderly/very young	Hypovolemia
	Malnourished	Shock
	Dehydrated	
	Diabetes mellitus	Hypoglycemia
Blood loss	Same as NPO, plus:	
	Coagulation disorders	Hemorrhage
	Aspirin	
	Anticoagulants	
	Antiplatelets	
	Tobacco use	
Biotransformation of anesthetic compounds	Renal disorders	Drug toxicity
	Hepatic disorders	
	Elderly	
	Alcohol or drug abuse	
Myocardial depression	Uncompensated heart disease	Dysrhythmias
	Hypertension	Hypotension
		Shock
Hypotension	Coronary artery disease	Shock
	Monoamine oxidase inhibitors	Stroke
	Phenothiazides	
Respiratory depression	Chronic obstructive pulmonary disease	Hypoxia
	History of smoking	Apnea
	Congestive heart failure	
	Obesity	
	Upper respiratory infection	
	Diuretics	
	"Mycin" medications	

TABLE 4-3. Intraoperative and Postoperative Implications of Preexisting Compromised Functions

Condition	Associated Compromised Functions	Intraoperative Implications	Postoperative Implications
Advanced age	↑Cardiac reserves	Cardiac failure ⟶	
	↑Peripheral resistance		Thrombosis
	↓Ability to increase cardiac output	Hypotension/shock ⟶	
	↓Lung capacity	Hypoxia	Pneumonia, atelectasis
	↑Residual volume	Electrolyte imbalances ⟶	
	↓Cough reflex ⟶		Respiratory infection
	↓Renal blood flow	Shock	
	↓Glomerular filtration	Impaired ability to excrete anesthetics ⟶	
	Enlarged prostrate ⟶		Urinary retention
	↓Gastric motility ⟶		Paralytic ileus, constipation
	↑Bone resorption	Fractures ⟶	
	Impaired ability to regulate temperature	Hypothermia	Hypo/hyperthermia
	↓Sound transmission	Difficulty hearing ⟶	
	↓Lens elasticity ⟶		Risk for falls
	↓Hepatic function	↓Excretion of medications = ↑toxicity	Impaired protein synthesis ↓phagocytosis
Obesity	Excess of adipose tissue (↓vascularity)	Larger incision	Delayed healing
		Prolonged anesthesia time	Dehiscence/evisceration
	Impaired mobility	↑Risk of injury (fall, skin)	Thrombosis
	↓Efficiency of respiratory muscles	Hypoventilation	Respiratory infection
	↓Gastric emptying time ⟶		Aspiration, pneumonia
Alcoholism	↓Hepatic function	↓Excretion of medications = ↑toxicity	Malnourishment
	↓Phagocytosis ⟶		Delayed healing
	Impaired protein synthesis	Cross-tolerance to anesthetics	Cross-tolerance to analgesics
	↓Adrenocortical response ⟶		Withdrawal symptoms

TABLE 4-4.   *Factors That Increase Fluid Loss and Decrease Fluid Intake*

Decreased Fluid Intake
Nothing by mouth
Nausea/vomiting
Imposed fluid restrictions
Fatigue, pain

Increased Fluid Loss
Vomiting
Blood loss
Burns
Fever
Ascites
Abnormal drainage (wound, drains)
Diarrhea
Diuretics
Bowel preparations (enema, medications)

Most clients anticipating surgery experience anxiety and fear. The uncertainties of surgery produce the anxiety; anticipated pain, incisions, and immobility can produce fear. Anxiety has been classified as mild, moderate, severe, and panic. (See Table 3-5 for more information.)

Anxiety can be differentiated into *state anxiety* and *trait anxiety. State anxiety* is the response to a stressful situation; *trait anxiety* refers to the variable interpretations persons make of threatening situations (Spielberger and Sarason, 1975). It is expected that clients and their families would have state anxiety. To help assuage this anxiety, the nurse should explore with the client and family their fears and concerns. Besides identifying sources of anxiety, the nurse also should assess possible avenues of support or comfort, asking questions such as, "What would provide you with more comfort before surgery?" and, "What do you usually do when you are under stress?"

Moderate anxiety is expected before surgery. Usually, clients with moderate anxiety are willing to share their concerns. Clients who demonstrate panic anxiety or verbalize that they will die in the operating room present a serious situation clinically. When faced with such a client the nurse should consult with the physician, who may want to consider postponing surgery.

Clients who are suffering, either physically or emotionally, can be best aided by a nonjudgmental listener who encourages them to express their feelings and conveys that it is acceptable to have such emotions. This behavior demonstrates sincerity and warmth to the client (Carpenito and Duespohl, 1985).

In order to communicate effectively, a nurse must first acknowledge and accept her or his own personal vulnerability. As human beings, nurses feel the emotions of sadness, fear, and frustration. To deny the existence of these feelings is to deny one's own humanity. The nurse has a responsibility to encourage clients to share, to indicate that she or he accepts clients' responses to situations, and to convey that she or he is emotionally involved. This emotional involvement is often quite difficult for nurses to incorporate into their nursing practice; however, pride and personal satisfaction soon replace all personal discomfort as nurses realize they make a positive dif-

ference in clients' surgical experiences (Carpenito and Duespohl, 1985).

A client who is suffering tends to respond positively to a nurse who accepts his or her response. For example, explaining that fear before surgery is normal to a client experiencing fear usually is comforting; sharing with a grieving family that you understand their loss does not eliminate the loss but does convey support. The ability to communicate effectively does not come automatically, however; it is a planned and learned art involving practice and caring.

PREOPERATIVE TEACHING

Preoperative teaching is defined as the supportive and educational actions the nurse takes to assist a surgical client in promoting his or her own health before and after surgery. The client's requirements for nursing assistance lie in the areas of decision-making, acquisition of knowledge and skills, and behavioral changes (Glass, McGraw, and Smith, 1982).

Preoperative teaching should be a combination of emotional support and information-giving (Glass, McGraw, and Smith, 1982). Studies have shown that clients who receive structured information regarding what they will feel, see, hear, and smell, in addition to what will happen, report less anxiety during surgical procedures (Johnson, 1978; Felton, 1985; King and Tarsitano, 1982). For example, explaining the sensations involved in intravenous catheter insertion rather than limiting the instruction to "an IV will be in your arm" helps reduce the client's anxiety associated with unexpected sensations.

The advent of new, more effective instructional technology and the reduced lengths of stay require that the nurse use a variety of strategies to achieve outcome criteria. Retention of information is increased when the teaching–learning process involves a variety of senses (Cannon, 1989). Learning also is enhanced by the client's active involvement and provisions for practice; for example, it helps to encourage the client to practice coughing, deep breathing, and leg exercises during the teaching sessions.

Many of these strategies can be used in group classes. Group sessions are time- and cost-effective, allowing one nurse to provide general information to a group of clients experiencing a similar event, e.g., new diagnosis of diabetes mellitus, upcoming coronary surgery. They also provide an opportunity for clients and families to share their concerns. Many people find it comforting to know that others are undergoing a similar experience.

Group sessions can be scheduled on a regular basis, e.g., from 7 to 8 PM Sunday through Thursday. Staff nurses from several units can rotate teaching sessions. At these sessions, the nurses can do the following:

☐   Elicit questions and concerns
☐   Evaluate achievement of outcome criteria
☐   Provide additional information

Keep in mind that all clients who attend group classes also must receive one-on-one teaching. A staff nurse on the client's unit can reinforce the teaching and elicit questions from the client or family after the group session.

Providing the client with instruction and opportunities to practice preoperatively can enhance his or her participation in postoperative care. Moreover, family members who are involved in preoperative teaching sessions can later be enlisted to coach the client in necessary postoperative care measures, such as coughing and deep breathing exercises.

Today, many clients are admitted the same day as surgery and most others have reduced lengths of stay, minimizing the time available for client teaching. In response to increasing time constraints, nursing departments have developed various simple, quick teaching programs aimed at ensuring positive outcome criteria; for example, brochures on postoperative care routines for a specific type of surgery and group classes for same-day surgery clients held the week before surgery is scheduled.

PREOPERATIVE NURSING RECORD

Figure 4-1 presents a preoperative assessment/care plan that the nurse completes the evening before surgery or, if this is not possible, on the morning of surgery. This form also can be used in a same-day surgical setting. This record helps the nurse collect essential preoperative data. Section I outlines specific areas concerning medical and surgical history, informed consent, and laboratory or diagnostic studies. Section II is a combination of assessment and plan of care. Content areas relating to present status and risk factors are specified in the left-hand column. If the data indicate no anticipated problems or identify no specific risk factors, they are recorded in the assessment column only. If the data present a problem or a risk factor for a potential problem, they are recorded under the diagnosis/plan column and the diagnostic statement is checked, as are the contributing or risk factors. If the nurse has identified additional contributing or risk factors, they can be written in. The diagnoses identified on this form are both nursing diagnoses and collaborative problems.

Each of the nursing diagnoses or collaborative problems identified has corresponding standards of care that specifically direct the nurse to reduce or eliminate, monitor, or report the problem. These standards of care are in addition to the generic standards of care that have been identified by the American Association of Operating Room Nurses (AAORN). Table 4-5 is an example of a generic standard of care for a client experiencing anxiety. Under this standard, the only documentation required is whether an unusual response is observed (item 13).

Policies that require nurses to copy from standards of care further reduce the nurse–client interaction time. Copying from a printed sheet does not produce an individualized plan. Rather, it would be more prudent to require only specific interactions to be handwritten. Space is provided under each diagnosis on the assessment form so that the nurse can add any additional interventions beyond the standard when indicated. Figure 4-2 illustrates some additional interventions added for a client by the nurse prior to surgery. Any additional interventions provided by the nurse but not identified preoperatively should be recorded on the progress or nurse's notes, not on the care plan. Remember, a care plan is written only if another nurse will be responsible for providing the care; a nurse should not write a care plan just for herself or himself to follow.

If the nurse has not identified any specific diagnoses, she or he places a checkmark before this statement at the end of the form:

TABLE 4-5. Standard of Care for the Operating Room for a Patient With Moderate Anxiety

Goal

Verbalize specific fears/concerns

Plan

1. Encourage ventilation of concerns/fears
2. Answer questions related to nursing management
3. Direct questions related to medical care to physician
4. Complete room preparations prior to patient entry
5. Minimize noise/traffic
6. Orient to operating room; repeat information to allow retention
7. Remain with patient through induction
8. Continue psychological monitoring
9. Give clear, concise explanations
10. Convey caring, supportive attitude
11. Keep spotlight off until patient is asleep
12. Remove dentures/glasses/ hearing aid in operating room suite
13. Document unexpected responses

Problems requiring addendum nursing interventions are not present at this time. Follow standard of care for perioperative nursing care.

The nurse completing the preoperative section then signs in the space indicated.

When a nurse cannot visit all postoperative clients, she or he should select certain clients according to preoperative assessment findings, with clients having problems or risk factors validated before surgery receiving top priority. During the postoperative visit, the nurse assesses whether the interventions provided have prevented or reduced the problems.

THE POSTANESTHESIA RECOVERY PERIOD

During the immediate postoperative period, a client is extremely vulnerable to physiological complications resulting from the effects of anesthetics on respiratory and circulatory function. Throughout the client's stay in the postanesthesia recovery room (PAR), the nurse should monitor the client at least every 15 to 20 minutes.

Level I Standards of Care should include the nursing diagnoses and collaborative problems that are present in most clients in PAR. Table 4-6 lists the collaborative problems and nursing diagnoses commonly seen in post surgical clients in PAR. The nurse should record assessments and usual interventions on the PAR flow record. Unusual data or events will be recorded on the progress note.

Level II standards in the PAR would refer to additional standard care needed after a specific surgery, e.g., mastectomy. Level II standards could also address a single diagnosis. For example, if the preoperative assessment indicates that a client recovering from a hip-pinning operation has a nursing diagnosis of Altered Thought Processes related to unknown etiology (as manifested by repetitive questions of "Where am I?" or "Why am I here?"), the PAR nurse would continually need to orient the client to the environment and to the reasons for the hip

Section I Preoperative Phase

Date _____

Diagnosis _____

Surgeon _____

Procedure scheduled and date _____

Age _____ Weight _____ Height _____

I.D. band on   Yes _____   No _____

H & P done   Yes _____   No _____

Medical clearance   Yes _____   No _____

Pre-op instruction done   Bedside _____   Group _____

Consent signed

   Scheduled procedure   Yes _____   No _____

   Blood   Yes _____   No _____

   Other   Yes _____   No _____

   (Specify) _____

_____ Chart incomplete   _____ Patient not available for visit

Lab/Diagnostic Studies

	Normal	Abnormal	No Results	Not Ordered
Hct				
HgB				
K				
Na				
PT/PTT				
Calcium				
VDRL				
HIV				
Cultures				
Glucose				
Chest X-ray				
EKG				
Type and cross units				
Urinalysis				
Other				

Medical Problems and Surgical History

Previous surgical experience?   Yes _____   No _____

  Specify: _____

Past problems with anesthesia?   Individual   Yes _____   No _____

                         Family   Yes _____   No _____

Existing medical problems: (check)

_____ Diabetes   _____ Cardiac disease   _____ Arthritis

_____ Hypertension   _____ Cancer   _____ Respiratory

_____ Hematologic   _____ Hepatic   _____ AIDS

_____ Seizures   _____ CVA   _____ Renal

_____ Other _____

Section II Perioperative Nursing Record

ASSESSMENT	DIAGNOSIS/PLAN

I. Ability to Communicate
Verbal
☐ Appropriate
 	
Language spoken
☐ English
☐ Spanish
☐ Other (specify) _____
 	
Hearing
☐ Appropriate
	Impaired Verbal Communication related to
	  ☐ Inability to speak secondary to (specify) _____
	  ☐ Inability to communicate in English
	
	Impaired communication related to
	  ☐ Deafness
	  ☐ Impaired hearing
	  ☐ Diminished level of consciousness

Figure 4-1. Preoperative nursing assessment/care plan.

(continued)

ASSESSMENT	DIAGNOSIS/PLAN
II. Risks for Injury	
1. Level of consciousness ☐ Alert	Potential for Injury related to ☐ Confusion ☐ Drowsiness ☐ Nonresponsive state
2. Weight _____ Height _____ ☐ Within normal limits (WNL) within 15% of ideal wt.	Potential for Injury: Fall related to ☐ Obesity > 15%
3. Allergies ☐ None reported	☐ Drug allergy (specify) _____
4. Therapeutic devices ☐ None present	☐ IV, Foley, drains, casts (circle or specify) _____

5. Skin integrity
   Presence of lesions/edema
   ☐ None
   ☐ Deferred
	Impaired Skin Integrity related to
	
	☐ Lesions ☐ Edema
	   (specify size and location) _____

Allergies (refer to 3)
   ☐ None reported
	Potential Impaired Skin Integrity related to
	☐ Allergy to metal, chemicals, cleansers, adhesives (circle or
	   specify) _____

Weight ☐ Within 15% of ideal weight	☐ Cachexia ☐ Obesity
Circulatory status ☐ WNL	☐↓Circulation secondary to (specify) _____

6. Understanding of surgical experience
   ☐ Satisfactory
   ☐ Unable to evaluate
	Anxiety related to
	☐ Lack of understanding of (specify) _____

7. Emotional status
   Anxiety level
   ☐ Mild
	Anxiety/fear:
	☐ Moderate ⎫
	☐ Severe ⎬ related to impending surgical experience and:
	☐ First surgical experience
	☐ History of negative surgical experience (own, relative, specify)
	_____
	☐ Specify _____

8. Risk for hemorrhage
   History of hematologic disorder
   ☐ None reported
	Potential Complication: Hemorrhage
	
	☐ History of hematologic disorder (specify) _____

Presence of medications that increase risk ☐ None	☐ Aspirin therapy ☐ Anticoagulants ☐ None
9. History of: Substance use:	Potential Complication: Cardiac, Hepatic, Respiratory, Hemorrhage

Alcohol use
   ☐ None reported
	☐ Alcohol use
	   ___ drinks day/wk.

Smoking
   ☐ None reported
   ☐ <1/2 pk/day
	☐ ___ pk/day

Street drugs ☐ None reported	☐ (Specify) _____
Anesthesia problems (individual, family) ☐ None reported	

10. Support system
   ☐ Available identity: _____
   ☐ Can be notified at no. _____
	Support System
	☐ Unavailable
	☐ No support system

11. Other problems
   ☐ None identified
	☐ (Specify) _____
	☐ Problems requiring addendum nursing interventions are not present
	   at this time. Follow standard of care for perioperative nursing care.
	
	_____ R.N.

Figure 4-1 *(continued)*

ASSESSMENT	DIAGNOSIS/PLAN
I. Ability to Communicate Verbal ☒ Appropriate Language spoken ☒ English ☐ Spanish ☐ Other (specify) _____ Hearing ☐ Appropriate	Impaired Verbal Communication related to ☐ Inability to speak secondary to (specify) _____ ☐ Inability to communicate in English Impaired communication related to ☐ Deafness ☒ Impaired hearing ☐ Diminished level of consciousness *Speak into left ear.*
II. Risks for Injury 1. Level of consciousness ☒ Alert 2. Weight __140__ Height __5'6"__ ☒ Within normal limits (WNL) within 15% of ideal wt. 3. Allergies ☒ None reported 4. Therapeutic devices ☐ None present 5. Skin integrity Presence of lesions/edema ☒ None ☐ Deferred Allergies (refer to 3) ☒ None reported Weight ☐ within 15% of ideal weight	Potential for Injury related to ☐ Confusion ☐ Drowsiness ☐ Nonresponsive state Potential for Injury: Fall related to ☐ Obesity > 15% ☐ Drug allergy (specify) _____ ☒ (IV) Foley, drains, casts (circle or specify) _____ Impaired Skin Integrity related to ☐ Lesions ☐ Edema (specify size and location) _____ Potential Impaired Skin Integrity related to ☐ Allergy to metal, chemicals, cleansers, adhesives (circle or specify) _____ ☐ Cachexia ☐ Obesity

Figure 4-2. Preoperative nursing record.

pain. The standardized care plan for Altered Thought Processes would contain the usual nursing interventions indicated. Interventions for specific nursing diagnoses should be recorded, as should the client's status.

Figure 4-3 illustrates how the nurse can record nursing diagnoses and collaborative problems that frequently occur in the PAR, and Figure 4-4 presents a nursing record form for documenting the client's status and nursing interventions in the PAR.

Before discharge or transfer from the PAR to the nursing unit, the client must meet preestablished criteria. The criteria used in many PAR discharge protocols include those listed below:

☐ Ability to turn head
☐ Extubated with clear airway
☐ Conscious, easily awakened
☐ Vital signs stable (blood pressure within 20 mm Hg of client's baseline)
☐ Dry, intact dressing
☐ Urine output at least 30 mL/hr
☐ Patent, functioning drains, tubes, and IV lines
☐ Anesthesiologist's approval for discharge (Luczum, 1984)

Exceptions for these discharge criteria can be made if the transfer is to intensive care, or if the surgeon or anesthesiologist has evaluated the client and approved discharge (Luczum, 1984).

POSTOPERATIVE DOCUMENTATION

Because most clients on a surgical unit have recently undergone surgery, they share many of the same nursing diagnoses and collaborative problems. For example, most postoperative clients have the following nursing diagnoses:

☐ Altered Comfort
☐ Potential Altered Respiratory Function
☐ Potential for Infection

They also have the following collaborative problems:

☐ Potential Complication: Urinary retention
☐ Potential Complication: Hemorrhage
☐ Potential Complication: Hypovolemia
☐ Potential Complication: Thrombophlebitis
☐ Potential Complication: Paralytic ileus.

TABLE 4-6. *Common Collaborative Problems and Nursing Diagnoses for Post-General Surgery Clients in the Postanesthesia Recovery Room*

Collaborative Problems

Potential complication: Respiratory
Potential complication: Hypo/hypervolemia
Potential complication: Hemorrhage
Potential complication: Cardiac

Nursing Diagnoses

Potential for Aspiration related to somnolence and increased secretions secondary to intubation
Anxiety related to acute pain secondary to surgical trauma to tissue and nerves
Potential for Injury related to somnolence secondary to anesthesia
Potential Hypothermia related to exposure to cool OR temperature

---

A general care plan for clients and families experiencing surgery, incorporating these and other "generic" nursing diagnoses and collaborative problems, is presented in Appendix II.

Because these "generic" diagnoses and collaborative problems are not specific to a particular client but rather are applicable to most clients undergoing surgery, the nurse should not write care plans based on them. Time constraints stemming from dramatically reduced lengths of stay for surgical clients mandate that a nurse not waste valuable nursing time writing routine care plans (e.g., postoperative respiratory preventive measures). Nurses should use Kardexes to communicate frequency of routine monitoring and treatments. Handwritten care plans should represent only those addendum individualized interventions that a client requires for treatment of priority diagnoses.

SAME-DAY SURGERY

In same-day surgery (also known as outpatient or ambulatory surgery), the client is admitted the morning of surgery and discharged later that day, when stable, to recover at home.

Besides same-day surgery clients, many clients undergoing major surgery now are admitted the morning of surgery, although they remain in the hospital for days to recover. (Many hospitals currently report that 60% to 70% of their surgical clients are admitted the morning of surgery.) For this reason, departments of nursing and selected nursing areas must have systems in place to address the nursing process efficiently even when client contact time is limited. A nurse's accountability for assessment, diagnosis, planning, implementation, and evaluation does not diminish merely because the client is not hospitalized the day before surgery.

A client scheduled to undergo surgery should be assessed in selected areas. The nurse can accomplish this assessment through various methods:

☐ Scheduling an assessment interview the same day that preoperative screening tests are performed
☐ Requesting that the client or a family member complete a preoperative assessment form and mail it to the same-day surgery nursing unit or bring it the morning of surgery
☐ Conducting a telephone interview 1 or 2 days before surgery
☐ Conducting the assessment and interview the morning of surgery

If assessment has been conducted by telephone or mail, the nurse still must assess certain areas on the morning of surgery. Figure 4-5 presents a short-stay nursing record. On this record, Section I includes the areas to be assessed before surgery; Section II is designated for postoperative care and status documentation. The nurse should also complete a preoperative diagnosis summary record (Fig. 4-6). This summary record also can be used for clients coming from in-house units. All of this information should be communicated to the OR/PAR staff.

Because another shift will not care for a same-day surgery client, writing an individualized care plan is unnecessary. Instead, care plans in short-stay units can be standardized. Appendix III presents a generic standard of care for same-day surgical clients. The nurse documents delivery of care primarily on a flow record. If the client has additional diagnoses or interventions to address, the nurse records these addendum diagnoses or interventions as a progress note, not as part of a care plan. Discharge planning should be addressed in the standardized care plan under the diagnosis Potential Altered Health Maintenance.

Potential for Aspiration related to: ☐ Anesthesia ☐ Surgery
Data: ☐ Airway in place ☐ Uncuffed ET ☐ Deflated ET Cuff
Intervention: ☐ Close observation ☐ Removal of airway/ET tube ☐ Position on side: ☐ (L) ☐ (R) ☐ _____
Evaluation: ☐ Pulse oximeter readings ☐ ABGs ☐ Lung sounds ☐ Chest   RN: _____

PC: Cardiac ☐ Dysrhythmia ☐ COPD/CHF ☐ Hyper/Hypotension
Data: ☐ ECG monitor ☐ Swan-Ganz ☐ Dyspnea ☐ Tachycardia ☐ Bradycardia
☐ Hypotension ☐ Hypertension ☐ Abnormal lung sounds
Intervention: ☐ Adjust IV rate ☐ Analgesic given ☐ HOB → ☐ Notify MDA ☐ Trendelenberg
Evaluation: ☐ BP > 90 systolic ☐ Stable cardiac rhythm/rate ☐ Pre- and post-op SPO$_2$ within 2–3 percentage points   RN: _____

Figure 4-3. Documentation example for postanesthesia care unit. *(Developed by Cecilia A. Cathey, RN, and nursing staff in PACU, St. Cloud Hospital, St. Cloud, Minnesota. Used with permission.)*

			Adm	15	30	45	60	75	90	Out

Date:

Time in:

Adm RN:

Surgical Procedure:

Anesthesiologist/CRNA:

Pre-op Medication

Time:

General / Anesthetic / Spinal

Length HR   MIN

BP/pulse pre-op

O₂ Therapy

Nasal Prongs	Flow	On	Off

INTAKE

IV in OR:

Blood in OR:

On adm:

Add on:

IV DC @

Total intake:

OUTPUT

EBL:

NG:

Urine:

Foley: Secured

Other:

Total output:

Pulse ● **Respiration** O **Diastolic** ∧ **Systolic** ∨

240 220 200 180 160 140 120 100 80 60 40 20 10 5

TIME

Temperature

PAR SCORE

Able to move 4 extremities on command = 2
Able to move 2 extremities on command = 1   Activity
Able to move 0 extremities on command = 0

Can cough or cry on command = 2
Breathing easily   = 1   Respirations
Airway requires attention   = 0

BP ± 20% of preanesthesia level   = 2
BP ± 20–50% of preanesthesia level = 1   Circulation
BP ± 50% of preanesthesia level   = 0

Fully awake and oriented = 2
Arouses when called   = 1   Consciousness
No response when called = 0

Normal skin appearance = 2
Pale, dusky, blotchy   = 1   Color
Cyanotic   = 0

TOTALS

Position:
S—Supine   P—Prone   H—Head of bed   F—Foot of bed
RS—Right side   Tr—Trendelenberg   LS—Left side

Noninvasive monitor—extremity checked

Cardiac monitor   NSR____ or:

Requires chin lift or hyperextension to maintain airway

Requires nasal/oral airway or E.T. tube   DC @

Respirations deep, rhythmical s̄ effort

Respirations shallow, rhythmical s̄ effort

     or:

Breath sounds clear to auscultation

Palpable/Doppler peripheral pulses

Regular apical or radial pulses

Capillary filling in fingers/toes   3 seconds

Skin warm and dry

Absence of bleeding, hematoma, or edema at op site

Dressing dry s̄ evidence of drainage

Tubes and drains patent s̄ excessive drainage

Absence of apparent nausea or vomiting

Absence of apparent pain or discomfort

Absence of palpable bladder distention

Spinal sensory level

IV site without redness or swelling

IV infusing well   site

Initials of RN   Yes = ✓   No = —

Figure 4-4. Sample PAR nursing record.
(continued)

_____
_____
_____
_____
_____
_____
_____
_____
_____
_____
_____
_____
_____
_____
_____
_____
_____
_____

Initials	Signatures		Time		Initials
		Medications			

Laboratory Reports:

Allergies:

Isolation required: _____ Yes _____ No

Care classification: ☐ Emergency after hours   Anesthesiologist:

I-Requires one RN for 50% of stay (1:2)	II-Requires one RN for ↑50% of stay (1:1)	III-Requires ↑one RN for 50% of stay (2:1)

Discharge: Yes = ✔ No = —

Discharge criteria met: _____

Instructed to deep breath/cough: _____

Instructed to stay in bed and call for assistance: _____

Instructed to call for pain/nausea medication: _____

Instructed on food/fluid intake: _____

Appears to understand: _____

Family member/friend present: _____

Special instructions: _____

_____

Side rails up: _____ Bed in low position: _____

Call light within range: _____

Dentures: _____

Vital signs on arrival to unit: _____

_____

Transferred to care of: _____

_____

Time: _____ PACU Nurse: _____

Signature receiving nurse: _____

Figure 4-4 *(continued)*

Section I: Preoperative

Date: _____

Time of Arrival on Unit:

_____ A.M.
_____ P.M.

Via: ☐ Ambulatory
☐ Wheelchair
☐ Stretcher

Accompanied by:
☐ Member of family
☐ Friend
☐ Unaccompanied

Name and phone number of person driving client home
Name: _____
Phone no.: _____
Waiting room: _____ Yes _____ No

Patient Has?

	No	Yes
Hearing aid	☐	☐
Eye glasses	☐	☐
Contact lenses	☐	☐
Artificial eye	☐	☐
Prosthesis	☐	☐
Wig or hair piece	☐	☐

Dentures
None ☐
Partial ☐
Upper ☐
Lower ☐
Denture cup ☐
Removed ☐

Medical Problems and Surgical History

Previous surgical experience? Yes_____ No _____
Specify: _____

Past problems with anesthesia? Individual Yes_____ No _____
Family Yes_____ No _____

Existing medical problems: (Circle)
_____ Diabetes _____ Cardiac disease _____ Arthritis _____ Seizures
_____ Hypertension _____ Cancer _____ Respiratory _____ CVA
_____ Hematologic _____ Liver _____ AIDS _____ Renal
_____ Other _____

Allergies   Medications (Include time of last dose.)
_____   _____
_____   _____
_____   _____

☐ No known allergies

Vital signs: Temperature _____ Respiration _____
BP _____ Pulse _____ Height _____ Weight _____ Actual/Reported

Diet: Skin:
Last solid food _____ A.M.   No Yes
P.M.   Rash ☐ ☐ _____
A.M.   Bruises ☐ ☐ _____
Last liquids _____ P.M.   Cuts ☐ ☐ _____
Scars ☐ ☐ _____
Lesions ☐ ☐ _____
Other ☐ ☐ _____

Abnormal lab work _____ No _____ Yes Called to _____

Abnormal X-ray results _____ No _____ Yes Called to _____

Pre-op teaching done _____ Video _____ Printed _____ Bedside
Operative permit signed _____ Yes _____ No
Identification band on _____ Yes _____ No
PAT studies done _____ Yes _____ No
H & P done _____ Yes _____ No

Time	Premedication given	Site	By

Figure 4-5. Same-day surgery nursing record.
(continued)

NOTES:

_____
_____
_____
_____
_____

_____ R.N.
Signature of Admitting Nurse

Section II: Postoperative

Graphic Chart

Name: _____

Time: _____

	260
RESP o	240
	220
	200
	180
PULSE.	160
	140
	120
DIAS <	100
	80
	60
SYST >	40
	20
TEMP	
URINE	
STOOLS	

Date _____ Time _____ A.M. P.M.

Operation _____
_____

Dressings _____
_____

Other _____

Medications given:

Time	Medication	Site	By

Nourishment _____
Amt _____
Tolerated _____ Yes _____ No

Activity tolerated
_____ HOB 60°   _____ Time
_____ Dangle   _____ Time
_____ OOB chair   _____ Time

Section III: Discharge Summary

Discharge Status:

BP _____ Pulse _____ Respiration _____ Temperature _____
IV D/c'd: Time _____ Amt absorbed _____
Voided _____ Yes _____ No
Dressing intact/dry _____ Yes _____ No
Pain tolerable _____ Yes _____ No
Prescriptions given _____ No _____ Yes List: _____
General instruction sheets given _____ Client _____ Other _____
_____ Instruction sheet given _____ Client _____ Other _____
Instructed to call for appointment _____ Yes _____ No
Accompanied by _____ Family _____ Friend _____ Unaccompanied in taxi

Notes: (Unusual events, interactions)

_____
_____
_____
_____
_____

Discharged by _____ R.N.

Figure 4-5 (continued)

Impaired Communication related to
☐ Deafness
☐ Impaired hearing
☐ Diminished level of consciousness
☐ Inability to speak secondary to (specify) _____
☐ Inability to communicate in English

Potential for Infection Transmission related to
☐ HIV positive
☐ Hepatitis: Type _____
☐ Other _____

Potential for Injury related to
☐ Confusion
☐ Drowsiness
☐ Nonresponsive state
☐ Obesity > 15%
☐ IV, Foley, drains, casts (circle or specify) _____

Impaired Skin Integrity related to
☐ Lesions   ☐ Edema
   (specify size and location) _____

Potential Impaired Skin Integrity related to
☐ Allergy to metal, chemicals, cleansers, adhesives (circle or
   specify) _____
☐ Cachexia
☐ Obesity
☐ ↓ Circulation secondary to (specify) _____

Anxiety related to
☐ Lack of understanding of (specify) _____

Anxiety/fear:
☐ Moderate ⎫
☐ Severe   ⎬ related to impending surgical experience and:
☐ First surgical experience
☐ History of negative surgical experience (own, relative, specify)
   _____

☐ Specify _____

Potential Complication: Hemorrhage
☐ History of hematologic disorder (specify) _____
☐ Aspirin therapy
☐ Anticoagulants
☐ None

Potential Complication: Cardiac, Hepatic, Respiratory, Hemorrhage
☐ Alcohol use
   ___ drinks day/wk.
☐ Smoking
   ___ pk/day
☐ Street drugs (specify) _____

Support System
☐ Unavailable
☐ No support system
☐ (Specify) _____

Allergies
☐ None reported
☐ Unable to determine
☐ List: _____

Other Significant Data/Comments
_____
_____
_____
_____
_____
_____
_____
_____

☐ Problems requiring specific nursing interventions are not present at
   this time. Follow standard of care for perioperative nursing care.

_____ R.N.

Figure 4-6.   Preoperative diagnosis summary record.

Summary

Surgery produces both expected and unexpected responses in clients. Through vigilant assessment, the nurse identifies those clients at high risk for complications and those who are responding negatively to the surgical experience.

Because many events occur in a short time span for a surgical client, documentation in the perioperative phases must be concise but specific. The described documentation reflects the use of the nursing process by the nurse preoperatively and postoperatively, with attention to professional standards and efficiency.

References/Bibliography

Cannon, C. (1989). Knowledge deficit. In L.J. Carpenito. *Nursing diagnosis: Application to clinical practice* (3rd ed.). Philadelphia: J.B. Lippincott.

Carpenito, L.J., & Duespohl, T.A. (1985). *A guide to effective clinical instruction* (2nd ed.). Rockville, MD: Aspen Systems.

Constantian, M.B. (1980). *Pressure ulcers: Principles and techniques of management.* Boston: Little, Brown.

Felton, G. (1985). Preoperative teaching. In G. Bulechek & J. McClosky. *Nursing interventions: Treatments for nursing diagnoses.* Philadelphia: W.B. Saunders.

Glass, G.R., McGraw, B. & Smith, M.L. (1982). *Meta-analyses in social research.* Beverly Hills, CA: Sage Publications.

Johnson, J.E. (1978). Sensory information, instruction in a coping strategy, and recovery from surgery. *Research in Nursing and Health, 1,* 14–17.

King, I., & Tarsitano, B. (1982). The effect of structured and unstructured preoperative teaching: A replication. *Nursing Research, 31*(6), 324–329.

Luczum, M.E. (1984). *Postanesthesia nursing: A comprehensive guide.* Rockville, MD: Aspen Systems.

McConnell, E. (1987). *Clinical considerations in perioperative nursing.* Philadelphia: J.B. Lippincott.

Spielberger, C., & Sarason, I. (Eds.). (1975). *Stress and anxiety,* Vol. I. Washington DC: Hemisphere.

UNIT II

Clinical Nursing Care Plans

Unit II comprises care plans for 82 clinical situations. The 39 care plans in Section 1 focus on persons experiencing medical conditions; the 24 care plans in Section 2 focus on care of persons experiencing surgery; and the 19 care plans in Section 3 address the care of individuals undergoing diagnostic studies or therapeutic procedures. These care plans represent the nursing diagnoses and collaborative problems that are known to occur frequently in these clinical situations and to be of significant importance. It is critical to note that each nursing diagnosis must be confirmed or ruled out on the basis of the data collected about a specific client.

COMPONENTS OF EACH CARE PLAN

Definition

Each care plan begins with a description of the clinical situation. This information is provided to highlight certain aspects of the condition or situation or to summarize a knowledge base for the reader.

Time Frame

A client's response to certain situations or conditions can vary depending upon when the event occurs in the health–illness continuum. For example, a client with newly diagnosed diabetes mellitus will have different responses than a client with an exacerbation. Therefore, each care plan designates a time frame. The focus of the care plans in this book is the initial diagnosis. The nurse can also use the care plan if a client is readmitted for the same condition; however, the nurse will need to re-evaluate the client and his needs.

Diagnostic Cluster

A diagnostic cluster represents a set of nursing diagnoses and collaborative problems that are predicted to be present and of significant importance in a selected clinical situation. There are, of course, many nursing diagnoses and collaborative problems that clients can experience. The diagnostic cluster represents those with high predictability. However, the client may have priority nursing diagnoses or collaborative problems that are not listed in the diagnostic cluster for a given situation. Therefore, these diagnostic clusters serve to assist the nurse in creating the initial care plan. As the nurse interacts with and assesses the client, more specific diagnoses, goals, and interventions can be added.

In addition, collaborative problems and nursing diagnoses not detailed in the care plan are listed under the heading "Refer to." These are included in the diagnostic cluster to give the nurse a complete picture of clinical care.

Discharge Criteria

Discharge criteria are the behaviors that are desired in order to maintain or achieve maximum functioning after discharge.

The discharge needs of clients and families can necessitate two types of nursing actions: teaching the client and family to manage the situation at home, and referring the client and family to agencies for assistance with continuing care and management at home. The discharge criteria cited in each care plan represent those that a staff nurse can usually achieve with a client or family during a typical length of stay.

Many of the care plans use the nursing diagnosis "Potential Altered Health Maintenance related to insufficient knowledge of _____" or "Potential Impaired Home Maintenance Management related to _____." These two diagnoses apply to a client and/or family who are at risk for problems after discharge because of a *potential* response to discharge. The plan of care for these diagnoses aims at preventing them from happening. For these two diagnoses, then, the discharge criteria also represent the outcome criteria. In other words, the outcome criteria—measurable behaviors that represent a favorable status—are that the client meets discharge criteria. Therefore, no outcome criteria are cited for these two diagnoses. Instead, the nurse is referred to the discharge criteria.

Collaborative Problems

Each care plan describes and discusses nursing care for one or more physiological complications that the nurse jointly treats with medicine. These collaborative problems have both physician- and nursing-prescribed interventions associated with them. The independent nursing interventions consist of monitoring the client for the onset of the complication or for its status if it is occurring. Other independent nursing interventions may include positioning, activity restrictions, etc. Keep in mind that collaborative problems are not physiological nursing diagnoses. Physiological nursing diagnoses that nurses independently treat are listed in the care plan as nursing diagnoses, e.g., Impaired Skin Integrity.

You will note that collaborative problems do not have outcome criteria. Outcome criteria are not useful in assisting the nurse to evaluate the effectiveness of nursing interventions for collaborative problems. For example, consider the collaborative problem "Potential Complication: Increased intracranial pressure." Appropriate outcome criteria might be as follows: The client will be alert and oriented, and the pupils will be equal and react to light accommodation. If the client's sensorium changes and the pupils respond sluggishly to light, will these data accurately evaluate the effectiveness of nursing care? The answer, of course, is no. Instead, they evaluate the client's clinical status, which is the result of many factors.

Outcome criteria are used to assist the nurse in evaluating whether the care plan should be continued, revised, or discontinued. The outcome criteria in the example above clearly do not serve this purpose. What they do is set forth monitoring criteria that can be added to the care plan as established norms for evaluating the client's condition, e.g., normal range for urine output, blood pressure, or serum potassium. These are clearly not client goals. Certain nursing goals will serve to evaluate the effectiveness of nursing actions for collaborative problems, since nurses are accountable for detecting early changes in physiological status and managing these episodes. Thus, collaborative problems on the care plans in Unit II will have associated nursing goals. Refer to Chapter 1 of this book and to Chapter 2 in Carpenito (1989) for a more thorough discussion of collaborative problems.

Related Physician-Prescribed Interventions

This section is provided as reference material. It outlines physician-prescribed interventions for the specific condition or situation. These interventions have established systems and guidelines for delivery and communication. Physician-prescribed interventions do not treat nursing diagnoses. Along with nursing-prescribed interventions, they do treat collaborative problems.

Nursing Diagnoses

Each care plan has at least two actual or potential nursing diagnoses. Keep in mind that the nurse should have validation for the diagnosis before the care plan is initiated. Actual nursing diagnoses are validated by the presence of the appropriate major signs and symptoms. Potential nursing diagnoses are validated by the presence of the appropriate risk factors.

Outcome Criteria

The outcome criteria outlined for each nursing diagnosis consist of measurable behaviors of the client or family that represent a favorable status. Because a potential nursing diagnosis represents a situation that a nurse can prevent, the outcome criteria for that diagnosis represent a health status that the nurse will aim to maintain, thereby preventing the situation from occurring. The following is an example of a potential nursing diagnosis and its corresponding outcome criterion:

> Potential Impaired Skin Integrity related to immobility
> Outcome Criterion: Will demonstrate continued intact skin

If the outcome criteria are associated with an *actual* nursing diagnosis, they represent a behavior or status that the nurse will assist the client to achieve. The following is an example of an actual nursing diagnosis and its corresponding outcome criterion.

> Impaired Skin Integrity related to immobility
> Outcome Criterion: Will demonstrate evidence of granulation tissue

Focus Assessment Criteria

Each nursing diagnosis section begins with focus assessment criteria. Focus assessment criteria direct the nurse's assessment toward specific data collection. This data will help to better evaluate the client's present status or response. The data listed in each care plan are clinically significant for the given situation. A discussion of and rationale for this clinical significance accompany each assessment criteria.

Rationale

A supporting rationale is presented for each nursing intervention for both collaborative problems and nursing diagnoses. The rationale explains why the intervention is appropriate and why it will produce the desired response. Rationales may be scientific principles derived from the natural, physical, and behavioral sciences, or they may be drawn from the humanities and nursing research. The rationales for client teaching interventions also include why the teaching is needed and why the specific content is taught.

Documentation

Each nursing diagnosis or collaborative problem section ends with a list of where the nurse will most appropriately document the care given. For some diagnoses, responsible documentation is recorded on a flow record, e.g., vital signs or urine output. For others, the nurse records a progress note. Teaching can be recorded on a teaching flow record or on a discharge summary record. Policies for documentation are determined by the department of nursing. This section can serve to assist departments of nursing in formulating their documentation policies. It is unnecessary to record a progress or nursing note on every diagnosis on the care plan. Flow records can be used to document such routine or standard care as repetitive assessment results and even interventions for most collaborative problems and many nursing diagnoses.

Addendum Diagnoses

Frequently the nurse will identify and validate the presence of a potential or actual diagnosis that is not included in the given care plan for the situation or diagnostic cluster. The nurse can refer to the index of nursing diagnoses and collaborative problems in the back of this book to retrieve information about the identified diagnosis. For example, Mr. Jamie has had a myocardial infarction; the nurse initiates the care plan for an individual experiencing an MI. In addition, Mr. Jamie is immobile. The nurse can find "Potential for Disuse Syndrome related to immobility" in the index and retrieve the information about that diagnosis. Then, the diagnosis, goals, and interventions can be added as additional or addendum diagnoses.

Reference

Carpenito, L.J. (1989). *Nursing diagnosis: Application to clinical practice* (3rd ed.). Philadelphia: J.B. Lippincott.

Section 1

Medical Conditions

Cardiovascular and Peripheral Vascular Disorders

Congestive Heart Failure

Congestive heart failure (CHF) is a syndrome that occurs when the heart is unable to pump sufficient blood for metabolic needs. Symptoms vary depending on whether heart failure is left-sided or right-sided. Left-sided failure can result from hypertension, myocardial ischemia or infarction, and aortic valve disease; right-sided failure from pulmonary diseases, pericarditis, and tricuspid or pulmonary stenosis.

▲ **Time Frame**

Initial diagnosis (non-intensive care unit or ICU)
Exacerbation of chronic condition

▲ **Discharge Criteria**

Before discharge, the client or family will:

1. Describe the rationales for prescribed treatments
2. Demonstrate the ability to count pulse rate correctly
3. State the causes of symptoms and describe their management
4. State the signs and symptoms that must be reported to a health care professional

Collaborative Problems

Potential Complications:	Refer to:
Hypoxemia	
Deep Vein Thrombosis	Myocardial Infarction
Cardiogenic Shock	Myocardial Infarction
Hepatic Failure	Cirrhosis

Nursing Diagnoses

Potential Altered Health Maintenance related to lack of knowledge of low-salt diet, drug therapy (diuretic, digitalis), activity program, signs and symptoms of complications	Chronic Obstructive Pulmonary Disease
Activity Intolerance related to insufficient oxygen for activities of daily living	
Altered Nutrition: Less Than Body Requirements related to nausea; anorexia secondary to venous congestion of gastrointestinal tract and fatigue	Chronic Obstructive Pulmonary Disease
Altered Peripheral Tissue Perfusion related to venous congestion secondary to right-side heart failure	Cirrhosis
Anxiety related to breathlessness	Chronic Obstructive Pulmonary Disease
Sleep Pattern Disturbance related to nocturnal dyspnea and inability to assume usual sleep position	Chronic Obstructive Pulmonary Disease
Potential Fluid Volume Excess: Edema related to decreased renal blood flow secondary to right-side heart failure	Cirrhosis
Powerlessness related to progressive nature of condition	Chronic Obstructive Pulmonary Disease

Collaborative Problem

▲ **Nursing Goal**

The nurse will manage and minimize hypoxemic episodes.

Potential Complication: Hypoxemia

Interventions

1. Monitor for signs and symptoms of hypoxia:
   a. Increased and irregular pulse rate
   b. Increased respiratory rate
   c. Decreased urine output (less than 30 mL/hr)
   d. Changes in mentation
   e. Cool, moist, cyanotic, mottled skin
   f. Decreased capillary refill time

Rationale

1. Decreased cardiac output leads to an insufficient supply of oxygenated blood to meet the metabolic needs of tissues. Decreased circulating volume/cardiac output can result in hypoperfusion of the kidneys and decreased tissue perfusion, with a compensatory response of decreased circulation to extremities and increased pulse and respiratory rates. Changes in mentation may result from cerebral hypoperfusion.

Interventions

2. Monitor for signs and symptoms of acute pulmonary edema:
   a. Severe dyspnea
   b. Tachycardia
   c. Adventitious breath sounds
   d. Persistent cough
   e. Productive cough with frothy sputum
   f. Cyanosis
3. Cautiously administer IV fluids. Consult with the physician if the ordered rate exceeds 125 mL/hr. Be sure to include additional IV fluids—e.g., antibiotics—when calculating the hourly allocation.
4. Assist the client with measures to conserve strength, such as resting before and after activities, e.g., meals.

Related Physician-Prescribed Interventions

Medications

Digitalis glycosides
Diuretics
Potassium supplements
Vasodilators

Sympathomimetics
Bipyridines
Anticoagulants

Intravenous Therapy

Nonsaline solutions with replacement electrolytes

Laboratory Studies

Electrolytes
BUN, creatinine
Liver function studies (SGOT, LDH)

Coagulation studies
Arterial blood gas analysis

Diagnostic Studies

Chest x-ray film
ECG

Nuclear imaging scan
Echocardiography

Therapies

Emergency protocols (cardiac shock, dysrhythmias)
Fluid restrictions
Sodium-restricted diet
Oxygen via cannula

Rotating tourniquets (in extreme cases)
Pacemaker insertion (in selected cases)
Rehabilitation therapy

Rationale

Vasoconstriction and venous congestion in dependent areas (e.g., limbs) produce changes in skin and pulses.
2. Circulatory overload can result from the reduced size of the pulmonary vascular bed. Hypoxia causes increased capillary permeability, which in turn causes fluid to enter pulmonary tissue, producing the signs and symptoms of pulmonary edema.

3. Circulatory overload can be caused by failure to regulate IV fluids carefully.

4. Adequate rest reduces oxygen consumption and decreases the risk of hypoxia.

▲ Documentation

Flow records
  Vital signs
  Intake and output
  Assessment data
Progress notes
  Change in physiological status
  Interventions
  Client response to interventions

Nursing Diagnosis

▲ Outcome Criteria

The outcome criteria for this diagnosis represent those associated with discharge planning. Refer to discharge criteria.

Potential Altered Health Maintenance related to insufficient knowledge of low-salt diet, activity program, drug therapy (diuretic, digitalis), and signs and symptoms of complications

Focus Assessment Criteria	Clinical Significance
1. Readiness and ability to learn and retain information	1. A client or family that does not achieve goals for learning will require a referral for assistance postdischarge.

Interventions

1. Teach the client and family about the condition and its causes.

Rationale

1. Teaching reinforces the need to comply with prescribed treatments (diet, activity, and medications).

Interventions	*Rationale*
2. Explain the need to adhere to a low-sodium diet, as prescribed. Consult with a nutritionist, as necessary.	2. Excess sodium intake increases fluid retention, which in turn increases vascular volume and cardiac workload.
3. Explain the actions of prescribed medications, which typically include digitalis preparations or diuretics. Digitalis increases the stroke volume of the heart, which reduces congestion and diastolic pressure. Diuretics decrease the reabsorption of electrolytes, particularly sodium, thus promoting water loss.	3. Such explanations can help increase client compliance and reduce errors in self-administration.
4. Teach the client how to count his or her pulse rate.	4. Pulse-taking can detect an irregular rhythm or a high (>120) or low (<60) rate, which may indicate a drug side effect or disease complication.
5. Teach the client to weigh himself or herself daily and to report a gain of 2 or more pounds.	5. Daily weights can help detect fluid retention early, enabling prompt treatment to prevent pulmonary congestion.
6. Explain the need to increase activity gradually and to rest if dyspnea and fatigue occur.	6. Regular exercise, such as walking, can improve circulation and increase cardiac stroke volume and cardiac output. Dyspnea and fatigue indicate hypoxemia resulting from overexertion.

7. Instruct the client and family to report the following signs and symptoms to a health care professional:
  a. Loss of appetite
  b. Visual disturbances
  c. Shortness of breath
  d. Persistent cough
  e. Edema in the ankles and feet
 	
  f. Muscle weakness or cramping
	7. Early detection of these signs and symptoms and prompt intervention can reduce the risk of severe drug side effects or worsening CHF.
	  a,b. These are common side effects of digitalis.
	
	  c,d. These indicate a worsening of CHF.
	
	  e. Edema indicates circulatory overload secondary to decreased cardiac output.
	  f. Muscle weakness and cramping may indicate hypokalemia secondary to increased potassium excretion from diuretic therapy.

8. Provide information about or initiate referrals to community resources, e.g., the American Heart Association, home health agencies.	8. Such resources may be able to provide the client and family with needed assistance in home management and self-care.

▲ Documentation

- Discharge summary record
  - Client teaching
  - Outcome achievement or status
  - Referrals, if indicated

References/Bibliography

Cameron, K., (1987). Chronic illness and compliance. *Journal of Advanced Nursing, 12*(6), 671–676.

Carrieri, V.K., & Janson-Bjerklies, S. (1989). The sensation of dyspnea. *Heart and Lung, 13*(4), 436–445.

Curgian, L.M. (1985). Nutrition in chronic respiratory disease. *Rehabilitation Nursing, 10*(4), 22–23.

DeVito, A.J. (1985). Rehabilitation of patients with chronic obstructive pulmonary disease. *Rehabilitative Nursing, 10*(2), 12–15.

Poindexter, S.M. (1986). Nutrition in congestive heart failure. *Nutritional Clinical Practice, 1*(2), 83–88.

Shenkman, B. (1985). Factors contributing to attrition rates in a pulmonary rehabilitation program. *Heart and Lung, 14*(1), 53–58.

Myocardial Infarction

Myocardial infarction (MI) describes myocardial tissue that has been destroyed because of inadequate blood supply. The causes of inadequate blood supply can be narrowing or occlusion of the coronary artery from atherosclerosis, embolus, or thrombus; or decreased coronary blood flow from shock or hemorrhage.

Diagnostic Cluster

▲ Time Frame
Initial diagnosis
Postintensive care
Recurrent episodes

▲ Discharge Criteria
Before discharge, the client or family will:

1. State the cause of cardiac pain and the rationales for medication therapy and activity and dietary restrictions
2. Demonstrate accuracy in taking pulse
3. Identify personal risk factors that are modifiable
4. Describe at-home activity restrictions
5. Describe self-administration of daily and p.r.n. medications
6. Describe the signs and symptoms that must be reported to a health care professional
7. Verbalize the follow-up care needed and the community resources available
8. Describe appropriate actions to take in the event problems occur

Collaborative Problems

Potential Complications:
Dysrhythmias
Cardiogenic Shock
Congestive Heart Failure
Thromboembolism
Recurrent Myocardial Infarction

Nursing Diagnoses

Anxiety/Fear (individual, family) related to unfamiliar situation status, unpredictable nature of condition, negative effect on life style, possible sexual dysfunction

Grieving related to actual or perceived losses secondary to cardiac condition

Anxiety related to Acute Pain secondary to cardiac tissue ischemia

Potential Colonic Constipation related to decreased peristalsis secondary to medication effects, decreased activity, and change in diet

Activity Intolerance related to insufficient oxygenation for activities of daily living (ADL) secondary to cardiac tissue ischemia

Potential Altered Health Maintenance related to lack of knowledge of hospital routines, treatments, conditions, medications, diet, activity progression, signs and symptoms of complications, reduction of risks, follow-up care, community resources

Collaborative Problems

▲ Nursing Goal
The nurse will manage and minimize cardiac complications.

Potential Complication: Dysrhythmias
Potential Complication: Cardiogenic shock
Potential Complication: Congestive heart failure
Potential Complication: Thromboembolism
Potential Complication: Recurrent MI

Interventions

1. Monitor for signs and symptoms of dysrhythmias:
   a. Abnormal rate, rhythm
   b. Palpitations, syncope
   c. Cardiac emergencies (arrest, ventricular fibrillation)

Rationale

1. Myocardial ischemia results from reduced oxygen to myocardial tissue. Ischemic tissue is electrically unstable, causing dysrhythmias such as premature ventricular contractions, which can lead to ventricular fibrillation and death.

Interventions

2. Maintain oxygen therapy as prescribed.

3. Monitor for signs and symptoms of cardiogenic shock:
   a. Increasing pulse rate with normal or slightly decreased blood pressure
   b. Urine output less than 30 mL/hr
   c. Restlessness, agitation, change in mentation
   d. Increasing respiratory rate
   e. Diminished peripheral pulses
   f. Cool, pale, or cyanotic skin
   g. Thirst
4. Monitor for signs and symptoms of congestive heart failure and decreased cardiac output:
   a. Gradual increase in heart rate
   b. Increased shortness of breath
   c. Diminished breath sound, rales
   d. Decreased systolic blood pressure
   e. Presence of or increase in S3 or S4 gallop
   f. Peripheral edema
   g. Distended neck veins
5. Monitor for signs and symptoms of thromboembolism:

   a. Diminished or absent peripheral pulses

   b. Unusual warmth/redness or cyanosis/coolness

   c. Leg pain
   d. Sudden severe chest pain, increased dyspnea

   e. Positive Homan's sign

6. Monitor for signs and symptoms of recurrent MI:
   a. Sudden, severe chest pain with nausea/vomiting
   b. Increased dyspnea
   c. Increased ST elevation and abnormal Q waves on the ECG
7. Apply antiembolic stockings.

8. Encourage the client to perform leg exercises but to avoid isometric exercises.

Rationale

2. Supplemental oxygen therapy increases the circulating oxygen available to myocardial tissue.
3. Shock can be caused by severe pain or greatly reduced cardiac output secondary to severe tissue hypoxia. The compensatory response to decreased circulatory volume aims to increase blood oxygen levels by increasing heart and respiratory rates and to decrease circulation to extremities (marked by decreased pulses and cool skin). Diminished oxygen to the brain causes changes in mentation.

4. Congestive heart failure is caused by myocardial ischemia, which reduces the ability of the left ventricle to eject blood, thus decreasing cardiac output and increasing pulmonary vascular congestion. This causes fluid to enter pulmonary tissue, producing rales, productive cough, cyanosis, and possibly signs and symptoms of respiratory distress.

5. Prolonged bed rest, increased blood viscosity and coagulability, and decreased cardiac output contribute to thrombus formation.
   a. Insufficient circulation causes pain and diminished peripheral pulse.
   b. Unusual warmth and redness points to inflammation; coolness and cyanosis indicate vascular obstruction.
   c. Leg pain results from tissue hypoxia.
   d. Obstruction to pulmonary circulation causes sudden chest pain and dyspnea.
   e. In a positive Homans' sign, dorsiflexion of the foot causes pain as a result of insufficient circulation.

6. These signs and symptoms indicate myocardial tissue deterioration with increasing hypoxia.

7. Antiembolic stockings reduce venous stasis and promote venous return.
8. Leg exercises promote venous return. Isometric exercises greatly increase blood pressure and heart rate as sustained muscle tension impairs blood flow.

▲ **Documentation**

Graphic/flow record
   Vital signs
   Intake and output
   Rhythm strips
Progress notes
   Status of client
   Unusual events

Related Physician-Prescribed Interventions

Medications

Vasodilators, antianginals
Beta-blockers
Calcium channel blockers
Analgesics
Sedatives/hypnotics

Antidysrhythmics
Stool softeners
Anticoagulants
Diuretics

Intravenous Therapy

IV access for medication administration

Related Physician-Prescribed Interventions (continued)

Laboratory Studies

Cardiac enzymes/isoenzymes
Electrolytes
White blood count
Sedimentation rate
Chemistry profile

Arterial blood gas analysis
Cholesterol
Triglycerides
Coagulation studies

Diagnostic Studies

ECG
Chest x-ray film
Echocardiogram
Nuclear imaging studies
Magnetic resonance imaging

Stress test
Coronary arteriography
Cardiac catheterization
Digital subtraction angiography

Therapies

Oxygen via cannula
Therapeutic diet (low-salt, low-saturated fats, low-cholesterol)

Pacemaker insertion (selected cases)
Cardiac rehabilitation program

Nursing Diagnoses

▲ Outcome Criteria

The client or family will:

1. Verbalize fears related to the disorder
2. Share concerns about the disorder's effects on normal functioning, role responsibilities, and life style

Anxiety/Fear (individual, family) related to unfamiliar situation, unpredictable nature of condition, or negative effects on life style

Focus Assessment Criteria	*Clinical Significance*

1. Anxiety level
2. Present coping response (client and family):
  a. Denial
  b. Anger
  c. Depression
  d. Guilt
	1,2. All persons experience some type of emotional reaction post-MI. The client's and family's perception of the effects of MI (financial, physical, psychological, spiritual, and social) determine the nature and extent of the reaction.

Interventions

1. Assist the client to reduce his or her anxiety:
   a. Provide reassurance and comfort.
   b. Convey a sense of understanding and empathy.
   c. Encourage the client to verbalize any fears and concerns regarding MI and its treatment.
   d. Identify and support effective coping mechanisms.
2. When the client's anxiety is at a mild to moderate level, take the opportunity to teach about procedures, home care, relaxation techniques, and so on.
3. Encourage family and friends to verbalize their fears and concerns to staff members.

4. Provide the client and family with valid reassurance and reinforce positive coping behavior.
5. Encourage the client to use relaxation techniques, such as guided imagery and relaxation breathing.
6. Contact the physician immediately if the client's anxiety is at the severe or panic level.

▲ Documentation

Progress notes
    Present emotional status
    Response to interventions

7. Refer also to the nursing diagnosis Anxiety in the Generic Care Plan, Appendix I, for general assessment and interventions.

Rationale

1. An anxious client has a narrowed perceptual field with a diminished ability to learn. The client may experience symptoms caused by increased muscle tension and disrupted sleep patterns. Anxiety tends to feed upon itself, trapping the client in a spiral of increasing anxiety, tension, and emotional and physical pain.

2. Some fears are based on inaccurate information and can be relieved by providing accurate information. A client with severe or panic anxiety does not retain learning.
3. Verbalization allows sharing and provides the nurse with an opportunity to correct misconceptions.
4. Praising the client for effective coping can reinforce future positive coping responses.
5. Relaxation techniques enhance the client's sense of control over his or her body's response to stress.
6. Severe anxiety interferes with client learning and compliance, and also increases the heart rate.

The client will:

1. Express grief
2. Describe the meaning of loss
3. Report an intent to discuss feelings with significant others

Grieving related to actual or perceived losses secondary to cardiac disease

Focus Assessment Criteria

1. Signs and symptoms of grief reaction, such as crying, anxiety, fear, withdrawal, restlessness, decreased appetite, and decreased independence in activities

Clinical Significance

1. Losses related to function, livelihood, and possibly life invariably provoke a grief response. This grief response can be profound, depending on how the client perceives the condition to interfere with personal goals.

Interventions

1. Provide the client with opportunities to ventilate his or her feelings:
   a. Discuss the loss openly.
   b. Explain that grief is a normal reaction to a loss.
   c. Explore the client's perception of the loss.
2. Encourage the client to use coping strategies that have helped in the past.

3. Promote grief work—the adaptive process of mourning—with each response.
   a. Denial:
      • Explain the presence of denial in the client or a family member to the other members.
      • Do not push the person to move past denial without emotional readiness.
   b. Isolation:
      • Convey acceptance by allowing expressions of grief.
      • Encourage open, honest communication to promote sharing.
      • Reinforce the person's sense of self-worth by allowing privacy when desired.
      • Encourage a gradual return to social activities (e.g., support groups, church activities, etc.).
   c. Depression:
      • Reinforce the person's sense of self-esteem.
      • Identify the level of depression and tailor your approach accordingly.
      • Use empathetic sharing; acknowledge the grief (e.g., "It must be very difficult for you.").
      • Identify any signs of suicidal ideation or behavior (e.g., frequent statements of intent, revealed plan).
   d. Anger:
      • Encourage verbalization of anger.
      • Explain to other family members that the person's anger represents an attempt to control his or her environment more closely because of the inability to control the loss.
   e. Guilt:
      • Acknowledge the person's expressed self-view.

Rationale

1. Frequent contact by the nurse indicates acceptance and may facilitate trust. Open communication can help the client work through the grieving process.

2. This strategy helps the client to refocus on problem-solving and enhances his or her sense of control.
3. Responses to grief vary among clients. The nurse must recognize and accept each client's individual response, to intervene appropriately.

Interventions

- Encourage the person to focus on positive aspects.
- Avoid arguing with the person about what he should have done differently.

  f. Fear:
  - Focus on the present reality, and maintain a safe and secure environment.
  - Help the person explore reasons for his or her fears.

  g. Rejection:
  - Reassure the person by explaining that this response is normal.
  - Explain this response to other family members.

  h. Hysteria:
  - Reduce environmental stressors, e.g., limit staff, minimize external noise.
  - Provide a safe, private area to display grief in his or her own fashion.

4. Promote family cohesiveness:
   a. Support the family at its level of functioning.
   b. Encourage family members to evaluate their feelings and to support one another.

Rationale

4. A grieving person often isolates himself physically and especially emotionally. Repression of feelings interferes with family relationships.

▲ **Documentation**

Progress notes
   Present emotional status
   Interventions
   Client's and family's response to interventions

▲ **Outcome Criteria**

The client will:

1. Report episodes of pain
2. Report pain relief after initiation of pain relief measures

Anxiety related to acute pain secondary to cardiac tissue ischemia

Focus Assessment Criteria	*Clinical Significance*
1. Site, onset, precipitating factors, description of pain (e.g., crushing, radiating, constricting) 2. Associated behaviors, such as restlessness	1,2. Cardiac pain results from decreased oxygen of myocardial tissue; hypoxia is caused by narrowed or blocked coronary arteries. Treatment focuses on reducing pain, decreasing energy expenditure, and dilating the coronary arteries.

Interventions

1. Instruct the client to report a pain episode immediately.
2. Administer analgesics per physician's order. Document administration and the degree of relief the client experiences.
3. Instruct the client to rest during a pain episode.
4. Reduce environmental distractions as much as possible.
5. After the acute pain phase passes, explain the cause of the pain and possible precipitating factors (physical and emotional).
6. If possible, obtain and evaluate a 12-lead ECG or rhythm strip during pain episodes.
7. Explain and assist with noninvasive pain relief measures such as these:
   a. Positioning
   b. Distraction (activities, breathing exercises)
   c. Massage
   d. Relaxation exercises

Rationale

1. Less medication generally is required if it is administered early in a pain episode.
2. Severe, persistent pain unrelieved by analgesics may indicate impending or extending infarction.
3. Activity increases the body's oxygen needs, which can exacerbate cardiac pain.
4. Environmental stimulation can increase the heart rate and may exacerbate myocardial tissue hypoxia, increasing pain.
5. Calm explanation may reduce the client's stress associated with fear of the unknown.
6. Cardiac monitoring may help differentiate variant angina from extension of the infarction.
7. These measures can help prevent painful stimuli from reaching higher brain centers by replacing the painful stimuli with another stimulus. Relaxation reduces muscle tension, decreases the heart rate, may improve stroke volume, and enhances the client's sense of control over the pain.

▲ **Documentation**

Graphic/flow record
   Medication administration
Progress notes
   Unsatisfactory pain relief
   Status of pain

Potential Colonic Constipation related to decreased peristalsis secondary to medication effects, decreased activity, and change in diet

Focus Assessment Criteria	*Clinical Significance*
1. Bowel patterns prehospitalization: frequency, use of aids (laxatives, enemas)	1. This assessment identifies whether the client had optimal bowel habits before hospitalization.

Interventions

1. Provide for privacy during defecation and instruct the client to do the following:
   a. Use the call bell if chest pain occurs.
   b. Avoid straining by exhaling during defecation.
   c. Assume the normal semi-squatting position on the toilet, if not contraindicated.
2. Explain the possible causes of constipation and its effects on cardiac rhythm (vagal stimulation). Explain that immobility, change in usual diet, and embarrassment can contribute to constipation, and that narcotics reduce neural innervation, which controls peristalsis.
3. Administer stool softeners, as ordered.

4. Promote factors that contribute to optimal elimination.
   a. Balanced diet:
      • Review a list of high-fiber foods; e.g., fresh fruits with skins on, bran, nuts and seeds, whole-grain breads and cereals, cooked fruits and vegetables, fruit juices.
      • Discuss the client's dietary preferences.
      • Instruct the client to eat about 800 g of fruits and vegetables (e.g., about four pieces of fresh fruit and a large salad) daily.
   b. Adequate fluid intake:
      • Encourage the client to drink at least 2 liters (8 to 10 glasses) of water daily, unless contraindicated.
      • Discuss the client's fluid preferences.
      • Set up a regular schedule for fluid intake.
   c. Regular time for elimination:
      • Identify the client's normal defecation pattern before onset of constipation.
      • Review the client's daily elimination routine.
      • Establish a regular time for defecation as part of a new routine, taking into account daily schedule, availability of facilities, and other factors.
      • Suggest that he attempt defecation about an hour after a meal and remain in the bathroom for a sufficient length of time.
   d. Simulation of the client's home environment:
      • Use the toilet instead of a bedpan or commode, if possible.

Rationale

1. Vagal stimulation caused by breath holding or straining during defecation increases intrathoracic pressure, which decreases venous return to the heart. Release of pressure results in increased venous return, thus increasing cardiac workload.

2. Teaching preventive measures and the hazards of certain behaviors may increase compliance and reduce complications.

3. Stool softeners increase the wetting efficiency of intestinal water, which softens the fecal mass and aids elimination.

4.

   a. A well-balanced, high-fiber diet stimulates peristalsis.

   b. Sufficient fluid intake, at least 2 liters a day, is necessary to maintain a normal elimination pattern and promote proper stool consistency.

   c. Taking advantage of normal circadian rhythms can help establish normal elimination patterns.

   d. A comfortable, relaxed environment can promote regular bowel movements.

Interventions

- Offer a bedpan or commode if the client cannot use the toilet.
- Assist the client into position on the toilet, bedpan, or commode, if necessary.
- Provide privacy: close the door or draw curtains around the bed, play a TV or radio to mask sounds, provide a room deodorizer.
- Enhance comfort (e.g., provide reading material as a diversion) and ensure safety (e.g., make sure a call bell is readily available.

  e. Optimal positioning:
- Assist the client as necessary to assume a normal semi-squatting position on the toilet or commode.
- Assist the client onto the bedpan if necessary, and raise the head of the bed to high Fowler's position or the permitted elevation.
- Stress the importance of avoiding straining during defecation.

  f. Regular activity:
- Explain the beneficial effects of daily activity on elimination.
- Assist with ambulation if necessary.

Rationale

e. Proper positioning during defecation attempts uses the abdominal muscles and the force of gravity to enhance defecation.

f. Activity influences elimination by improving abdominal muscle tone and stimulating appetite and peristalsis.

▲ **Documentation**

Graphic/flow record
  Bowel movements
  Bowel sounds

▲ **Outcome Criteria**

The client will:

1. Identify factors that increase cardiac workload
2. Demonstrate cardiac tolerance (marked by stable pulse, respirations, and blood pressure) to activity increases

Activity Intolerance related to insufficient oxygenation for activities of daily living (ADL) secondary to cardiac tissue ischemia

Focus Assessment Criteria	*Clinical Significance*
1. Degree of activity progression	1,2. A post-MI client must be monitored carefully to determine the rate at which activity can safely progress.
2. Physiological response to activity	

Interventions

1. Increase the client's activity each shift, as indicated:
   a. Allow the client's legs to dangle first; support the client from the side.
   b. Elevate the bed to the high position and raise the head of the bed.
   c. Increase the client's time out of bed by 15 minutes each shift.
   d. Allow the client to set his or her rate of ambulation.
   e. Set an increased ambulation distance goal for each shift.
   f. Increase activity when pain is at a minimum or after pain relief measures take effect.
   g. Increase the client's self-care activities from partial to complete self-care, as indicated.
2. Monitor the client's vital signs:

Rationale

1. Gradual activity progression, directed by the client's tolerance, enhances physiological functioning and reduces cardiac tissue hypoxia.

2. Tolerance to increased activity depends on the client's ability to adapt to the physiological requirements of the increased activity. Adaptation requires optimal cardiovascular, pulmonary, neurological, and musculoskeletal function.

Interventions

a. Prior to activity (ambulation, morning care)
b. Immediately after activity
c. After the client has rested for 3 minutes

3. Assess for abnormal responses to increased activity, such as the following:
   a. Decreased pulse rate
   b. Decreased or no change in systolic blood pressure
   c. Excessive increase or decrease in respiratory rate
   d. Failure of pulse to return to near resting rate within 3 minutes after activity
   e. Confusion, vertigo, uncoordinated movements
4. Plan adequate rest periods according to the client's daily schedule.
5. Identify and acknowledge the clients' progress.

6. Take steps to increase the quality and quantity of the client's sleep and rest periods. Make provisions for at least 2 hours of uninterrupted sleep at night.
7. Instruct the client on how to monitor his or her physiological response to activities postdischarge.
8. Teach the client how to conserve energy during ADLs, at work, and during recreational activities:
   a. Explain the need for rest periods both before and after certain activities.
   b. Instruct the client to stop an activity if fatigue or other signs of cardiac hypoxia occur.
   c. Instruct the client to consult with the physician or nurse practitioner before increasing activity after discharge.

Rationale

The expected immediate physiological response to activity includes the following:
a. Increased pulse rate and strength
b. Increased systolic blood pressure
c. Increased respiratory rate and depth
After 3 minutes, the pulse should return to within 10 beats per minute of the client's resting pulse rate.

3. Abnormal responses indicate intolerance to increased activity.

4. Rest periods provide the body with intervals of low energy expenditure.
5. Providing incentive can help promote a positive attitude and decrease the client's sense of frustration associated with dependency.
6. A person must complete an entire sleep cycle (70–100 minutes) to feel rested.

7. This self-monitoring can detect early signs and symptoms of hypoxia.

8. Energy conservation prevents oxygen requirements from exceeding a level that the heart can meet.

▲ **Documentation**

Graphic/flow record
　Vital signs
　Ambulation (time, amount)
Progress notes
　Abnormal or unexpected response to increased activity

▲ **Outcome Criteria**

The outcome criteria for this diagnosis represent those associated with discharge planning. Refer to discharge criteria.

Potential Altered Health Maintenance related to lack of knowledge of condition, hospital routines, treatments, medications, diet, activity progression, signs and symptoms of complications, reduction of risks, follow-up care, and community resources

Focus Assessment Criteria	*Clinical Significance*
1. Client's knowledge of and/or experiences with cardiac disorders	1. A client's knowledge and personal experiences can deter or improve compliance.
2. Readiness and ability to learn	2. A client who does not achieve goals for learning requires a referral for assistance postdischarge.

Interventions

1. Explain the pathophysiology of MI using teaching aids appropriate for the client's educational level (e.g., pictures, models, written materials).

Rationale

1. Such explanations reinforce the need to comply with instructions on diet, exercise, and other aspects of the treatment regimen.

Interventions	*Rationale*

2. Explain the risk factors for MI that can be eliminated or modified:
  a. Obesity
	2. Focusing on factors that can be controlled can reduce the client's feelings of powerlessness.
	  a. Obesity increases peripheral resistance and cardiac workload.

b. Tobacco use	b. Smoking causes tachycardia and raises blood pressure from its vasoconstrictive effects.
c. Diet high in fat or sodium	c. A high-fat diet contributes to plaque formation in arteries; excessive sodium intake increases water retention.
d. Sedentary life style	d. A sedentary life style leads to poor collateral circulation.
e. Excessive alcohol intake	e. Alcohol is a potent vasodilator; subsequent vasoconstriction increases cardiac workload.
f. Hypertension	f. Hypertension with increased peripheral resistance damages the arterial intima, contributing to arteriosclerosis.
3. Teach the client the importance of stress management through relaxation techniques and regular, appropriate exercise.	3. Although the exact effect of stress on coronary artery disease is not clear, the release of catecholamines elevates systolic blood pressure, increases cardiac workload, induces lipolysis, and promotes platelet clumping (Underhill, 1982).

4. Teach the client how to assess the radial pulse and instruct him or her to report any of the following symptoms:
  a. Dyspnea
  b. Chest pain unrelieved by nitroglycerin
  c. Unexplained weight gain or edema
  d. Unusual weakness
  e. Irregular pulse or any unusual change
	4. These signs and symptoms may indicate myocardial ischemia and vascular congestion (edema) secondary to decreased cardiac output.

5. Instruct the client to report side effects of prescribed medications, which may include diuretics, digitalis, or beta adrenergic blocking agents.	5. Recognizing and promptly reporting medication side effects can help prevent serious complications, e.g., hypokalemia.
6. Reinforce the physician's explanation for the prescribed therapeutic diet. Consult with a dietitian if indicated.	6. Repetitive explanations may help improve compliance with the therapeutic diet.

7. Explain the need for activity restrictions and how activity should progress gradually. Instruct the client to do the following:
  a. Increase activity gradually
  b. Avoid isometric exercises and lifting objects weighing more than 30 lb
  c. Avoid jogging, heavy exercise, and sports until the physician advises otherwise
  d. Consult with the physician on when to resume work, driving, sexual activity, recreational activities, and travel (plane or car)
  e. Take frequent 15- to 20-minute rest periods, four to six times a day, for 1 to 2 months
  f. Perform activities at a moderate, comfortable pace; if fatigue occurs, stop and rest 15 minutes, then continue
	7. Increasing activity gradually allows cardiac tissue to heal and accommodate to increased demands. Overexertion increases oxygen consumption and cardiac workload.

8. When the physician allows the client to resume sexual activity, teach the client to do the following: a. Avoid sexual activity in extremes of temperature, immediately after meals (wait 2 hours), when intoxicated, when fatigued,	8. To meet the increased myocardial oxygen demands resulting from sexual activity, the client should avoid all situations that cause vasoconstriction and vasodilation.

Interventions

Rationale

       with an unfamiliar partner or in an unfamiliar environment, and with anal stimulation

    b. Rest before engaging in sexual activity (mornings are the best time) and after activity

    c. Terminate sexual activity if chest pain or dyspnea occurs

    d. Take nitroglycerine before sexual activity, if prescribed

    e. Use usual positions unless they increase exertion

9. Reinforce the necessity of follow-up care.

10. Provide information on community resources, such as the American Heart Association, self-help groups, counseling, and cardiac rehabilitation groups.

9. Proper follow-up is essential to evaluate if and when progression of activities is advisable.

10. Such resources can provide additional support, information, and follow-up assistance that the client may need postdischarge.

▲ Documentation

Discharge summary record
   Discharge instructions
   Follow-up instructions
   Status at discharge (pain, activity, wound)
   Achievement of goals (individual or family)

References/Bibliography

Derenowski, J.M. (1988). The relationship of social support systems, health locus of control, health value orientation and wellness motivation in the postmyocardial infarction patient during three phases of rehabilitation, *Progress in Cardiovascular Nursing, 3*(4), 143–52.

Gawlinski, A. (1989). Nursing care after AMI: A comprehensive review. *Critical Care Nurse Quarterly, 12*(2), 64–70.

Misinski, M. (1988). Pathophysiology of acute myocardial infarction: A rationale for thrombolytic therapy. *Heart and Lung* (Suppl.), *17*(6), 743–50.

Riffle, K.L., et al. (1988). The relationship between perception of supportive behaviors of others and wives' ability to cope with initial myocardial infarctions in their husbands. *Rehabilitation Nursing, 13*(6), 310–315.

Sirles, A.T., et al. (1989). Cardiac disease and the family: Impact, assessment and implications. *Journal of Cardiovascular Nursing, 3*(2), 23–32.

Underhill, S., Woods, S., Sivarajan, E., & Halpenny, C. (1982). *Cardiac Nursing.* Philadelphia: J.B. Lippincott.

Wiggins, N.C. (1989). Education and support for the newly diagnosed cardiac family: A vital link in rehabilitation. *Journal of Advanced Nursing, 14*(1), 63–67.

Deep Venous Thrombosis

A clot in a deep vein (rather than a superficial vein), deep venous thrombosis can result from hemoconcentration due to fluid loss or dehydration, decreased circulation due to decreased metabolism or injury, or pressure on the vein from several possible sources (e.g., use of leg holders during surgery or use of a knee-gatch.

Diagnostic Cluster

▲ **Time Frame**

Initial diagnosis
Recurrent acute episodes

▲ **Discharge Criteria**

Before discharge, the client or family will do the following:

1. Identify factors that contribute to thrombosis recurrence
2. Relate the signs and symptoms that must be reported to a health care professional
3. Verbalize an intent to implement life style changes

Collaborative Problems	Refer to:
Potential Complications:	
Pulmonary Embolism	
Chronic Leg Edema	Venous Stasis Ulcers
Chronic Stasis Ulcers	Venous Stasis Ulcers

Nursing Diagnoses

Pain related to impaired circulation	
Potential Impaired Skin Integrity related to chronic ankle edema	
Potential Altered Health Maintenance related to lack of knowledge of prevention of recurrence of deep vein thrombosis and signs and symptoms of complications	
Potential Colonic Constipation related to decreased peristalsis secondary to immobility	Immobility or Unconsciousness
Potential Altered Respiratory function related to immobility	Immobility or Unconsciousness

Collaborative Problems

▲ **Nursing Goal**

The nurse will manage and minimize episodes of pulmonary embolism.

Potential Complication: Pulmonary Embolism

Interventions

1. Monitor respiratory function.

2. If the client is on anticoagulant therapy, monitor prothrombin time (PT) and partial thromboplastin time (PTT).

3. Instruct the client to maintain strict bed rest with the legs elevated above the heart.
4. Explain the rationale for anticoagulant therapy and for immobilization.
5. Avoid massaging the affected extremity.
6. Instruct the client to report (and save) any pink-tinged sputum.
7. Monitor for signs and symptoms of pulmonary embolism:
   a. Sudden chest pain
   b. Tachycardia
   c. Dyspnea
   d. Pallor
   e. Agitation
   f. Decreased pO_2

Rationale

1. Assessment should establish a baseline for subsequent comparisons to detect any changes.
2. Anticoagulant therapy may cause thrombocytopenia. PT and PTT values greater than two times normal (control) can produce bleeding and hemorrhage.
3. The recumbent position promotes venous drainage.
4. The client's understanding of the need for treatments may improve compliance.
5. Massage may dislodge the clot.
6. Blood-tinged sputum may indicate pulmonary bleeding.
7. These signs and symptoms may indicate a blockage in the pulmonary arterial system caused by a clot originating in a peripheral vein.

Interventions

8. Instruct the client to report any chest pain immediately.
9. Monitor leg edema, pain, and inflammation. Measure leg circumference 10 cm below and above knee. Report any increases immediately.
10. If you suspect an increase in the thrombosis, request a venous Doppler exam done by the vascular lab.

11. Prepare the client for insertion of a vena caval filter if thrombosis continues to propagate during heparin therapy.

Rationale

8. Early reporting enables prompt evaluation and treatment.
9. These measures help track the progression of the clot and inflammation.

10. Propagation of a thrombosis from the calf to the thigh increases the risk of a pulmonary embolus; Doppler exam can detect thrombosis propagation.
11. Occasionally, a venous thrombosis continues to propagate despite heparin therapy, e.g., if a malignancy alters the clotting mechanism. The only way to prevent the clot from traversing the vena cava to the lungs is to insert a vena caval filter, which provides a mechanical barrier.

▲ *Documentation*

Flow records
  Position in bed and activity restrictions
  Leg measurements and changes in measurement, color, or pain
Progress notes
  Client teaching

Related Physician-Prescribed Interventions

Medications
  Anticoagulants   Antipyretics
  Analgesics
Intravenous Therapy
  Continuous or intermittent intravenous
Laboratory Studies
  Hematocrit   Coagulation studies
Diagnostic Studies
  Magnetic resonance imaging   Contrast venography
  Noninvasive vascular studies (Doppler, oscillometry, plethysmography)
Therapies
  Compression stockings   Moist heat
  Elastic support hose

Nursing Diagnoses

▲ *Outcome Criteria*

The client will report an improvement of pain after pain relief measures.

Pain related to impaired venous return

Focus Assessment Criteria

1. Pain
   a. Description
   b. Location
   c. Duration
   d. Aggravating factors
   e. Alleviating factors
   f. Accompanying signs and symptoms

Clinical Significance

1. A baseline assessment of pain enables evaluation of the client's response to pain relief measures.

Interventions

1. Elevate the affected leg higher than the heart to promote venous drainage.

2. Explain the need to avoid aspirin to relieve pain if the client is on anticoagulant therapy.
3. Refer to the General Surgery care plan, Appendix II, for additional interventions.

Rationale

1. Venous pain usually is aggravated with leg in the dependent position and is slightly relieved with the leg elevated.
2. Aspirin prolongs clotting time.

▲ *Documentation*

Medication administration record
  Type, route, dosage of all medications
Progress notes
  Unsatisfactory relief from pain relief measures

▲ **Documentation**

Flow record
    Present condition of ankles
    Client teaching
    Client's response to teaching

Potential Impaired Skin Integrity related to chronic ankle edema

Focus Assessment Criteria	Clinical Significance
1. Client's understanding of deep venous thrombosis and sequelae	1. The client's understanding of possible complications may encourage compliance with restrictions and exercises.
2. Condition of skin on ankles	2. A baseline assessment enables detection of any changes in status.

Interventions	Rationale
1. Teach the client about the vulnerability of the skin on the ankles to the effects of chronic venous insufficiency.	1. Postphlebitis syndrome, caused by incompetent valves in deep veins, results in edema, altered pigmentation, and stasis dermatitis.
2. Teach the client to avoid situations that impede circulation to the legs, e.g., sitting for long periods.	2. Impeded circulation to the legs can promote recurrence of deep venous thrombosis.
3. Teach the client to perform leg exercises every hour, when advisable.	3. Leg exercises promote the muscle pumping effect on the deep veins, improving venous return.
4. If ankle edema occurs, encourage the use of elastic stockings for support.	4. Elastic stockings reduce venous pooling by exerting even pressure over the leg and increase flow to deeper veins by reducing the caliber of the superficial veins.
5. Teach the client to report any ankle injury or lesion immediately.	5. Decreased circulation can cause a minor injury to worsen and become a serious one.
6. Instruct the client to report his history of thrombosis at all future hospitalizations.	6. A high-risk client should alert nursing and medical staff so preventive measures can be initiated.

▲ **Outcome Criteria**

The outcome criteria for this diagnosis represent those associated with discharge planning. Refer to the discharge criteria.

Potential Altered Health Maintenance related to lack of knowledge of prevention of recurrence of deep vein thrombosis and signs and symptoms of complications

Focus Assessment Criteria	Clinical Significance
1. Knowledge of the pathology of deep venous thrombosis and preventive measures	1. This assessment guides client and family teaching.
2. Readiness and ability to retain information	2. A client or family that does not achieve goals for learning would require a referral for assistance postdischarge.

Interventions	Rationale

1. Explain relevant venous anatomy and physiology, including:
   a. Leg vein anatomy
   b. Function of venous valves
   c. Importance of muscle pumping action
	1,2. This teaching helps reinforce the need to comply with instructions (restrictions, exercises).

2. Teach the pathophysiology of deep venous thrombosis, including:
   a. Effect of thrombosis on valves
   b. Hydrostatic pressure in venous system
   c. Pressure transmitted to capillary system
   d. Pressure in subcutaneous tissue	

3. Teach preventive measures:
 	
   a. Initiating a regular exercise program (e.g., walking or swimming)
	3. These measures can help prevent subsequent episodes of deep venous thrombosis.
	   a. Exercise increases muscle tone and promotes the pumping effect on veins.

Interventions

    b. Avoiding immobility

    c. Elevating the legs whenever possible

    d. Using elastic support stockings (*Note,* these stockings should be checked by a health care professional to ensure proper fit.)

    e. Using extra means of support if exposed to additional risk; e.g., ace wraps or compression pump if prolonged immobility is necessary

4. If the client is being discharged on anticoagulant therapy, refer to the Anticoagulant Therapy care plan for more information.

5. Explain the need to do the following:

    a. Maintain a fluid intake of 2500 mL a day unless contraindicated

    b. Stop smoking

    c. Maintain ideal weight

    d. Avoid garters, girdles, and knee-high stockings.

6. Teach the client and family to watch for and promptly report these symptoms:

    a. Diminished sensation in legs or feet

    b. Coldness or bluish color in legs or feet

    c. Increased swelling or pain in legs or feet

    d. Sudden chest pain or dyspnea

Rationale

    b. Immobility increases venous stasis.

    c. Elevation reduces venous pooling and promotes venous return.

    d. The use of over-the-counter support stockings is controversial; improperly fitted stockings may produce a tourniquet effect.

    e. External elastic compression or a compression pump can provide the external pressure during a long period of immobility and help prevent venous pooling.

4. Low-dose heparin therapy has been proven to be of value in preventing deep venous thrombosis in clients for whom it is not contraindicated.

5. These practices help decrease the risk of recurrence:

    a. Adequate hydration prevents increased blood viscosity.

    b. Nicotine is a potent vasoconstrictor.

    c. Obesity increases compression of vessels.

    d. Garters, girdles, and knee-high stockings constrict vessels, causing venous pooling.

6. Early detection enables prompt intervention to prevent serious complications.

    a,b,c. These changes in the legs and feet may point to an extension of the clot with resulting compromised circulation and inflammation.

    d. Sudden chest pain or dyspnea may indicate a pulmonary embolism.

▲ **Documentation**

Discharge summary record
    Client teaching
    Outcome achievement or status

References/Bibliography

Ansari, A. (1986). Acute and chronic pulmonary thromboembolism; current perspectives. Part II: Etiology, pathology, pathogenesis and pathophysiology. *Clinical Cardiology, 9*(9), 449–456.

Dalen, J.E., Paraskos, J.A., Ockene, I.S., Alpert, J.S., & Hirsh, J. (1986). Venous thromboembolism: scope of the problem. *Chest, 89*(5), 370–373.

Langsfeld, M., Hershey, F.B., Thorpe, L., Auer, A.I., Binnington, H.B., Hurley, J.J., & Woods, J.J. (1987). Duplex B-mode imaging for the diagnosis of deep venous thrombosis. *Archives of Surgery, 122*(5), 587–591.

Lindner, D.J., Edwards, J.M., Phinney, E.S., Taylor, L.M., & Parker, J.M. (1986). Long-term hemodynamic and clinical sequelae of lower extremity deep vein thrombosis. *Journal of Vascular Surgery, 4*(5), 436–442.

Maxwell, R.S., & Greenfield, L.J. (1987). Effects of pulmonary embolism on survival of patients with Greenfield vena caval filters. *Surgery, 101*(4), 389–393.

Hypertension

Defined as persistent elevated blood pressure above 140/90 mm Hg in persons under age 50 and above 160/95 mm Hg in persons over 50 years of age, hypertension is the major cause of coronary heart disease, cerebrovascular accident, and renal failure. Sustained hypertension and accompanying increased peripheral resistance cause a disruption in the vascular endothelium, forcing plasma and lipoproteins into the intimal and subintimal layers of the vessel and causing plaque formation (atherosclerosis). Increased pressure also causes hyperplasia of smooth muscle, which scars the intima and results in thickened vessels with narrowed lumena (Underhill et al., 1989).

Diagnostic Cluster

▲ Time Frame

Initial diagnosis

▲ Discharge Criteria

Before discharge, the client will:

1. Demonstrate blood pressure self-measurement
2. Identify risk factors for hypertension
3. Explain the action, dosage, side effects, and precautions for all prescribed medications
4. Verbalize nutritional factors associated with hypertension
5. Relate an intent to comply with life style changes and prescriptions postdischarge
6. Describe the signs and symptoms that must be reported to a health care professional

Collaborative Problems

Potential Complications:
Retinal Hemorrhage
Cerebral Vascular Accident
Cerebral Hemorrhage
Renal Insufficiency

Nursing Diagnoses

Potential Noncompliance related to negative side effects of prescribed therapy versus the belief that treatment is not needed without the presence of symptoms

Potential Altered Health Maintenance related to lack of knowledge of condition, diet restrictions, medications, risk factors, and follow-up care

Collaborative Problems

▲ Nursing Goal

The nurse will manage and minimize vascular complications.

Potential Complication: Retinal Hemorrhage
Potential Complication: Cerebrovascular Accident
Potential Complication: Cerebral Hemorrhage
Potential Complication: Renal Insufficiency

Interventions

1. Monitor for symptoms of retinal hemorrhage: visual defects, including blurring, spots, and loss of visual acuity.
2. Monitor for signs and symptoms of cerebrovascular accident (CVA):
   a. Orientation or memory deficits
   b. Weakness
   c. Paralysis
   d. Mobility, speech, or sensory deficits.
3. Monitor for signs and symptoms of cerebral hemorrhage:
   a. Sudden severe occipital headache
   b. Diplopia
   c. Ataxia
   d. Nystagmus

Rationale

1. Evidence of blood vessel damage in the retina indicates similar damage elsewhere in the vascular system.
2. In the brain, sustained hypertension causes progressive cerebral arteriosclerosis and ischemia. CVA follows an interruption of cerebral blood supply caused by cerebral artery occlusion or rupture, resulting in sensory and motor deficits.

3. Cerebral hemorrhage involves a focal area of bleeding into brain tissue from a ruptured intracerebral artery. Also, as a matter of differentiation from cerebral occlusion, resulting deficits from hemorrhage never are rapidly reversible, as may occur with occlusion lesions.

Interventions

    e. Pupils small but reactive to light

4. Monitor for early signs and symptoms of renal insufficiency:

    a. Decreased serum protein level

    b. Sustained elevated urine specific gravity

    c. Elevated urine sodium levels

    d. Sustained insufficient urine output (<30 mL/hr)

    e. Increased BUN, serum creatinine, potassium, phosphorus, and ammonia levels, and decreased creatinine clearance

Rationale

4. With decreased blood supply to the nephrons, the kidney loses some ability to concentrate and form normal urine.

    a. Further structural abnormalities may cause the vessels to become more permeable and allow leakage of protein into the renal tubules.

    b,c. Decreased ability of the renal tubules to reabsorb electrolytes causes increased urine sodium levels and increased urine specific gravity.

    d. Decreased glomerular filtration rate, eventually causes insufficient urine output and stimulates renin production, which results in increased blood pressure in an attempt to increase blood flow to the kidneys.

    e. Decreased renal function impairs the excretion of urea and creatinine in the urine, thus elevating BUN and creatinine levels.

▲ **Documentation**

Graphic/flow record
    Vital signs
    Intake and output
    Laboratory values
Progress notes
    Status of client
    Unusual events
    Changes in behavior

Related Physician-Prescribed Interventions

Medications
    Diuretics
    Beta-adrenergic inhibitors
    Vasodilators
    Angiotensin-converting enzyme inhibitors

Intravenous Therapy
    Not indicated

Laboratory Studies
    Hemoglobin/hematocrit
    Thyroid studies
    BUN/creatinine
    Aldosterone (serum, urine)
    Serum glucose
    Serum potassium, calcium
    Serum cholesterol, triglycerides
    Urinalysis
    Urine UMA
    Uric acid
    Urine steroids

Diagnostic Studies
    ECG
    Intravenous pyelography
    Chest x-ray film
    Computed tomography (CT) scan

Therapies
    Sodium restricted diet

Nursing Diagnoses

▲ **Outcome Criteria**

The client will:

1. Verbalize feelings related to following the prescribed regimen

2. Identify sources of support for assisting with compliance

3. Verbalize the potential complications of noncompliance

Potential Noncompliance related to negative side effects of prescribed therapy versus the belief that treatment is not needed without the presence of symptoms

Focus Assessment Criteria

1. Client's perception of hypertension

Clinical Significance

1. The client's understanding of the seriousness of hypertension is critical to compliance.

Interventions

1. Identify any factors that may predict client noncompliance, such as these:

    a. Lack of knowledge

Rationale

1. Identifying any barriers to compliance enables the nurse to plan interventions to eliminate these barriers and improve compliance.

Interventions

    b. Noncompliance in the hospital
    c. Failure to perceive the seriousness or chronicity of hypertension
    d. Belief that the condition will go away
    e. Belief that the condition is hopeless
2. Emphasize to the client the potentially life-threatening consequences of noncompliance. (Refer to Collaborative Problems for more information.)
3. Point out that blood pressure elevation typically produces no symptoms.
4. Discuss the likely effects of a future stroke, renal failure, or coronary disease on significant others (spouse, children, grandchildren)
5. Include the client's significant others in teaching sessions, whenever possible.

6. Emphasize to the client that ultimately it is his or her choice whether or not to comply with the treatment plan.

7. Instruct the client to check or have someone else check his blood pressure at least once a week, and to keep an accurate record of readings.
8. Explain the possible side effects of antihypertensive medications (e.g., impotence, decreased libido, vertigo); instruct the client to consult the physician for alternative medications should these side effects occur.
9. If the cost of antihypertensive medications is a burden for the client, consult with social services.

Rationale

2. This emphasis points out the seriousness of hypertension, which may encourage the client to comply with treatment.

3. Absence of symptoms often encourages noncompliance.

4. This discussion emphasizes the potential impact of the client's hypertension on his significant others, which may encourage compliance.

5. Significant others also should understand the possible consequences of noncompliance, to encourage them to assist the client in complying with treatment.

6. Helping the client understand that he or she is responsible for compliance may enhance the client's sense of control and self-determination, which may help improve compliance.

7. Weekly blood pressure readings are needed to evaluate the client's response to treatments and life style changes.

8. A client who experiences these side effects may be tempted to discontinue medication therapy on his own.

9. The client may require financial assistance, to prevent noncompliance due to financial reasons.

▲ **Documentation**

Discharge summary record
    Client teaching
    Response to interventions

▲ **Outcome Criteria**

The outcome criteria for this diagnosis represent those associated with discharge planning. Refer to discharge criteria.

Potential Altered Health Maintenance related to lack of knowledge of condition, diet restrictions, medications, risk factors, and follow-up care

Focus Assessment Criteria	*Clinical Significance*
1. Client's ability and readiness to retain information	1. A client or family that does not achieve learning goals requires a referral for assistance postdischarge.

Interventions

1. Discuss blood pressure concepts using terminology the client and significant other(s) can understand:
    a. Normal values
    b. Effects of sustained high blood pressure on the brain, heart, kidneys, and eyes
    c. Control versus cure
2. Teach the client blood pressure self-measurement, or teach significant other(s) how to measure the client's blood pressure.
3. Explain the relationship between nutritional factors and blood pressure control, particularly the water-retaining properties of sodium. Teach the client or significant other(s) to read labels

Rationale

1. This teaching reinforces the need to comply with treatment and life style changes.

2. Self-monitoring is more convenient and may improve compliance.

3. Sodium controls water distribution throughout the body. An increase in sodium causes an increase in water, thus increasing circulating volume and raising blood pressure.

Interventions

and package information on foods and over-the-counter (OTC) medications. Refer to a dietitian, if indicated.
4. Provide the client or significant other(s) with medication guidelines and drug information cards for all prescribed medications. Explain the following:
   a. Dosage
   b. Action
   c. Side effects
   d. Precautions.
5. Alert the client and significant other(s) to OTC medications that are contraindicated, such as these:
   a. High-sodium medications (Maalox, Bromo-seltzer, Rolaids)
   b. Decongestants, e.g., Vicks Formula 44

   c. Laxatives, e.g., Phospho-soda

6. Explain the risk factors that can be eliminated or modified:

   a. Smoking

   b. High-fat or high-sodium diet

   c. Stress

   d. Obesity

7. Stress the importance of follow-up care.
8. Teach the client and significant other(s) to report these symptoms:
   a. Headaches, especially on awakening
   b. Chest pain
   c. Shortness of breath
   d. Weight gain or edema
   e. Changes in vision
   f. Frequent nosebleeds
   g. Side effects of medications

Rationale

4. This teaching conveys to the client side effects that should be reported and precautions that should be taken.

5. Over-the-counter medications commonly are viewed as harmless, when in fact many can cause complications.
   a. High-sodium content medications promote water retention.
   b. Decongestants act as vasoconstrictors, which raise blood pressure.
   c. Some laxatives contain high levels of sodium.
6. Understanding the risk factors that can be controlled may help improve the client's sense of control over the disorder and enhance compliance.
   a. Tobacco acts as a vasoconstrictor, which raises blood pressure.
   b. A high-fat diet contributes to plaque formation and narrowing of vessels; a high-sodium diet promotes water retention.
   c. Stress causes a sympathetic response that raises blood pressure.
   d. Obesity increases peripheral resistance and cardiac workload, raising blood pressure.
7. Follow-up care can help detect complications.
8. These signs and symptoms may indicate elevated blood pressure or other cardiovascular complications.

▲ **Documentation**

Discharge summary record
   Status of goal attainment
   Status at discharge
   Discharge instructions
   Referrals

References/Bibliography

Brunner, L., & Suddarth, D.S. (1986). *The Lippincott manual of nursing practice* (4th ed). Philadelphia: J.B. Lippincott.
Chobanian, A.V. (1982). Hypertension. *Clinical Symposia, 34*(5).
Lectch, C.J., & Tinker, R.V. (1978). *Primary care.* Philadelphia: F.A. Davis.
Papadopoulos, C. (1987). Cardiovascular drugs and sexuality: A cardiologist's review. *Archives of Internal Medicine, 140,* 1341.
Rudy, E. (1984). *Advanced neurological and neurosurgical nursing.* St. Louis: C.V. Mosby.
Stevenson, J.B., & Lumstead, G.S. (1984). Sexual dysfunction due to antihypertensive agents. *Drug Intelligence and Clinical Pharmacy, 18,* 113.
Thompson, J., McFarland, G., Hirsch, J., Tucker, S., & Bowers, A. (1986). *Clinical nursing.* St. Louis: C.V. Mosby.
Underhill, S., Woods, S., Sivarajan, E., & Halpenny, C. (1989). *Cardiac nursing* (2nd ed.). Philadelphia: J.B. Lippincott.

Peripheral Arterial Disease (Atherosclerosis)

Atherosclerosis obliterans, a progressive disease, is the leading cause of obstructive arterial disease of the extremities in persons over age 30. At least 95% of arterial occlusive disease cases are atherosclerotic in origin.

The World Health Organization describes atherosclerosis as "a variable combination of changes in the intima of arteries, consisting of the focal accumulation of lipids, complex carbohydrates, blood and blood products, fibrous tissue, and calcium deposits and associated with medial changes." It is characterized by specific changes in the arterial wall as well as the development of an intraluminal plaque. Atherosclerosis can lead to myocardial infarction, renal hypertension, stroke, and amputation.

The known risk factors for atherosclerosis include hyperlipidemia, smoking history, hypertension, diabetes mellitus, and a family history of strokes or heart attacks, especially at an early age. Altering modifiable risk factors has been shown to reduce significantly the chances of progressing to the morbid consequences of this disease. Teaching the risk factors and modifying behaviors that reduce risk factors are important components of nursing interventions for atherosclerotic disease.

Diagnostic Cluster

▲ Time Frame
Initial diagnosis

▲ Discharge Criteria
Before discharge, the client or family will:
1. List common risk factors for atherosclerosis
2. State specific activities to manage claudication
3. Describe principles and steps of proper foot care
4. Describe any life style changes indicated (e.g., cessation of smoking, low-fat diet, regular exercise program)
5. Lower low-density lipoprotein (LDL) cholesterol to less than 160 mg/dL, or less than 130 mg/dL if coronary heart disease or two risk factors are present
6. Relate the signs and symptoms that must be reported to a health care professional
7. Identify community resources available for assistance

Collaborative Problems

Potential Complications:
Stroke
Ischemic Ulcers
Acute Arterial Thrombosis
Hypertension

Nursing Diagnoses

Activity Intolerance related to claudication
Potential for Injury related to effects of orthostatic hypotension
Potential Altered Health Maintenance related to lack of knowledge of condition, management of claudication, risk factors, foot care, and treatment plan

Refer to:

Hypertension

Collaborative Problems

▲ **Nursing Goal**

The nurse will manage and minimize circulatory complications.

Potential Complication: Stroke
Potential Complication: Ischemic Ulcers
Potential Complication: Acute Arterial Thrombosis

Interventions

1. Teach the client about the signs and symptoms of transient ischemic attack (TIA) and the importance of reporting to the physician if they occur.
   a. Dizziness, loss of balance, or fainting
   b. Changes in sensation or motor control in arms or legs
   c. Numbness in face
   d. Speech changes
   e. Visual changes or loss of vision
   f. Temporary loss of memory
2. Assess for ischemic ulcers. Report ulcers or darkened spots of skin to the physician.

3. Reinforce teaching of foot care. (Refer to the nursing diagnosis Potential Altered Health Maintenance, page 81, for more information.)
4. Monitor peripheral circulation (pulses, sensation, skin color). Report any changes immediately.

Rationale

1. The risk of stroke increases in clients who have had a TIA. Disruption of cerebral circulation can result in motor or sensory deficits.

2. Atherosclerosis causing arterial stenosis and subsequent decreased tissue perfusion interferes with and may prevent healing of skin ulcers. Darkened spots of skin distal to arterial stenosis may indicate tissue infarctions related to ischemia.
3. Protection from skin loss may preserve tissue by preventing access to infective agents.

4. In acute arterial thrombosis, loss of sensation occurs first with accompanying pain associated with ischemia. This may be followed by a decrease in motor function.

▲ **Documentation**

Flow record
    Assessment results
Progress notes
    Changes in condition

Related Physician-Prescribed Interventions

Specific interventions also depend on how atherosclerosis affects circulation and renal, cerebral, and cardiac function. Refer to specific care plan (e.g., hypertension, renal failure) for more information.

Medications
Vasodilators   Pentoxifylline
Adrenergic blocking agents

Intravenous Therapy
Not indicated

Laboratory Studies
Cholesterol/triglycerides   Hemoglobin/hematocrit

Diagnostic Studies
Doppler ultrasonic flow   Angiography
Oscillometry   Digital subtraction angiography
Exercise test   Plethysmography

Therapies
Angioplasty (selected)   Diet low in salt, saturated fats, cholesterol

Nursing Diagnoses

▲ *Outcome Criteria*

The client will:

1. Identify activities that cause claudication
2. State why pain occurs with activity
3. Develop a plan to increase activity and decrease claudication

Activity Intolerance related to claudication

Focus Assessment Criteria	*Clinical Significance*

1. Client's daily activity:
  a. Need for ambulation for employment, e.g., mail carrier
  b. Sources of relaxation, daily activities
2. Degree of activity necessary to cause claudication:
  a. Walking distance at a certain pace
  b. Duration of exercise
3. Client's learned behavior to reduce or eliminate symptoms.
 	
4. Presence of obesity or tobacco use
	1. This assessment determines the extent to which the condition affects the client's life style.
	2. Depending on the extent of circulatory compromise, the client may be taught measures to allow maximum tissue perfusion and prevent any further compromise.
	3. Conservative self-care management may increase the time that the client is able to deal with the condition before seeking an operation.
	4. Obesity increases peripheral vascular resistance and smoking causes vasoconstriction, both of which reduce circulation to the legs.

Interventions

1. Teach the client about the physiology of blood supply in relation to activity and the pathophysiology of claudication.
2. Reassure the client that activity does not harm the claudicating tissue.

3. Plan activities to include a scheduled ambulation time:
   a. Institute a daily walking regimen of at least 30 minutes.
   b. Teach the client to "walk into" the pain, to pause when claudication occurs, and then to continue as soon as discomfort disappears.
4. Assist the client to reduce or eliminate modifiable risk factors:
   a. If obesity is a problem, develop a weight loss plan; consult with a dietitian.

   b. If the client smokes, explain the relationship between smoking and claudication, refer him to a smoking cessation program, and help him identify activities to substitute for smoking, e.g., breathing exercises, stress reduction for coping problems.
5. Provide information on pentoxifylline (Trental), if prescribed by the physician. Explain the following:
   a. Drug action
   b. The drug does not reduce the need for other activities to reduce risk factors.
   c. He should not expect an immediate effect, because it takes from 4 to 6 weeks of therapy to determine effectiveness.

Rationale

1. The client's understanding of the condition may promote compliance with restrictions and the exercise program.
2. The client may be tempted to discontinue activity when pain occurs in an attempt to avoid further injury.
3. A regimented exercise program can help develop collateral blood flow and ameliorate claudication.

4. Controlling or eliminating certain risk factors can help prevent claudication.
   a. Weight reduction reduces the workload on the muscles of the legs, which provide a pumping motion on vessels.
   b. Found to be the most important risk factor in the development of claudication in the Framingham Heart Study, smoking produces carbon monoxide, which increases tissue hypoxia. Nicotine causes vasospasms that last up to 1 hour after exposure.
5. Pentoxifylline reportedly improves red blood cell flexibility and decreases blood viscosity.

▲ *Documentation*

Discharge summary record
  Client teaching
  Outcome achievement or status
  Referrals

Potential for Injury related to effects of orthostatic hypotension

Focus Assessment Criteria	*Clinical Significance*
1. History of dizziness, lightheadedness, falling, medication use (e.g., vasodilators, antihistamines), other medical conditions	1. Clinical disorders and pharmacologic agents may be associated with orthostatic hypotension.
2. Bilateral brachial blood pressure (blood pressure taken in the supine position followed immediately by blood pressure taken in the standing position). *Note,* if brachial pressures differ, use the arm with the higher pressure.	2. A significant difference between the supine and standing blood pressure readings confirms orthostatic hypotension.

Interventions

1. Teach the client about the nature of orthostatic hypotension and its probable causes. Explain that the change to an upright position normally causes a decrease in venous return and cardiac output (caused by venous pooling) of 500 mL to 1 liter of blood in the legs. The corresponding drop in blood pressure stimulates baroreceptors, causing venous and arterial constriction and an increase in heart rate through increased sympathetic activity.

2. If brachial pressures differ between arms, explain the need to use one arm consistently for blood pressure measurement.

3. Instruct the client to avoid prolonged bed rest.

4. Teach the client to maintain adequate hydration, especially in summer months or in hot, dry climates.

5. Refer the client to a physician if you suspect that a prescribed medication may be responsible for the symptoms.

6. Teach the client to rise from the supine to the standing position in stages, first with one leg dependent, then the other.

7. Instruct the client to avoid hot baths or showers.

8. If a pressure (40 to 50 mm Hg) support garment (waist-high stocking) is prescribed, teach the client how to use it properly. Instruct him to put on the garment early in the day and to avoid sitting while wearing it.

9. Teach the client to sleep with pillows under his head.

Rationale

1. The client's understanding of orthostatic hypotension may help him modify behavior to reduce the frequency and severity of episodes.

2. Use of the arm with the higher pressure gives a more accurate assessment of the mean blood pressure.

3. Prolonged bed rest increases venous pooling.

4. Adequate hydration is necessary to prevent dehydration and resulting decreased circulating volume.

5. Certain medications—e.g., vasodilators, antihistamines—can precipitate orthostatic hypotension.

6. Gradual position change allows the body to compensate for venous pooling.

7. External heat may dilate the superficial vessels sufficiently to shunt blood from the brain, causing neurological symptoms.

8. This device reduces venous pooling by applying constant pressure over the leg surface. Elastic compression garments are easier to put on in the morning, before gravity causes increased edema. Bending at the groin and the knee causes constriction of the garment and increases pressure.

9. Decreasing the contrast between the supine and upright positions helps decrease the amount of intravascular fluid shift with position changes.

Potential Altered Health Maintenance related to lack of knowledge of condition, management of claudication, risk factors, foot care and treatment plan

Focus Assessment Criteria	*Clinical Significance*
1. Readiness and ability to retain learning	1. A client or family that does not achieve learning goals requires a referral for assistance postdischarge.
2. History of claudication and distance the client can walk before onset	2. Claudication is disabling when it restricts life style or earning ability.

Interventions

1. Explain the relationship of certain risk factors to the development of atherosclerosis:
   a. Smoking causes arterial vasoconstriction and can lead to postoperative graft failure. Chemicals present in tobacco irritate the endothelial lining and stimulate the proliferation of atherosclerotic plaque.
   b. In hypertension, increased intravascular pressure stimulates the proliferation of plaque.
   c. A client with poorly controlled diabetes tends to have arterial disease in the small vessels of the legs and feet.
   d. Hyperlipidemia promotes the progression of atherosclerosis. (Refer to the Cerebrovascular Accident care plan for additional teaching points.)
   e. Obesity coupled with high cholesterol and a sedentary life style increases the potential for atherosclerosis.
   f. Cold exposure increases the risk of damage to tissues with a compromised arterial blood flow. Older people with decreased sensation and blood flow should be taught to avoid cold temperatures.
   g. A sedentary life style aggravates the peripheral vascular and coronary artery disease of atherosclerosis.
2. Discuss and plan weight reduction, if necessary. Consult with a dietitian, if necessary, for dietary teaching, and refer the client to a weight loss program if appropriate.
3. Help the client quit smoking, if necessary. Refer him to a smoking cessation program, and provide support while he is withdrawing from nicotine.
4. Explain the importance of regular exercise, e.g., walking.
5. Explain the risks that atherosclerotic disease poses to feet:
   a. Diabetes-related peripheral neuropathy and microvascular disease

   b. Pressure ulcers

Rationale

1. Understanding that modifying or eliminating certain factors can reduce the risk of atherosclerosis can encourage the client to comply with the therapeutic regimen.

2. A decrease in body weight reduces the blood carried by the legs, thus reducing energy expenditure and oxygen demand.

3. Clients who smoke have been found to have a statistically higher incidence of atherosclerosis and bypass graft failure than those who do not smoke.
4. Maintaining a regular exercise program helps reduce the risk and severity of atherosclerosis.
5. The client's understanding may encourage compliance with necessary life style changes.
   a. The atherosclerotic process is accelerated in diabetes. Diabetic neuropathy prevents the client from feeling ischemic or injured areas.
   b. Healing of open lesions requires approximately ten times the blood supply than does keeping intact tissue alive. A client without an ulcer may just be able to use

Interventions

6. Teach foot care measures.
   a. Daily inspection
      • Use a mirror.
      • Look for corns, calluses, bunions, scratches, redness, blisters.
      • If vision is poor, have a family member or other person inspect the feet.
   b. Daily washing
      • Use warm, not hot, water, to avoid burning insensitive tissue. (Check the water temperature with the hand or elbow before immersing feet.)
      • Avoid prolonged soaking, which may macerate tissue.
      • Dry well, especially between the toes.
   c. Proper foot hygiene
      • Cut nails straight across; use an emery board to smooth edges.
      • Avoid using any chemicals on corns or calluses; they can cause an injury that will not heal.
      • Avoid using antiseptics such as iodine, which can damage healthy tissue.
      • If feet are dry, apply a thin coat of lotion. Avoid getting lotion between the toes; the skin between the toes does not require extra lubrication and macerates easily.
7. Teach the client to:
   a. Avoid hot water bottles and heating pads
   b. Wear wool socks to warm feet at night
   c. Never warm foot covering before going out in cold weather (wool socks and lined boots)
   d. Avoid walking barefoot
8. Instruct the client to wear well-fitting leather shoes (he may require shoes made with extra depth), always to wear socks with shoes, to avoid sandals with straps between the toes, and to inspect the insides of his shoes daily for worn areas, protruding nails, or other objects.
9. Teach the client to:
   a. Wear socks that fit well
   b. Avoid socks with elastic bands
   c. Avoid sock garters
   d. Avoid crossing the legs
10. Emphasize the importance of visiting a podiatrist for nail/callus/corn care if the client has poor vision or any difficulty with self-care.
11. Explain that if the client cannot inspect his own feet, he should arrange for another person to inspect his feet regularly.
12. Identify available community resources.

▲ **Documentation**
Discharge summary record
   Client teaching
   Outcome achievement or status
   Referrals when indicated

Rationale

the foot; an ulcer in the foot may necessitate amputation.
6. Daily foot care can reduce tissue damage and help prevent further injury and infection.

7. These precautions help reduce the risk of injury.

8. Well-fitting shoes help prevent injury to skin and underlying tissue.

9. Tight garments and certain leg positions constrict leg vessels, further reducing circulation.

10. The client may require assistance with foot care to ensure adequate care and prevent self-inflicted injuries.
11. Daily inspection helps ensure early detection of skin or tissue damage.

12. Community resources can assist the client with weight loss, smoking cessation, diet, and exercise programs.

References/Bibliography

American Heart Association. (1986). *Stroke: Warning signs.* Dallas: AHA.

Barker, L.R., Burton, J.R., et al. (1986). *Principles of ambulatory medicine.* Baltimore: Williams and Wilkins, 1263–1267.

Boozer, M., & Craven, R.F. (1981). Nursing care of the patient with chronic occlusive peripheral artery disease. *Cardiovascular Nursing, 15,* 13.

Clyne, C.A.C., et al. (1982). Smoking ignorance and peripheral vascular disease. *Archives of Surgery, 117,* 1062.

Doyle, J.E. (1981). If your patient's legs hurt, the reason may be arterial insufficiency, *Nursing 81, 11,* 74.

Eickhoff, J.M., & Engell, H.C. (1982). Local regulation of blood flow and the occurrence of edema after arterial reconstruction of the lower limbs. *Annals of Surgery,* 195:474.

Expert Panel. (1988). Report of the national cholesterol education program expert panel on detection, evaluation, and treatment of high blood cholesterol in adults. *Archives in Internal Medicine, 148,* 36–69.

Helden, E.R. (1987). The cholesterol enigma. *Journal of the Society for Peripheral Vascular Nursing, 4,* 5–7.

Hubner, C. (1987). Exercise therapy and smoking cessation for intermittent claudication. *Journal of Cardiovascular Nursing, 1*(2), 50–58.

Imparato, A.M., Kim, G.E., Davidson, T., et al. (1975). Intermittent claudication: Its natural course. *Surgery, 78,* 795.

Jasinkowski, N. (1982). The unique needs of a distal bypass patient. *RN, 45,* 44.

Juergens, J.L., & Spittell, J.A., Jr. (1980). *Textbook of peripheral vascular disease.* Philadelphia: W.B. Saunders, 20–27.

Kannel, W.B., D'Agnostino, R.B., & Belanger, A.L. (1987). Fibrinogen, cigarette smoking and risk of cardiovascular disease: Insights from the Framingham Study. *American Heart Journal, 13,* 1006–1010.

Kannel, W.B., & McGee, D.L. (1985). Update on some epidemiologic features of intermittent claudication: The Framingham Study. *Journal of the American Geriatrics Society, 33*(1), 13–18.

Roberts, W.C. (1987). Frequency of systemic hypertension in various cardiovascular diseases. *The American Journal of Cardiology, 60*(9), 1E–8e.

Tifft, C.P., & Chobanian, A.V. (1985). Evaluation and treatment of orthostatic hypotension. *Practical Cardiology, 11*(5), 103–117.

Wolf, P.A., D'Agnostino, R.B., Kannel, W.B., Bonita, R., & Belanger, A.J. (1988). Cigarette smoking as a risk factor for stroke: The Framingham Study. *JAMA, 259*(7), 1025–1029.

Raynaud's Syndrome

Raynaud's syndrome is an episodic, reversible, vasospastic ischemia of the digits, most commonly occurring in the fingers but occasionally affecting the toes. The sequence of events is as follows: Cold induces vasospasm with occlusion of the arterioles and veins, producing blanching. If the veins relax faster than the arterioles, the digits become cyanotic; the final rubor color results from hypoxia-induced vasodilatation (Campbell and LeRoy, 1986).

Primary Raynaud's syndrome exists as an isolated episode. Secondary Raynaud's syndrome occurs in association with a disease or condition that causes changes in the digital circulation. Conditions commonly associated with Raynaud's syndrome include rheumatoid arthritis, dermatomyositis–polymyositis, scleroderma, systemic lupus erythematosis, arteritis, atherosclerosis, hypothyroidism, and malignancy. Environmental risk factors include prolonged use of vibrating tools and exposure to chemical irritants. Women are affected five times more frequently than men.

Diagnostic Cluster

▲ Time Frame

Initial diagnosis

▲ Discharge Criteria

Before discharge, the client or family will:

1. State the risk factors that cause vasoconstriction
2. State the need to avoid or modify exposure to cold environment
3. Verbalize an intent to institute life style changes to reduce risk factors
4. Identify signs and symptoms that must be reported to a health care professional

---

Collaborative Problems

Potential Complication:
Acute Arterial Occlusion

Nursing Diagnoses

Fear related to potential loss of work secondary to work-related aggravating factors

Acute Pain related to ischemia secondary to acute vasospasm

Potential Altered Health Maintenance related to insufficient knowledge of condition, risk factors, and self-care

---

Collaborative Problems

▲ Nursing Goal

The nurse will manage and minimize episodes of arterial occlusion.

▲ Documentation

Flow records
  Assessments (before, during, and after acute episodes)
Discharge summary record
  Client teaching and evaluation of learning

Potential Complication: Acute arterial occlusion

Interventions

1. Review the client's history for episodes of Raynaud's syndrome.

2. Assess the physical characteristics of involved digit(s):
   a. Color: white, if the episode has just occurred; bluish/purple, if the episode is hours old
   b. Temperature: involved digit(s) feel cold
   c. Pulsation of digital vessels (via Doppler flow meter): may be absent during episode
3. Teach the client how to assess digital circulation and to report unusual or progressive signs.

Rationale

1. A client who has experienced repeated attacks of increasing frequency and duration may have an underlying disease. Disease progression eventually may involve arterial occlusion.
2. A baseline assessment provides the criteria for subsequent evaluation to assess progression.

3. Early detection of occlusions enables prompt intervention to prevent serious ischemia.

Related Physician-Prescribed Interventions

Medications
Vasodilators   Calcium channel-blockers
Antihypertensives

Intravenous Therapy
None indicated

Laboratory Studies
None indicated

Diagnostic Studies
Allen test   Digital plethysmography
Doppler evaluation   Peripheral arteriography

Therapies
None indicated

Nursing Diagnoses

▲ **Outcome Criteria**

The client will identify the source of fear and take measures to alleviate that fear.

Fear related to potential loss of work secondary to work-related aggravating factors

Focus Assessment Criteria	*Clinical Significance*

1. Client's job or occupation for:
  a. Chronic exposure to cold environment
  b. Use of vibrating tools
	1. Modification of job or occupation may be necessary to reduce the risk factors and reduce the symptoms.

Interventions	*Rationale*

1. Assist the client to identify the focus of his fear:
  a. Inability to perform job
  b. Inability to find another position
  c. Likelihood that he will lose his job
	1. Open, honest dialogue may help initiate constructive problem-solving and can instill hope.

2. Assist the client to identify alternatives to his present position:
  a. Alteration in present job
  b. Different position in the same company
  c. Different position in a different company
3. Refer the client for career counseling.
	2,3. The client may need assistance to determine realistic options and to promote effective coping.

▲ **Documentation**

Progress notes
  Interactions with client
Discharge summary record
  Referrals

▲ **Outcome Criteria**

The client will do the following:

1. Report relief of acute pain through management of acute vasospasm
2. Relate methods to increase tissue perfusion

Acute Pain related to ischemia secondary to acute vasospasm

Focus Assessment Criteria	*Clinical Significance*
1. Pain location and characteristics 2. Client's understanding of the cause of the pain	1,2. This assessment establishes a baseline for subsequent assessments and interventions, including client teaching.

Interventions	*Rationale*
1. Discuss the cause of the pain with the client. Explain that cold induces vasospasm, which occludes arterioles and veins, causing tissue hypoxia and pain.	1. Understanding the cause of pain helps the client plan ways to prevent it.
2. Teach the client to avoid cold exposure to the hands and feet:	2. Avoiding cold stimulus that produces the vasoconstrictive response can prevent unnecessary discomfort. Gloves may help prevent cold fingers from absorbing heat from warm fingers and causing spread of symptoms. Chilling of the entire body may cause vasospasm in the fingers and toes as a result of compensatory responses to raise the core temperature.

Interventions

Rationale

  a. Wear gloves (preferably wool) during all periods of cold exposure, no matter how brief—even to remove frozen food from a freezer.
  b. Avoid holding cold drinks in an unprotected hand.
  c. Wear warm, lined footwear and wool socks during all periods of cold exposure.
  d. Avoid getting the feet wet in cold temperatures.
  e. Avoid exposing the entire body to cold at one time.

3. Teach the client techniques to warm or rewarm extremities slowly after chilling:
  a. Place the hands or feet in another warm part of body, e.g., hands under arms, feet in warm hands
  b. Warm by placing into warm (not hot) water (105°F).

4. Discuss the possible use of medications with the attending physician.

3. Rapid warming or rewarming may cause the veins to dilate faster than arterioles, producing cyanosis.

4. Certain medications may relieve symptoms. For example, calcium channel-blockers relax spasm-prone blood vessels by slowing the flow of calcium into cells; guanethidine interferes with the release of norepinephrine from the sympathetic neuroeffector junction.

5. Teach the client relaxation techniques.

5. Relaxation may help dilate peripheral blood vessels and relieve symptoms.

▲ **Documentation**

Progress notes
    Episodes of pain, precipitating factors
    Pain relief measures implemented
    Client's response to these measures

6. Teach the client measures to raise core body temperature:
  a. Take warm showers.
  b. Drink warm milk or broth.

6. Increasing the core temperature can reduce vasospasms. Measures that have been used by the clients successfully but have not yet been studied on a large scale include activities that counter sympathetic response, such as warming the sympathetic ganglia of the back, shoulders, and upper thorax.

▲ **Outcome Criteria**

The outcome criteria for this diagnosis represent those associated with discharge planning. Refer to discharge criteria.

Potential Altered Health Maintenance related to lack of knowledge of condition, risk factors, and self-care

Focus Assessment Criteria	*Clinical Significance*
1. Client's readiness to learn and ability to retain information	1. A client who does not achieve learning goals may need referrals for follow-up assistance.

Interventions

Rationale

1. Teach the client about Raynaud's syndrome and explain its relationship to other disorders, including arthritis, arteritis, scleroderma, polymyositis, atherosclerosis, hypothyroidism, and lupus erythematosus.

2. Inform the client of risk factors:
  a. Exposure to cold temperatures
  b. Vibration against involved digits
  c. Vasoconstrictive medications
  d. Nicotine
  e. Caffeine

3. Teach the client to avoid cold exposure to the hands and feet:

1. The client's understanding of the condition can reinforce the need to comply with restrictions and life style changes.

2. The client's understanding of risk factors enables modification of these factors.

3. Avoiding cold stimulus that produces the vasoconstrictive response can prevent unnecessary

Interventions

    a. Wear gloves (preferably wool) during all periods of cold exposure, no matter how brief—even to remove frozen food from a freezer.

    b. Avoid holding cold drinks in an unprotected hand.

    c. Wear warm, lined footwear and wool socks during all periods of cold exposure.

    d. Avoid getting the feet wet in cold temperatures.

    e. Avoid exposing the entire body to cold at one time.

4. Teach the client measures to protect the fingers and toes from injury, e.g., testing wash water for temperature, taking care around sharp objects.

5. Encourage the client to avoid smoking cigarettes, pipes, or cigars. Refer him to a community agency for assistance with smoking cessation, if necessary.

6. Encourage the client to avoid caffeine-containing drinks and foods such as caffeinated coffee, tea, cocoa, colas, and chocolate.

Rationale

discomfort. Gloves may help prevent cold fingers from absorbing heat from warm fingers and causing spread of symptoms. Chilling of the entire body may cause vasospasm in the fingers and toes as a result of compensatory responses to raise the core temperature.

4. Diminished sensation in fingers and toes increases the risk of injury. Cuts, burns, bruises, or needle pricks may cause vasospasm or an injury that might prove difficult to heal.

5. Tobacco smoking causes cutaneous vasoconstriction. Nicotine acts as a sympathetic stimulus provoking a vasoconstrictive response.

6. Caffeine-containing drinks and foods act as vasoconstrictive agents.

▲ **Documentation**

Discharge summary record
    Client teaching
    Evaluation of outcome
    achievement and status

References/Bibliography

Arneklo-Nobin, B. (1983). *The white cold hand: Physiologic, angiographic and pharmacologic study on the hand circulation with special reference to Raynaud's phenomenon.* University of Lund, Sweden.

Belch, J.J.F., Drury, J., McLaughlin, K., O'Dowd, A., Anderson, J., Sturrock, R.D., & Forbes, C.D. (1987). Abnormal biochemical and cellular parameters in the blood of patients with Raynaud's phenomenon. *Scottish Medical Journal, 32,* 12–14.

Campbell, P.M., & LeRoy, E.C. (1986). Raynaud phenomenon. *Seminars in Arthritis and Rheumatism, 16*(2), 92–103.

Caperton, E. (1983). Raynaud's phenomenon; role of diet pills and cold remedies, *Postgraduate Medicine, 73,* 6–10.

Craven, R.F., & Curry, T.D. (1981). When the diagnosis is Raynaud's. *AJN, 5,* 1007–1009.

Holmgren, K. (1981). Vascular laboratory evaluation of Raynaud's syndrome. *Bruit, 5,* 19–22.

Malamet, R., Wise, R.A., Ettinger, W.H., & Wigley, F.M. (1985). Nifedipine in the treatment of Raynaud's phenomenon. *The American Journal of Medicine, 78*(4), 602–608.

Porter, J.M., & Edwards, J.M. (1985). Raynaud's syndrome. Part 2: Treatment options. *Drug Therapy, 5,* 79–90.

Rivers, S.P., & Porter, J.M. (1983). Clinical approach to Raynaud's syndrome. *Vascular Diagnosis and Therapy, 6,* 1–2, 15–24.

Wigley, F.N., Wise, R.A., Malamet, R., & Scott, T.E. (1987). Nicardipine in the treatment of Raynaud's phenomenon, *Arthritis and Rheumatism, 30*(3), 281–286.

Venous Stasis Ulcers

A venous stasis ulcer is a skin lesion, usually occurring around the ankle or lower leg, caused by prolonged venous hypertension. Postphlebitis syndrome, also known as chronic venous insufficiency, refers to the sequence of events that generally precedes venous stasis ulcers. Postphlebitis syndrome results from a deep venous thrombosis that destroys the valves in the leg veins, rendering them incompetent. Blood return to the heart from the venous system is then accomplished through collateral circulation. With no valves to check the back flow during systole, gravitational force increases the pressure in the venous system, with the greatest increase at the most distal area, the ankle. This increased hydrostatic pressure forces fluid into the interstitial space and causes the capillary walls to rupture, producing the characteristic chronic ankle edema and darkened skin. Eventually, when the skin can no longer contain the fluid, it breaks and an ulcer begins. This may be precipitated by trauma to the edematous tissues.

Diagnostic Cluster

▲ Time Frame

Initial diagnosis
Acute exacerbations

▲ Discharge Criteria

Before discharge, the client or family will:

1. Describe the etiology of venous stasis and ulcer formation
2. Relate how to prevent injury and infection
3. Relate methods to decrease risk factors
4. Demonstrate correct use of therapeutic elastic stockings
5. Relate signs and symptoms that must be reported to a health care professional

Collaborative Problems

Potential Complication:
Cellulitis

Nursing Diagnoses

Potential Body Image Disturbance related to chronic open wounds and response of others to appearance
Chronic Pain related to ulcers and débridement treatments
Altered Health Maintenance related to lack of knowledge of condition, prevention of complications, risk factors, and treatment

Collaborative Problems

▲ Nursing Goal

The nurse will manage and minimize cellulitis.

Potential Complication: Cellulitis

Interventions

1. Monitor arterial circulation by taking peripheral pulses, assessing capillary refill time, and performing a Doppler examination, if necessary.
2. Monitor venous circulation by assessing the color and size of the leg. Look for patterns of change, such as increased swelling.
3. Assess the tissue surrounding the ulcer for signs and symptoms of cellulitis:
   a. Erythema
   b. Increased tenderness
   c. Increased local temperature
   d. Drainage

Rationale

1,2. Careful, regular assessment of arterial and venous circulation enables detection of changes.

3. Broken skin weakens the defense against infectious organisms, increasing the risk of cellulitis.

Interventions

4. Teach the client to perform dressing changes using sterile/clean technique.
5. Unless contraindicated, elevate the affected extremity to a level above the heart.

6. Treat the ulcer and any accompanying cellulitis with topical antibiotics or compresses, as ordered.

7. Teach the client the importance of maintaining overall good health through proper diet, adequate hydration, and regular exercise.

Rationale

4. Wounds must be protected from bacterial infection.
5. Elevation helps reduce edema, which interferes with healing by causing local congestion, thereby preventing return flow of blood and metabolic wastes.
6. Topical products may be ordered to cleanse and protect the local area. Systemic antibiotics are generally indicated when cellulitis occurs.
7. Overall good health increases the body's resistance to this type of infection.

▲ *Documentation*

Flow records
    Assessment findings
    Topical applications
    Leg positions

Related Physician-Prescribed Interventions

Medications

Enzymatic débridement   Non-narcotic analgesics
  ointment   Antibiotics
Dextranomer beads
Topical lidocaine
  (Xylocaine)

Intravenous Therapy
Not indicated

Laboratory Studies
Wound cultures

Diagnostic Studies
Doppler ultrasound   Venography
Arteriography

Therapies
Dressings

Nursing Diagnoses

▲ *Outcome Criteria*

The client will communicate feelings about his appearance.

Potential Body Image Disturbance related to chronic open wounds and response of others to appearance

Focus Assessment Criteria

1. Ability to express feelings about appearance
2. Ability to participate in dressing procedure

Clinical Significance

1,2. This information helps evaluate the client's present response and progress. Participation in self-care and planning indicates attempts to cope with body-image changes.

Interventions

1. Contact the client frequently and treat him with warm, positive regard.

2. Encourage the client to verbalize feelings about his appearance and perceptions of life style impacts.
3. Validate the client's perceptions and assure him that his responses are normal and appropriate.
4. Assist the client to identify positive self-attributes.

Rationale

1. Frequent contact by the care giver indicates acceptance and may facilitate trust. The client may be hesitant to approach the staff because of a negative self-concept.
2,3. The nurse's validation of the client's emotions and perceptions increases the client's self-awareness and promotes self-esteem.

4. The client may focus only on the change in self-image and not on the positive characteristics that contribute to the whole concept of

Interventions

5. Discuss and suggest ways that the client can cope with body-image changes:
   a. Cover the dressing.
   b. Change the dressing frequently to prevent odors.
   c. Plan activities that require standing or walking early in the day, when edema is decreased.
6. Assist the client with hygiene and grooming, as necessary.

7. Encourage the client to receive visitors.

Rationale

self. The nurse must reinforce these positive aspects and encourage the client to reincorporate them into his self-concept.
5. Open, draining, malodorous lesions are offensive to others. Teaching the client to control the odor and appearance of the ulcers promotes an improved self-concept and body image.

6. Participation in self-care and planning can help the client cope positively with body-image changes.
7. Maintaining social contacts during hospitalization helps reduce feelings of isolation and promotes self-esteem.

▲ **Documentation**

Progress notes
  Present emotional status
  Interventions
  Response to interventions

▲ **Outcome Criteria**

The client will:

1. Report decreased pain with dressing changes
2. Report an increased tolerance for the chronic pain occurring between dressing changes

Chronic Pain related to ulcers and débridement treatments

Focus Assessment Criteria	*Clinical Significance*
1. Pain occurrence and characteristics	1. This baseline assessment serves as a basis for subsequent assessments.
2. Present method of pain management and its effectiveness	2. The client is the expert on his pain and on the effectiveness of pain relief measures.

Interventions

1. Explain the etiology of the pain.

2. Reduce the pain associated with dressing changes by soaking dressings before removal, if necessary.

3. When possible, use dressings that prove the least painful, e.g., hydrocolloid with support.

4. Use topical analgesics if necessary and if ordered by the physician.

5. If the client desires systemic analgesics, instruct him to use aspirin or acetaminophen.

Rationale

1. In some clients, knowledge of the sensory expectations and the reason for the pain may reduce the anxiety associated with treatments.
2. Although removing a dry dressing from a draining wound is an effective method of debriding the ulcer, the process is painful. The advantage must be weighed against the discomfort.
3. A hydrocolloid dressing, such as Duoderm, reduces the pain associated with these ulcers by keeping the wound bed moist and preventing air from contacting exposed nerve endings.
4. Use of a topical analgesic such as lidocaine (Xylocaine) reduces the discomfort from the exposed nerve endings at the wound edges.
5. Venous ulcers can be very painful, and the client may request systemic analgesics. Because venous ulcers are a chronic problem, it is best to avoid narcotics to manage the pain. Peripherally acting analgesics, such as aspirin or acetaminophen, are more appropriate.

▲ **Documentation**

Medication administration record
  Type, dosage schedule, and
    administration route of all
    medications
Progress notes
  Unsatisfactory pain relief

▲ **Outcome Criteria**

The outcome criteria for this diagnosis represent those associated with discharge planning. Refer to the discharge criteria.

Potential Altered Health Maintenance related to lack of knowledge of condition, prevention of complications, risk factors, and treatments

Focus Assessment Criteria	*Clinical Significance*
1. Readiness to learn and ability to retain information	1. A client or family that does not achieve learning goals needs referrals for assistance postdischarge.

Interventions

1. Explain the etiology of chronic venous insufficiency, including the following:
   a. Simple physiology of venous system
   b. Pathology of venous insufficiency
   c. Etiology of venous ulcers
2. Teach the client to do these things:
   a. Wear heavy stockings and shoes
   b. Avoid activities that might risk trauma to the legs
   c. Protect the legs from edema by:
      • Avoiding constricting clothing such as garters and tight belts
      • Avoid crossing the legs
      • Elevating the feet above the level of the heart whenever possible
      • Avoiding sitting with the groin and knees bent at right angles
   d. Prevent the ulcer from expanding by:
      • Removing dressings gently to prevent trauma to tissue
      • Avoiding using tape on skin
      • Always washing hands before and after dressing change
3. Explain signs and symptoms to watch for and report:
   a. Increase in ulcer size
   b. Changes in drainage color, amount, and odor
   c. Inflammation of surrounding tissue
4. When the ulcer is healed, teach the client to wear the prescribed elastic compression whenever the legs are not elevated.

5. Instruct the client to have the stockings or bandages checked every 3 to 4 months.

6. Explain risk factors:

   a. Increased susceptibility to trauma to edematous tissue

   b. Factors precipitating deep vein thrombosis (DVT)
   c. Infection of open lesion

   d. Cellulitis of tissue surrounding the ulcer

Rationale

1. This knowledge may help the client plan or modify his own care in his home environment.

2. Knowledge of prognosis and prophylactic strategies assists the client in preventing, avoiding, or minimizing problems that occur with chronic venous insufficiency.

3. Early recognition and prompt reporting of signs and symptoms of infection increase the likelihood of infection control.

4. External elastic compression effectively protects the tissues from the internal pressure and osmotic forces. The compression must be prescribed by a physician and must be greater than the capillary filling pressure at the ankle.

5. Leg size may vary because of edema; a change in leg size necessitates a change in the elastic compression.

6. Understanding that certain risk factors can be eliminated or minimized may encourage the client to take steps to do so.
   a. Protecting tissue with compromised circulation from trauma may prevent lesion formation.
   b. Veins that have had a previous DVT are at a higher risk for subsequent DVT.
   c,d. Open lesions and cellulitis provide entry or growth for bacteria.

▲ **Documentation**

Discharge summary record
   Client teaching
   Outcome achievement or status

References/Bibliography

Angel, M.F., Ramasastry, S.S., Swartz, W.M., Basford, R.E., & Futrell, J.W. (1987). The causes of skin ulcerations associated with venous insufficiency: A unifying hypothesis. *Plastic and Reconstructive Surgery, 79*(2), 289–297.

Dodd, H., & Cockett, F.B. (1976). The post-thrombotic syndrome and venous ulceration. In *Pathology and surgery of the veins of the lower limb*. New York: Churchill Livingstone, 246–314.

Doyle, J.E. (1983). All leg ulcers are not alike; managing and preventing arterial and venous ulcers. *Nursing '83, 13*(1), 58–63.

Doyle, J.E. (1986). Treatment modalities in peripheral vascular disease. *Nursing Clinics of North America, 21*(2), 250–252.

Fahey, V.A. (1984). An in-depth look at deep vein thrombosis. *Nursing 84, 14,* 33–41.

Lindner, D.J., Edwards, J.M., Phinney, E.S., Taylor, L.M., & Porter, J.M. (1986). Long-term hemodynamic and clinical sequelae of lower extremity deep vein thrombosis. *Journal of Vascular Surgery, 4*(5), 436–442.

Raju, S. (1983). Venous insufficiency of the lower limb and stasis ulceration: changing concepts and management. *Annals of Surgery, 197*(6), 688–697.

Samson, R.H., Scher, L.H., Veith, F.J., Gupta, S.K., & Ascer, E. (1986). Photoplethysmographic evaluation of external compressive therapy for chronic venous ulceration. *Journal of Cardiovascular Surgery, 27,* 4–26.

Tretbar, L.L. (1987). Chronic venous insufficiency of the legs: pathogenesis of venous ulcers. *Journal of Enterostomal Therapy, 14,* 105–108.

Respiratory Disorders

Chronic Obstructive Pulmonary Disease

Chronic obstructive pulmonary disease (COPD) refers to a group of disorders that cause airway obstruction, including chronic bronchitis and emphysema. Chronic bronchitis involves excessive bronchial mucus production and cough caused by chronic inflammation of the bronchioles and hypertrophy and hyperplasia of the mucous glands. In emphysema, airway obstruction is caused by hyperinflation of the alveoli, loss of lung tissue elasticity, and narrowing of small airways. COPD most commonly results from chronic irritation by chemical irritants (industrial, tobacco), air pollution, or recurrent respiratory tract infection.

Diagnostic Cluster

▲ **Time Frame**

Acute episode (nonintensive care)

▲ **Discharge Criteria**

Before discharge, the client or family will:

1. Identify long- and short-term goals
2. Identify adjustments needed in order to maintain self-care
3. State how to prevent further pulmonary deterioration
4. State signs and symptoms that must be reported to a health care professional
5. Identify community resources that can provide assistance with home management

Collaborative Problems

Potential Complications:
Hypoxemia
Right-sided Heart Failure

Refer to:

Nursing Diagnoses

Ineffective Airway Clearance related to excessive and tenacious secretions

Activity Intolerance related to inadequate oxygenation for activities and fatigue

Anxiety related to breathlessness and fear of suffocation

Powerlessness related to feeling of loss of control and the restrictions that this condition places on life style

Sleep Pattern Disturbance related to cough, inability to assume recumbent position, environmental stimuli

Potential Altered Health Maintenance related to lack of knowledge of condition, treatments, prevention of infection, breathing exercises, risk factors, signs and symptoms of complications

Potential Altered Nutrition: Less Than Body Requirements related to anorexia secondary to dyspnea, halitosis, and fatigue

Pressure Ulcers

Collaborative Problems

▲ **Nursing Goal**

The nurse will minimize and manage cardiovascular complications.

Potential Complication: Hypoxemia
Potential Complication: Right-sided Heart Failure

Interventions

1. Monitor for signs of acid–base imbalance:
   a. Arterial blood gas (ABG) analysis: pH < 7.35 and PCO_2 > 46 mm Hg

Rationale

1.
   a. ABG analysis helps evaluate gas exchange in the lungs. In mild to moderate COPD, the client may have a normal $PaCO_2$ level because of chemoreceptors in the medulla responding to increased $PaCO_2$ by increasing ventilation. In severe COPD, the client cannot sustain this increased ventilation, and the $PaCO_2$ value increases.

Interventions

    b. Increased and irregular pulse
    c. Increased respiratory rate followed by decreased rate

    d. Changes in mentation

    e. Decreased urine output (< 30 mL/hr)
    f. Cool, pale, or cyanotic skin

2. Administer low flow (2 L/min) of oxygen as needed through a cannula.

3. Obtain a sputum sample for culture and sensitivity.

4. Eliminate smoke and strong odors in the client's room.
5. Monitor ECG for dysrhythmias secondary to altered ABGs.
6. Monitor for signs of right-sided congestive heart failure:
    a. Elevated diastolic pressure
    b. Distended neck veins
    c. Peripheral edema
    d. Elevated central venous pressure (CVP).

7. Refer to the Congestive Heart Failure care plan for additional interventions if right-sided failure occurs.

Rationale

b,c. Respiratory acidosis develops owing to excessive CO_2 retention. The client with respiratory acidosis from chronic disease at first increases heart rate and respiration in an attempt to compensate for decreased oxygenation. After a while, the client breathes more slowly and with prolonged expiration. Eventually, his respiratory center may stop responding to the higher CO_2 levels, and breathing may stop abruptly.

    d. Changes in mentation result from cerebral tissue hypoxia.

e,f. The compensatory response to decreased circulatory oxygen is to increase blood oxygen by increasing heart and respiratory rate and to decrease circulation to the kidneys and to the extremities (marked by decreased pulses and skin changes).

2. This measure increases circulating oxygen levels. Higher flow rates increase carbon dioxide retention. The use of a cannula rather than a mask reduces the client's fears of suffocation.

3. Sputum culture and sensitivity determine whether an infection is contributing to symptoms.

4. Irritants to the respiratory tract can exacerbate symptoms.
5. ABG alterations may precipitate cardiac dysrhythmias.
6. The combination of arterial hypoxemia and respiratory acidosis acts locally as a strong vasoconstrictor of pulmonary vessels. This leads to pulmonary arterial hypertension, increased right ventricular systolic pressure, and, eventually, right ventricular hypertrophy and failure.

▲ **Documentation**

Flow record
    Vital signs
    Intake and output
    Assessment data
Progress notes
    Change in status
    Interventions
    Client's response to interventions

Related Physician-Prescribed Interventions

Medications
Bronchodilators
Corticosteroids (oral, inhaled)
Sympathomimetics (inhaled)

Adrenergics
Antimicrobials
Antitussives (nonnarcotic)

Intravenous Therapy
Not indicated

Laboratory Studies
ABG analysis
Serum albumin
Sputum culture

Electrolytes
Liver function studies

Diagnostic Studies
Chest x-ray film
Bronchography

Pulmonary function tests
Stress test

Therapies
Intermittent positive-pressure breathing (IPPB)
Low oxygen through a cannula

Chest physiotherapy
Ultrasonic nebulizer

Nursing Diagnoses

Ineffective Airway Clearance related to excessive and tenacious secretions

▲ Outcome Criteria

The client will:

1. Demonstrate effective coughing and increased air exchange in lungs
2. Relate strategies to decrease tenacious secretions

Focus Assessment Criteria	Clinical Significance
1. Ability to maintain upright position	1. A nonupright position causes abdominal organs to shift to the chest, preventing sufficient lung expansion to produce an effective cough.
2. Cough (productive, painful, effective)	2. The cough must be effective to remove secretions.
3. Sputum (color, character, amount, odor)	3. The secretions must be sufficiently liquid to enable expulsion.

Interventions

1. Instruct the client on the proper method of controlled coughing:
   a. Breathe deeply and slowly while sitting up as high as possible.
   b. Use diaphragmatic breathing.
   c. Hold the breath for 3 to 5 seconds and then slowly exhale as much as possible through the mouth. (The lower rib cage and abdomen should sink down.)
   d. Take a second breath, hold, and cough from the chest (not from the back of the mouth or throat) using two short, forceful coughs.
2. Teach the client measures to reduce the viscosity of secretions:
   a. Maintain adequate hydration; increase fluid intake to 2 to 3 quarts a day if not contraindicated by decreased cardiac output or renal disease.
   b. Maintain adequate humidity of inspired air.
3. Auscultate the lungs before and after the client coughs.
4. Encourage or provide good mouth care after coughing.

Rationale

1. Uncontrolled coughing is tiring and ineffective, leading to frustration.
   a. Sitting high shifts the abdominal organs away from the lungs, enabling greater expansion.
   b. Diaphragmatic breathing reduces the respiratory rate and increases alveolar ventilation.
   c,d. Increasing the volume of air in lungs promotes expulsion of secretions.

2. Thick secretions are difficult to expectorate and can cause mucus plugs, which can lead to atelectasis.

3. This assessment helps evaluate the effectiveness of the client's cough effort.
4. Good oral hygiene promotes a sense of well-being and prevents mouth odor.

▲ Documentation

Progress notes
Effectiveness of cough
Description of sputum

Activity Intolerance related to fatigue and inadequate oxygenation for activities

▲ Outcome Criteria

The client will:

1. Demonstrate methods of effective coughing, breathing, and conserving energy
2. Identify a realistic activity level to achieve or maintain

Focus Assessment Criteria	Clinical Significance
1. Tolerance to activities of daily living (ADLs) and physiological response to activity, i.e., pulse rate, blood pressure, respirations	1–2. Activity tolerance hinges on the client's ability to adapt to the physiological requirements of increased activity. Adaptation requires optimal cardiopulmonary, vascular, neurological, and musculoskeletal function.
2. Aggravating factors (environmental or emotional)	

Interventions

1. Explain activities and factors that increase oxygen demand:
   a. Smoking

Rationale

1. Smoking, extremes in temperature, and stress cause vasoconstriction, which increases cardiac workload and oxygen requirements. Excess

Interventions

  b. Extremes in temperature
  c. Excessive weight
  d. Stress
 2. Provide the client with ideas for conserving energy:
  a. Sit whenever possible when performing ADLs, e.g., on a stool when showering.
  b. Pace activities throughout the day.
  c. Schedule adequate rest periods.
  d. Alternate easy and hard tasks throughout the day.
 3. Gradually increase the client's daily activities as tolerance increases.

 4. Teach the client effective breathing techniques, such as diaphragmatic and pursed-lip breathing.

 5. Maintain supplemental oxygen therapy, as needed.
 6. Provide emotional support and encouragement.

 7. After activity, assess for abnormal responses to increased activity:
  a. Decreased pulse rate
  b. Decreased or unchanged systolic blood pressure
  c. Excessively increased or decreased respiratory rate
  d. Failure of pulse to return to near resting rate within 3 minutes after activity
  e. Confusion, vertigo, uncoordinated movements
 8. Plan adequate rest periods according to the client's daily schedule.

Rationale

weight increases peripheral resistance, which also increases cardiac workload.

 2. Excessive energy expenditure can be prevented by pacing activities and allowing sufficient time to recuperate between activities.

 3. Sustained moderate breathlessness from supervised exercise improves accessory muscle strength and respiratory function.
 4. Diaphragmatic breathing deters the shallow, rapid, inefficient breathing that usually accompanies COPD. Pursed-lip breathing slows expiration, keeps alveoli inflated longer, and provides some control over dyspnea.
 5. Supplemental oxygen increases circulating oxygen levels and improves activity tolerance.
 6. Fear of breathlessness may impede increased activity.
 7. Intolerance to activity can be assessed by evaluating cardiac, circulatory, and respiratory status.

 8. Rest periods allow the body a period of low energy expenditure, increasing activity tolerance.

▲ **Documentation**

Progress notes
 Activity level
 Physiological response to activity (vital signs)

▲ **Outcome Criteria**

The client will:

1. Verbalize feelings of anxiety
2. Demonstrate breathing techniques to decrease dyspnea

Anxiety related to breathlessness and fear of suffocation

Focus Assessment Criteria	*Clinical Significance*
1. Anxiety level	**1.** Anxiety increases respiratory and heart rates, resulting in increased oxygen requirements.
2. Knowledge of breathing techniques	**2.** This assessment guides client teaching.

Interventions

 1. Provide a quiet, calm environment when the client is experiencing breathlessness.
 2. Do not leave the client alone during periods of acute breathlessness.
 3. During periods of acute breathlessness do the following:
  a. Open curtains and doors
  b. Eliminate unnecessary equipment
  c. Limit visitors
  d. Eliminate smoke and odors

Rationale

 1. Reducing external stimuli promotes relaxation.

 2. The client needs reassurance that help is available if needed.
 3. These measures may help reduce feelings of suffocation.

▲ **Documentation**

Progress notes
 Acute anxiety episodes
 Interventions
 Client's response to interventions

Interventions	Rationale
4. Encourage the client to use breathing techniques, especially during times of increased anxiety. Coach him through the breathing exercises.	4. Concentrating on diaphragmatic or pursed-lip breathing slows the respiratory rate and gives the client a sense of control.

▲ **Outcome Criteria**

The client will:

1. Identify personal strengths
2. Identify factors that he can control

Powerlessness related to feelings of loss of control and life style restrictions

Focus Assessment Criteria	Clinical Significance
1. Understanding of disease process 2. Perception of control 3. Effects on life style	1–3. A client's response to loss of control depends on the meaning of the loss, individual patterns of coping, personal characteristics, and responses of others.

Interventions	Rationale

1. Explore the effects of the condition on the following:
  a. Client's occupation
  b. Leisure and recreational activities
  c. Role responsibilities
  d. Relationships
	1. Illness can negatively affect the client's self-concept and ability to achieve goals. Specifically, in COPD, dyspnea can interfere with the client's ability to work and play.

2. Determine the client's usual response to problems.	2. To plan effective interventions, the nurse must determine whether the client usually seeks to change his own behaviors to control problems or whether he expects others or external factors to control problems.
3. Help the client identify personal strengths and assets.	3. Attempts should be made to discourage the client from focusing only on limitations.
4. Assist in identifying energy patterns and in scheduling activities around these patterns.	4. A review of the client's daily schedule can help the nurse and client to plan activities that promote feelings of self-worth and dignity and to schedule appropriate rest periods to prevent exhaustion.
5. Discuss the need to accept help from others and to delegate some tasks.	5. The client may need assistance to prevent exhaustion and hypoxia.
6. Help the client seek support from other sources, e.g., self-help groups, support groups.	6. The client may benefit from opportunities to share similar experiences and problem-solving with others in the same situation.

▲ **Documentation**

Progress notes
  Interactions with the client

Sleep Pattern Disturbance related to cough, inability to assume recumbent position, environmental stimuli

▲ **Outcome Criteria**

The client will report a satisfactory balance of rest and activity.

Focus Assessment Criteria	Clinical Significance
1. Usual sleep requirements	1. Sleep requirements vary with age, life style, activity, and stress level.
2. Usual bedtime routines, environment, and sleeping position	2. Bedtime rituals, a familiar environment, and comfortable positioning help relaxation and promote sleep.
3. Quantity and quality of sleep	3. Only the client can determine his satisfaction with the quantity and quality of sleep.

Interventions	Rationale

1. Explain the sleep cycle and its significance:
  a. Stage I: Transitional stage between wakefulness and sleep (5% of total sleep)
  b. Stage II: Asleep but easily aroused (50%–55% of total sleep)
	1. A person typically goes through four or five complete sleep cycles each night. If the person awakens during a sleep cycle, he may not feel rested in the morning.

Interventions

Rationale

    c. Stage III: Deeper sleep; arousal is more difficult (10% of total sleep)

    d. Stage IV: Deepest sleep; metabolism and brain waves slow (10% of total sleep).

2. Discuss individual differences in sleep requirements based on these factors:

    a. Age

    b. Activity level

    c. Life style

    d. Stress level

3. Promote relaxation:

    a. Provide a dark, quiet environment.

    b. Allow choices regarding pillows, linens, covers.

    c. Provide comforting bedtime rituals as necessary.

    d. Ensure good room ventilation.

    e. Close the room door, if the client desires.

4. Plan procedures to limit sleep disturbances. Allow the client at least 2-hour segments of uninterrupted sleep.

5. Explain why hypnotics or sedatives should be avoided.

6. If desired, elevate the head of the bed on 10-inch blocks or use a gatch with pillows under the arms.

7. Take measures to control coughing:

    a. Avoid giving the client cold or hot liquids at bedtime.

    b. Consult the physician for antitussives, if indicated.

8. Teach the client measures to promote sleep:

    a. Eat a high-protein snack before bedtime, e.g., cheese, milk.

    b. Avoid caffeine.

    c. Attempt to sleep only when feeling sleepy.

    d. If sleeping difficulty occurs, leave the bedroom and engage in a quiet activity, such as reading, in another room.

    e. Try to maintain the same sleep habits 7 days a week.

9. Assist with a usual bedtime routine, e.g., personal hygiene, snack, music.

---

2. The usual recommendation of 8 hours of sleep every night actually has no scientific basis. A person who can relax and rest easily requires less sleep to feel refreshed. With aging, total sleep time generally decreases, especially Stage IV sleep, and Stage I sleep time increases.

3. Sleep is difficult until relaxation is attained. The hospital environment can impair relaxation.

4. Generally, a person must complete an entire sleep cycle (70–100 minutes) four to five times a night to feel rested.

5. These medications lose their effectiveness after a week; increasing dosages carries the risk of dependence.

6. This can enhance relaxation and sleep by giving the lungs more room for expansion through reducing upward pressure of abdominal organs.

7. These measures help prevent cough stimulation and disruption of sleep.

8.

    a. Digested protein produces tryptophan, which has a sedating effect.

    b. Caffeine stimulates metabolism and deters relaxation.

    c. Frustration increases if sleep is attempted when not sleepy or relaxed.

    d. The bedroom should be reserved specifically for sleep.

    e. Irregular retiring and arising patterns can disrupt the biological clock, exacerbating sleep difficulties.

9. Following a familiar bedtime routine may help promote relaxation and aid sleep.

▲ **Outcome Criteria**

The outcome criteria for this diagnosis represent those associated with discharge planning. Refer to discharge criteria.

▲ **Documentation**

Progress notes
    Sleep patterns (amount, awakenings)
    Client's evaluation of sleep quantity and quality

Potential Altered Health Maintenance related to lack of knowledge of condition, treatments, prevention of infection, breathing exercises, risk factors, signs and symptoms of complications

Focus Assessment Criteria	*Clinical Significance*
1. Readiness and ability to learn and retain information	1. Episodes of cerebral hypoxia can prevent retention of learning. A client who does not achieve goals for learning requires a referral for assistance postdischarge.

Interventions	*Rationale*
1. Help the client formulate and accept realistic short- and long-term goals.	1. This may help the client realize that he has much control over his life and can make choices to improve the quality of his life.
2. Teach about the diagnosis and treatment regimen.	2. Understanding may help encourage compliance and participation in self-care.
3. Teach measures to help control dyspnea and infections:	3.
a. Eat a well-balanced diet.	
b. Take sufficient rest periods.	
c. Gradually increase activity.	a,b,c. These practices promote overall good health and increase the resistance to infection.
d. Avoid exposure to the following:	d. Exposure to these respiratory irritants can cause bronchospasm and increase mucus production. Smoking destroys the ciliary cleansing mechanism of the respiratory tract. Heat raises body temperature and increases the body's oxygen requirements, possibly exacerbating symptoms.
• Smoke	
• Dust	
• Severe air pollution	
• Extremely cold or warm temperatures	
4. Teach and have the client demonstrate breathing exercises (Walsh):	4. A client with COPD typically breathes shallowly from the upper chest. Breathing exercises increase alveolar ventilation and reduce respiratory rate.
a. Incentive spirometer	a. Incentive spirometry encourages deep, sustained inspiratory efforts.
b. Diaphragm exercise: Place fingers on the lower ribs; inhale, pushing out against light pressure of fingers.	b. Expanding and contracting the diaphragm muscle can help strengthen it.
c. Lung apex exercises: Apply light pressure just below the clavicle as you inhale. While exhaling, apply pressure to the sternum with the heel of your hand.	c. Counterpressure forces the client to breathe harder, which strengthens muscles and aerates lung apexes.
d. Posterior lung exercises: Lie on your side, and have someone else place both hands over your lower thorax and apply pressure as you exhale.	d. Breathing against gravity and counterpressure strengthens respiratory muscles.
e. Lateral lower rib area exercises: Exhale completely, then have another person apply pressure to the lower rib cage area with both hands as you inhale. During exhalation, tighten the abdomen as the other person again applies pressure.	e. Complete exhalation promotes maximum expansion of the rib cage.
5. Teach and evaluate the technique of postural drainage:	5. The force of gravity helps loosen and drain secretions.
a. Assume a dependent position to drain the involved lung area, using pillows or a reclining chair.	
b. Cough and expectorate secretions while in the dependent position.	
c. Hold the position for 10 to 15 minutes.	
6. Advise the client not to perform breathing exercises shortly before or after eating.	6. The exertion associated with breathing exercises may reduce appetite. Performing the exercises after eating may cause vomiting.
7. Explain the hazards of infection and ways to reduce the risk:	7. A client with COPD is prone to infection due to inadequate primary defenses, i.e., decreased ciliary action and stasis of secretions. Minor respiratory infections can cause serious problems in a client with COPD. Chronic debilitation and retention of secretions (which provide a medium for microorganism growth) put the client at high risk for complications.
a. Avoid contact with infected persons.	
b. Receive immunization against influenza and bacterial pneumonia.	
c. Take antibiotics as prescribed if sputum becomes yellow or green.	

Interventions

d. Adhere to chest physiotherapy, medications, and hydration schedule.
e. Cleanse all equipment well.

8. Instruct the client to report the following:
a. Change in sputum characteristics or failure of sputum to return to usual color after 3 days of antibiotic therapy
b. Elevated temperature

c. Increase in cough, weakness, or shortness of breath
d. Increased confusion or drowsiness

e. Weight loss

f. Weight gain or swelling in ankles and feet

9. Teach the proper use of a hand-held nebulizer and oxygen therapy.
10. Teach methods to conserve energy. See the nursing diagnosis Fatigue in the Inflammatory Joint Disease care plan, page 297, for more information.
11. Provide information about or initiate referrals to community resources, such as the American Lung Association, self-help groups, Meals-on-Wheels, and home health agencies.

Rationale

8.
a. Sputum changes may indicate an infection or resistance of the infective organism to the prescribed antibiotic.
b. Circulating pathogens stimulate the hypothalamus to elevate body temperature.
c. Hypoxia is chronic; exacerbations must be detected early to prevent complications.
d. Cerebral hypoxia can produce confusion or drowsiness.
e. Inadequate intake can result from dyspnea, fatigue, medication side effects, and anorexia secondary to hypoxia and sputum production.
f. These signs may indicate fluid retention secondary to pulmonary arterial hypertension and decreased cardiac output.
9. Accurate instructions can help prevent medication overdose or oxygen dependence.
10. Energy conservation helps prevent exhaustion and exacerbation of hypoxia.

11. These resources can provide the client with needed assistance with home management and self-care.

▲ Documentation

Discharge summary record
    Client teaching
    Outcome achievement or status
    Referrals, if indicated

References/Bibliography

Curgian, L.M., et al. (1988). Enhancing sexual performance in COPD. *Nurse Practitioner, 13*(6), 34–38.
Dougherty, S. (1988). The malnourished respiratory patient. *Critical Care Nursing, 8*(4), 13–22.
Hahn, K. (1989). Sexuality and COPD. *Rehabilitation Nursing, 14*(4), 191–195.
Hunter, S.M. (1987). Educating clients with COPD. *Home Healthcare Nurse, 5*(6), 41–43.
Johnson, A.P. (1988). The elderly and COPD. *Journal of Gerontology Nursing, 14*(12), 20–24.
Renfroe, K.L. (1988). Effect of progressive relaxation on dyspnea and state anxiety in patients with chronic obstructive pulmonary disease. *Heart and Lung, 17*(4), 408–413.
Traver, G.A. (1988). Measures of symptoms and life quality to predict emergent use of institutional health care resources in chronic obstructive airways disease. *Heart and Lung, 17*(6), 689–697.

Pneumonia

An inflammatory process of the lung parenchyma, usually in the bronchioles and alveolar sacs, pneumonia can be caused by bacteria, viruses, fungi, parasites, inhalation of chemicals, aspiration of gastric contents, or accumulation of fluids in lung bases. Pneumonia is the most common infectious cause of death in the United States. One fourth to one third of the clients hospitalized with pneumococcal pneumonia develop bacteremia. About 50% of all pneumococcal pneumonias occur in persons over age 60.

Diagnostic Cluster

▲ **Time Frame**

Acute episode

▲ **Discharge Criteria**

Before discharge, the client or family will:

1. Describe how to prevent infection transmission
2. Describe rest and nutritional requirements
3. Describe methods to reduce the risk of recurrence
4. State signs and symptoms that must be reported to a health care professional

Collaborative Problems

Potential Complications:	Refer to:
Respiratory Insufficiency	
Septic Shock	
Paralytic Ileus	

Nursing Diagnoses

Potential Altered Oral Mucous Membrane related to mouth breathing, frequent expectorations, and decreased fluid intake secondary to malaise	
Potential Altered Health Maintenance related to lack of knowledge of condition, infection transmission, prevention of recurrence, diet, signs and symptoms of recurrence, and follow-up care	
Activity Intolerance related to insufficient oxygenation for ADL	Chronic Obstructive Pulmonary Disease
Potential Altered Nutrition: Less than Body Requirements related to anorexia, dyspnea, and abdominal distention secondary to air swallowing	Cirrhosis
Ineffective Airway Clearance related to pain, increased tracheobronchial secretions, and fatigue	Chronic Obstructive Pulmonary Disease

Collaborative Problems

▲ **Nursing Goal**

The nurse will manage and minimize complications of pneumonia.

Potential Complication: Respiratory Insufficiency
Potential Complication: Septic Shock
Potential Complication: Paralytic Ileus

Interventions

1. Monitor for signs and symptoms of hyperthermia:
   a. Fever of 103° F or above
   b. Chills
   c. Tachycardia
   d. Signs of shock: restlessness or lethargy, confusion, decreased systolic blood pressure

2. Provide cooling measures, e.g., reduced clothing and bed linen, tepid baths, increased fluids, hypothermia blanket

Rationale

1. Bacteria can act as a pyrogen by raising the hypothalamic thermostat through the production of endogenous pyrogens, which may mediate through prostaglandins. Chills can occur when the temperature set-point of the hypothalamus changes rapidly. High fever increases metabolic needs and oxygen consumption. The impaired respiratory system cannot compensate, and tissue hypoxia results.

2. Reduction of body temperature is necessary to lower metabolic rate and reduce oxygen consumption.

Interventions

3. Monitor respiratory status and assess for signs and symptoms of inflammation:
   a. Increased respiratory rate
   b. Fever, chills (sudden or insidious)
   c. Productive cough
   d. Diminished or absent breath sounds
   e. Pleuritic pain
   f. Tachycardia
   g. Marked dyspnea
   h. Cyanosis

4. Monitor for signs and symptoms of septic shock:
   a. Subnormal body temperature
   b. Hypotension
   c. Decreased level of consciousness
   d. Weak, rapid pulse
   e. Rapid, shallow respirations
   f. Cold, clammy skin
   g. Oliguria

5. Monitor for signs and symptoms of paralytic ileus:
   a. Absence of bowel movements
   b. Absent bowel sounds
   c. Abdominal rigidity and distention
   d. Nausea and vomiting

6. Administer cough suppressants or expectorants as ordered by the physician.

7. Maintain oxygen therapy, as prescribed, and monitor its effectiveness.

8. Provide respiratory physiotherapy (e.g., percussion, postural drainage) to move thick, tenacious secretions along the tracheobronchial trees.

Rationale

3. Tracheobronchial inflammation, impaired alveolar capillary membrane function, edema, fever, and increased sputum production disrupt respiratory function and alter the blood's oxygen-carrying capacity.

4. Septic shock may develop in a client with pneumonia if treatment is delayed or if the organism causing the pneumonia is very virulent and drug resistant. An elderly client has an increased risk of other complicating illnesses and may exhibit only subtle signs of septic shock.

5. Paralytic ileus can result from anorexia and decreased food intake or from increased insensible fluid loss due to hyperthermia and hyperventilation. Abdominal distention is aggravated by "air hunger"—mouth-breathing due to hypoxia.

6. Dry, hacking cough interferes with sleep and saps energy. Cough suppressants should be used judiciously, however, because complete depression of the cough reflex can cause atelectasis by preventing the movement of tracheobronchial secretions.

7. Oxygen therapy may help prevent restlessness if the client is becoming dyspneic, and it also may help prevent pulmonary edema. Because the client is no longer gasping for air, the risk of abdominal distention is decreased. Frequent arterial blood gas (ABG) analysis is essential to detect depressed ventilatory drive.

8. Exudate in the alveoli and bronchospasms caused by an increase in bronchopulmonary secretions can decrease ventilatory effort and impair gas exchange.

▲ **Documentation**

Medication administration record
   Type, dosage, route of all
      medications
Flow record
   Vital signs
   Assessments
Progress notes
   Cooling measures employed
   Effects on temperature

Related Physician-Prescribed Interventions

Medications
Antimicrobials
Bronchodilators
Expectorants

Analgesics (non-narcotic)
Mucolytics

Intravenous Therapy
Supplemental, as needed

Laboratory Studies
ABG analysis
Sputum cultures/Gram stain
Complete blood count

Serologic tests
Sedimentation rate
Electrolytes

Diagnostic Studies
Chest x-ray film

Therapies
Continuous positive airway pressure (CPAP)
Oxygen via cannula

Ultrasonic nebulizer

Nursing Diagnoses

▲ **Outcome Criteria**

The client will exhibit intact, moist oral mucous membranes.

Potential Altered Oral Mucous Membrane related to mouth breathing, frequent expectorations, and decreased fluid intake secondary to malaise

Focus Assessment Criteria	Clinical Significance
1. Overall condition and moisture of the oral cavity and lips	1. These assessment data serve as a baseline for continuous evaluation.
2. Ability to perform oral care	2. The client may need assistance in performing essential oral care.
3. Hydration status	3. Dehydrated oral mucosa is more vulnerable to injury.

Interventions	Rationale
1. Discuss the importance of frequent oral hygiene.	1. Regular oral hygiene removes microorganisms, decreasing the risk of infection.
2. Encourage frequent rinsing of the mouth with water and discourage mouth breathing.	2. Dry oral mucosa causes discomfort and increases the risk of breakdown and infection. Mouth breathing causes loss of oral moisture.
3. Teach the client to avoid mouthwashes containing alcohol and lemon-glycerin swabs.	3. These agents cause drying of mucous membranes.

4. Monitor hydration status:
    a. Oral intake
    b. Parenteral therapy
    c. Intake and output
    d. Urine specific gravity
	4. Proper hydration must be maintained to liquify secretions and prevent drying of oral mucosa.

5. If the mouth or lips are sore, instruct the client to avoid acidic and very hot or cold foods.	5. These foods can irritate oral mucosa.
6. Encourage the client to avoid alcohol and tobacco use.	6. Alcohol and tobacco can irritate oral mucosa.
7. Encourage the client to lubricate the lips every 2 hours or as needed.	7. Proper lip care replaces moisture and reduces cracking.

▲ **Documentation**

Flow record
    Oral assessment
    Oral care
Discharge summary record
    Client teaching

▲ **Outcome Criteria**

The outcome criteria for this diagnosis represent those associated with discharge planning. Refer to the discharge criteria.

Potential Altered Health Maintenance related to lack of knowledge of condition, infection transmission, prevention of recurrence, diet, signs and symptoms of recurrence, and follow-up care

Focus Assessment Criteria	Clinical Significance
1. Readiness and ability to learn and retain information	1. Malaise and other factors may impede the ability to learn. If learning goals are not achieved, a referral may be needed for post-discharge assistance.

Interventions	Rationale
1. Explain the pathophysiology of pneumonia using teaching aids (e.g., illustrations, models) appropriate for the client's or family's educational level.	1. The client's understanding of the disease process and its possible complications may encourage compliance with the therapeutic regimen.
2. Explain measures to prevent the spread of infection:	2. Although pneumococcal pneumonia is not highly communicable, during the acute phase the client should refrain from visiting with persons predisposed to pneumonia, e.g., elderly or seriously ill persons, those with sickle cell disease, postsurgical patients, or persons with chronic respiratory disease.

Interventions

    a. Cover the nose and mouth when sneezing or coughing.

    b. Dispose of used tissues in a paper bag; when the bag is half full, close it securely and place it in a larger disposal unit.

    c. Wash hands frequently.

3. Explain measures to prevent infectious recurrence:

    a. Complete the entire course of prescribed antibiotic therapy and report any side effects.

    b. Keep scheduled follow-up medical appointments.

    c. Continue deep breathing exercises for 6 to 8 weeks during the convalescent period.

    d. Plan rest periods during morning and afternoon.

    e. Obtain influenza and pneumococcal immunizations if the client has a chronic respiratory condition, is elderly, or is immunosuppressed.

4. Encourage adequate hydration, with intake of 300 mL per day if not contraindicated.

5. Encourage adequate, nutritious food intake and use of high-protein supplements, if necessary.

6. Encourage the client to avoid smoking.

7. Instruct the client and family to report any signs or symptoms occurring after initiation of

Rationale

3. A client with pneumonia commonly has an underlying chronic disease; impaired host defenses increase the risk of recurrence.

    a. Because most clients notice a decrease in symptoms after 72 hours of treatment, they sometimes do not recognize the importance of continuing their antibiotic as prescribed. Antibiotics should be continued until completed and a follow-up x-ray film confirms that infection has subsided.

    b. Even though clinical signs may be absent, particularly in older clients, a chest x-ray film is necessary to confirm absence of pneumonia. This also allows further evaluation, as some clients with lung cancer initially present with pneumonia.

    c. Deep breathing increases alveolar expansion and thus facilitates movement of secretions from the tracheobronchial tree with coughing. Routine planned deep breathing and coughing sessions increase vital capacity and pulmonary compliance.

    d. Increased metabolism results from hyperthermia and from the body's defense mechanisms for fighting infection. More energy is expended as the lungs work harder to perfuse the tissues of the body adequately. These factors result in increased physical fatigue.

    e. Because bacterial pneumonia may occur as a complication of influenza, yearly influenza immunization is recommended. The currently used pneumococcal vaccine (Pneumovax) confers a very high rate of immunity, because it contains 23 of the most common pneumococcal organisms. Pneumovax should be administered only on a one-time basis.

4. Insensible fluid losses from hyperthermia and productive cough predispose the client to dehydration, particularly an elderly client.

5. Increased metabolism raises the client's calorie requirements; however, dyspnea and anorexia sometimes prevent adequate caloric intake. High-protein supplements provide increased calories and fluids if anorexia and fatigue from eating interfere with food intake.

6. Chronic smoking destroys the tracheobronchial ciliary action, the lungs' first defense against infection. It also inhibits alveolar macrophage function and irritates the bronchial mucosa.

7. Pneumonia may be resistant to the prescribed antibiotic, or secondary infection with organ-

▲ **Documentation**

Graphic/flow record
 Discharge instructions
 Follow-up instructions
Progress notes
 Status at discharge
 Outcome achievement or status

Interventions

treatment, e.g., thickening of respiratory secretions, return or persistence of fever, increased chest pain, or malaise.

8. Encourage the client to avoid factors that lower resistance to pneumonia—e.g., overexertion, chilling, and excessive alcohol intake—particularly during the convalescent period.

Rationale

isms not susceptible to prescribed antibiotic may have occurred.

8. A client who has had one episode of pneumonia is at increased risk for recurrence. Any upper respiratory infection may lead to bacterial invasion in the lower respiratory tract.

References/Bibliography

Leedom, J.M. et al. (1988). Pneumonia in compromised patients. *Patient Care, 22*(3), 153–165.

Pugliese, G. et al. (1987). Nosocomial bacterial pneumonia: An overview. *American Journal of Infectious Control, 15*(6), 249–265.

Summer, W.R. et al. (1989). Nosocomial pneumonia: Characteristics of the patient interaction. *Respiratory Care, 34*(2), 116–124.

Yannelli, B. et al. (1988). Infection control in critical care . . . Winthrop University hospital infectious disease symposium. *Heart and Lung, 17*(6), 596–600.

Metabolic and Endocrine Disorders

Cirrhosis

A set of changes in liver tissue characterized by the nodular regeneration of parenchymal cells and scar tissue formation, cirrhosis is divided into three types: (1) Laennec's portal cirrhosis, which results from chronic alcohol toxicity and the accompanying malnutrition; (2) postnecrotic cirrhosis, which involves scar tissue resulting from acute viral hepatitis; and (3) biliary cirrhosis, in which scarring results from chronic biliary obstruction. In all types, the fibrosis or scarring interferes with normal liver function and portal blood flow. Impaired portal blood flow causes venous congestion in the spleen and gastrointestinal (GI) tract.

Diagnostic Cluster

▲ Time Frame
Initial diagnosis
Recurrent acute episodes

▲ Discharge Criteria
Before discharge, the client or family will:
1. Describe the causes of cirrhosis
2. Describe activity restrictions and nutritional requirements
3. State actions that reduce anorexia, edema, and pruritus at home
4. State the signs and symptoms that must be reported to a health care professional

Collaborative Problems

Potential Complications: **Refer to:**
Hemorrhage
Hypokalemia
Portal Systemic Encephalopathy
Drug Toxicity (opiates, short-acting barbiturates, major
  tranquilizers)
Renal Failure

Nursing Diagnoses

Altered Nutrition: Less Than Body Requirements, related to anorexia, impaired protein, fat, glucose metabolism and impaired storage of vitamins (A, C, K, D, E)

Pruritus related to accumulation of bilirubin pigment and bile salts

Fluid Volume Excess related to portal hypertension, lowered plasma colloidal osmotic pressure, and sodium retention

Potential Altered Health Maintenance related to lack of knowledge of pharmacological contraindication, nutritional requirements, signs and symptoms of complications, and risks of alcohol ingestion

Pain related to liver enlargement and ascites   Pancreatitis

Diarrhea related to excessive secretion of fats in stool secondary   Pancreatitis
  to liver dysfunction

Potential for Infection related to leukopenia secondary to   Leukemia
  enlarged, overactive spleen and hypoproteinemia

Collaborative Problems

▲ Nursing Goal
The nurse will manage and minimize complications of cirrhosis.

Potential Complication: Hemorrhage
Potential Complication: Hypokalemia
Potential Complication: Portal Systemic Encephalopathy
Potential Complication: Drug Toxicity
Potential Complication: Renal Failure

Interventions

1. Monitor for hemorrhage by assessing the following:
   a. Vital signs
   b. Hematocrit and hemoglobin
   c. Stools, for occult blood
   d. Prothrombin time
2. Teach the client to report unusual bleeding (e.g., in the mouth after brushing teeth) and ecchymotic areas.
3. Monitor for signs and symptoms of hypokalemia:
   a. Low serum potassium levels
   b. Irregular pulse
   c. Nausea and vomiting
   d. Abdominal cramping
   e. Hypoactive bowel sounds
4. Monitor for portal systemic encephalopathy by assessing the following:
   a. General behavior
   b. Orientation to time and place
   c. Speech patterns
   d. Laboratory values: blood pH and ammonia levels
5. Assess for side effects of medications.
6. Avoid administering narcotics, sedatives, and tranquilizers and exposing the client to ammonia products.
7. Monitor for renal failure by assessing the following:
   a. Intake and output
   b. Urine specific gravity
   c. Laboratory values: serum sodium level
8. Monitor for hypertension.

9. Teach the client and family to report signs and symptoms of complications:
   a. Increased abdominal girth

   b. Rapid weight loss or gain

   c. Bleeding

   d. Tremors

   e. Confusion

Rationale

1. Liver dysfunction results in impaired synthesis of clotting factors, which increases the risk of bleeding. Obstructed hepatic blood flow results in dilated vessels prone to hemorrhage, e.g., esophageal varices.

2. Mucous membranes are more prone to injury because of their great surface vascularity.

3. Overproduction of aldosterone causes sodium and water retention and increased potassium excretion.

4. Liver dysfunction results in high serum ammonia levels, possibly leading to hepatic coma.

5,6. Liver dysfunction results in decreased metabolism of certain medications (e.g., opiates, sedatives, tranquilizers), increasing the risk of toxicity from high drug blood levels.
7. Obstructed hepatic blood flow results in decreased blood to the kidneys, impairing glomerular filtration and leading to fluid retention and decreased urinary output.

8. Fluid retention and overload can cause hypertension.
9. Early detection allows prompt intervention to help prevent progression of complications.
   a. Increased abdominal girth may indicate worsening portal hypertension.
   b. Rapid weight loss points to negative nitrogen balance; weight gain, to fluid retention.
   c. Bleeding indicates decreased prothrombin time and clotting factors.
   d. Tremors result from impaired neurotransmission due to failure of the liver to detoxify enzymes that act as false neurotransmitters.
   e. Confusion results from cerebral hypoxia caused by high serum ammonia levels due to the liver's impaired ability to convert ammonia to urea.

▲ **Documentation**

Flow records
    Weight
    Vital signs
    Stools for occult blood
    Abdominal girth
    Urine specific gravity
    Intake and output
Progress notes
    Evidence of bleeding
    Evidence of tremors or confusion

Related Physician-Prescribed Interventions
Medications
    Vitamin/mineral supplement   Vasodilators
    Digestive enzymes   Potassium
    Diuretics
Intravenous Therapy
    Hyperalimentation

Related Physician-Prescribed Interventions (continued)

Laboratory Studies

Serum bilirubin and albumin	BUN
SGOT, SGPT, LDH	Serum ammonia
Alkaline/phosphatase	Serum glucose
Globulins	Electrolytes
CBC	Urine urobilinogen
Prothrombin time	

Diagnostic Studies

Liver scan	Percutaneous transhepatic portography
Liver biopsy	Chest x-ray film
Esophagoscopy	

Therapies

Diet (high-calorie, low-fat, moderate-protein, low-salt)	Oxygen via cannula
	Paracentesis
Fluid restrictions	

Nursing Diagnoses

▲ Outcome Criteria

The client will:

1. Describe the reasons for nutritional problems
2. Relate which foods are high in protein and calories
3. Gain weight (specify amount) without increased edema
4. Explain the rationale for sodium restrictions

Altered Nutrition: Less Than Body Requirements, related to anorexia, impaired protein, fat and glucose metabolism, and impaired storage of vitamins (A, C, K, D, E)

Focus Assessment Criteria	*Clinical Significance*
1. Intake (caloric count, type of food, supplements)	1. Intake must be evaluated because of the effects of cirrhosis on metabolism, vitamin storage, and appetite.
2. Weight (daily)	2. Daily weights are indicated to evaluate nitrogen balance.
3. Abdominal girth (daily)	3. Hepatic congestion causes ascites, which can be evaluated by abdominal girth measurements.
4. Laboratory values: serum albumin and protein levels	4. A decrease in plasma proteins results from decreased hepatic synthesis of plasma proteins.

Interventions	*Rationale*
1. Discuss the causes of anorexia, dyspepsia, and nausea. Explain that obstructed hepatic blood flow causes GI vascular congestion, resulting in gastritis and diarrhea or constipation, and that impaired liver function causes metabolic disturbances (fluid, electrolyte, glucose metabolism), resulting in anorexia and fatigue.	1. Helping the client understand the condition can reduce anxiety and may help improve compliance.
2. Teach and assist the client to rest before meals.	2. Fatigue further decreases the desire to eat.
3. Offer frequent small feedings (six per day plus snacks).	3. Increased intra-abdominal pressure from ascites compresses the GI tract and reduces its capacity.
4. Restrict liquids with meals and avoid fluids 1 hour before and after meals.	4. Fluids can overdistend the stomach, decreasing appetite and intake.
5. Maintain good oral hygiene (brush teeth, rinse mouth) before and after ingestion of food.	5. Accumulation of food particles in the mouth can contribute to foul odors and taste, which diminish appetite.

Interventions

6. Arrange to have foods with the highest protein/calorie content served at the time the client feels most like eating.
7. Teach the client measures to reduce nausea:
   a. If possible, avoid the smell of food preparation, and try eating cold foods, which have less odor.
   b. Loosen clothing when eating.
   c. Sit in fresh air when eating.
   d. Avoid lying down flat for at least 2 hours after eating. (A client who must rest should sit or recline so his head is at least 4 inches higher than his feet.)
8. Limit foods and fluids high in fat.

9. Explain the need to increase intake of foods high in the following elements:
   a. Vitamin B$_{12}$ (eggs, chicken, shellfish)
   b. Folic acid (green leafy vegetables, whole grains, meat)
   c. Thiamine (legumes, beans, oranges)
   d. Iron (organ meats, dried fruit, green vegetables, whole grains)
10. Teach the need to take water-soluble forms of fat-soluble vitamins (A, D, and E).
11. Explain the risks of alcohol ingestion.

12. Consult with the physician if the client does not consume sufficient nutrients.

Rationale

6. This increases the likelihood of the client consuming adequate amounts of protein and calories.
7. Venous congestion in the GI tract predisposes to nausea.

8. Impaired bile flow results in malabsorption of fats.
9. Vitamin intake must be increased to compensate for decreased metabolism and storage of vitamins due to liver tissue damage.

10. Impaired bile flow interferes with absorption of fat-soluble vitamins.
11. Alcohol is toxic to the liver and decreases appetite, contributing to inadequate intake.
12. High-protein supplements, total parenteral nutrition, or tube feedings may be needed.

▲ **Documentation**

Flow records
  Weight
  Intake (type, amount)
  Abdominal girth

▲ **Outcome Criteria**

The client will verbalize decreased pruritus.

Pruritus related to accumulation of bilirubin pigment and bile salts

Focus Assessment Criteria	*Clinical Significance*
1. Skin condition 2. Factors that aggravate or relieve pruritus	1,2. Obstruction of bile flow causes deposition of bile salts in the skin, where they act as an irritant, causing itching.

Interventions

1. Maintain hygiene without causing dry skin:
   a. Give frequent baths, using cool water and mild soap (castile, lanolin) or a soap substitute.
   b. Blot skin dry; do not rub.
2. Prevent excessive warmth by maintaining cool room temperatures and low humidity, using light covers with a bed cradle, and avoiding overdressing.
3. Advise against scratching; explain the scratch–itch–scratch cycle. Instruct the client to apply firm pressure to pruritic areas instead of scratching.
4. Consult with the physician for a pharmacological treatment (e.g., antihistamines, antipruritic lotions), if necessary.

Rationale

1. Dryness increases skin sensitivity.

2. Excessive warmth aggravates pruritus by increasing sensitivity through vasodilation.

3. Scratching stimulates nerve endings, aggravating pruritus.

4. If pruritus is unrelieved or if the skin is excoriated from scratching, topical or systemic medications are indicated.

▲ **Documentation**

Progress notes
  Unrelieved pruritus
  Excoriated skin

▲ **Outcome Criteria**

The client will:

1. Relate actions that decrease fluid retention
2. List foods high in sodium

Fluid Volume Excess related to portal hypertension, lowered plasma colloidal osmotic pressure, and sodium retention

Focus Assessment Criteria	Clinical Significance
1. Diet (sodium and protein content)	1. A diet high in sodium and low in protein can contribute to edema formation.
2. Presence of edema	2. A baseline assessment of edema enables ongoing assessment for changes.

Interventions	Rationale
1. Assess the client's diet for inadequate protein or excessive sodium intake.	1,2. Decreased renal flow results in increased aldosterone and ADH secretion, causing water and sodium retention and potassium excretion.

2. Encourage the client to decrease salt intake. Teach the client to take the following actions:
  a. Read food labels for sodium content
  b. Avoid convenience foods, canned foods, and frozen foods
  c. Cook without salt and use spices (e.g., lemon, basil, tarragon, mint) to add flavor
  d. Use vinegar in place of salt to flavor soups, stews, etc. (e.g., 2–3 teaspoons of vinegar to 4–6 quarts, according to taste)	

3. Ascertain with the physician whether the client may use a salt substitute. Avoid those containing ammonium.	3. Ammonium elevates serum ammonia levels and may contribute to hepatic coma.

4. Take measures to protect edematous skin from injury:
  a. Inspect the skin for redness and blanching.
  b. Reduce pressure on skin, e.g., pad chairs and footstools.
  c. Prevent dry skin by using soap sparingly, rinsing off soap completely, and using a lotion to moisten skin.
	4. Edematous skin is taut and easily injured. Dry skin is more vulnerable to breakdown and injury.

▲ **Documentation**

Progress notes
    Presence of edema

▲ **Outcome Criteria**

The outcome criteria for this diagnosis represent those associated with discharge planning. Refer to the discharge criteria.

Potential Altered Health Maintenance related to lack of knowledge of pharmacological contraindications, nutritional requirements, signs and symptoms of complications, and risks of alcohol ingestion

Focus Assessment Criteria	Clinical Significance
1. Client's or family's readiness and ability to learn and retain information	1. A client or family that does not achieve the goals for learning requires a referral for assistance postdischarge.

Interventions	Rationale
1. Teach the client or family about the condition and its causes and treatments.	1. This teaching reinforces the need to comply with the therapeutic regimen, including diet and activity restrictions.
2. Explain portal system encephalopathy to the family. Teach them to observe for and report any confusion, tremors, night wandering, or personality changes.	2. The development of encephalopathy typically is first noted by family members.
3. Explain the need for adequate rest and avoidance of strenuous activity.	3. As the liver repairs itself, physical activity depletes the body of the energy needed for healing. Adequate rest is needed to prevent relapse.

Interventions

4. Explain the need for diet high in protein and calories and low in salt. (Refer to the nursing diagnosis Altered Nutrition on page 112 for specific interventions.)
5. Explain the hazards of certain medications, including narcotics, sedatives, tranquilizers, and ammonia products.
6. Teach the client or family to watch for and report signs and symptoms of complications:

    a. Bleeding (gums, stools)

    b. Hypokalemia (muscle cramps, nausea, vomiting)

    c. Confusion, altered speech patterns

    d. Increasing severity of symptoms

    e. Rapid weight loss or gain

7. Explain the need to avoid alcohol.

8. Stress the importance of follow-up care and laboratory studies.

Rationale

4. Protein and caloric requirements are greater when tissue is healing.

5. Certain drugs are hepatoxic. Impaired liver function slows metabolism of some drugs, causing levels to accumulate.
6. Progressive liver failure affects hematopoietic function and electrolyte and fluid balance, causing potentially serious complications that require prompt intervention.

    a. Bleeding indicates decreased prothrombin time and clotting factors.
    b. Hypokalemia results from overproduction of aldosterone, which causes sodium and water retention and potassium excretion.
    c. Confusion and altered speech patterns result from cerebral hypoxia due to high serum ammonia levels caused by the liver's impaired ability to convert ammonia to urea.
    d. Exacerbation of symptoms indicates progressive liver damage.
    e. Rapid weight loss points to negative nitrogen balance; weight gain, to fluid retention.

7. Alcohol increases hepatic irritation and may interfere with recovery.
8. Timely follow-up enables evaluation of liver function and early detection of relapse or recurrence.

▲ **Documentation**

Flow records
    Client teaching
    Referrals when indicated
Progress notes
    Unachieved outcomes

References/Bibliography

Anderson, E.D. (1986). The cirrhotic process in the alcoholic. *Critical Care Quarterly, 8*(4), 74–78.
Fredette, S.L. (1984). When the liver fails. *American Journal of Nursing, 84*(1), 64–67.
Hall, P. (1985). *Alcoholic liver disease.* New York: John Wiley & Sons.
Schiff, L., & Schiff, E.R. (1987). *Diseases of the liver* (6th ed). Philadelphia: J.B. Lippincott.

Diabetes Mellitus

Diabetes mellitus is a syndrome characterized by hyperglycemia. The American Diabetes Association (ADA) classifies diabetes as Type I (insulin-dependent/juvenile onset), Type II (noninsulin-dependent/adult onset), and other types (gestational diabetes, impaired glucose tolerance, and secondary diabetes). Although the etiology, clinical course, and treatments differ among types, the common denominator is hyperglycemia. Between 5% and 10% of clients with diabetes have Type I, which requires insulin injections. Type II, which may result from a decrease in insulin production or an insensitivity of cells to insulin, accounts for 90% to 95% of cases.

Diagnostic Cluster

▲ Discharge Criteria

Before discharge, the client or family will:

1. Define diabetes as a chronic disease requiring a lifelong treatment regimen of diet, exercise, and, in some cases, medication
2. State the causes, signs and symptoms, and treatment of hypoglycemia and hyperglycemia
3. Demonstrate the procedure for blood glucose self-monitoring
4. State the type, dosage, duration of action, and potential side effects of the insulin that the client requires, if applicable
5. Demonstrate the proper technique for drawing up and administering insulin, if applicable
6. State the caloric level of the prescribed meal plan and the percentages of carbohydrates, protein, and fat
7. State the relationship of exercise to weight control, insulin activity, and blood glucose level
8. Explain the importance of proper foot care for diabetics
9. Describe self-care measures during illness, including the need to increase the frequency of blood glucose monitoring
10. Describe four potential complications of diabetes and four factors that may increase the risk of complications
11. State a plan for blood glucose monitoring at home
12. State an intent to wear diabetes identification at all times
13. List three community resources available for diabetics

Collaborative Problems

Potential Complications:
Ketoacidosis (DKA)
Hyperosmolar, Hyperglycemic, Nonketotic (HHNK) Coma
Hypoglycemia
Infections
Vascular Problems
Neuropathy
Retinopathy
Nephropathy

Nursing Diagnoses

Fear (client, family) related to diagnosis of diabetes, potential complications of diabetes, insulin injection, negative effect on life style

Potential Ineffective Coping (client, family) related to chronic disease, complex self-care regimen, and uncertain future

Altered Nutrition: More Than Body Requirements related to intake in excess of activity expenditures, lack of knowledge, and ineffective coping

Potential for Injury related to decreased tactile sensation, diminished visual acuity, and hypoglycemia

Potential Altered Sexuality Patterns (male) related to erectile problems secondary to peripheral neuropathy or psychological conflicts

Potential Sexual Dysfunction (female) related to frequent genitourinary problems, physical and psychological stressors of diabetes

Powerlessness related to the future development of complications of diabetes (blindness, amputations, kidney failure, painful neuropathy)

Potential Noncompliance related to complexity and chronicity of prescribed regimen

Potential Altered Health Maintenance related to insufficient knowledge of condition, self-monitoring of blood glucose, medications, ADA exchange diet, treatment of hypoglycemia, weight control, sick day care, exercise program, foot care, signs and symptoms of complications, and community resources

Collaborative Problems

▲ **Nursing Goals**

The nurse will manage and mini-mize:
Abnormal blood sugar episodes
Vascular complications

Potential Complication: Diabetic Ketoacidosis (DKA)
Potential Complication: Hyperosmolar Hyperglycemia Nonketotic (HHNK) Coma
Potential Complication: Hypoglycemia
Potential Complication: Infections
Potential Complication: Vascular Problems
Potential Complication: Neuropathy
Potential Complication: Retinopathy
Potential Complication: Nephropathy

Interventions

1. Monitor for signs and symptoms of ketoaci-dosis:
   a. Blood glucose > 300 mg/dL
   b. Positive plasma ketone, acetone breath
   c. Headache
   d. Kussmaul's respirations
   e. Anorexia, nausea, vomiting
   f. Polyuria, polydipsia
   g. Decreased serum sodium, potassium, phos-phates
   h. Dehydration, masked by dry mucous mem-branes, poor skin turgor

2. Monitor for signs and symptoms of hyperos-molar, hyperglycemic, nonketotic (HHNK) coma:
   a. Blood glucose 600–2000 mg/dL
   b. Serum sodium normal or elevated
   c. Serum potassium normal or elevated
   d. Serum osmolality > 350 mOsm/kg
   e. Hypotension
   f. Dehydration
   g. Altered sensorium

3. Monitor cardiac function and circulatory sta-tus:
   a. Rate, rhythm
   b. Skin color
   c. Capillary refill
   d. Peripheral pulses
   e. Serum potassium

4. Monitor for signs and symptoms of hypoglyce-mia:
   a. Blood glucose < 70 mg/dL
   b. Pale, moist, cool skin
   c. Tachycardia, diaphoresis
   d. Jitteriness, irritability
   e. Headache, slurred speech
   f. Incoordination
   g. Drowsiness
   h. Visual changes
   i. Hunger, nausea, abdominal pain

5. Monitor for signs and symptoms of infection:
   a. Red, painful, warm skin
   b. Furunculosis
   c. Carbuncles
   d. Upper respiratory tract infection (URTI)
   e. Urinary tract infection (UTI)
   f. External otitis

Rationale

1. When insulin is not available, blood glucose levels rise and the body metabolizes fat and protein for energy-producing ketone bodies. Excessive level of ketone bodies causes head-aches, nausea, vomiting, and abdominal pain. Respiratory rate and depth increase in order to increase CO_2 excretion and reduce acidosis. Glucose inhibits water reabsorption in the renal glomerulus, leading to osmotic diuresis with loss of water, sodium, potassium, and phosphates.

2. HHNK coma is a state of excessive hypergly-cemia precipitated by chronic disease and in-fections. HHNK coma occurs in Type II insu-lin-resistant diabetics who are markedly dehydrated. Ketones usually are not present. Glucose inhibits water reabsorption in the renal glomerulus, leading to osmotic diuresis with loss of water, sodium, potassium, and phosphates. Cerebral impairment is due to in-tracellular dehydration in the brain.

3. Severe dehydration can cause reduced cardiac output and compensatory vasoconstriction. Cardiac dysrhythmias can result from potas-sium imbalances.

4. Hypoglycemia (insufficient glucose levels) can be caused by too much insulin, too little food, or excessive physical activity. When blood glucose falls rapidly, the sympathetic system is stimulated to produce adrenaline, which causes diaphoresis, cool skin, tachycardia, and jitteriness. When blood glucose falls slowly, the central nervous system is depressed, caus-ing headache, slurred speech, incoordination, drowsiness, and visual changes. Lack of avail-able glucose can cause hunger and gastroin-testinal distress.

5. The rapid diagnosis and treatment of infection in a patient with diabetes is necessary, because infection is a leading cause of metabolic ab-normalities leading to diabetic coma.

Interventions

6. Monitor for signs and symptoms of macrovascular complications and assess for risk factors for cardiovascular complications:
   a. Family history of heart disease
   b. Male over age 40
   c. Cigarette smoking
   d. Hypertension
   e. Hyperlipidemia
   f. Obesity
   g. Uncontrolled diabetes
7. Monitor for signs and symptoms of retinopathy:
   a. Blurred vision
   b. Black spots
   c. "Cobwebs"
   d. Sudden loss of vision

8. Teach the client to have an annual ophthalmological examination.

9. Monitor for signs and symptoms:
   a. Peripheral neuropathy
      • Pain
      • Decreased sensation
      • Decreased deep tendon response (Achilles, patella)
      • Decreased vibratory sense
      • Charcot's foot ulcer
      • Decreased proprioception
      • Paresthesia
   b. Automatic neuropathy
      • Orthostatic hypotension
      • Impotence
      • Abnormal sweating
      • Bladder paralysis
      • Nocturnal diarrhea
      • Gastroparesis
10. Monitor for signs and symptoms of nephropathy
    a. Hypertension
    b. Proteinuria, bacteriuria, casts
    c. Elevated WBC count
    d. RBC in urine
    e. Fever
    f. Flank pain
    g. Chills
    h. Stress incontinence
    i. Blood urea nitrogen (BUN) and creatinine
11. Monitor for proteinuria:
    a. Consult with physician for a 24-hour urine test.

Rationale

6. Diabetes is often associated with severe degenerative vascular changes. Lesions of the blood vessels not only strike diabetics at an earlier age than nondiabetics but also tend to produce more severe pathological changes. Early atherosclerotic changes are probably caused by high blood glucose and high lipid levels that are characteristic of persistent hyperglycemia. Atherosclerosis in turn leads to premature cardiac artery disease.
7. Diabetic retinopathy does not cause visual symptoms until a fairly advanced stage has been reached—usually macular edema or proliferative retinopathy. Five thousand new cases of blindness related to diabetes occur yearly in the United States. Incidence and severity of retinopathy is thought to be related to the duration and the degree of control of diabetes.
8. Early detection of diabetic retinopathy can enable timely laser treatments to shrink abnormal vessels.
9. Among the most common and perplexing complications of diabetes, neuropathy can be one of the earliest complications to develop and may even be present upon diagnosis. Sensory symptoms usually predominate and include numbness, tingling, and pain or loss of sensation. Current treatments include improved control of blood glucose and use of antidepressant drugs.

10. In diabetic nephropathy, the capillary basement membrane thickens owing to chronic filtering of high glucose blood. The membrane also becomes more permeable, causing increased loss of blood proteins in urine. These increased filtration requirements increase the pressure in renal blood vessels, contributing to sclerosis.

11. Clinical manifestations of diabetic nephropathy typically do not occur until late in the disease. Proteinuria is often the first sign of the disorder. A 24-hour urine test is much more sensitive than a urinalysis to the presence of microalbumin. The 24-hour urine test measures values below 550 mg/dL, whereas a urinalysis only measures albumin above 550 mg/dL. Therefore, decreased kidney function is identified sooner, and more aggressive ther-

Interventions

Rationale

▲ *Documentation*

Flow records
  Vital signs
  Urine specific gravity
  Blood glucose level
Progress notes
  Signs of infection or injury
  Changes in sensation
  Other client complaints
  Abnormal laboratory values

12. Instruct the client on the importance of controlling hypertension.

13. Teach the client about the risk factors that may precipitate renal damage:
  a. Hypertension
  b. Neurogenic bladder
  c. Urethral instrumentation
  d. Urinary tract infection
  e. Nephrotoxic drugs

apy may be initiated if the 24-hour urine collection is part of the management plan.
12. Blood pressure control is the most important therapy to prevent or ameliorate renal damage.
13. Making the client aware of risk factors can help reduce their occurrence and reduce renal impairment.

Related Physician-Prescribed Interventions

Medications
  Oral antidiabetic agents   Insulin

Intravenous Therapy
  Not indicated

Laboratory Studies
  Serum glucose   Serum osmolality
  Plasma acetone   Electrolytes
  Free fatty acids   Glucose tolerance test

Diagnostic Studies
  Not indicated unless complications are suspected,
    e.g., renal insufficiency, retinopathy

Therapies
  ADA diet

Nursing Diagnoses

▲ *Outcome Criteria*

The client will:
1. Effectively communicate feelings regarding the diagnosis of diabetes
2. Identify two methods to achieve psychological equilibrium

Fear (individual, family) related to diagnosis of diabetes, potential complications of diabetes, insulin injection, or negative effects on life style

Focus Assessment Criteria

1. Client's level of anxiety:
  a. Mild anxiety
    • Broad perceptual field
    • Absence of facial and muscle tension
    • Feelings of safety
    • Intact learning ability
  b. Moderate anxiety
    • Narrowed perceptual field
    • Intact problem-solving ability
    • Increased respiratory and heart rates, shakiness
  c. Severe anxiety
    • Distorted sense of time
    • Survival response
    • Inattentiveness
    • Greatly reduced perception
    • Hyperventilation, headaches, dizziness
  d. Panic anxiety
    • Inability to learn
    • Distorted perception
    • Lapses in recall of thoughts
    • Impaired communication
    • Vomiting
    • Possibly violent behavior

Clinical Significance

1. Anxiety varies in intensity depending on how the client perceives the severity of the threat and on the success or failure of his efforts to cope with his feelings.

Focus Assessment Criteria	*Clinical Significance*
2. Client's stressors 3. Client's past experiences related to diabetes 4. Client's specific concerns or fears	2–4. A client with diabetes typically is justifiably afraid of many things, such as pain, complications, and dependency. The client may be able to express some of these fears and not others, or may express some fears indirectly.
5. Available support systems	5. Additional support is needed; sources can be family, friends, and health care professionals.

Interventions	*Rationale*

1. Assist the client in reducing anxiety:
  a. Provide reassurance and comfort.
  b. Stay with the client during periods of high anxiety.
  c. Identify and support effective coping mechanisms.
  d. Always speak to the client in a calm and soothing voice.
  e. Convey a sense of understanding and empathy.
  f. Encourage the client to verbalize any fears or concerns.
	1. An anxious client has a narrowed perceptual field and impaired ability to learn. The client may experience symptoms caused by increased muscle tension. Diminished ability to sleep restfully may cause the client to overreact to stressful situations. Anxiety tends to feed on itself, catching the client in a widening spiral of anxiety, tension, and emotional and physical pain.

2. Provide current, accurate information on the disease process and self-care measures.	2. Some fears are based on inaccurate information and thus can be relieved by providing accurate information.
3. Encourage family and friends to verbalize their fears and concerns to staff. Involve them in teaching sessions.	3. A client who feels well supported in life is able to cope more effectively with stressful situations. A diabetic client in particular needs support from health care professionals, peers, and family. Lack of support increases anxiety and fear.
4. Provide valid reassurance and reinforce positive behavior.	4. Emphasizing successes may promote effective coping.
5. Encourage the client to practice relaxation techniques.	5. Relaxation gives the client a sense of control over his body's response to stress.

▲ **Documentation**

Progress notes
  Present emotional status
  Response to nursing actions
  Participation in self-care

▲ **Outcome Criteria**

The client will:
1. Verbalize feelings about diabetes
2. Describe situations that cause stress
3. List several methods of stress reduction
4. Identify appropriate resources

Potential Ineffective Coping (client, family) related to chronic disease, complex self-care regimens and uncertain future

Focus Assessment Criteria	*Clinical Significance*

1. Life event changes
2. Emotional resources
  a. Intimacy
  b. Social integration
  c. Ability to solve problems and make decisions
  d. Values and beliefs
  e. Goals, hopes, and desires
3. External resources
  a. Peers and friends
  b. Family
  c. Financial situation
  d. Education
  e. Work
4. Life style (effects on or changes in)
5. Communication skills
	1–5. Chronic disease invariably affects the emotional composition of the client and all those with whom he intimately interacts. Emotional stress is a significant factor in impairment of metabolic homeostasis. A thorough psychosocial assessment is the first step in developing an individualized and effective care plan.

Interventions

1. Explore with the client and significant others (together and in separate sessions) the actual or perceived effects of the disease on the following:
   a. Finances
   b. Occupation (sick time)
   c. Time, life style
   d. Energy
   e. Relationships
   f. Control
2. Assist the client and significant others in identifying previous coping strategies that proved successful.

3. Encourage the client to participate in his plan of care.

4. Encourage the client to discuss plans to incorporate diabetes into his life style.

5. Encourage strong family support.

6. Provide an environment in which the client can function independently to some degree without assistance.
7. Encourage the client to join support groups.

8. Advise the client to subscribe to journals about diabetes (e.g., *Diabetes Forecast, Diabetes Self-Management*) and give the client a list of resources including organizations, current books, and suppliers of diabetic products.

Rationale

1. Common frustrations associated with diabetes stem from problems involving the disease itself, the treatment regimen, and the health care system. Recognizing that these problems are common indicates a need to use the technique of anticipatory guidance to prevent the associated frustrations.

2. Coping methods vary and often are related to the client's perception of a stressful situation. Some avoid the situation; others confront it, seek more information, or rely on religious beliefs or other coping mechanisms for support.
3. The client's participation in self-care and planning indicates attempts to cope positively with the situation.
4. Evidence that the client will pursue his goals and maintain his life style reflects positive adjustment and adequate self-esteem.
5. Family support often is a significant contributing factor to a client's acceptance of diabetes.
6. Self-care reduces feelings of dependency and loss of control.

7. Sharing with persons in a similar situation can provide opportunities for mutual support and problem-solving.
8. Clients vary greatly in the resources they have available. Making use of available resources improves the client's ability to cope with the disorder.

▲ **Documentation**

Progress notes
   Interactions
   Participation in self-care
   Referrals

▲ **Outcome Criteria**

The client will:

1. State an intent to follow a prescribed diet in which caloric intake is sufficient to decrease or maintain weight
2. Verbalize the value of decreasing weight related to control of blood glucose

Altered Nutrition: More than Body Requirements related to intake in excess of activity expenditures, lack of knowledge, or ineffective coping

Focus Assessment Criteria

1. Height, weight, age, sex
2. Occupation, educational level, economic level, cultural heritage
3. Nutritional history and current meal plan
4. History of weight loss or weight gain
5. Social history:
   a. Resistance associated with obesity
   b. Person responsible for shopping
   c. Cooking facilities at home
   d. Meals eaten away from home
   e. Person who prepares meals at home
   f. Whether the client lives alone or eats alone
   g. Available support systems
6. Exercise regimen:
   a. Frequency
   b. Type of exercise
   c. Employment activity
7. A 3- to 5-day food intake diary

Clinical Significance

1–11. The primary goal in diabetic management is weight reduction and achievement of ideal body weight. Weight loss alone may improve the abnormalities of glucose intolerance, insulin secretion, and insulin use. Moderate weight loss (20 to 40 lb) often produces a major and persistent reduction in blood glucose level. The client's experiences, beliefs, and activities have a profound influence on eating behaviors and exercise. Only through behavior modification can the client achieve long-term success in weight maintenance. Without significant alterations in life style, resumption of previous eating habits and return of obesity almost invariably occur.

▲ Documentation

Flow records
　Height and weight
Progress notes
　Nutritional history
　Written contract stating spe-
　　cific goals and rewards
　Graphs showing weight loss
　　or gain

Focus Assessment Criteria

8. Emotional connotation of food to the client
9. Client's motivation to follow the prescribed meal plan
10. Client's attitudes, beliefs, and behaviors related to eating and exercise
11. Laboratory study results: blood glucose, glycosylated hemoglobin levels

Clinical Significance

Interventions

1. Refer to the Obesity care plan for specific interventions and rationales.

▲ Outcome Criteria

The client will:

1. Verbalize three risks that may cause injury related to decreased tactile sensation and diminished vision
2. State the relationship of injury to hypoglycemia
3. Identify three methods of coping with diminished tactile sensation and vision

Potential for Injury related to decreased tactile sensation, diminished visual acuity, and hypoglycemia

Focus Assessment Criteria

1. Visual acuity and position sense
2. Ability to differentiate objects through tactile stimulation
3. Ability to perform activities of daily living (home and work)
4. Judgment
5. History of falls or injuries, or fear of falling
6. Use of assistive devices
7. Onset, severity, and frequency of hypoglycemia
8. Client's knowledge of "hypoglycemia unawareness"

Clinical Significance

1–6. Visually handicapped clients differ from one another as much as members of any group. The potential for injury may be nonexistent in one client but a major problem for another. An individualized assessment can identify the client's specific needs.

7,8. The sudden onset of hypoglycemia or low blood glucose may cause injury. A diabetic client known to have "hypoglycemic unawareness" is at increased risk of injury owing to a defect in the body's defense system that impairs the ability to feel the usual warning symptoms associated with hypoglycemia, e.g., hunger, weakness, tingling, and dizziness. Such a client may progress from alertness to unconsciousness very rapidly.

▲ Documentation

Discharge summary record
　Client teaching
　Status of outcome achieve-
　　ment

Interventions

1. Advise the client to monitor blood glucose level closely.

2. Teach the client's significant other(s) to prepare and administer glucagon.

3. Refer to the nursing diagnosis Potential Altered Health Maintenance for additional teaching points.

Rationale

1. Careful monitoring of blood glucose level can detect a change before it results in serious hypoglycemia.
2. Glucagon can be administered in a severe case of hypoglycemia to raise the blood glucose level quickly.

▲ Outcome Criteria

The client will:

1. Discuss his present sexual patterns
2. Describe available community resources

Potential Altered Sexuality Patterns (male) related to erectile problems secondary to peripheral neuropathy or psychological conflicts

Focus Assessment Criteria

1. Sexual activity:
   a. Frequency
   b. Satisfaction
   c. Libido
   d. Erectile problems

Clinical Significance

1,2,3. Assessment of sexual activity and relationships enables the nurse to initiate discussions of possible sexual concerns and problems.

Focus Assessment Criteria	*Clinical Significance*
2. Relationship with partner(s)	
3. Cultural influences	
4. Conflicts (e.g., in values, body image, self-esteem)	4,5. Psychogenic impotence is characterized by abrupt onset, occurrence of nocturnal emissions, and preserved capacity for masturbation. The client's knowledge of the high incidence of impotence in diabetes may trigger psychogenic impotence.
5. Emotional status (e.g., anxious, depressed, irritable)	
6. Use of prescribed medications, other drugs, and alcohol	6. Drugs must be assessed as a cause of impotence. Most commonly identified drugs are antihypertensives, antidepressants, and phenothiazines. Alcohol use may cause impotence by impairing neural reflexes.
7. Presence of peripheral neuropathy	7. Neuropathy may cause impotence.

Interventions	*Rationale*
1. Discuss the common effects of diabetes on male sexuality. Explain that sexual dysfunction is a complex problem that may result from physiological or psychological difficulties. Diabetics are more prone to sexual dysfunction because the disease damages the nervous and circulatory system and also has an impact on the psyche.	1. Explaining the causes can help the client differentiate between physiological and psychogenic impotence and may help him overcome the problem.
2. Clearly convey that you are willing to discuss the client's feelings and concerns; project an attitude of concern and empathy.	2. Open, honest dialogue can reduce the client's embarrassment and his reluctance to share his fears and concerns.
3. If the client is physiologically unable to sustain an erection sufficient for intercourse, discuss the possible use of penile prostheses.	3. Penile implants provide the erection needed for intercourse without altering sensations or the ability to ejaculate.
4. Reaffirm the need for closeness and expressions of caring; involve the client's partner in touching and other means of sexual expression.	4. Sexual pleasure and gratification are not limited to intercourse. Other expressions of sexuality and caring may prove even more meaningful and gratifying.
5. If necessary, refer the client to a sexual therapist or mental health counselor for information, evaluation, or treatment of sexual problems.	5. The client may need specialized evaluation and treatment.

▲ **Documentation**

Progress notes
 Assessment data
 Interactions
 Referrals

▲ **Outcome Criteria**

The client will:
1. Express feelings about her sexual patterns
2. Relate an intent to share her feelings with her partner

Potential Sexual Dysfunction (female) related to frequent genitourinary problems and physical and psychological stressors associated with diabetes

Focus Assessment Criteria	*Clinical Significance*

1. Sexual patterns
  a. Libido
  b. Satisfaction with sex role
  c. Frequency of activity
  d. Discomfort during intercourse
	1. Assessment of sexual patterns and satisfaction enables the nurse to initiate discussions of the client's sexual problems or concerns.

2. Relationship with partner(s)	2–6. Diabetes, like any chronic disease, affects a client's life physically, emotionally, and financially, which can in turn negatively affect sexual function. Diabetes also has a genetic component, which may affect sexuality and family planning decisions.
3. Conflicts (e.g., in values, body image, self-esteem)	

Focus Assessment Criteria	Clinical Significance
4. Emotional status (e.g., anxious, depressed, irritable) 5. Pregnancy and contraception history 6. Cultural influences	

Interventions	Rationale
1. Discuss the effects of diabetes on female sexuality. Explain that poor control of blood glucose seems to be the major contributing factor to decreased sexual satisfaction.	1. Helping the client understand the causes of sexual dysfunction may reduce her guilt and anxiety.
2. Encourage the client to verbalize her concerns; listen attentively with a nonjudgmental attitude.	2. This can help reduce the client's embarrassment and reluctance to share concerns.
3. Explain the importance of planned pregnancies.	3. Family planning is essential for the diabetic woman. Research has shown that tight control of blood glucose before conception and throughout pregnancy helps ensure a positive outcome.

4. Teach the client measures to prevent perineal irritation, vaginitis, and urinary tract infection (UTI).
  a. Maintain good hygiene.
  b. Wear only cotton panties or those with a cotton crotch.
  c. Avoid tight jeans.
  d. Use only a water-soluble vaginal lubricant.
  e. Maintain a high fluid intake.
	4. Vaginitis and UTI occur more often in diabetic women than in nondiabetic women. Elevated blood glucose levels enhance bacterial growth in the vagina and urinary tract.

5. Encourage regular physical exercise—at least 3 times a week for 30 minutes each session.	5. Regular exercise can promote a sense of well-being and positively affect self-esteem, which may enhance the client's sense of sexuality.
6. If necessary, refer the client to a sexual therapist or mental health counselor for information, evaluation, or treatment of sexual problems.	6. The client may need specialized evaluation and treatment.

▲ **Documentation**

Progress notes
  Assessment data
  Interactions
  Referrals

▲ **Outcome Criteria**

The client will:
1. Identify risk factors for complications that can be controlled
2. Participate in decisions regarding care

Powerlessness related to the future development of complications of diabetes, e.g., blindness, amputations, kidney failure, and neuropathy

Focus Assessment Criteria	Clinical Significance
1. Client's understanding of the disease process 2. Client's perception of control 3. Perceived effects on life style	1–3. Assessing these factors provides information on the client's response to loss of control, perception of the loss, individual coping patterns, personal characteristics, and response to others.

Interventions	Rationale

1. Explore the client's perception of the effects of diabetes on the following:
  a. Occupation
  b. Role responsibilities
  c. Relationships
	1. As a chronic disease commonly causing serious complications or premature death and requiring a complex lifelong therapeutic regimen, diabetes commonly triggers feelings of vulnerability and lack of control and affects the client's life style, personality, and overall emotional well-being.

2. Determine the client's usual response to problems.	2. Discussions help to determine whether the client usually seeks to change his own behaviors to control problems or expects others or external factors to control problems.

Interventions

3. Assist the client in identifying his strengths and assets.
4. Help the client identify usual energy patterns and discuss the need to schedule activities around these patterns. With the client, identify those activities that are personally important and schedule them when energy normally is high.
5. Advise the client to participate in a regular exercise program.
6. Stress the value of sharing feelings with family and friends.
7. Help the client seek support from other sources, e.g., self-help groups, support groups.

Rationale

3. The client may need assistance to discourage focusing only on personal limitations.
4. Identifying when certain activities are best performed may allow their continuation. This can help promote feelings of self-worth and dignity.

5. Regular exercise improves carbohydrate metabolism and enhances feelings of well-being.
6. Open, honest dialogue may help enlist the support of others.
7. Opportunities to share feelings, experiences, and problem-solving strategies with others in a similar situation can be very useful.

▲ *Documentation*

Progress notes
    Participation in self-care and decisions
    Emotional status
    Interactions

▲ *Outcome Criteria*

The client will:

1. State the risks and benefits of following the prescribed treatment regimen
2. Enter into a contract with the health care provider to set mutual goals for a treatment regimen

Potential Noncompliance related to the complexity and chronicity of the prescribed therapeutic regimen

Focus Assessment Criteria

1. Health care beliefs related to diabetes:
   a. Susceptibility
   b. Consequences
   c. Value of treatment
   d. Risks and benefits of treatment
2. Current coping mechanisms
3. Quality of support systems and of the social and economic environment
4. Knowledge of the disease process and self-care skills
5. Failure to progress, persistence of symptoms, or exacerbation of symptoms
6. Laboratory test results pointing to probable noncompliance with the therapeutic regimen
7. Avoidance of teaching and learning situations
8. Statements indicating unacceptability of the therapeutic regimen, side effects, or health care providers

Clinical Significance

1–8. Diabetes is a complex illness requiring major adaptations—both psychological and physiological—for effective management. The success of the therapeutic regimen depends largely on the client's lifelong commitment to daily self-management.

Interventions

1. Identify and correct any misconceptions the client has regarding diabetes and its management.
2. Teach the client the necessary information using the teaching strategies of selectivity, brevity, and written reinforcement.
3. Identify specific discrete goals within the therapeutic regimen that the client can strive for and realistically achieve.
4. Encourage the client to enter into a contract to accomplish a mutual goal.
5. Provide incentives to encourage compliant behavior and future life challenges.

Rationale

1. The client's beliefs about health, diabetes, and its treatment strongly influence the likelihood of his compliance with the therapeutic regimen.
2. These strategies enhance teaching and learning and may help improve compliance.
3. Advising the client to take small steps toward a large goal may be the most effective strategy for improving compliance.
4. Contracting—a written agreement between two people—has been used successfully in health care to increase client compliance.
5. This encourages the client to determine his own goals and rewards, which may help improve compliance.

Interventions

6. Assist the client by identifying and coordinating life style modifications that require additional resources. Whenever possible, alter the therapeutic regimen to fit the client's individual circumstances. Areas of modification commonly include the following:
   a. Diet
   b. Medications, including insulin delivery systems
   c. Exercise

Rationale

6. This strategy teaches skills of self-management for future life challenges. The greater the modification of the client's life style, the inconvenience, and the cost, the lower the likelihood of his compliance with the prescribed regimen.

▲ **Documentation**

Discharge summary record
   Client teaching
Progress notes
   Interactions

▲ **Outcome Criteria**

The outcome criteria for this diagnosis represent those associated with discharge planning. Refer to the discharge criteria.

Potential Altered Health Maintenance related to insufficient knowledge of condition, self-monitoring of blood glucose, medications, ADA exchange diet, treatment of hypoglycemia, weight control, sick day care, exercise program, foot care, signs and symptoms of complications, and community resources

Focus Assessment Criteria

1. Current knowledge and home management of diabetes
2. Contributing factors:
   a. Anxiety
   b. New diagnosis
   c. Lack of previous instruction
3. Community, family, and economic resources
4. Attitudes, feelings, and concerns related to diabetes
5. Readiness and ability to learn
6. Dexterity, vision

Clinical Significance

1–5. These assessment criteria help identify factors that may interfere with learning. A client or family that does not achieve goals for learning requires a referral for assistance postdischarge.

6. The management of diabetes mellitus requires dexterity to perform insulin injections, when indicated, and good vision to perform foot inspections and blood glucose monitoring. A client with any limitations in these areas may need assistance.

Interventions

1. Instruct the client and family on the etiology of diabetes and on the triad of diabetes treatment: diet, exercise, and medications.
2. Explain the potential complications of diabetes:
   a. Chronic
      • Coronary artery disease (CAD)
      • Peripheral vascular disease (PVD)
      • Retinopathy
      • Neuropathy
      • Nephropathy
      • Ulcers
      • Amputations
   b. Acute
      • Hypoglycemia
      • Diabetic ketoacidosis (DKA)
      • Hyperglycemic, hyperosmolar, nonketotic coma (HHNK)
3. Teach the signs and symptoms of hyperglycemia:
   a. Polyuria
   b. Polydipsia

Rationale

1. This teaching can encourage compliance and preparation for self-care.

2. Explaining possible complications can stress the importance of compliance and regular check-ups, e.g., eye examinations

3. Elevated blood glucose causes severe dehydration due to osmotic diuresis. Serum potassium is elevated because of hemoconcentration. Because carbohydrates are not metabolized, the

Interventions

    c. Polyphasia
    d. Fatigue
    e. Blurred vision
    f. Weight loss
4. Teach the possible causes of hyperglycemia:
    a. Increased food intake
    b. Decreased insulin
    c. Decreased exercise
    d. Infection
    e. Poor absorption of insulin
5. Teach about the Somogyi phenomenon (rebound hyperglycemia) and how to prevent it.

6. Discuss the need to monitor blood glucose versus urine glucose. Explain the following:
    a. Urine glucose levels depend on the renal threshold (180–300 mg/dL)
    b. Negative urine glucose does not indicate normal blood glucose; glucose "spills" into urine at a minimum of 180 mg/dL.
    c. There is a poor correlation between urine glucose levels and blood glucose levels.
    d. Urine glucose cannot warn of impending hypoglycemia.
    e. Blood glucose gives immediate, accurate results, enabling timely adjustment of food, exercise, and insulin.
7. Recommend a specific product for self-monitoring of blood glucose (SMBG), based on the client's motivation, physical ability, and financial resources.
8. Provide initial and follow-up assistance to help the client master the SMBG procedure.
9. If the client desires to purchase a SMBG device:
    a. Assist client to obtain third-party reimbursement for SMBG supplies.
    b. Share a resource list of distributors of SMBG products.
    c. Provide literature on the rationale and procedure for SMBG.
    d. As a cost-saving measure, recommend that strips be cut in half lengthwise for visual interpretation.
10. Teach the client to record all SMBG results in a log book.

11. Explain the need to increase the frequency of testing when sick, when a meal is delayed, and before strenuous exercise.
12. Assist the client to identify the name, dosage, action, and side effects of prescribed insulin.

Rationale

client remains hungry and loses weight despite intake.

4. Increased food intake requires an increase in insulin or an increase in exercise; otherwise hyperglycemia will ensue. Infection increases insulin requirements. Insufficient or poorly absorbed insulin results in hyperglycemia.

5. Caused by excessive administration of insulin to treat the hyperglycemic episode, rebound hyperglycemia involves the release of glucocorticoids and catecholamines as a hormonal response to hypoglycemia. This release promotes gluconeogenesis and glycogenesis, which in turn lead to hyperglycemia (rebound).
6. Because urine testing is noninvasive and inexpensive, the client may need incentives to perform SMBG. SMBG has made euglycemia a realistic goal for some diabetics. Although not a panacea, SMBG has begun the trend toward "tight control"—particularly for an intelligent, highly motivated client who desires optimal control and leads an active life style. Research has shown an improvement in blood glucose control as a direct result of SMBG and a direct association between blood glucose control and the frequency of testing.

7. All SMBG testing devices require manual dexterity and fair visual acuity; some also require good color vision.

8. Follow-up evaluation is needed to ensure correct technique.
9. The client may be able to reduce the expense through comparative shopping and third-party reimbursement.

10. Daily records help in evaluating patterns in relation to intake, insulin administration, and activities.
11. These situations may change dietary or insulin requirements.

12. A client needs to understand his prescribed insulin in order to make appropriate decisions about adjusting insulin, eating, and exercising.

Interventions	*Rationale*
13. Monitor for the effectiveness of insulin therapy.	13. Blood glucose monitoring is used to identify periods of hypoglycemia or hyperglycemia.
14. Advise the client about drugs that interact with blood glucose and about over-the-counter (OTC) sugar-free drugs (cough syrups, throat lozenges, etc.).	14. Understanding drug interactions can help the client avoid drugs that may cause a serious decrease or increase in blood glucose. For example, oral hypoglycemic agents, insulin, glucagon, aspirin, and beta-adrenergic blockers decrease blood glucose; corticosteroids, birth control pills, diuretics, and cold remedies containing decongestants increase blood glucose.
15. Explain the need to adhere to the prescribed diet and exercise program.	15. Diet and exercise therapy are essential to treating all types of diabetes.

16. Discuss alternative methods of injecting insulin:
  a. Jet injectors (needle-less)
  b. External insulin pumps
	16. Jet injectors offer the client freedom from needles but are expensive (about $600) and require weekly cleaning. Insulin pumps are even more expensive ($2000–$3000) and are appropriate only for highly motivated Type I diabetics (who have no endogenous insulin). The pump requires the client's constant attention and participation. Blood glucose must be monitored four to six times a day to allow appropriate decisions about the amount of insulin required.

17. Teach the client and evaluate return demonstrations of the following:
  a. Measuring the dose
  b. Mixing insulins, if applicable
  c. Double-checking correct dose and insulin expiration date
  d. Preparing the injection site
  e. Injecting the insulin
	17. Return demonstration allows the nurse to evaluate the client's ability to administer insulin unassisted.

18. Explain the need to rotate injection sites among arms, thighs, abdomen, and buttocks.	18. Using the same area repetitively can cause atrophy (depressions in skin) or scarring (hypertrophy).
19. Teach proper storage of insulin at home and during travel. Throw away bottles that have been exposed to extreme temperatures or direct sunlight for a long period.	19. The vial of insulin currently being used may be stored at room temperature. Spare vials of insulin are safely kept in the refrigerator. Insulin may not be frozen.
20. Strongly advise the client to have an individualized meal plan developed by a Registered Dietitian (RD).	20. A proper nutrient balance represents one aspect of diet therapy aimed at maintaining normal blood glucose level. The ADA recommends 50% to 60% carbohydrates, 12% to 20% protein, and 30% fats.
21. Explain the goals of dietary therapy for the client after consultation with a RD.	21. Reinforcing the goals of dietary therapy may help improve compliance.
22. Help the client to identify problem situations that may interfere with following his meal plan.	22. Noncompliance may be avoided by problem-solving before noncompliance occurs.

23. Assist the client in planning and implementing his ADA meal plan:
  a. Provide a resource list of current printed material.
  b. Suggest that he use the *ADA Cookbook* or another cookbook that specifies food exchanges: *Eat and Stay Thin, Better Homes and Gardens Cookbook.*
  c. Suggest that he carry a pocket guide or card.
	23. This intervention may increase compliance and reduce complications.

Interventions

Rationale

   d. Assist with planning a restaurant meal that follows his ADA meal plan and considers the portion sizes.

   e. Stress the importance of preparing food as recommended, e.g., broiling instead of frying.

   f. Reinforce the importance of limiting foods high in saturated fats and salt.

   g. Encourage increased dietary fiber intake within dietary guidelines.

24. Encourage the client to subscribe to a diabetes journal such as *Diabetes Forecast* or *Diabetes Self-Management.*

25. Assist the client to make a list of favorite "legal foods."

26. Stress the importance of six-month consultations with an RD.

27. Explain the complication of hypoglycemia and its signs and symptoms to client and family. Insulin reaction, insulin shock, and hypoglycemia are all synonymous for low blood glucose (< 70 mg/dL). Hypoglycemia may result from a combination of three things: too much insulin, too little food, or too vigorous an increase in activity. Reactions occur suddenly (in a matter of minutes), usually just before meal times, during or after exercise, and when injected insulin is at its peak action. Common signs and symptoms are listed below:

   a. Mild hypoglycemia (sympathetic nervous system)
- Pallor
- Diaphoresis
- Weakness
- Hunger
- Perioral paresthesias
- Tachycardia/palpitations
- Peculiar starving expression
- Outer trembling/inner nervousness

   b. Severe hypoglycemia (central nervous system)
- Headache
- Hypothermia
- Incoherent speech
- Lack of motor coordination
- Mental confusion
- Severe lethargy
- Unconsciousness
- Coma/convulsions

28. Teach the client measures to prevent hypoglycemia:

   a. Check blood glucose level routinely.

   b. Comply with the prescribed meal plan.

   c. Check blood glucose before exercise or strenuous activity.

   d. Check with a health care provider for guidelines to decrease insulin or increase food before exercise or strenuous activity.

24. These publications provide up-to-date information on meal planning.

25. Teaching what is permitted emphasizes the positive rather than the negative aspects of treatment.

26. Periodic sessions with an RD enables evaluation of diet and daily blood sugar readings.

27. Early detection of hypoglycemia enables prompt intervention to prevent serious, possibly fatal, reaction.

28. Regular SMBG can help minimize severe fluctuations.

Interventions

    e. Be aware of changes in daily routines that may precipitate hypoglycemia.

    f. Always carry some form of glucose in the same pocket or purse.

    g. Plan food intake carefully when drinking alcohol.

    h. Always wear diabetes identification.

29. Teach self-management of hypoglycemia:

    a. Treat hypoglycemia with or without symptoms based on the following chart:

Blood Glucose Level	Treatment
50–69 mg/dL	One fruit exchange
< 50 mg/dL	Two fruit exchanges

    • Additional fruit exchanges should be taken every 15 minutes until blood glucose level is >69 mg/dL.

    • If hypoglycemia occurs at night or after significant exercise and after a blood glucose level >69 mg/dL is established, eat ½ bread and ½ meat exchange.

    • Recheck blood glucose 1 hour after the first blood glucose reading >69 mg/dL.

    b. Teach that a slowly digested carbohydrate (e.g., 3 saltines, ½ oz cheese, 1 cup plain nonfat yogurt, ¼ cup cereal with milk) may be needed after 10 g of a fast-acting source (e.g., small box of raisins, ½ cup fruit juice, 4 to 5 dried fruit pieces, ½ cup regular [not diet] soda) if the client must wait an hour or longer before the next meal.

    c. Discuss commercial products available for treating hypoglycemia:

      • Dextrosol tablets (Orange Medical)

      • Glucose tablets (B-D)

      • Monoject gel (Sherwood)

      • Glutose liquid (Paddock)

      • Glucagon injection (Eli Lilly)

    d. Encourage the client to teach family members and friends how to prepare and administer glucagon to treat severe hypoglycemia.

30. Teach the importance of achieving and maintaining normal weight for height. (Refer to the Obesity care plan, for specific strategies.)

31. Explain how illness can influence blood glucose levels.

32. Teach the client to monitor blood glucose and urine for ketones at least every 4 hours.

33. Teach the client to increase carbohydrate intake when ill, according to this ADA exchange system:

    a. *Milk exchange* = 12 g carbohydrates

Rationale

29. Self-management of hypoglycemia is critical. Slowly digested carbohydrates help maintain blood glucose at proper levels until mealtime. Commercial hypoglycemic agents are especially useful if the client refuses to eat or is semiconscious. Glucagon causes glycogenolysis in the liver if adequate stores of glycogen are present. If the client is in critical condition and has been in a coma for some time, the glycogen stores probably have already been utilized, and IV glucose is the only treatment that will be effective.

30. An obese client has fewer available insulin receptors. Weight loss restores the number of insulin receptors on cells and also increases energy level and exercise tolerance.

31. Anticipating the effects of illness on the blood glucose level can alert the client to take precautions (e.g., increase insulin dosage) when ill.

32. Early detection of ketones in urine can enable prompt intervention to prevent serious ketoacidosis.

33. Illness often causes loss of appetite. Liquids or semi-soft foods may be substituted for the client's normal diet. An insulin-dependent diabetic should try to maintain a consistent car-

Interventions

    1 cup skim milk
    1 cup plain yogurt
    ½ cup ice cream
  b. *Bread exchange* = 15 g carbohydrates
    1 slice bread or toast
    ½ English muffin
    ½ bagel
    ½ cup cooked cereal
    6 saltines
    6 pretzels
    20 oyster crackers
  c. *Fruit exchange* = 15 g carbohydrates
    ½ cup orange juice
    ½ cup apple cider
    ½ cup unsweetened applesauce
    ½ cup ginger ale or cola (not diet)

  Note: Vegetables contain 5 g carbohydrates per serving; meats and fats have no carbohydrate content. Carbohydrate contents of other foods include:
  ½ cup regular Jello = 24 g carbohydrate
  2 level tsp. sugar = 8 g carbohydrate
  1 can chicken noodle soup = 15 g carbohydrate

34. Instruct the client to notify a health care professional if he cannot eat, is vomiting, or has diarrhea.

35. Explain the benefits of regular exercise:
  a. Improved fitness
  b. Psychological benefits—e.g., enhanced ability to relax, increased self-confidence, improved self-image
  c. reduction of body fat
  d. weight control

36. Explain the effects of exercise on glucose utilization

37. Explain the rationale for not exercising when blood glucose level exceeds 300 g/dL or when ketones are present.

38. Instruct the client to seek the advice of a health care provider before beginning an exercise program.

39. Teach the client to avoid injecting insulin into a body part that is about to be exercised.

40. Encourage the client to exercise with others, or at least where other informed persons are nearby, and always to wear diabetic identification.

41. Explain how to reduce serious hypoglycemic episodes related to exercise:
  a. Carry a source of sugar in his pocket.
  b. Have glucagon available whenever he participates in intense exercise

Rationale

bohydrate intake, which will supply readily available glucose so the body will not burn fat for energy, which produces ketones.

34. Immediate interventions are required to prevent dehydration and hypoglycemia.

35,36. Emphasizing the benefits of exercise may help improve compliance with the prescribed exercise regimen.

37. Exercise is contraindicated when blood glucose level exceeds 300 mg/dL, because exercise causes a rise in blood glucose and a resulting increase in ketone production, as hepatic production of glucose becomes disproportionately greater than the use of insulin.

38. Exercise may be contraindicated in the presence of certain complications, e.g., severe nephropathy, proliferative retinopathy.

39. Insulin absorption is increased in a body part that is exercised, which alters the insulin's usual action.

40. This ensures that assistance is available should hypoglycemia occur.

41. Proper timing of exercise, monitoring of blood glucose, and adjusting food or insulin decrease the risk of exercise-induced hypoglycemia. In the event of a severe reaction, a semiconscious or unconscious client may require

Interventions	*Rationale*
c. Identify a relative or friend who is willing and able to inject glucagon if needed. d. Monitor blood glucose before and after exercise. e. Exercise when blood glucose level tends to be higher, such as shortly after a meal.	glucagon. Instructing others in the preparation and injection of glucagon may save an unnecessary trip to the hospital.
42. Explain that because diabetics are at high risk for foot problems, the client should watch for and promptly report any injuries to or changes in the feet.	42. Foot lesions in diabetics are the result of peripheral neuropathy, peripheral vascular disease, superimposed infection, or a combination of these complications. Feet that are deformed, insensitive, and ischemic are prime targets for lesions and are susceptible to trauma.
43. Teach the importance of daily foot care and inspection.	43. Treatment is often delayed, because the diabetic is not aware of the injury until it has spread through the foot and possibly to the bone. The infected tissue kills healthy tissue, causing gangrene. Decreased vascular circulation prevents healing and may lead to amputation. An estimated 50% of all amputations due to diabetes complications could be prevented with early detection and prompt treatment.
44. Teach the client measures to prevent foot damage: a. Maintain normal blood glucose and cholesterol levels. b. Remove shoes and socks at every office visit. c. Contact a health care provider at the first sign of a problem, e.g., tenderness, redness, drainage. d. Trim toenails properly or seek professional care, and seek professional care on a regular basis if corns, calluses, or ingrown toenails are present. e. Make foot care and inspection part of a daily routine. f. Avoid exposing the feet to extremes of heat and cold. g. Wear warm, natural fiber socks and well-made, properly fitting shoes. h. Avoid smoking.	44. A diabetic's feet are more prone to injury because of decreased circulation: a. This reduces conditions (i.e., hyperglycemia) that contribute to microorganism growth. b. This helps remind the health care provider to examine the client's feet. c. Early detection and prompt treatment can prevent worsening of complications. d. Proper toenail trimming can prevent injury from incorrect self-care. e. Daily inspection can detect early changes. f. These precautions help prevent burns and vasoconstriction. g. Warm socks and good shoes absorb perspiration and help prevent corns, calluses, and blisters. h. The nicotine in tobacco causes blood vessels to contract and decreases the blood flow to the feet.
45. Teach the client and family to watch for and report the following: a. Unexplained fluctuations in blood and urine glucose b. Unexplained ketoacidosis episodes c. An injury (e.g., cut, scratch, burn) that does not show signs of healing in 24 hours d. Change in vision e. Vomiting or diarrhea that lasts more than 8 hours f. Signs of infection (e.g., elevated temperature, productive cough)	45. a,b. Severe blood glucose fluctuations or ketoacidosis episodes can be life-threatening and require careful investigation. c. Early treatment can prevent serious infections. d. Visual changes may indicate retinal vessel hemorrhage. e. Specific treatments may be needed to prevent dehydration. f. Infection may necessitate medication adjustments.

Interventions

46. Provide informational materials or referrals to groups that can assist the client to maintain goals and manage diabetes:
  a. American Diabetes Association
  b. Support groups
  c. Diabetes journals such as *Diabetes Forecast, Diabetes Self-Management,* and *Clinical Diabetes*
  d. Films "Focus on Feelings" and "Focus on Families" (from Oracle)

Rationale

46. A client who feels well supported is able to cope more effectively with life's stressors. A chronically ill person with multiple stressors needs to identify or develop an effective support system. Consisting of people, activities, and events, a support system helps a client achieve goals and manage stress. Knowing a friend or neighbor with diabetes, participating in a walk-a-thon for the ADA, and reading about a person who is coping successfully with diabetes are examples of support systems.

▲ **Documentation**

Discharge summary record
  Client teaching
  Status of outcome achievement
  Referrals

References/Bibliography

Bergman, M. (1987). *Principles of diabetes management.* New York: Medical Examination Publishing Company.

Brodoff, B., & Bleicher, S. (Eds.). (1982). *Diabetes mellitus and obesity.* Baltimore: Williams & Wilkins.

Brunner, L., & Suddarth, D. (1982). *The Lippincott manual of nursing practice* (3rd ed.). Philadelphia: J.B. Lippincott.

Davidson, J. (1986). *Clinical diabetes mellitus: A problem oriented approach.* New York: Thieme, Inc.

Ellenberg, M., Rifkin, H. (Eds.). (1983). *Diabetes mellitus theory and practice* (3rd ed.). New York: Medical Examination Publishing Company.

Espenshade, J.E. (1982). *Staff manual for teaching patients about diabetes mellitus.* Chicago: American Hospital Association.

Etzwiler, D., Fraz, N., Hollander, P., & Joynes, J. (1987). *Learning to live well with diabetes* (revised). Minnetonka, MN: International Diabetes Center.

Franz, M., Krosnick, A., Maschak-Carey, B., Parker, T., & Wheeler, F. (1986). *Goals for diabetes education.* VA: American Diabetes Association.

Gordon, M. (1982). *Manual of nursing diagnosis.* New York: McGraw-Hill.

Kojak, G. (1982). *Clinical diabetes mellitus.* Philadelphia: W.B. Saunders.

Kozier, B. (1983). *Fundamentals of nursing concepts and procedures* (2nd ed.). CA: Addison-Wesley.

Marble, A., Krall, L., Bradley, R., Christlieb, A., & Soeldner, J. (Eds.). (1985). *Joslins' diabetes mellitus* (12th ed.). Philadelphia: Lea & Febiger.

Staff (1985). *Nursing diagnosis standard care plans.* MI: Harper-Grace Hospitals.

Poole, D. (1986). Type II diabetes mellitus update: Diagnosis and management. *Nurse Practitioner, 11*(8), 26–41.

Rifkin, H., & Raskin, P. (Eds.). (1981). *Diabetes mellitus,* Vol. V. Bowie, MD: R.J. Brady.

Rifkin, H. (Eds.). (1984). *The physician's guide to type II diabetes (NIDDM) diagnosis and treatment.* VA: American Diabetes Association.

Tucker, S., Breeding, M., Canobbio, M., Paquette, E., Wells, M., Willmann, M. (1984). *Patient care standards* (3rd ed.). St. Louis: C.V. Mosby.

Scardina, R. (1983). Diabetic foot problems: Assessment and prevention. *Clinical Diabetes 1,* 1–7.

Hepatitis (Viral)

Hepatitis is an inflammation of the liver usually caused by one of two types of viruses, type A or type B. Type A hepatitis is a virus transmitted by fecal–oral contamination. Type B or serum hepatitis is transmitted by contaminated blood. Type A has a sudden onset, whereas type B has an insidious onset. Although most cases of hepatitis resolve completely, some individuals have a resulting chronic hepatitis that can be debilitating.

Diagnostic Cluster

Collaborative Problems

	Refer to:
Potential Complications:	
Progressive Liver Degeneration	Cirrhosis
Portal Systemic Encephalopathy	
Hypokalemia	Cirrhosis
Hemorrhage	Cirrhosis
Drug Toxicity	Cirrhosis
Renal Failure	Cirrhosis

Nursing Diagnoses

Potential for Infection Transmission related to contagious nature of virus A (gastrointestinal secretions) and virus B (serum)	
Potential Altered Health Maintenance related to lack of knowledge of condition, rest requirements, precautions to prevent transmission, nutritional requirements, and contraindications	
Altered Nutrition: Less Than Body Requirements related to anorexia, epigastric distress, and nausea	Cirrhosis
Pruritus related to accumulation of bilirubin pigment and bile salts	Cirrhosis
Pain related to swelling of inflamed liver	Pancreatitis

▲ **Discharge Criteria**

Before discharge, the client or family will:

1. Describe the modes of disease transmission
2. State signs and symptoms that must be reported to a health care professional

Collaborative Problems

▲ **Nursing Goal**

The nurse will detect hepatic complications.

▲ **Documentation**

Flow records
  Intake and output
Progress notes
  Evaluation of signs and symptoms

Potential Complication: Progressive Liver Degeneration

Interventions

1. Monitor for signs of progressive liver degeneration:
   a. Failure of hepatitis symptoms to resolve (e.g., jaundice, epigastric discomfort, clay-colored stools)
   b. Failure of liver enzyme levels and coagulation tests to return to normal

Rationale

1. Hepatitis A usually is cured but sometimes progresses to acute liver necrosis. Hepatitis B has a mortality rate of 10%, with another 10% developing chronic hepatitis (Brunner and Suddarth, 1989).

Related Physician-Prescribed Interventions

Medications

Antiemetics
Antacids
Vitamins

Antidiarrheals
Antihistamines

Intravenous Therapy

Total parenteral therapy

Protein hydrolysates

Related Physician-Prescribed Interventions (continued)

Laboratory Studies

Liver function tests   Alkaline phosphatase
SGOT   Serum albumin
Complete blood cell count

Diagnostic Studies

Liver scan

Therapies

Dietary restrictions depending on fat   Bed rest
  and protein tolerance

Nursing Diagnoses

▲ Outcome Criteria

The client will:

1. Remain in isolation until noninfectious
2. Demonstrate meticulous handwashing during hospitalization

Potential for Infection Transmission related to contagious nature of virus A (gastrointestinal secretions) and virus B (serum)

Focus Assessment Criteria	Clinical Significance

1. Mode of transmission:
  a. Airborne
  b. Contact (droplet, contaminated objects)
  c. Vehicle-borne (needles, blood)
  d. Vector-borne (animal, insects)
	1. Appropriate precautions depend on the mode of transmission.

Interventions	Rationale

1. Initiate appropriate isolation precautions:
  a. Type A (infectious):
    • Gowns and gloves when contact with feces is anticipated
  b. Type B (serum):
    • Gowns and gloves when contact with blood and body fluids is anticipated
    • Avoid recapping needles; dispose of immediately in designated container
  c. Type non-A, non-B:
    • Gowns and gloves when there is anticipated contact with blood and body fluids
    • Avoid recapping needles; dispose of immediately in designated container.
	1. Type A hepatitis can be transmitted through fecal–oral contamination for 7 days after onset of jaundice. Type B hepatitis and Type non-A, non-B hepatitis can be transmitted through contact with blood or body fluids until the client is HBsAg-negative. Needle-stick injuries commonly occur when the nurse is recapping the needle after use.

2. Use appropriate techniques for disposal of infectious waste, linen, and body fluids and for cleaning contaminated equipment and surfaces.	2. These techniques help protect others from contact with infectious materials and prevent disease transmission.
3. Refer the infection control practitioner for follow-up with the appropriate Health Department.	3. This referral is necessary to identify the source of exposure and other possibly infected persons.
4. Explain the importance of frequent handwashing to the client, family and other visitors, and health care personnel.	4. Handwashing removes the organism, which breaks the chain of infection transmission.

▲ Documentation

Flow records
  Isolation precautions required
Discharge summary record
  Client teaching

▲ Outcome Criteria

The outcome criteria for this diagnosis represent those associated with discharge planning. Refer to the discharge criteria.

Potential Altered Health Maintenance related to lack of knowledge of condition, rest requirements, precautions to prevent transmission, nutritional requirements, and activity restrictions

Focus Assessment Criteria	Clinical Significance
1. Client's or family's readiness and ability to learn and retain information	1. A client or family that does not achieve the goals for learning requires a referral for assistance postdischarge.

Interventions

1. Explain the mode of infection transmission to the client and family. (Refer to the nursing diagnosis Potential for Infection Transmission for more information.)
2. Explain to contacts—family, peers—that they should receive hepatitis B vaccine or immune globulin.

3. Explain the need to rest and avoid strenuous activity.

4. Explain the need for diet high in protein and calories. (Refer to the nursing diagnosis Altered Nutrition in the Cirrhosis entry, page 112, for more information.)
5. Explain the hazards of certain medications—narcotics, sedatives, tranquilizers—and ammonia-containing products.

6. Teach the client and family to watch for and report signs and symptoms of complications:
   a. Unusual bleeding (e.g., gums, stools)

   b. Hypokalemia (manifested by muscle cramps, nausea, vomiting)

   c. Confusion, altered speech patterns

   d. Increasing severity of symptoms

   e. Rapid weight loss or gain

7. Explain the importance of avoiding alcohol.

8. Stress the importance of follow-up care and laboratory studies.

Rationale

1. Understanding how infection can be transmitted is the first step in prevention.

2. For their protection, family and associates should receive active or passive immunization for the hepatitis B virus. (Not indicated for hepatitis A.)
3. As the liver repairs itself, excessive physical activity depletes the body of the energy needed for healing. Adequate rest is needed to prevent relapse.
4. Protein and caloric requirements increase during periods of tissue healing.

5. Certain drugs are hepatoxic. Moreover, in hepatitis, impaired liver function slows drug metabolism, causing drug levels to accumulate in the body.
6. Early recognition and reporting enables prompt intervention to prevent serious complications.
   a. Bleeding indicates decreased prothrombin time and clotting factors.
   b. Overproduction of aldosterone causes sodium and water retention and potassium excretion.
   c. Neurological impairment results from cerebral hypoxia due to high serum ammonia levels caused by the liver's impaired ability to convert ammonia to urea.
   d. Worsening symptoms indicate progressive liver damage.
   e. Rapid weight loss points to negative nitrogen balance; weight gain, to fluid retention.
7. Alcohol increases hepatic irritation and may interfere with recovery.
8. Follow-up care enables evaluation of liver function and detection of relapse or recurrence.

▲ **Documentation**

Discharge summary record
  Client teaching
  Outcome achievement
  Referrals, when indicated

References/Bibliography

Berk, J. (ed.). (1985). *Gastroenterology,* Vol. 7. Philadelphia: W.B. Saunders.
Brunner, L., & Suddarth, D. (1989). *Textbook of medical-surgical nursing* (6th ed.). Philadelphia: J.B. Lippincott.
Dong, B., Barton, E., & Mancini, B. (1979). Viral hepatitis. *Nursing Practice, 9*(3), 27–32.
Valenti, W. (1986). Hepatitis B prevention. *Infection Control, 7*(2), 74–77.

Hypothyroidism

In hypothyroidism, thyroid gland dysfunction results in a deficiency of thyroid hormones thyroxine (T_4) and triiodothyronine (T_3). These hormones are responsible for maintaining body metabolism.

Diagnostic Cluster

▲ *Time Frame*
Initial diagnosis

▲ *Discharge Criteria*
Before discharge, the client or family will:

1. Describe dietary restrictions
2. Relate the importance of adhering to the medication schedule
3. Describe risk factors
4. Relate signs and symptoms that must be reported to a health care professional
5. Identify community resources available for assistance

Collaborative Problems

Potential Complications:
Metabolic
Atherosclerotic Heart Disease
Acute Organic Psychosis
Hematologic

Refer to:

Nursing Diagnoses

Altered Comfort related to cold intolerance secondary to decreased metabolic rate

Potential Altered Health Maintenance related to insufficient knowledge of condition, treatment regimen, signs and symptoms of complications, dietary management, pharmacological therapy, and contraindications

Altered Nutrition: Less Than Body Requirements related to intake greater than metabolic needs secondary to slowed metabolic rate

Corticosteroid Therapy

Colonic Constipation related to decreased peristaltic action secondary to decreased metabolic rate and decreased physical activity

General Surgery

Collaborative Problems

▲ *Nursing Goal*
The nurse will manage and minimize complications of hypothyroidism.

Potential Complication: Metabolic
Potential Complication: Atherosclerotic heart disease
Potential Complication: Hematologic
Potential Complication: Acute organic psychosis

Interventions

1. Monitor metabolic function

   a. Cardiac
      • Decreased cardiac output
      • Low blood pressure, decreased pulse
   b. Respiratory

Rationale

1. Deficiencies in circulating hormones reduce metabolism, thus affecting all body systems. The severity of signs and symptoms is dependent on the duration and degree of thyroid hormone deficiency.

   a. Cardiac tissue changes, decreased stroke volume, and heart rate reduce cardiac output.
   b. Hypoventilation occurs partly because of monopolysaccharide deposits in respiratory system, with subsequent decreased vital capacity. Hypercarbia also further decreases the respiratory rate.

Interventions	Rationale
c. Neurologic • Paresthesias of fingers and toes • Changes in affect, mentation, short-term memory, delusions • Slowed, slurred speech	**c.** Paresthesias result from direct metabolic changes on nerves and interstitial edema of surrounding tissues. Changes in affect, mentation, short-term memory, and delusions are caused by cerebral edema, resulting from changes in adrenal gland affecting water retention, and by cerebral hypoxia, resulting from decreased cerebral blood flow. Speech problems result from edema in the cerebellar region of the brain.
d. Musculoskeletal • Muscle weakness • Pathologic fractures	**d.** Muscle weakness and stiffness are caused by mucoprotein edema separating muscle fibers. Pathologic fractures result from impaired calcium transport and utilization caused by decreased calcitonin levels (produced by thyroid gland).
e. Gastrointestinal • Constipation • Impaired digestion	**e.** GI tract motility is decreased because of mucoproteins in the interstitial spaces. Poor food digestion occurs throughout the GI tract because of mucosal atrophy and decreased production of hydrochloric acid.
f. Hormonal • Hypoglycemia • Increased thyroid-stimulating hormone (TSH) • Decreased T_3, T_4 • Menorrhagia or amenorrhea, decreased libido	**f.** Hypoglycemia results from changes in the adrenal cortex. Increased TSH usually confirms the diagnosis of primary hypothyroidism, which accounts for approximately 90% of cases of hypothyroidism. Levothyroxine (T_4) and triiodothyronine (T_3) are produced and distributed by the thyroid gland; T_4 is responsible for maintaining a steady metabolic rate. Altered levels of sexual hormones in early hypothyroidism result in prolonged heavy menstrual periods and changes in libido. Prolonged hypothyroidism leads to amenorrhea, anovulation, and infertility resulting from effects of myxedema on luteinizing hormone.
g. Integumentary • Thickened, dry skin • Yellowish skin color in absence of jaundiced sclera • Thin, brittle nails with transverse grooves • Coarse, dry hair with beginning hair loss (e.g., eyebrows).	**g.** Hyperkeratosis, an overgrowth of the horny layer of the epidermis, occurs with subsequent decrease in activity of sweat glands and resulting skin dryness. Monopolysaccharide accumulation in subcutaneous tissue results in thickened skin. Low-density lipoprotein, the primary plasma carrier of carotene, increases with low levels of thyroid hormone, resulting in yellowed skin. Dry skin, hair loss, and nail changes result in altered cell replication resulting from decreased thyroid hormones.
2. Monitor for myxedema coma.	**2.** Myxedema coma may result from untreated progressive myxedema. It carries a 50% mortality rate.
3. Monitor a myxedematous client for signs and symptoms of myocardial ischemia and infarction after initiating thyroid hormone replacement: **a.** Abnormal rate or rhythm **b.** Palpitations **c.** Syncope **d.** Cardiac emergencies, e.g., arrest, ventricular fibrillation	**3.** As oxygen requirements increase with increased metabolism, angina may result if the client has atherosclerosis or coronary artery disease caused by reduced lipid metabolism with monopolysaccharide deposits in the myocardium.

Interventions

4. Monitor for signs and symptoms of atherosclerotic heart disease:
   a. Elevated blood pressure
   b. Vertigo
   c. Chest pain

5. Monitor for signs and symptoms of acute organic psychosis:
   a. Agitation
   b. Acute anxiety
   c. Paranoia
   d. Delusions
   e. Hallucinations

6. Monitor for signs and symptoms of anemia:
   a. Fatigue
   b. Hypoxia
   c. Easy bruising
   d. Confusion

7. Monitor for signs of abnormal bleeding:
   a. Petechiae
   b. Bleeding gums
   c. Ecchymotic areas
   d. Blood in urine, stool, or emesis

8. Avoid administering sedatives and narcotics or reduce dosage to one half or one third the regular dose.

Rationale

4. Atherosclerosis can occur rapidly in a client with hypothyroidism, because the protein-bound iodine and T₄ levels are low and blood cholesterol levels are high. Sometimes a decrease in atherosclerosis occurs after thyroid hormone replacement is initiated. However, excessive doses of thyroid hormone replacement initially may result in vascular occlusion due to atherosclerosis.

5. Often, a client with severe behavioral symptoms has an underlying psychiatric disorder that may not improve and actually may be exacerbated by thyroid hormone therapy.

6. Normochromic, normocytic anemia results from a decrease in erythrocyte mass as a compensatory response to decreased oxygen demand.

7. Thyroid hormone deficiencies cause increased capillary fragility, prolonged clotting time, and decreased platelet adhesiveness.

8. Slowed breakdown of these medications prolongs high circulating levels, resulting in heightened responses and possibly respiratory depression.

▲ Documentation

Flow records
    Vital signs
    Intake and output
    Rhythm strips
Progress notes
    Unusual events

Related Physician-Prescribed Interventions

Medications
Thyroid hormone

Intravenous Therapy
Not indicated

Laboratory Studies
Serum T₄, T₃   Thyroglobulin
Resin T₃ uptake   Protein-bound iodine
Thyroid stimulating hormone

Diagnostic Studies
Radioactive iodine uptake   EKG
Thyroid scan

Therapies
Weight loss diet

Nursing Diagnoses

▲ Outcome Criteria

The client will:
1. Report episodes of cold intolerance
2. Report improved tolerance to cold after body heat retention measures are employed

Altered Comfort related to cold intolerance secondary to decreased metabolic rate

Focus Assessment Criteria:	*Clinical Significance*

1. Presence of discomfort
  a. Description
  b. Site
  c. Onset
  d. Precipitating factors
2. Body temperature
3. Skin color and temperature
	1–3. A baseline assessment aids the nurse in planning interventions and client teaching.

Interventions

1. Monitor for signs of hypothermia:
   a. Rectal temperature <36° C (96° F)
   b. Decreased pulse and respiration rate
   c. Cool skin
   d. Blanching, redness, or pallor
   e. Shivering
2. Explain measures to prevent chilling:
   a. Increase temperature in the living environment.
   b. Eliminate drafts.
   c. Use several blankets at night.
   d. Protect from cold exposure, e.g., wear several layers of clothing and wool hats, socks, and gloves.
3. Explain the need for gradual rewarming after cold exposure, avoiding application of external heat to rewarm rapidly.

4. Encourage the client to avoid cigarette smoking.

Rationale

1. Decreased circulating thyroid hormones reduce the metabolic rate; the resulting vasoconstriction increases the risk of hypothermia.

2. Chilling increases the metabolic rate and puts increased stress on the heart.

3. Vascular collapse can result from a rapid increase in metabolic rate and subsequent strain on the heart from increased myocardial oxygen requirements.
4. Smoking further increases the vasoconstriction caused by a decreased metabolic rate, increasing susceptibility to cold in peripheral areas.

▲ **Documentation**

Flow records
    Vital signs, including rectal temperature
Discharge summary record
    Client teaching
    Outcome achievement

▲ **Outcome Criteria**

The outcome criteria for this diagnosis represent those associated with discharge planning. Refer to the discharge criteria.

Potential Altered Health Maintenance related to insufficient knowledge of condition, treatment regimen, signs and symptoms of complications, dietary management, pharmacological therapy, and activity restrictions

Focus Assessment Criteria	*Clinical Significance*
1. Client's or family's readiness and ability to learn and retain information	1,2. Depressed mentation and short attention span can prevent retention of learning. A client or family that does not achieve goals for learning requires a referral for assistance postdischarge.
2. Concerns regarding the effects of the condition on the client's life style	

Interventions

1. Explain the pathophysiology of hypothyroidism, using teaching aids appropriate to the client's or family's educational level (e.g., pictures, slide-tapes, models).
2. Explain risk factors that can be eliminated or modified:

   a. Exposure to cold
   b. Tobacco use
   c. Regular alcohol intake
   d. High-fat diet

   e. Stressors, e.g., emotional stress, infections

3. Instruct the client and family to observe for and report signs and symptoms of disease complications:
   a. Progression of disease signs and symptoms
   b. Behavioral changes, e.g., agitation, confusion, delusions, paranoia, hallucinations
   c. Angina
   d. Extreme fatigue
   e. Seizure activity
   f. Edema in the feet and ankles

Rationale

1. Presenting relevant and useful information in an easily understandable format greatly decreases learning frustration and may help increase compliance.
2. The client's understanding that certain risk factors can be controlled may help improve compliance with the therapeutic regimen.
   a,b,c. Exposure to cold, as well as tobacco and alcohol use, increase vasoconstriction.

   d. Decreased thyroid hormone levels increase blood lipids.
   e. Stress produces an increase in metabolic rate in hypothyroidism.
3. Early detection and reporting of complications enables prompt treatment.

Interventions	*Rationale*
4. Reinforce explanations for therapeutic diet. Consult dietitian when indicated.	4. Understanding the reasons for the therapeutic diet may encourage the client to comply with it.
a. Low-calorie diet	**a.** A low-calorie diet compensates for a decreased metabolic rate.
b. Small portions of nutritious foods	**b.** Small portions compensate for impaired digestion secondary to decreased production of hydrochloric acid.
c. Avoid excessive fluid intake	**c.** Limited fluid intake may help reduce fluid retention secondary to increased capillary permeability.
d. Fiber	**d.** Increased fiber intake can help increase GI motility.
e. Avoid soybeans, white turnips, cabbage, and peanuts	**e.** These foods interfere with thyroid hormone production.
5. Explain why precautions are required when taking certain medications:	5. Understanding that the delayed metabolism of medications can cause sustained elevated levels may encourage the client to adhere to the dosage schedule.
a. Phenothiazides, sedatives, narcotics, anesthetics: Chemical reactions are slowed, causing delayed breakdown of medications and prolonged high circulating levels, resulting in increased somnolence.	
b. Insulin: Thyroid hormones may increase blood glucose levels.	
c. Digitalis, indomethacin, anticoagulants: Delayed metabolism can potentiate their effects.	
d. Dilantin: Lowers circulating T_4 levels.	
6. Explain that side effects of thyroid hormone therapy can produce signs and symptoms similar to those of hyperthyroidism:	6. Excessive dosage can cause hyperthyroidism and a too-rapid metabolic rate. These signs and symptoms tend to be less exaggerated in an elderly client than in a younger one.
a. Tachycardia	
b. Increased respiratory rate	
c. Restlessness, irritability	
d. Heat intolerance	
e. Increased perspiration	
f. Diarrhea	
7. Teach the client to observe for symptoms of a too-rapid change in metabolic rate:	7. The client must begin the medication regimen slowly so that dysrhythmias and angina do not significantly increase cardiac workload.
a. Headaches	
b. Palpitations	
c. Angina	
8. Explain the importance of continuing daily medication and periodic laboratory testing throughout the rest of the client's life. Explain the following:	8. Fluctuations in drug blood levels produce signs and symptoms of hypothyroidism.
a. The client should take thyroid hormone at the same time each day.	
b. T_3 and T_4 testing should be done periodically to check thyroid hormone blood levels.	
9. Reinforce the need for follow-up care.	9. Follow-up enables evaluation for signs of hypothyroidism or hyperthyroidism.

▲ **Documentation**

Discharge summary record
   Discharge instructions
   Follow-up instructions
   Status at discharge
   Achievement of goals (family or individual)

References/Bibliography

Gambert, S., & Brensinger, J.F. (1983). Assessing thyroid function in the elderly. *Nurse Practitioner, 8*(7), 38–43.

McMillian, J.Y. (1988). Preventing myxedema coma in the hypothyroid patient. *Dimensions in Critical Care Nursing, 7*(3), 136–145.

Sawin, C.T. (1985). Hypothyroidism. *Medical Clinics of North America, 69*(5), 989–1004.

Obesity

Obesity is a complex problem involving social, psychological, and metabolic issues. Most commonly, obesity is caused by overeating and insufficient exercise. Behavioral characteristics common to obese persons include the following:

- Response to external cues rather than internal cues as to when to eat or stop eating
- Eating in response to feelings of depression, elation, loneliness, sadness, or boredom
- Excessive eating in a short time span, followed by feelings of remorse
- Inactivity or underactivity (Mellin, Slinkard, and Irwin, 1982)

Diagnostic Cluster

▲ Discharge Criteria

Before discharge, the client or family will:

1. Relate caloric, nutritional, and exercise requirements
2. State condition of home behavioral management of inappropriate food consumption or energy expenditure
3. Relate community resources or professionals to contact after discharge

Nursing Diagnoses

Altered Health Maintenance related to imbalance between caloric intake and energy expenditure

Ineffective Individual Coping related to increased food consumption secondary to response to external stressors

Nursing Diagnoses

▲ Outcome Criteria

The client will:

1. Identify eating and exercise patterns
2. Describe the relationship between metabolism, intake, and exercise
3. Lose weight as contracted in an outpatient program
4. Prepare and shop for a nutritionally sound diet
5. Adhere to an exercise program

Altered Health Maintenance related to imbalance between caloric intake and energy expenditure

Focus Assessment Criteria

1. Height, weight, and vital signs
2. Medical problems; presence of risk factors
3. Food intake and exercise history
4. Dieting and body weight history, including recent gains or losses
5. Factors contributing to excessive caloric intake:
   a. Knowledge deficit related to balanced nutritional intake
   b. Inappropriate response to external cues (e.g., urge rather than hunger, boredom, stress, anger, guilt)
   c. Lack of initiative or motivation
   d. Imbalance in nutritive composition of diet (e.g., excessive fat or simple carbohydrate intake)
   e. Cultural or familial factors
   f. Poor eating habits, (e.g., eating fast foods, eating on the run, skipping meals)
6. Factors contributing to inadequate energy expenditure:

Clinical Significance

1–8. To help ensure success, when planning a weight reduction program, all factors contributing to the client's obesity should be identified.

Focus Assessment Criteria	*Clinical Significance*
a. Knowledge deficit of the importance of exercise in weight reduction and maintenance b. Inadequate exercise program c. Sedentary life style or occupation d. Fatigue e. Lack of initiative or motivation f. Activity intolerance g. Poor time management, prioritization, or planning 7. Support or sabotage from family and friends in weight reduction efforts 8. Client's current desire and readiness (physiological and psychological) to comply with a controlled caloric intake and exercise program	
9. Rule out an eating disorder—i.e., anorexia nervosa or bulimia—or other conditions requiring treatment by other health care professionals.	9. Certain conditions or weight loss modes may require specific therapies beyond the scope of nursing, e.g., bulimia, conditions requiring special diets, conditions requiring carefully planned exercise, and weight loss through a protein-sparing modified fast requiring careful laboratory monitoring.

Interventions	*Rationale*
1. Increase the client's awareness of how body weight is affected by the balance between food intake and activity. Explain that successful weight reduction and maintenance hinge on achieving a balance between reduced caloric intake and increased caloric expenditure through regular exercise. To determine the number of calories the client should consume daily to reach and maintain his or her ideal weight, multiply the client's ideal weight in pounds by 11, if female, or 12, if male. One pound of fat roughly equals 3500 calories. Thus, to lose 2 lb/week, the client must cut 7000 calories from his or her current weekly intake. Exercise caloric expenditure charts may be used to determine the calories burned during various activities.	1. Weight loss goals may be achieved through a combination of reduced caloric intake and increased caloric expenditure through exercise. Any increase in physical activity increases energy output and caloric deficits in a person following a reduced-calorie dietary regimen.
2. Help the client develop a safe, realistic weight loss program that considers these factors: a. Amount of loss desired b. Duration of program c. Cost d. Nutritional soundness e. Compatibility with life style	2. Realistic goals increase the likelihood of success. Successes give the client an incentive to continue the program.
3. Help the client identify environmental factors that contribute to poor eating patterns by discussing the following: a. Friends, family, coworkers: What are their habits? Would they be supportive? b. What types of foods are found in the home? At parties? At work? In the lunch room?	3. Helping the client identify external factors may increase his internal motivation to overcome them.

Interventions   *Rationale*

    c. In what type of leisure or recreational activities does the client engage? Is the client sedentary?

    d. What route(s) does the client take to and from work? Does the client pass by fast food restaurants?

    e. Who does the housework? Gardening and yardwork? Errands?

    f. How much television does the client watch?

    g. Has the client responded to any advertisements for rapid weight loss programs or devices?

4. Instruct the client to keep a diary for 1 week that includes these things:
    a. Food intake and exercise
    b. Location and times of meals
    c. Emotions during mealtimes
    d. Person(s) with whom the client ate
    e. Any skipped meals
    f. Snacks

5. Discuss the hazards of the following activities:
    a. Eating while doing another activity, such as watching TV or reading
    b. Eating while standing up, which can give the illusion of not eating a meal
    c. Eating out of boredom, stress, or another psychological reason
    d. Eating because everyone else is eating

6. Teach the client the basics of balanced nutritional intake, including supportive measures:
    a. Choose a diet plan that encourages high intake of complex carbohydrates and limited fat intake. Recommended U.S. dietary goals are 30% of total calories from fat, 12% from protein, 48% from complex carbohydrates, and 10% from simple carbohydrates.
    b. Be aware that method of preparation also affects total calorie and fat content. For example, a chicken-fried steak is a protein with a high fat content, owing to its method of preparation (frying).
    c. Try to obtain as many fat calories as possible from fruits and vegetables instead of from meat and dairy products.
    d. Eat more chicken and fish, which contain less fat and total calories per ounce than red meat.
    e. Limit high-fat salad dressings, especially dressing containing mayonnaise (216–308 calories per 2-ounce serving).
    f. Avoid fast foods, which have a high fat and total calorie content.
    g. When dining in a restaurant, make special requests, e.g., serve salad dressing on the side, omit sauce from entree.
    h. Plan meals in advance.

4. Such a diary helps the client become aware of his food intake patterns.

5. Certain situations may be identified as cues that trigger inappropriate eating.

6. Successful weight loss and long-term maintenance can be achieved through a diet low in fat and high in complex carbohydrates.

Interventions   *Rationale*

    i. If attending a party or dining out, plan your eating ahead of time and stick to it.

    j. When food shopping, prepare a shopping list and adhere to it.

    k. Involve the family in meal planning for better nutrition.

    l. Buy the highest quality ground beef to limit fat content. (Ground round has about 10% fat; regular hamburger, 25% fat.)

    m. Choose a wide variety of appropriate foods to reduce feelings of deprivation.

    n. Avoid eating at family-style buffets, which increase the chance of overeating.

    o. Drink 8 to 10 glasses (8 oz) of water daily, to help excrete the by-products of weight loss (cellular breakdown).

    p. Measure foods and count calories; keep records.

    q. Read food labels and note ingredients, composition, and total calories per serving. Choose "lite" products when possible. Be aware that many prepared foods have hidden ingredients, such as salt and saturated fats, and that some so-called "natural" foods, such as granola, are high in fat and sugar.

    r. Eat slowly and chew food thoroughly.

    s. Experiment with spices, fat substitutes, and low-calorie recipes.

    t. Chew gum while preparing meals, to deter eating while cooking.

7. Discuss the benefits of exercise:

    a. Reduces caloric absorption

    b. Acts as an appetite suppressant

    c. Increases metabolic rate and caloric expenditure

    d. Preserves lean muscle mass

    e. Increases oxygen uptake

    f. Improves self-esteem and decreases depression, anxiety, and stress

    g. Aids restful sleep

    h. Improves body posture

    i. Provides fun, recreation, and diversion

    j. Increases resistance to degenerative diseases of middle and later years, e.g., cardiovascular disorders

7. A significant amount of lean mass (muscle), up to 30%, can be lost on a calorie-restricted diet. Exercise minimizes this loss. Exercise also contributes to an overall feeling of well-being, which can positively influence self-esteem during dieting.

8. Help the client develop a safe, realistic exercise program, considering the following factors:

    a. Personality and life style

    b. Time availability

    c. Occupation: sedentary or active

    d. Safety: e.g., sports injuries, environmental hazards

    e. Cost of club membership or equipment

    f. Age, physical size, and physical condition

8,9. The client is more likely to comply with a regular exercise program that is convenient and enjoyable. A gradually progressing exercise program minimizes discomfort and injury, encouraging compliance.

9. Discuss beginning an exercise program. Instruct the client to consult with a physician

Interventions

Rationale

before starting, if indicated. Advise the client
as follows:
  a. Start slow and easy.
  b. Choose activities that exercise many parts
     of the body.
  c. Choose activities that are vigorous enough
     to cause "healthful fatigue."
  d. Do reading, consult with experts, and talk
     with friends and co-workers who exercise.
  e. Develop a regular exercise program and
     chart progress.
  f. Add supplemental activities, e.g., park far
     away and walk, work on garden, walk up
     stairs, spend weekends at leisure activities
     that require walking, such as festivals or
     art fairs.
  g. Eliminate time- and energy-saving devices
     when practicable.
  h. Work up to ½ to 1 hour of exercise per
     day at least four days per week.
  i. Avoid lapses of more than 2 days between
     exercise sessions, to maintain optimum
     conditioning.

10. Teach the client about the risks of obesity:
  a. Metabolic abnormalities
  b. Arteriosclerosis
  c. Hypertension
  d. Left ventricular hypertrophy
  e. Diabetes mellitus
  f. Gallbladder disease
  g. Increased risk of complications of surgery
  h. Respiratory disease
  i. Increased risk of cancer, e.g., breast, colon
  j. Increased risk of accident and injury

10. The client must understand that obesity is a
multiple-system health hazard. A diet high in
fat and simple cholesterol contributes to atherosclerosis, diabetes, gallbladder disease,
breast cancer, and colon cancer. A sedentary
life style decreases muscle tone and strength;
compromised mobility and balance increase
the risk of falls and injury. Fatty tissue is less
vascular and more susceptible to infection. Increased peripheral resistance causes increased
cardiac workload, which raises blood pressure.
Excessive abdominal fatty tissue compromises
diaphragmatic movement, which can lead to
hypoventilation.

11. Discuss the value of weekly goals versus the
larger weight loss goal, e.g., will walk 2 days
for 20 minutes each day.

11. Weekly goals enable achievement and foster
compliance. Unsatisfactory habits can be tar-
geted (e.g., the client doubles eating time by
actively slowing consumption) and healthy
habits can be promoted (e.g., the client eats
plain popcorn as an evening snack). Since
weight loss may vary from week to week, a
primary focus on pounds lost may be discouraging.

▲ **Documentation**

Progress notes
  Client teaching
  Planning:
    Weight loss goal
    Exercise (type, frequency)
    Weekly goals

▲ **Outcome Criteria**

The client will:
1. Identify stressors and effective response patterns
2. When in an outpatient program, adhere to the diet and
   exercise program

**Ineffective Individual Coping related to increased food consumption secondary to
response to external stressors**

Focus Assessment Criteria	*Clinical Significance*
1. Personal stressors	1–3. Often, obesity is facilitated or aggravated by inappropriate responses to external cues, particularly stressors. This response triggers an ineffective coping pattern in which the client eats in response to stress cues rather than to physiological hunger.

Focus Assessment Criteria	*Clinical Significance*
2. Stressors contributing to the eating behavior	
3. Effective and ineffective responses to stressors	
4. Coping strengths	**4–8.** The client's insight into his or her eating problem is a critical factor in predicting the success of treatment.
5. Cultural or familial patterns that enhance or impair positive outcomes	
6. Insight into eating in response to external rather than internal cues	
7. Motivation to alter destructive patterns	
8. Ability to distinguish "urges" from physiologic hunger	

Interventions	*Rationale*

1. Assist the client to do the following:
  a. Alter ways of thinking, e.g., think of "cheating" as "off-target behavior"; "eating" as "energy intake"; "exercise" as "energy consumption"
  b. Reduce fears of loss of control, e.g., learn to take a taste without fear of a binge
  c. Take risks and reward successes
  d. Identify potential problem areas and have a definite plan for getting back "on target"
  e. Understand that weight management simply involves balancing energy intake and energy consumption
  f. Observe role models and understand that persons who maintain their weight are not "just lucky"
  g. Examine personal meanings for eating and food other than as a means to meet physiological needs and sustain life
	1. Our society places a high priority on thinness and typically labels obese persons as undesirable and undisciplined. These measures attempt to alter the client's attitude toward obesity, weight reduction, and exercise.

2. Encourage and assist the client to do the things below:
  a. Contract reduction and exercise programs with realistic goals
  b. Keep intake and exercise records
  c. Hang an admired photograph on the refrigerator
  d. Increase knowledge about weight loss and exercise by talking with health-conscious friends, relatives, and associates
  e. Make new friends who are health-conscious and active
  f. Get a friend to go on the program also or to serve as a support person
  g. Reward himself or herself for progress
  h. Keep in mind that self-image and behavior are learned and can be unlearned
  i. Build a support system of people who value growth and appreciate him or her as an individual
  j. Be aware of rationalization, e.g., a lack of time may actually be poor prioritization
  k. Keep a list of positive outcomes
	2. Significant weight loss takes many months. These activities help increase the client's interest and maintain motivation throughout the long program.

3. If possible, involve the client's family in the weight-reduction project. Determine whether or not support is present.	**3.** Family support is important. If support is not present, open discussions are needed to elicit their support.

Interventions

4. Instruct the client to limit body measurements and weighing to once per week.

5. Encourage the client to avoid persons who may sabotage weight loss attempts, if possible.
6. Teach the client to do the following:
   a. Distinguish between an urge and actual hunger
   b. Use distraction, relaxation, and guided imagery
   c. Make a list of external cues or situations that lead to off-target behavior
   d. List constructive actions to substitute for off-target behavior, e.g., take a walk
   e. Post the list of alternative behaviors on the refrigerator
   f. Adhere to the list and reward himself or herself when appropriate
   g. Reevaluate whether the plan is realistic every 1 or 2 weeks

Rationale

4. Fluctuations in body weight are common, especially in females, owing to water retention. Daily weights are misleading and often disheartening; body measurements provide a better indicator of losses. Moreover, consistent exercising results in lean muscle mass gain. Because muscle weighs more than fat, this may be reflected as a weight gain on the scale.
5. Certain persons and relationships may be threatened by the client's weight loss.
6. Identification and reduction of inappropriate or destructive responses to stressors can be the critical factor for successful weight loss and maintenance.

▲ **Documentation**

Progress notes
   Interactions

References/Bibliography

Brody, J. (1981). *Jane Brody's nutrition book.* New York: W.W. Norton.

Bray, G.A. (Ed.). (1979). *Obesity in America.* Washington, D.C.: DHEW Publication No. NIH 19–359.

Brownell, K.D., Heckerman, C.L., Westlake, R.I., Hayes, S.C., & Monti, P.M. (1978). The effect of couples training and partner co-operativeness in the behavioral treatment of obesity. *Behavior Research and Therapy, 16,* 323–333.

Brownell, K.D., & Stunkard, A.J. (1980). Exercise in the development and control of obesity. In: A.J. Stunkard (Ed.), *Obesity.* Philadelphia: W.B. Saunders.

Danforth, E. (1985). Diet and obesity. *American Journal of Clinical Nutrition, 41,* 1132–1145.

Fernstein, A.R. (1960). The treatment of obesity: An analysis of methods, results and factors that influence success. *Journal of Chronic Diseases, 11,* 349–393.

Franklin, B.A., & Rubenfire, M. (1980). Losing weight through exercise. *JAMA, 244,* 377–379.

Fox, S.M., Naughton, J.R., & Haskell, W.L. (1971). Physical activity in prevention of coronary heart disease. *Annals of Clinical Research, 3,* 404–432.

Mellin, L., Slinkard, L.A., & Irwin, C.E. (1982). Behavior associated with obesity in white female adolescents. Paper presented at the Society for Adolescent Medicine Annual Meeting, New York.

Pitta, P., Alpert, M., & Perelle, A. (1980). Cognitive stimulus-control program for obesity with emphasis on anxiety and depression reduction. *International Journal of Obesity, 4,* 227–233.

Sheldahl, L.M. (1986). Special ergometric techniques and weight reduction. *Medicine and Science in Sports and Medicine, 18,* 25–28.

Smith, G.S., & Delprato, D.L. (1976). Stimulus control of covert behaviors (urges). *Psychological Record, 26,* 461–466.

Stern, F.M. (1978). Imagery procedures in weight control. *Obesity/Bariatric Medicine, 7,* 60–64.

Storlie, J., & Jordan, H.A. (Eds.). (1984). *Behavioral management of obesity.* New York: Spectrum Publications, 137–150.

Stunkard, A.J. (1983). Biological and psychological factors in obesity. In R.K. Goodstern (Ed.). *Eating and weight disorders.* New York: Springer-Verlag, 1–31.

Wadden, T.A., Stunkard, A.J., & Brownell, K.D. (1983). Very low caloric diets: Their efficacy, safety and future. *Annals of Internal Medicine, 99,* 675–684.

Warwick, M., & Garrow, J.S. (1981). The effect of addition of exercise to a regime of dietary restriction on weight loss, nitrogen balance, resting metabolic rate and spontaneous physical activity in three obese women in a metabolic ward. *International Journal of Obesity, 5,* 25–32.

Wilson, G.T., & Brownell, K.D. (1978). Behavior therapy for obesity: Including family members in the treatment process. *Behavior Therapy, 9,* 943–945.

Wooley, S.C., Wooley, O.W., & Dyrenforth, S.R. (1979). Theoretical, practical, and social issues in behavioral treatments of obesity. *Journal of Applied Behavior Analysis, 12,* 3–25.

Pancreatitis

Inflammation of the pancreas can be caused by gallstones (acute) or long-term alcohol use (chronic). Regardless of the cause, inflammation results from autodigestion attributed to obstruction of the pancreatic duct and hypersecretion of pancreatic exocrine enzymes.

Diagnostic Cluster

▲ Time Frame
Initial diagnosis
Recurrent acute episode

▲ Discharge Criteria
The client or family will:
1. Explain the causes of symptoms
2. Describe signs and symptoms that must be reported to a health care professional
3. Relate the importance of adhering to dietary restrictions and avoiding alcohol
4. If alcohol abuse is present, admits to the problem
5. Relate community resources available for alcoholism

Collaborative Problems

Potential Complications:
Hypovolemia/Shock
Hypocalcemia
Hyperglycemia
Delirium Tremens

Nursing Diagnoses

Pain related to nasogastric suction, distention of pancreatic capsule, and local peritonitis

Diarrhea related to excessive excretion of fats in stools secondary to insufficient pancreatic enzymes

Altered Nutrition: Less Than Body Requirements related to vomiting, anorexia, impaired digestion secondary to decreased pancreatic enzymes

Ineffective Denial related to acknowledgment of alcohol abuse or dependency

Potential Altered Health Maintenance related to lack of knowledge of disease process, treatments, contraindications, dietary management, and follow-up care

Collaborative Problems

▲ Nursing Goals
The nurse will manage and minimize episodes of:
Hypovolemia
Hypocalcemia
Hyperglycemia
Delirium tremens

Potential Complication: Hypovolemia/Shock
Potential Complication: Hypocalcemia
Potential Complication: Hyperglycemia
Potential Complication: Delirium Tremens

Interventions

1. Monitor for signs and symptoms of hypovolemia and shock:
   a. Increasing pulse rate, normal or slightly decreased blood pressure
   b. Urine output < 30 mL/hr
   c. Restlessness, agitation, change in mentation
   d. Increasing respiratory rate
   e. Diminished peripheral pulses
   f. Cool, pale, or cyanotic skin
   g. Thirst

Rationale

1. Hypovolemia related to pancreatitis can have several origins, including decreased oral intake, NPO status, and excess fluid loss through nasogastric tube drainage or vomiting. In addition, pancreatic enzymes destroy vessel walls, resulting in bleeding. Plasma shifts secondary to increased vascular permeability resulting from the inflammatory response also contribute to hypovolemia. The compensatory response to decreased circulatory volume is to increase blood oxygen by increasing heart and respiratory rates and to decrease circulation to the extremities, causing decreased pulse and cool

Interventions

2. Monitor fluid status:
   a. Intake (parenteral, oral)
   b. Output/loss (urinary, nasogastric tube, drainage, vomiting)
3. Monitor for signs and symptoms of hypocalcemia:
   a. Change in mental status
   b. Cardiac dysrhythmias
   c. Numbness, tingling of fingers, toes
   d. Muscle cramps
   e. Seizures
4. Monitor glucose levels in blood and urine.

5. Monitor for signs and symptoms of hyperglycemia:
   a. Early signs
      • Polyurea
      • Polydipsia
   b. Later manifestations (ketoacidosis)
      • Polyphagia
      • Fruity breath odor
      • Weakness
      • Warm, flushed, dry skin
      • Hypotension
      • Blood glucose > 300 mg/dL
6. Monitor for signs and symptoms of alcohol withdrawal:
   a. Tremors
   b. Diaphoresis
   c. Anorexia, nausea, vomiting
   d. Increased heart rate and respiratory rate
   e. Agitation
   f. Hallucinations (visual or auditory)
   g. Delirium tremens (grand mal seizures, disorientation to time and place, panic level of anxiety, visual hallucinations)
7. Consult with a physician for sedation in appropriate dosage to control symptoms.
8. Take measures to reduce stimulation:
   a. Keep a night line on.
   b. Reduce noise.
   c. Turn off bright lights.
   d. Lower the volume of TV and radio.
   e. Speak slowly in short sentences.
9. Do not leave the client alone.

▲ **Documentation**

Flow records
  Vital signs
  Intake and output
Progress notes
  Behavior, orientation
  Changes in physiological
    status
  Actions taken
  Response

Rationale

skin. Diminished oxygen to the brain causes changes in mentation.
2. Fluid shifts, nasogastric suctioning, and NPO status can disrupt fluid balance in a high-risk client. Stress can produce sodium and water retention.
3. Calcium binds with free fats, which are excreted owing to the lack of lipase and phospholipase, which are needed for digestion. Low serum calcium levels produce increased neural excitability, resulting in muscle spasms (cardiac, facial, extremities) and central nervous system irritability (seizures).
4. Injury to pancreatic beta cells decreases insulin production; injury to pancreatic alpha cells increases glucagon production.
5. Without insulin, cells cannot utilize glucose. Protein and fats are then metabolized, producing ketones. Ketoacidosis results, with the lungs and kidneys attempting to return the pH to normal. Increased urine excretion causes losses of water, sodium, potassium, magnesium, calcium, and phosphate. Respiration increases to reduce CO_2 levels.

6. Because chronic alcohol abuse can cause pancreatitis, the nurse must be alert for the signs even when the client denies alcoholism. Signs of alcohol withdrawal begin 24 hours after the last drink and can continue for 1 to 2 weeks.

7. Alcohol withdrawal often requires large doses of sedatives to prevent seizures.
8. Reducing stimuli can help reduce client anxiety.

9. High levels of panic and anxiety can herald acts of violence or suicide. Even when anxiety decreases, the risk for suicide often still remains.

Related Physician-Prescribed Interventions
Medications

Antibiotic therapy	Replacement enzymes
Vitamins	Analgesics
Insulin	Antacids
Anticholinergics	Tranquilizers/sedatives

Related Physician-Prescribed Interventions (Continued)

Intravenous Therapy
  Fluid/electrolyte replacement
Laboratory Studies
  Serum amylase   *Serum calcium and potassium*
  Urine amylase   *Triglycerides*
  Serum lipase, bilirubin   *LDH, SGOT*
  Serum albumin, protein   *Prothrombin time*
  Alkaline phosphates   *Coagulation studies*
  Serum glucose   *Cultures (blood, urine)*
Diagnostic Studies
  CT scan   *Upper GI series*
  Endoscopy
Therapies
  Nothing by mouth (NPO)   *Low-fat diet*
  Gastric suction

▲ **Outcome Criteria**

The client will report a progressive reduction of pain and relief after pain relief measures.

Pain related to nasogastric suction, distention of pancreatic capsule, and local peritonitis

Focus Assessment Criteria	*Clinical Significance*

1. Source of pain:
  a. Epigastric area
  b. Back, chest
  c. Flatus
  d. Nasogastric tube
	1. Determining the source and nature of the pain helps guide interventions.

2. Severity of pain based on a pain scale of 0 to 10 (0 = absence of pain; 10 = worst pain), rated:
  a. At its best
  b. At its worst
  c. After each pain relief measure
	2. A client with chronic pain may exhibit no outward signs. A rating scale provides a good method to measure the subjective experience of pain.

3. Physical signs of acute pain:
  a. Increased heart rate and respiratory rate
  b. Elevated blood pressure
  c. Restlessness
  d. Facial grimacing
  e. Guarding
	3. Some clients are reluctant to admit pain.

Interventions	*Rationale*
1. Collaborate with the individual to determine what methods could be used to reduce the pain's intensity.	1. The client has the most intimate and accurate knowledge of his pain.

2. Relate to the individual your acceptance of his response to pain:
  a. Acknowledge the presence of his pain.
  b. Listen attentively to his descriptions of the pain.
  c. Convey that you are assessing his pain because you want to understand it better.
	2. A client who must try to convince health care providers that he has pain experiences increased anxiety, which may increase the pain.

3. Provide accurate information and clear up any misconceptions the client may have: a. Explain the cause of the pain, if known.	3. A client who is prepared for a painful experience through an explanation of the actual sensations that he will feel tends to experience less

Interventions

    b. Relate how long the pain should last, if known.

    c. If indicated, provide accurate information on the risk of addiction to pain medications.

4. Provide nasogastric tube care, if appropriate:

    a. Explain that the tube is used to reduce gastric contents, which reduces pancreatic secretions.

    b. Apply a water-soluble lubricant around the nares to prevent irritation.

    c. Turn the client every 2 hours, to alternate the pressure of the tube on the esophageal mucosa.

    d. Provide frequent oral care with gargling; avoid alcohol-based mouthwashes, which dry mucosa.

5. Explain the need for bed rest.

6. Intervene to reduce accumulated gas, as indicated:

    a. Encourage frequent position changes, which can stimulate peristalsis.

    b. Advise the client to avoid gas-producing foods and fluids (e.g., soda, cabbage, beans, onions).

    c. Use a rectal tube as needed to expel flatus.

    d. If possible, administer non-narcotic analgesics. (Narcotics increase gas accumulation by decreasing peristalsis.)

    e. Encourage the client to experiment with positions to expel gas; e.g., side-lying with knees drawn up to the chest, prone.

7. Explain the need for the following:

    a. Advance diet slowly and avoid large meals, to reduce pancreatic activity

    b. Take antacids to neutralize gastric acid

    c. Restrict dietary fats (e.g., fried foods, ice cream, whole milk, nuts, gravies, meat fat, bacon), which require pancreatic enzymes for digestion

Rationale

stress than a client who receives vague or no explanations. Addiction is a psychological phenomenon involving the regular use of narcotics for emotional, not medical, reasons.

4. These interventions can reduce some of the discomfort associated with nasogastric tube use.

5. Rest decreases metabolism, reduces gastric secretions, and allows available energy to be used for healing.

6. Gas accumulation can be very painful.

7. The pain of pancreatitis may be reduced through modifications in eating habits.

▲ **Documentation**

Medication administration record
    Type, route, and dosage of all medications
Progress notes
    Status of pain
    Degree of relief from pain-relief measures

▲ **Outcome Criteria**

The client will:

1. Describe factors that cause diarrhea

2. Explain the rationales for interventions

3. Experience fewer episodes of diarrhea

Diarrhea related to excessive excretion of fats in stools secondary to insufficient pancreatic enzymes

Focus Assessment Criteria	*Clinical Significance*
1. Frequency, consistency, odor, and amount of stools	**1.** Decreased pancreatic enzyme secretion impairs protein and fat digestion. Undigested fats are excreted in the stool, increasing the fat content of stool to 50% to 90% compared to the normal value of approximately 20%. Steatorrhea—foul-smelling, frothy, frequent stools—results.

Interventions

1. Maintain an odor-free patient environment:
   a. Empty bedpan or commode immediately.
   b. Change soiled linen.
   c. Provide room deodorizer.
2. Provide good perianal care. Apply ointment (such as A and D Ointment) to protect tissue.
3. Instruct the client to avoid the following items:
   a. Hot or cold liquids
   b. Foods containing fat or fiber (e.g., milk, fruits)
   c. Caffeine
4. Instruct the client to report episodes of steatorrhea after discharge.

Rationale

1. Fecal odor causes embarrassment and self-consciousness and increases the stress of living with pancreatitis.

2. Frequent stools of increased acidity can irritate perianal skin.
3. Cold liquids can induce cramping; hot liquids can stimulate peristalsis. Fat and fiber increase peristalsis, and caffeine stimulates intestinal motility.

4. Steatorrhea may indicate worsening pancreatitis.

▲ **Documentation**

Flow records
   Intake and output
   Frequency of stools
   Consistency of stools

▲ **Outcome Criteria**

The client will:

1. Describe reasons for dietary restrictions
2. Weigh within norm for height and age

Altered Nutrition: Less than Body Requirements related to vomiting, anorexia, impaired digestion secondary to decreased pancreatic enzymes

Focus Assessment Criteria	*Clinical Significance*
1. Weight, intake	1. Pancreatitis can negatively affect nutrition because of decreased intake and impaired digestion. Weight can serve as an indicator of nitrogen balance. The diet's adequacy in meeting nutritional requirements also must be evaluated.
2. Stools (amount, characteristics)	2. Steatorrhea indicates impaired digestion.
3. Complaints of nausea, vomiting, stomatitis, gastritis, flatus	3. These symptoms can adversely affect eating patterns.
4. Laboratory values: BUN; serum albumin, protein, and cholesterol; hematocrit; hemoglobin	4. Presence of insufficient pancreatic enzymes in the GI tract results in insufficient protein catabolism and decreased protein absorption, producing decreased levels of BUN, serum albumin, cholesterol, and transferrin. Decreased transferrin (a protein) causes inadequate iron absorption and transport, resulting in decreased hematocrit hemoglobin.

Interventions

1. Promote foods that stimulate eating and increase calorie consumption.
2. Maintain good oral hygiene before and after meals.

3. Offer small, frequent feedings.

4. Determine what time of the day the client's appetite is greatest, and plan the most nutritious meal for this time.
5. Explain the need for a high-carbohydrate, low-protein, low-fat diet.

6. Explain the need to avoid alcohol, caffeine, and spicy foods.

Rationale

1. Appetite is negatively influenced by nausea and fear of pain associated with eating.
2. Good oral hygiene decreases microorganisms that can cause foul taste and odor, inhibiting appetite.
3. Small, frequent feedings can reduce malabsorption and distention by decreasing the amount of protein metabolized at one time.
4. This can help ensure intake of nutrients needed for cell growth and repair.

5. A diet low in protein and fat reduces the secretion of secretin and cholecystokinin, thus decreasing autodigestion and destruction of pancreatic cells.
6. Alcohol produces hypersecretion of protein in pancreatic secretions, which causes protein plugs and obstructs pancreatic ducts. Caffeine and spicy foods increase gastric and pancreatic secretions.

▲ **Documentation**

Flow records
   Intake (amount, type, time)
   Weight
   Output (urine, stool, vomitus)

Ineffective Denial related to acknowledgment of alcohol abuse or dependency

▲ **Outcome Criteria**

The client will:

1. State recognition of the need for treatment
2. Express a sense of hope

Focus Assessment Criteria	*Clinical Significance*
1. Alcohol use (reported by client or family) 2. Occupational functioning 3. Family and social functioning 4. Previous rehabilitation attempts	1–4. It is necessary to determine how alcohol use interferes with functioning and the client's desire and ability to acknowledge the need for help.

Interventions

1. Approach the client in a nonjudgmental manner. Be aware of your own feelings regarding alcoholism.

2. Help the client understand that alcoholism is an illness, not a moral problem.

3. Assist the client to examine how drinking has affected relationships, work, etc. Ask how he or she feels when not drinking.
4. Encourage significant others to discuss with the client how alcohol has affected their lives.
5. Focus on how the client can avoid alcohol and recover, not on reasons for drinking.

6. Explain that inpatient treatment programs or self-help groups are critical for assistance in recovering. Specific treatment programs include lectures, psychotherapy, peer assistance, recreational therapy, and support groups.
7. If sanctioned, schedule interactions with recovering alcoholics.
8. If sanctioned, schedule a visit with an expert from a detoxification program for ongoing treatment.
9. Refer the family to Al-Anon and Al-Ateen, as appropriate.

Rationale

1. The client probably has been reprimanded by many and is distrustful. The nurse's personal experiences with alcohol may increase or decrease her empathy for the client.
2. Historically, alcoholics have been viewed as immoral and degenerate. Acknowledgment of alcoholism as a disease can increase the client's sense of trust.
3. During an acute episode of pancreatitis, the client may be more likely to acknowledge his or her drinking problem.
4. Confrontation with family and peers may help to break down the client's denial.
5. The client may try to focus on the reasons for using alcohol in an attempt to minimize the problem's significance.
6. Participation in a structured treatment program greatly increases the chance of successful recovery from alcoholism.

7. Recovering alcoholics provide honest, direct confrontation with the realities of alcoholism.
8. A sense of hope can be promoted by affording the client direct contact with an expert who can help.
9. The client's family needs assistance to identify enabling behavior and strategies for dealing with a recovering or existing alcoholic.

▲ **Documentation**

Progress notes
  Dialogues
Discharge summary record
  Client teaching
  Outcome achievement
  Referrals

▲ **Outcome Criteria**

The outcome criteria for this diagnosis represent those associated with discharge planning. Refer to discharge criteria.

Potential Altered Health Maintenance related to lack of knowledge of disease process, treatments, contraindications, dietary management, and follow-up care

Focus Assessment Criteria	*Clinical Significance*
1. Client's readiness and ability to learn and retain information	1. A client who does not achieve the goals for learning requires a referral for assistance postdischarge.

Interventions

1. Explain causes of acute and chronic pancreatitis.

2. Teach the client to report these symptoms:
   a. Steatorrhea
   b. Severe back or epigastric pain
   c. Persistent gastritis, nausea, or vomiting

Rationale

1. Inaccurate perceptions of health status usually involve misunderstanding of the nature and seriousness of the illness, susceptibility to complications, and the need for restrictions for control of illness.
2. These signs and symptoms can indicate worsening of inflammation and increased malabsorption. Elevated temperature could indicate infection or abscess formation.

Interventions

▲ **Documentation**
Discharge summary record
 Client teaching
 Outcome achievement
 Referrals, if indicated

   d. Weight loss
   e. Elevated temperature
3. Explain the relationship of hyperglycemia to pancreatitis; teach the client to observe for and report signs and symptoms.

Rationale

3. Early detection and reporting enables prompt intervention to prevent serious complications.

References/Bibliography

Adinaro, D. (1987). Liver failure and pancreatitis: Fluid and electrolyte concerns. *Nursing Clinics of North America, 22*(4), 843–852.

Jeffers, C. (1989). Complications of acute pancreatitis/CE quiz. *Critical Care Nurse, 9*(4), 9.

Moorhouse, M.E., et al. (1988). Acute pancreatitis. *Journal of Emergency Nursing, 14*(6), 387–391.

Gastrointestinal Disorders

Gastroenteritis

An inflammation of the stomach and intestines, gastroenteritis can be caused by bacterial or viral pathogens. Most commonly, infection results from ingestion of food contaminated with *Staphylococcus* or *Salmonella* microorganisms. The infecting organisms penetrate the epithelial cells in the small intestine and colon, triggering an inflammatory response.

Diagnostic Cluster

▲ Time Frame
Acute episode

▲ Discharge Criteria
Before discharge, the client or family will:
1. Describe the causes of gastroenteritis and its transmission
2. Identify dietary restrictions that promote comfort and healing
3. State signs and symptoms of dehydration
4. State signs and symptoms that must be reported to a health care professional

Collaborative Problems

Potential Complication:
Fluid/Electrolyte Imbalance

Nursing Diagnoses

Potential Fluid Volume Deficit related to losses secondary to vomiting and diarrhea

Altered Comfort related to abdominal cramping, diarrhea, and vomiting secondary to vascular dilatation and hyperperistalsis

Potential Altered Health Maintenance related to lack of knowledge of condition, dietary restrictions, and signs and symptoms of complications

Collaborative Problems

▲ Nursing Goal
The nurse will manage and minimize episodes of fluid and electrolyte imbalance.

▲ Documentation
Flow records
  Intake and output
  Stools (amount, consistency)

Potential Complication: Fluid/Electrolyte Imbalances

Interventions

1. Monitor for signs and symptoms of dehydration:
   a. Dry skin and mucous membrane
   b. Elevated urine specific gravity
   c. Thirst
2. Carefully monitor intake and output.

3. Monitor for electrolyte imbalances:
   a. Sodium
   b. Chloride
   c. Potassium

Rationale

1. Rapid propulsion of feces through the intestines decreases water absorption. Low circulatory volume causes dry mucous membranes and thirst. Concentrated urine has an elevated specific gravity.
2. Intake and output records help detect early signs of fluid imbalance.
3. Rapid propulsion of feces through the intestines decreases electrolyte absorption. Vomiting also causes electrolyte loss.

Related Physician-Prescribed Interventions

Medications
  Antidiarrheals

Intravenous Therapy
  Fluid/electrolyte replacement

Laboratory Studies
  Stool cultures   Stool examination for blood, bacteria, parasites

Diagnostic Studies
  Not indicated

Therapies
  Diet as tolerated (e.g., clear fluids, full fluids, bland soft)

Nursing Diagnoses

▲ Outcome Criteria

The client will have a urine specific gravity between 1.010 and 1.025.

Potential Fluid Volume Deficit related to losses secondary to vomiting and diarrhea

Focus Assessment Criteria	Clinical Significance
1. Vital signs: blood pressure, temperature, pulse, respirations 2. Skin turgor, mucous membranes, urine output 3. Consistency and frequency of stools 4. Laboratory studies: electrolytes, urine specific gravity, BUN	1–4. These assessments provide baseline data for comparison with subsequent assessment findings.

Interventions

1. Monitor for early signs and symptoms of fluid volume deficit
   a. Dry mucous membranes (lips, gums)
   b. Amber urine
   c. Specific gravity > 1.025
2. Administer parenteral antiemetic medications, as ordered, parenterally
3. Give the client sips of weak tea, carbonated drinks, or tap water.
4. Monitor intake and output, making sure that intake compensates for output.

▲ Documentation

Flow records
   Vital signs
   Intake and output
   Daily weights
   Medications
   Vomiting episodes

5. Weigh the client daily.

Rationale

1. Decreased circulating volume causes drying of tissues and concentrated urine. Early detection enables prompt fluid replacement therapy to correct deficits.

2. Antiemetics prevent vomiting by inhibiting stimuli to the vomiting center.
3. Small amounts of clear liquids are more easily tolerated by irritated gastric mucosa.
4. Output may exceed intake, which already may be inadequate to compensate for insensible losses. Dehydration may increase the glomerular filtration rate, making output inadequate to clear wastes properly and leading to elevated BUN and electrolyte levels.
5. Accurate daily weights can detect fluid loss.

▲ Outcome Criteria

The client will:

1. Report a reduction in abdominal cramping
2. List foods to avoid

Altered Comfort related to abdominal cramps, diarrhea, and vomiting secondary to vascular dilatation and hyperperistalsis

Focus Assessment Criteria	Clinical Significance
1. Complaints of abdominal cramps, diarrhea, vomiting 2. Factors that may precipitate symptoms	1,2. This assessment helps evaluate the client's status and identify possible sources of irritation.

Interventions

1. Encourage the client to rest in the supine position with a warm heating pad on the abdomen.
2. Encourage frequent intake of small amounts of cool clear liquids (e.g., dilute tea, flat ginger ale, jello water): 30 to 60 mL every ½ to 1 hour.
3. Eliminate unpleasant sights and odors from the client's environment.
4. Instruct the client to avoid these items:
   a. Hot or cold liquids
   b. Foods containing fat or fiber (e.g., milk, fruits)
   c. Caffeine
5. Protect the perianal area from irritation.

▲ Documentation

Flow records
   Intake and output
   Tolerance of intake
   Stools (frequency, characteristics, consistency)
   Bowel sounds

Rationale

1. These measures promote GI muscular relaxation and reduce cramping.
2. Small amounts of fluids do not distend the gastric area and thus do not aggravate symptoms.

3. Unpleasant sights or odors can stimulate the vomiting center.
4. Cold liquids can induce cramping; hot liquids can stimulate peristalsis. Fats also increase peristalsis, and caffeine increases intestinal motility.

5. Frequent stools of increased acidity can irritate perianal skin.

▲ *Outcome Criteria*

The outcome criteria for this diagnosis represent those associated with discharge planning. Refer to the discharge criteria.

Potential Altered Health Maintenance related to lack of knowledge of condition, dietary restrictions, and signs and symptoms of complications

Focus Assessment Criteria	*Clinical Significance*
1. Knowledge of causative agents of gastroenteritis	1–3. This assessment helps determine the content and focus of client teaching.
2. Readiness for learning and possible barriers that might interfere	
3. Support person(s) who will assist the client	

Interventions

1. Discuss the disease process in understandable terms; explain the following:
   a. Causative agents
   b. Reason for enteric precautions
   c. Preventive measures
   d. Importance of scrupulous hand washing
2. Explain dietary restrictions:
   a. High-fiber foods (e.g., bran, fresh fruit)
   b. High-fat foods (e.g., whole milk, fried foods)
   c. Very hot or cold fluids
3. Teach the client and family to report these symptoms:
   a. Inability to retain fluids
   b. Dark amber urine persisting for more than 12 hours
4. Explain the importance of maintaining a balance between oral fluid intake and fluid output.
5. Explain the benefits of rest and encourage adequate rest.
6. Explain preventive measures:
   a. Proper food storage/refrigeration
   b. Proper cleaning of kitchen utensils, especially wooden cutting boards
   c. Handwashing before and after handling food

Rationale

1. The client's understanding may increase compliance with dietary restrictions and hygiene practices.

2. These foods can stimulate or irritate the intestinal tract.

3. Early detection and reporting of the signs of dehydration enable prompt interventions to prevent serious fluid or electrolyte imbalances.

4. Vomiting and diarrhea can rapidly cause dehydration.
5. Inactivity reduces peristalsis and allows the GI tract to rest.
6. The most common cause of gastroenteritis is ingestion of bacteria-contaminated food.

▲ *Documentation*

Discharge summary record
  Discharge instructions
  Progress toward goal attainment
  Status at discharge

References/Bibliography

Given, B., & Simmons, S.J. (1984). *Gastroenterology in clinical nursing* (4th ed.). Philadelphia: J.B. Lippincott.
Lamy, P.P. (1985). Treating GI upset in older adults. *Journal of Gerontology Nursing, 11*(7), 40–42.
Spollett, G. (1989). Irritable bowel syndrome: Diagnosis and treatment. *Nurse Practitioner, 14*(8), 32–44.

Inflammatory Bowel Disease

Comprising both Crohn's disease and ulcerative colitis, inflammatory bowel disease (IBD) causes inflammation of the intestinal lining and wall. As a result of increased blood flow to the tissues, the bowel becomes swollen and painful. Ulcers may form on the intestine lining and may penetrate deep into the damaged wall. Inflammation and ulcers also may narrow the intestinal lumen, interfering with passage of intestinal contents. Most cases of IBD are diagnosed in clients under age 30 (Myer, 1984).

Diagnostic Cluster

▲ Time Frame

Initial diagnosis
Recurrent acute episodes

▲ Discharge Criteria

Before discharge, the client or family will:

1. Discuss management of activities of daily living
2. State signs and symptoms that must be reported to a health care professional
3. Verbalize an intent to share feelings and concerns related to IBD with significant others
4. Identify available community resources or self-help groups

Collaborative Problems

Potential Complications:
Fluid/Electrolyte Imbalances
Intestinal Obstruction
Fistula/Fissure/Abscess
GI Bleeding
Anemia
Toxic Megacolon
Urolithiasis
Growth Retardation

Nursing Diagnoses

Chronic Pain related to intestinal inflammatory process
Altered Nutrition: Less Than Body Requirements related to dietary restrictions, nausea, diarrhea, and abdominal cramping associated with eating or painful ulcers of the oral mucous membrane
Diarrhea related to intestinal inflammatory process
Potential Ineffective Individual Coping related to chronicity of condition and lack of definitive treatment
Potential Altered Health Maintenance related to lack of knowledge of condition, diagnostic tests, prognosis, treatment, and signs and symptoms of complications

Related Care Plan

Corticosteroid Therapy

Collaborative Problems

▲ Nursing Goal

The nurse will detect and minimize complications of inflammatory bowel disease.

Potential Complication: **Fluid/Electrolyte Imbalances**
Potential Complication: **Intestinal Obstruction**
Potential Complication: **Fistula/Fissure/Abscess**
Potential Complication: **GI Bleeding**
Potential Complication: **Anemia**
Potential Complication: **Toxic Megacolon**
Potential Complication: **Urolithiasis**
Potential Complication: **Growth Retardation**

Interventions

1. Monitor laboratory values for electrolyte imbalances:
   a. Potassium level
   b. Sodium level
   c. Calcium level

Rationale

1. Chronic diarrhea and inadequate oral intake can deplete electrolytes. Small intestine inflammation impairs absorption of fluid and electrolytes.

Interventions

    d. Phosphorus level
    e. Magnesium level
    f. Zinc level
  2. Monitor for signs and symptoms of dehydration:
    a. Tachycardia
    b. Dry skin/mucous membrane
    c. Elevated urine specific gravity
    d. Thirst
  3. Monitor intake and output.

  4. Collect 24-hour urine samples weekly for evaluation of electrolytes, calcium, phosphates, urea, and nitrogen.
  5. Monitor for signs and symptoms of intestinal obstruction:
    a. Wavelike abdominal pain
    b. Vomiting (gastric juices, bile progressing to fecal material)
    c. Abdominal distention
    d. Change in bowel sounds (initially hyperactive progressing to none).
  6. If you suspect intestinal obstruction, withhold all food and fluids and notify the physician.

  7. Monitor for signs and symptoms of fistula, fissures, or abscesses:
    a. Purulent drainage
    b. Fecal drainage from vagina
    c. Increased abdominal pain
    d. Burning rectal pain following defecation
    e. Perianal induration, swelling, redness, and cyanotic tags
    f. Signs of sepsis (e.g., fever, increased WBC count)
  8. Monitor for signs and symptoms of GI bleeding:
    a. Decreased hemoglobin and hematocrit
    b. Fatigue
    c. Irritability
    d. Pallor
    e. Tachycardia
    f. Dyspnea
    g. Anorexia
  9. Monitor for signs of anemia:
    a. Decreased hemoglobin
    b. Decreased red blood cells
    c. B_{12} deficiency
    d. Folate deficiency

  10. Monitor for signs and symptoms of urolithiasis (refer to the Urolithiasis care plan if they occur):
    a. Flank pain
    b. Fever, chills

▲ **Documentation**

Flow records
  Abnormal laboratory values
  Vital signs
  Intake and output
  Bowel sounds
  Diarrhea episodes
  Vomiting episodes
  Drainage (wound, rectal, vaginal)
  Urine specific gravity

Rationale

  2. When circulating volume decreases, heart rate increases in an attempt to supply tissues with oxygen. Low circulatory volume causes dry mucous membranes and thirst. Concentrated urine has an elevated specific gravity.

  3. Intake and output monitoring provides early detection of fluid imbalance.
  4. This enables evaluation of electrolyte status and renal function.

  5. Inflammation and edema cause the obstruction. Intestinal contents are then propelled toward the mouth instead of the rectum.

  6. Avoidance of foods and fluids prevents further distention and prepares the GI tract for surgery.
  7. The inflammation and ulceration of Crohn's disease can penetrate the intestinal wall and form an abscess or fistula to other parts of the intestine or skin. Abscesses and fistulas may cause cramping, pain, and fever and may interfere with digestion. Sepsis may arise from seeding of the bloodstream from fistula tracts or abscess cavities.

  8. Chronic inflammation can cause erosion of vessels and bleeding.

  9. Anemia may result from GI bleeding, bone marrow depression (associated with chronic inflammatory diseases), and inadequate intake or impaired absorption of vitamin B_{12}, folic acid, and iron. Sulfasalazine therapy can cause hemolysis, which contributes to anemia.
  10. Severe diarrhea can lead to a decreased volume of concentrated urine. This, combined with intestinal bicarbonate loss and lowered pH, leads to the development of urate stones. With ileal resection or severe IBD, the calcium normally available to bind with oxalate binds instead with fatty acids, freeing dietary oxalate for absorption. Decreased urine volume enhances the precipitation of calcium oxalate in the kidney, predisposing to stone formation.

Interventions

11. Monitor an adolescent client for signs of growth retardation:
    a. Delayed bone growth
    b. Weight loss
    c. Delayed development of secondary sex characteristics

Rationale

11. Possible causes include decreased nutritional intake, loss of protein and nutrients by rapid passage through the GI tract, increased metabolic requirements secondary to bowel inflammation, and corticosteroid therapy (Hillemeier and McCallum, 1983).

Related Physician-Prescribed Interventions

Medications
Antidiarrheals
Immunosuppressants
Corticosteroids
Anticholinergics
Vitamins/minerals

Analgesics
Antibiotics
Bile acid sequestrants
Bulk-producing laxatives

Intravenous Therapy
Fluid/electrolyte replacement

Laboratory Studies
CBC
Serum electrolytes
Blood urea nitrogen
Creatinine

Serum protein electrophoresis
Sedimentation rate
Alkaline phosphatase

Diagnostic Studies
Colonoscopy
GI x-ray film

Biopsy

Therapies
Low-residue, high-protein diet

Nursing Diagnoses

▲ Outcome Criteria

The client will:
1. Relate that others acknowledge and validate the pain
2. Practice noninvasive pain relief measures to manage pain
3. Relate improvement of pain and an increase in ability to perform activities of daily living (ADLs)

Chronic Pain related to intestinal inflammatory process

Focus Assessment Criteria

1. Client's pain experience: intensity and tolerance

2. Factors that increase or decrease pain (e.g., eating, passing stool, flatus)

3. Effects of pain on client's life style and ability to perform ADLs
4. Knowledge of pain management techniques

Clinical Significance

1. Pain tolerance differs among clients and may vary in the same client in different circumstances.
2. Increased pain without relief from usual interventions may indicate complications such as intestinal obstruction or peritonitis.
3,4. This assessment may indicate the need for alternative pain management strategies.

Interventions

1. Acknowledge the presence of the client's pain.

2. Have the client rate pain intensity on a scale of 1 to 5 (1 = no pain; 5 = greatest pain possible), and his level of pain tolerance (1 = can tolerate; 5 = cannot tolerate at all).
3. Determine the relationship between eating and drinking and abdominal pain.

4. Determine the relationship between passage of stool or flatus and pain relief.

5. Determine the effects of chronic pain on the client's life style.

Rationale

1. Acknowledging and validating a client's pain may help reduce his anxiety, which can decrease pain.
2. Such a rating scale provides a good method of evaluating the subjective experience of pain.

3. The client may link eating or drinking to onset of abdominal pain, and may limit intake to avoid pain.
4. Pain not relieved by passage of feces or flatus may be a sign of intestinal obstruction or peritonitis.
5. Chronic pain can cause withdrawal, depression, anger, and dependency.

Interventions

6. Determine whether or not pain occurs during the night.

7. Provide for pain relief:
   a. Assist with position changes.

   b. Apply a warm heating pad to the abdomen—*except* during an acute flare-up of IBD.
   c. Encourage relaxation exercises.

   d. Encourage diversional activities such as family visits, telephone calls, and involvement in self-care.
   e. Administer prescribed anticholinergics to provide relief from cramping. Withhold if signs or symptoms of intestinal obstruction occur. Avoid narcotic analgesics.

8. Evaluate the effectiveness of the pain management plan.

Rationale

6. Abdominal cramps or a feeling of urgency to defecate may awaken the client at night. This usually occurs less often in Crohn's disease than in ulcerative colitis.

7.
   a. Repositioning may help move air through the bowel, relieving cramps.
   b. Warmth relaxes abdominal muscles.

   c. Relaxation may enhance the therapeutic effects of pain medication.
   d. Diversion may help distract the client from pain.

   e. Anticholinergic drugs decrease GI motility and help relieve cramping. Narcotic analgesics generally are discouraged because they mask the symptoms of life-threatening complications. Chronic use may also cause obstruction.

8. Frequent evaluation of pain relief enables adjustment of the regimen for maximum effectiveness. Failure to manage chronic pain may lead to depression.

▲ **Documentation**

Medication administration record
  Type, dosage, and route of all medications
Progress notes
  Pain descriptions
  Unsatisfactory relief from pain relief measures

▲ **Outcome Criteria**

The client will:

1. Verbalize understanding of nutritional requirements
2. Be in positive nitrogen balance as evidenced by weight gain of 2–3 lb/wk and by increased energy level and feelings of well-being

Altered Nutrition: Less Than Body Requirements related to dietary restrictions, nausea, diarrhea, and abdominal cramping associated with eating or painful ulcers of the oral mucosa

Focus Assessment Criteria

1. Appetite and energy level

2. Current body weight and history of recent weight loss

3. Food intolerances, if any

4. Condition of oral mucosa

5. Anthropometric measurements: mid-arm circumference, triceps skinfold

6. Relationship of eating to onset of nausea, diarrhea, or abdominal pain

Clinical Significance

1. A client with IBD typically suffers from malnourishment because of the malabsorption of nutrients in the bowel wall. In addition, the client tends to eat less because he associates nausea and abdominal cramping with food intake.

2. Weight loss is reported in 65% to 70% of clients with IBD. Weight loss may exceed 10 lb a month.

3. A client with IBD may have food intolerance to milk, fried or spicy foods, and foods high in fiber. In Crohn's disease, structural changes in the intestinal villi result in decreased absorption area and loss of the intestinal enzyme lactase.

4. A client with Crohn's disease is susceptible to painful aphthous ulcers of the mouth.

5. Anthropometric measurements help evaluate nutritional status. Mid-arm circumference measures somatic muscle mass; triceps skin fold estimates subcutaneous fat stored.

6. This assessment helps determine patterns and differentiate complications (intestinal obstruction and peritonitis).

Focus Assessment Criteria	*Clinical Significance*
7. Laboratory data:	**7.**
a. Serum albumin	**a.** Serum albumin levels reflect the body's protein status. Serum albumin takes about 3 weeks for protein repletion to be reflected. Clients with acute IBD have been shown to lose from two to 60 times the amount of albumin lost by healthy persons.
b. Serum transferrin and iron	**b.** Transferrin is the major transport protein for iron. Serum transferrin reflects protein repletion in 1 week.
c. Hemoglobin and hematocrit **d.** Total lymphocyte count	**c,d.** Protein malnutrition results in decreased WBC count and anemia.
e. Zinc, trace minerals	**e.** A client with IBD often has chronic zinc deficiency, manifested by anxiety, depression, alopecia, acrodermatitis, and diarrhea. Daily intravenous replacement improves these symptoms dramatically. Within hours, mental depression and anxiety are relieved, diarrhea responds to treatment, and the dermatitis begins resolving. Alopecia reverses within 2 weeks.

Interventions	*Rationale*

1. Administer total parenteral nutrition (TPN) therapy, as ordered, and intervene as follows:
  a. Teach long-term venous access catheter care. (Refer to the Long-Term Venous Access Devices care plan, page 572, for more information.)
	1.
	
	  a. TPN is the treatment of choice when weight loss, nutritional depletion, and symptoms of IBD are severe. In TPN, the client requires 45 to 50 Kcal and about 2 g of protein/kg of body weight/day to remain in positive nitrogen balance. This allows weight gain of about 8 oz/day. Clients with ulcerative colitis do not benefit from TPN therapy as greatly as do those with Crohn's disease.

b. Maintain NPO status.	**b.** NPO status decreases the mechanical, physical, and chemical activity of the bowel.
c. Provide psychosocial support and reassurance during bowel rest and TPN.	**c.** Prolonged NPO status is disturbing both socially and psychologically.
d. Assist the client to ambulate with an intravenous pole.	**d.** Ambulation enhances the client's sense of well-being and helps maintain or improve physical conditioning.

2. Wean the client from TPN feedings, when ordered:
  a. Use a relaxed, confident, consistent approach to TPN catheter care.
  b. Provide emotional support during the weaning process.
	2.
	
	  a,b. A client receiving TPN typically views the TPN catheter as his "lifeline." He may feel protective of it and question the expertise of the professional staff caring for it.

c. Reassure the client that weight loss during the first week off TPN is due to fluid loss.	**c.** A client generally loses 4 to 5 lb of fluid during the first week off TPN.
d. Help the client set realistic expectations for gaining weight after discontinuation of TPN.	**d.** The client may expect to gain weight on oral feeding at the same rate as when on TPN. This is not a realistic expectation, however.
e. Encourage use of high-protein drinks with meals.	**e.** Dietary supplements may be needed to meet nutritional requirements.

Interventions

    f. Arrange for a dietitian to spend time with the client.

3. Assist the client in resuming oral food intake:

    a. Encourage liquids with caloric value rather than coffee, tea, water, or diet soda.

    b. Assess the client's acceptance of and response to oral fluid intake.

    c. Start formula feedings in dilute form and progress to full strength as tolerated.

    d. Offer a variety of flavors of elemental feedings and keep them chilled.

    e. Assist with progression to soft, bland, and low-residue solids and encourage small frequent feedings high in calories, protein, vitamins, and carbohydrates.

    f. Teach the client to avoid raw fruits, vegetables, condiments, whole-grain cereals, gas-forming and fried foods, alcohol, and iced drinks.

    g. As ordered, supplement the client's diet with folic acid, ascorbic acid, iron, calcium, copper, and zinc.

Rationale

    f. Consultation may be needed to plan an adequate dietary regimen.

3. The client may need encouragement to resume oral intake, as he may resist for fear of pain.

    a. Calorie-rich liquids can help prevent malnutrition.

    b. The ability to absorb nutrients must be evaluated daily.

    c. If the client cannot tolerate a regular diet, elemental feedings may be ordered. They are better tolerated because they are residue-free, low in fat, nutritionally balanced, and digested mainly in the upper jejunum. They do not stimulate pancreatic, biliary, and intestinal secretions as does regular food.

    d. Elemental diets have an unpleasant odor and taste because of the amino acids present. Adding flavor and keeping them chilled increase their palatability.

    e. Gradual introduction of solid foods is needed to reduce pain and increase tolerance.

    f. These foods and liquids can irritate the GI tract.

    g. Mineral and electrolyte imbalances can result from poor absorption; replacement may be necessary.

▲ *Documentation*

Flow records
    Acceptance of food
    Tolerance of food
    Type and amount of food taken orally
    Daily weight
Progress notes
    Energy level

▲ *Outcome Criteria*

The client will:

1. Describe factors that cause diarrhea
2. Explain the rationales for interventions
3. Have fewer episodes of diarrhea
4. Verbalize signs and symptoms of dehydration and electrolyte imbalances

Diarrhea related to intestinal inflammatory process

Focus Assessment Criteria

1. Frequency, consistency, odor, and amount of stools
2. Onset of diarrhea in relationship to any of the following:
    a. Pain
    b. Eating
    c. Activity
    d. Stress
3. Urgency to expel stool
4. Flatus
5. Steatorrhea

6. Blood, mucus, or pus in stools

7. Serum albumin level

Clinical Significance

1–4. In IBD, an inflamed colon fails to reabsorb water and electrolytes, the rectum loses its capacity to retain a fluid load, and the small intestine may fail to absorb water, bile, salts, and lactose. All of these factors contribute to diarrhea. The severity of the diarrhea relates directly to the extent of bowel involvement.

5. Steatorrhea results from high unabsorbed fat content.
6. Blood, mucus, or pus in stools may indicate bleeding or abscess.
7. Hypoalbuminemia may be associated with severe diarrhea.

Interventions

1. Assess for the following:
    a. Decreased number of stools
    b. Increased consistency of stools
    c. Decreased urgency to expel stool

Rationale

1. Stool assessment helps evaluate the effectiveness of antidiarrheal agents and dietary restrictions.

Interventions	*Rationale*

2. Maintain an odor-free patient environment:
  a. Empty the bedpan or commode immediately.
  b. Change soiled linens.
  c. Provide a room deodorizer.
	2. Fecal odor can cause embarrassment and self-consciousness and can increase the stress of living with IBD.

3. Provide good perianal care.	3. Perianal irritation from frequent liquid stool should be prevented.
4. Decrease physical activity during acute episodes of diarrhea.	4. Decreased physical activity decreases bowel peristalsis.
5. Determine the relationship between diarrheal episodes and ingestion of specific foods.	5. Identification of irritating foods can reduce diarrheal episodes.

6. Observe for signs and symptoms of electrolyte imbalance:
  a. Decreased serum potassium
	6.
	
	  a. In osmotic diarrhea, impaired absorption of fluid by the intestines is caused by ingested solutes that cannot be digested, or by a decrease in intestinal absorption. Water and electrolytes are drawn into the intestine in greater quantities than can be absorbed, and the diarrheal fluid is high in potassium.

b. Decreased serum sodium	b. Secretory diarrhea occurs when the gut wall is inflamed or engorged or when it is stimulated by bile salts. The resulting diarrheal stool is high in sodium.

7. Replace fluid and electrolytes with oral fluid containing appropriate electrolytes:
  a. Gatorade, a commercial preparation of glucose-electrolyte solution
  b. Apple juice, which is high in potassium but low in sodium
  c. Colas, root beer, and ginger ale, which contain sodium but have a negligible potassium content
	7. The type of fluid replacement depends on the electrolyte(s) needed.

▲ **Documentation**

Flow records
  Intake and output
  Number of stools
  Consistency of stools
Medication administration record
  Frequency of p.r.n. antidiarrheal medication

▲ **Outcome Criteria**

The client will:
1. Verbalize factors that contribute to anxiety and stress
2. Verbalize methods to improve the ability to cope with the chronic condition

Potential Ineffective Individual Coping related to chronicity of condition and lack of definitive treatment

Focus Assessment Criteria	*Clinical Significance*

1. Emotional status and defense mechanisms:
  a. Independence or dependence
  b. Anger, denial of IBD
  c. Self-control, perfectionism, internal demands
  d. Self-confidence
  e. Perceived stressors and changes in health status
  f. Perceived coping status
	1. IBD is a life-disrupting illness that can dominate the lives of those it affects. The client may have heard that IBD is a "psychosomatic" disease and may misinterpret this to mean that it is all in his mind. He may have been told by family and caregivers that he could be symptom-free if he wished. This can lead to feelings of guilt and powerlessness.

2. Sleep disturbances:
  a. Changes in sleep patterns
  b. Cramping or diarrheal episodes during sleep hours
  c. Energy levels in evening and morning
	2. Some clients with IBD report inability to sleep because of being "wound up" and full of energy at bedtime. This may be related to use of corticosteroids in the treatment of IBD. Lack of sleep may contribute to a lack of ability to cope effectively with a chronic condition.

3. Family and social interactions
  a. Social participation
  b. Availability of and satisfaction with support systems
  c. Demands of others on client
  d. Demands of clients on others
	3. The ever-present risk of uncontrollable diarrhea can isolate the client and restrict the activities of all family members.

Interventions

1. Clear up misconceptions about IBD. Stress that psychological symptoms are a reaction to the IBD, not the cause of IBD.
2. Identify and minimize factors that contribute to anxiety:
   a. Explain all diagnostic tests, and support the client during each procedure.
   b. Do not label the client as "demanding" or a "big baby."
3. Allow the client to have some control over care. Demonstrate acceptance and concern when caring for the client.
4. Set appropriate limits if the client demands constant attention. Explain that frequent checks will be made at specified intervals to ensure that needs are met.
5. Set aside 15 to 30 minutes a day to allow the client time to verbalize fears and frustrations.
6. Reinforce effective coping strategies.

7. Involve family members or significant others in care, if possible.

8. Refer the client and family to the National Foundation for Ileitis and Colitis. (Each state has a chapter that offers self-help support groups for clients and families and annual conferences on coping with inflammatory bowel disease.)
9. Refer to the nursing diagnosis Ineffective Individual Coping in the Ostomy care plan for role-playing strategies to increase coping abilities.

Rationale

1. Correcting misconceptions may help reduce the guilt associated with this belief.

2. Understanding procedures can reduce anxiety. Labels lead to overt or subtle rejection by others and further exaggerate the client's feelings of helplessness and isolation.

3. A client with IBD typically feels as if he has lost control over other aspects of his life.

4. Demanding behavior is a sign of fear and dependency. If the client feels sure that the caregiver will return, he will feel more secure and be less demanding of time.
5. The nurse can use this time to help the client develop new, more effective coping strategies.
6. Reinforcement may promote continued use of effective coping strategies.
7. Family members and others play a very important role in supporting clients and helping them to cope with and accept their disease.
8. Discussing IBD with others with the same problem can reduce feelings of isolation and anxiety. Sharing experiences in a group led by professionals gives the client the benefit of others' experiences with IBD and interpretation of the experiences by health professionals.

▲ *Documentation*

Progress notes
　Participation in self-care
　Emotional status
　Interactions with staff and
　　significant others

▲ *Outcome Criteria*

The outcome criteria for this diagnosis represent those associated with discharge planning. Refer to the discharge criteria.

Potential Altered Health Maintenance related to lack of knowledge of condition, diagnostic tests, prognosis, treatment, or signs and symptoms of complications

Focus Assessment Criteria

1. Knowledge of intestinal signs and symptoms of IBD
2. Knowledge of extraintestinal signs and symptoms of IBD
3. Knowledge of diagnostic tests
4. Family history of IBD
5. Knowledge of etiology, prognosis, and treatment measures
6. Knowledge of potential complications

Clinical Significance

1–6. Assessing the client's and family's learning needs prior to teaching allows the nurse to determine the appropriate content and teaching methods and evaluate their readiness and ability to learn.

Interventions

1. Explain the diagnostic tests:

   a. Colonoscopy is done to explore the large intestine with a long, flexible tube. A clear liquid diet is maintained for 24–48 hours before the procedure, and a cleansing enema may be given before the examination. Medication is given to promote relaxation and aid insertion of the lubricated tube

Rationale

1. Explanations of what to expect can reduce the client's anxiety associated with the unknown.
   a. Colonoscopy may be used to diagnose the medical problem. Polyps can be removed and tissue collected for further study. The procedure may reduce the need for surgery.

Interventions   *Rationale*

into the anus. The procedure takes about 1
hour. The client may feel pressure and
cramping; breathing slowly and deeply may
help relieve discomfort.

b. GI x-ray films: The role of the barium
enema is to determine the extent of the disease early in its progression. It also helps
the endoscopist determine the configuration of the colon and indicates suspicious
areas that should be observed directly by
endoscopy.

c. Biopsy to differentiate ulcerative colitis and
Crohn's disease and to detect dysplasia

d. Blood tests:
- CBC
- Serum electrolytes
- BUN
- Creatinine
- Serum protein electrophoresis
- Sedimentation rate
- Alkaline phosphatase

b. Contrast studies of the colon using barium
have been used historically as a surveillance technique. The repetition of barium
enema every 6 to 12 months raises the
question of the effect of long-term radiation on intestinal mucosa that is already at
risk.

c. If dysplasia is found in multiple areas of
the colon, the patient is in a high-risk
group for developing carcinoma of the colon.

d. Bone marrow depression of blood cells may
be present with fulminating types of colitis.
The white blood count may be elevated and
the sedimentation rate increased. Electrolyte imbalance is common with severe
acute IBD. A decreased serum albumin and
negative nitrogen balance may result from
decreased protein intake and increased metabolic needs. Anemia may be caused by
iron deficiency or by chronic inflammation.

2. Explain the familial aspects of IBD. Although
the cause of IBD is unknown, 15% to 35% of
clients with IBD have a relative with the disorder; thus, it is considered a familial disorder.

3. Explain the possible etiology of IBD; theories
center on the body's immune system and include the following:
a. Hypersensitivity reaction in the gut
b. Autoimmune antibody–mediated damage to
the epithelial cells
c. Tissue deposition of antigen-antibody com-
plexes
d. Lymphocyte-mediated cytotoxicity
e. Impaired cellular immune mechanisms
Emotional and psychological factors have not
been identified or implicated in the etiology of
IBD. However, stress seems to provoke hyper-
reactivity of the colon in susceptible persons.

4. Discuss the prognosis of IBD. IBD typically is
a chronic illness with remissions and relapses.
In Crohn's diseases, the client is much more
likely to develop fistulas and abscesses. In ulcerative colitis, the client is more likely to develop toxic megacolon and carcinoma of the
colon. In ulcerative colitis, total colectomy and
ileostomy is considered a cure, because ulcerative colitis involves only the colon. Crohn's
disease can affect any portion of the intestinal
tract and tends to recur in the proximal bowel
even after colectomy.

5. Discuss the treatment of IBD:
a. Medical
- Medications

2,3 A client with IBD may have been led to believe that anxiety or psychological problems
caused the disorder. Dispelling this belief can
help the client accept the disorder and encourage compliance with treatment.

4. A client usually can deal with a frank and realistic discussion of the prognosis better than
with a lack of information about the prognosis.

5. Treatment of IBD is symptomatic.

Interventions

A. Sulfasalazine (the most commonly prescribed drug for IBD)

B. Metronidazole (Flagyl)

C. Corticosteroids

D. 6-Mercaptopurine

• Diet (Refer to the nursing diagnosis Altered Nutrition: Less Than Body Requirements in this care plan.)
• TPN and bowel rest (Refer to the nursing diagnosis Altered Nutrition: Less Than Body Requirements in this care plan.)
   b. Surgical
      • Bowel resection
         A. Total colectomy and ileostomy (Refer to the Ileostomy care plan.)
         B. Partial colectomy and colostomy (Refer to the Colostomy care plan.)
      • Incision, drainage, or resection of perianal fistulas and abscesses
6. Explain the potential complications of IBD (refer to the Collaborative Problems in this care plan for specific signs and symptoms):
   a. Fissures, fistulas, and perianal abscesses
   b. Anemia, which may result from either malabsorption of iron (Vitamin B_{12}) or folate deficiency
   c. Toxic megacolon, marked by a sharp increase in number of stools and flatus, bloody diarrhea, increasing abdominal pain and distention, and hypoactive or absent bowel sounds
   d. Intestinal obstruction or perforation
   e. Erythema nodosum or pyoderma gangrenosum: A condition exhibiting red, raised tender nodules, erythema nodosum occurs in 5% to 15% of clients with IBD. Pyo-

Rationale

A. It is thought that the 5-ASA component of sulfasalazine is therapeutic through its local anti-inflammatory effect on the intestinal mucosa. Sulfasalazine inhibits the absorption of ingested folate and may impair nutritional status, however.

B. Flagyl is used to correct abnormalities of absorption and to minimize the source of bacterial antigen contributing to the immune reaction of Crohn's disease. It is useful for perineal complications or in a client with a fistula.

C. Corticosteroids are used because of their anti-inflammatory and immunosuppressive effects. Oral doses are given and tapered gradually to decrease the risk of relapse. Hydrocortisone enemas can help control proctitis.

D. The medication 6-mercaptopurine may be used in a client with Crohn's disease who fails to respond to sulfasalazine and corticosteroid therapy. It provides immunosuppressive effects.

b. Surgical treatment is indicated only when medical treatment fails and the client becomes disabled.

6. The client's understanding of IBD complications can help ensure early detection and enable prompt treatment.

Interventions

derma gangrenosum—a deep, excruciatingly painful necrotizing lesion—may appear singly or in pairs.

f. Arthritis, migratory polyarthritis, or ankylosing spondylitis: The National Cooperative Crohn's disease study reported that 14% of clients studied had arthritis or arthralgia at the time of diagnosis.

g. Ocular lesions: Conjunctivitis, iritis, uveitis, or episceleritis occurs in 3% to 10% of clients with IBD.

h. Nephrolithiasis: Severe diarrhea can lead to decreased volume of concentrated urine. This, combined with intestinal bicarbonate loss and decreased pH, leads to the development of urate stones. With ileal resection or extensive IBD, the calcium normally available to bind with oxylate instead binds with fatty acids, freeing dietary oxylate for absorption. Decreased urine volume leads to increased precipitation of calcium oxylate in the kidneys.

i. Cholelithiasis: Gallstones occur in 30% to 35% of clients with Crohn's disease of the terminal ileum. The ileal dysfunction causes bile acid malabsorption and a decrease in the concentration of bile salts. The decrease in bile salt to cholesterol ratio predisposes to the precipitation of cholesterol stones.

j. Colon cancer: The incidence of colon cancer is 10 to 20 times greater in clients with ulcerative colitis than in the general population. The etiology of cancer in IBD is unknown. Close surveillance is needed, because cancer may mimic the signs and symptoms of IBD.

k. Growth retardation: Growth is impaired in 30% to 50% of young clients with IBD occurring before puberty. Possible causes include decreased nutritional intake, loss of protein and nutrients by rapid passage through the GI tract, increased metabolic requirements secondary to inflammatory bowel, and corticosteroid therapy.

7. Teach the importance of maintaining optimal hydration.

8. Teach measures to preserve perianal skin integrity:
   a. Use soft toilet tissue.
   b. Cleanse area with mild soap after bowel movements.
   c. Apply a protective ointment (e.g., A&D, Desitin, Sweet Cream).

9. Teach the client to report the following signs and symptoms:
   a. Increasing abdominal pain or distention

Rationale

7. Optimal hydration prevents dehydration and reduces the risk of renal calculi formation.

8. These measures can help prevent skin erosion from diarrheal irritation.

9. Early reporting enables prompt intervention to reduce the severity of complications.
   a. Increasing abdominal pain or distention may indicate obstruction or peritonitis.

Interventions

b. Persistent vomiting

c. Unusual rectal or vaginal drainage or rectal pain

d. Change in vision

e. Continued amber urine

f. Flank pain or ache

g. Heart palpitations

10. Provide information on available community resources, e.g., self-help groups, counseling

Rationale

b. Persistent vomiting may point to obstruction.

c. Unusual drainage or rectal pain may indicate abscesses or fistulas.

d. Vision changes may indicate ocular lesions.

e. Amber urine indicates dehydration.

f. Flank pain may indicate renal calculi.

g. Palpitations may point to potassium imbalance.

10. Communicating with others with IBD may help the client to cope better with the disorder's effects on his life style.

▲ *Documentation*

Discharge summary record
 Client teaching
 Outcome achievement or status
 Referrals, if indicated

References/Bibliography

Alterescu, V., & Alterescu, K.B. (1982). Medical management of IBD. In: D. Broadwell & B. Jackson (Eds.). *Principles of ostomy care.* St Louis: C.V. Mosby.

Brinson, R.R., Anderson, W.M., & Singh, M. (1987). Hypoalbuminemia-associated diarrhea in critically ill patients. *Journal of Critical Illness, 2*(9), 72–78.

Brooks, F.P. (1977). *Gastrointestinal pathophysiology.* New York: Oxford University Press.

Chan, A.T.H., & Fleming, C.R. (1983). Nutritional management in patients with Crohn's disease. *Internal Medicine for the Specialist, 4*(12), 65–77.

Das, K.M. (1983). Pharmacotherapy of inflammatory bowel disease: Sulfasalazine. *Postgraduate Medicine, 74*(6), 141–152.

Ferry, G.D., & Bartholemew, L.K. (1985). *Living with IBD.* New York: National Foundation for Ileitis & Colitis.

Frank, M.S., Brandt, L.J., & Bernstein, J. (1983). Pharmacotherapy of inflammatory bowel disease: Methonidazole. *Postgraduate Medicine, 74*(6), 155–160.

Given, B.A., & Simmons, S.J. (1984). *Gastroenterology in clinical nursing.* St Louis: C.V. Mosby.

Hillemeier, A.C., & McCallum, R.W. (1983). Inflammatory bowel disease: How to recognize and treat it in the adolescent. *Consultant, 23*(1), 37–52.

Korelitz, B. (1983). Pharmacotherapy of inflammatory bowel disease: 6-mercaptopurine. *Postgraduate Medicine, 74*(6), 165–172.

Lewicki, L.J., & Leeson, M.J. (1984). The multisystem impact on physiologic processes of inflammatory bowel disease. *Nursing Clinics of North America, 19*(1), 71–79.

McGarity, W.C. (1982). Ulcerative colitis and Crohn's disease: Pathology and surgical management. In D. Broadwell & B. Jackson (Eds.), *Principles of ostomy care.* St Louis: C.V. Mosby.

Myer, S.A. (1984). Overview of inflammatory bowel disease. *Nursing Clinics of North America, 19*(1), 3–9.

Russell, T.R. (1984). Surveillance for cancer in patients with ulcerative colitis. *Medical Times, 112*(2), 53–55.

Scherer, J.C. (1985). *Nurses' drug manual.* Philadelphia: J.B. Lippincott.

Simmons, M.A. (1984). Using the nursing process in treating inflammatory bowel disease. *Nursing Clinics of North America, 9*(1), 11–25.

Stotts, N.A., Fitzgerald, K.A., & Williams, K.R. (1984). Care of the patient critically ill with inflammatory bowel disease. *Nursing Clinics of North America, 12*(1), 61–69.

Tasman-Jones, C. (1983). Zinc deficiency complicating Crohn's disease. *Internal Medicine, 4*(12), 39–41.

Wilson, C. (1984). The diagnostic work-up for the patient with inflammatory bowel disease. *Nursing Clinics of North America, 19*(1), 51–59.

Wroblewski, J.J. (1985). Total parenteral nutrition: New hope for IBD patients. *Ostomy/Wound Management, 21*(7), 8–11.

Peptic Ulcer Disease

Peptic ulcer disease involves erosion in the mucosal wall of the stomach, pylorus, duodenum, or esophagus. The eroded areas are circumscribed and occur only in the areas of the gastrointestinal tract exposed to hydrochloric acid and pepsin. The erosion is caused by increased concentration or activity of acid-pepsin or by decreased mucosal resistance.

Diagnostic Cluster

▲ Time Frame
Initial diagnosis
Recurrent acute episodes

▲ Discharge Criteria
Before discharge, the client or family will:
1. Identify the causes of disease symptoms
2. Identify behaviors, substances, or foods that may alter gastric activity
3. Identify necessary adjustments to prevent ulcer formation
4. State signs and symptoms that must be reported to a health care professional
5. Relate community resources that can provide assistance with life style modifications

Collaborative Problems

Potential Complications:
Hemorrhage
Perforation
Pyloric Obstruction

Nursing Diagnoses

Acute/Chronic Pain related to lesions secondary to increased gastric secretions
Constipation/Diarrhea related to effects of medications on bowel function
Potential Altered Health Maintenance related to lack of knowledge of disease process, contraindications, signs and symptoms of complications, and treatment regimen

Collaborative Problems

▲ Nursing Goal
The nurse will manage and minimize complications of peptic ulcer disease.

Potential Complication: Hemorrhage
Potential Complication: Perforation
Potential Complication: Pyloric obstruction

Interventions

1. Monitor for signs and symptoms of hemorrhage and report promptly:
   a. Hematemesis
   b. Dizziness
   c. Generalized weakness
   d. Melena
   e. Increasing pulse rate with normal or slightly decreased blood pressure
   f. Urine output < 30 mL/hr
   g. Restlessness, agitation, change in mentation
   h. Increasing respiratory rate
   i. Diminished peripheral pulses
   j. Cool, pale, or cyanotic skin
   k. Thirst
2. Arrange for hemoglobin and hematocrit evaluation.

Rationale

1. Hemorrhage is the most common complication of peptic ulcer disease, occurring in 15% to 20% of clients. Signs and symptoms of hemorrhage may be insidious and present gradually or be quite demonstrative and massive. The compensatory response to decreased circulatory volume increases blood oxygen by increasing heart and respiratory rates and decreases circulation to extremities, marked by changes such as decreased pulse and cool skin. Diminished oxygen to the brain causes changes in mentation.

2. Hemoglobin and hematocrit levels determine blood loss status and enable typing and cross-matching for possible transfusion.

Interventions

3. Insert a nasogastric tube and prepare for iced saline lavage.

4. Monitor for signs and symptoms of perforation and report immediately:
   a. Sudden, severe abdominal pain
   b. Abdominal rigidity, absence of bowel sounds
   c. Extreme tenderness on palpation
   d. Acute vomiting
   e. Increasing pulse rate with normal or slightly decreased blood pressure
   f. Urine output < 30 mL/hr
   g. Restlessness, agitation, change in mentation
   h. Increasing respiratory rate
   i. Diminished peripheral pulses
   j. Cool, pale, or cyanotic skin
   k. Thirst
5. If perforation occurs, prepare for surgery according to standard protocols.
6. Monitor for signs and symptoms of pyloric obstruction and report promptly:
   a. Constipation
   b. Abdominal bloating
   c. Weight loss
   d. Epigastric pain after meals
   e. Cramping
   f. Nausea
   g. Vomiting of retained food
7. Withhold all oral foods and fluids if signs of bleeding, perforation, or obstruction occur.

Rationale

3. Nasogastric tube insertion may be done initially to determine the presence of fresh blood. Fresh blood generally calls for iced saline lavage.
4. Perforation is caused by erosion to the abdominal cavity or to adjacent structures. Peritonitis may develop from contaminated gastric juices in the peritoneal cavity.

5. Perforation necessitates emergency surgery.

6. Pyloric obstruction occurs when the area surrounding the pyloric sphincter becomes narrowed and stenosed because of scar tissue, edema, or muscle spasm.

7. Avoidance of oral intake prepares the bowel for surgery and decreases stimulus to the area.

▲ *Documentation*

Flow records
　Vital signs
　Intake and output
　Weight
　Gastric pH
　Stool characteristics
　Bowel sounds
Progress notes
　Unusual events

Related Physician-Prescribed Interventions

Medications
　Histamine-2 (H_2) receptor antagonists　　Anticholinergics
　Antacids
Intravenous Therapy
　None indicated
Laboratory Studies
　Serum pepsinogen I
Diagnostic Studies
　Fasting gastrin levels　　　　　　　Barium study
　Endoscopy
Therapies
　Diet as tolerated　　　　　　　　　Nasogastric suctioning

▲ *Outcome Criteria*

The client will:
1. Report symptoms of discomfort promptly
2. Verbalize increased comfort in response to treatment plan

Acute/Chronic Pain related to lesions secondary to increased gastric secretions

Focus Assessment Criteria

1. Pain characteristics: onset, duration, location, quality, quantity, and aggravating and alleviating factors
2. Pattern of discomfort in relation to food ingestion
3. Intake of substances that damage or irritate the mucosal barrier (e.g., alcohol, caffeine, tobacco, and certain foods and medications)

Clinical Significance

1–3. Contact of hydrochloric acid with exposed ulcer nerve endings presumably causes pain. The pain characteristically begins as an epigastric gnawing occurring 1½ to 3 hours after eating and frequently awakens the client during the night. The pain is commonly relieved by food or antacids.

Interventions

1. Explain the relationship between hydrochloric acid secretion and onset of pain.

2. Administer antacids, anticholinergics, and H₂ blockers as directed.
3. Encourage activities that promote rest and relaxation.
4. Help the client to identify irritating substances, e.g., fried foods, spicy foods, coffee.
5. Teach diversional techniques for stress reduction and pain relief.

6. Advise the client to eat regularly and to avoid bedtime snacks.

7. Encourage the client to avoid smoking and alcohol use.

8. Encourage the client to reduce intake of caffeine-containing beverages, if indicated.
9. Caution the client regarding the use of salicylates, unless otherwise recommended by the physician.
10. Teach the client the importance of continuing treatment even in the absence of pain.

Rationale

1. Hydrochloric acid (HCl) presumably is an important variable in the appearance of peptic ulcer disease. Because of this relationship, control of HCl secretion is considered an essential aim of treatment.
2. HCl secretion can be regulated by neutralizing it with various drug therapies.
3. Relaxation of muscles decreases peristalsis and decreases gastric pain.
4. Avoidance of irritating substances can help prevent the pain response.
5. The relationship between stress and peptic ulcer disease is based on the higher incidence of peptic ulcers in those with chronic anxiety.
6. Contrary to popular belief, certain dietary restrictions do not reduce hyperacidity. Individual intolerances must first be identified and used as a basis for restrictions. Avoidance of eating prior to bedtime may reduce nocturnal acid levels by eliminating the postprandial stimulus to acid secretion. During the day, regular amounts of food particles in the stomach help neutralize the acidity of gastric secretions.
7. Alcohol is a gastric irritant. Smoking has been associated with acid secretion and with delayed ulcer healing.
8. Gastric acid secretion may be stimulated by caffeine ingestion.
9. Salicylates irritate the mucosal lining and purportedly are ulcerogenic.
10. Dietary restrictions and medications must be continued for the prescribed duration. Pain may be relieved long before healing is complete.

▲ Documentation

Progress record
    Complaints of pain
    Response to treatment plan

Constipation or Diarrhea related to effects of medications on bowel function

▲ Outcome Criteria

The client will:

1. Describe the effects of medications on bowel function
2. Describe methods to reduce constipation

Focus Assessment Criteria	Clinical Significance
1. Bowel patterns before initiation of therapy	1–4. These assessments provide baseline data against which to compare subsequent assessments.
2. Usage of elimination aids, such as laxatives, fiber supplements, and enemas	
3. Intake and output	
4. Bowel function: daily amount, character, bowel sounds	

Interventions

1. Explain the side effects of medications and their relationship to bowel patterns.
2. Recommend alternating antacid medications to promote normal bowel function.

Rationale

1,2. Problems associated with antacid therapy are uncommon but should be monitored during the course of treatment. Antacids containing aluminum or calcium tend to be constipating; those with magnesium may promote a cathartic effect. Anticholinergic medications, such as propantheline (Pro-Banthine), have a generalized dehydrating effect.

Interventions

3. Encourage a fluid intake of at least 8 to 10 glasses per day.

4. Encourage foods and exercise that promote normal bowel activity but do not irritate gastric mucosa.
5. Refer to the generic care plan for surgical clients (Appendix II) for additional interventions for managing constipation.

Rationale

3. Sufficient fluid intake, at least 2 L daily, is necessary to maintain bowel patterns and promote proper stool consistency.
4. A well-balanced diet high in fiber content and exercise stimulates peristalsis.

▲ **Outcome Criteria**

The outcome criteria for this diagnosis represent those associated with discharge planning. Refer to discharge criteria.

Potential Altered Health Maintenance related to lack of knowledge of disease process, contraindications, signs and symptoms of complications, and treatment regimen

Focus Assessment Criteria	**Clinical Significance**
1. Knowledge level of therapeutic indications and requirements	1. Determining the client's or family's knowledge level helps guide teaching.
2. Readiness to learn and barriers that might impede teaching	2. A client or family that does not achieve goals for learning requires a referral for assistance postdischarge.

Interventions

1. Explain the pathophysiology of peptic ulcer disease using terminology and media appropriate to the client's and family's level of understanding.
2. Explain behaviors that can be modified or eliminated to reduce the risk of recurrence:
   a. Tobacco use
   b. Excessive alcohol intake
   c. Intake of caffeine-containing beverages and foods
3. If the client is being discharged on antacid therapy, teach the following:
   a. Chew tablets well and follow with a glass of water, to enhance absorption
   b. Lie down for ½ hour after meals to delay gastric emptying
   c. Take antacids 1 hour after meals to counteract the gastric acid stimulated by eating
   d. Avoid antacids high in sodium (e.g., Gelusil, Amphojel, Mylanta II); excessive sodium intake contributes to fluid retention and elevated blood pressure.
4. Discuss the importance of continued treatment even in the absence of overt symptoms.
5. Instruct the client and family to watch for and report these symptoms:
   a. Red or black stools
   b. Bloody or brown vomitus
   c. Persistent epigastric pain
   d. Sudden, severe abdominal pain
   e. Constipation (not resolved)
   f. Unexplained temperature elevation
   g. Persistent nausea or vomiting
   h. Unexplained weight loss

Rationale

1. Understanding helps reinforce the need to comply with restrictions and may improve compliance.

2. Caffeine and tobacco stimulate gastric acid secretion. Alcohol irritates gastric mucosa.

3. Proper self-administration of antacids can enhance their effects and minimize side effects.

4. Continued therapy is necessary to prevent recurrence or development of another ulcer.
5. These signs and symptoms may point to complications such as peritonitis, perforation, or GI bleeding. Early detection enables prompt intervention.

▲ **Documentation**

Discharge summary record
  Client teaching
  Status of goal achievements
  Referrals

Interventions	*Rationale*
6. Refer to community resources, if indicated (e.g., smoking cessation program, stress management class).	6. The client may need assistance with life style changes after discharge.

References/Bibliography

Bruckstien, A.H. (1986). Peptic ulcer disease: New concepts, new and current therapeutics. *Consultant, 26*(4), 157–168.

Hamilton, H. (1985). *Gastrointestinal disorders*. Springhouse: Springhouse Corp.

Koch, M.J. (1987). How to detect and heal lesions and relieve pain. *Consultant, 27*(5), 21–24.

Konopod, E. (1988). Stress ulceration: A stress complication in critically ill patients. *Heart and Lung, 17*(4), 339–348.

Rawls, D.E., & Dyck, W.P. (1984). Peptic ulcer: Previewing new drugs, reviewing current therapy. *Consultant, 24*(3), 85–103.

Staff. (1988). Access your care of the patient with peptic ulcer disease. *Nursing, 18*(4), 32.

Renal and Urinary Tract Disorders

Acute Renal Failure

Acute renal failure involves sudden loss of kidney function due to reduced renal blood flow or glomerular or tubular dysfunction. Renal blood flow can be reduced by hypotension, hypovolemia, or shock. Obstructed renal blood flow and tubular dysfunction also can be caused by calculi or tumors. Glomerular filtration reduction or tubular damage can result from precipitates—e.g., proteins and hemoglobin released from injured muscles in burns or infection—that become concentrated in kidney tubules. Some nonsteroidal anti-inflammatory medications impair renal blood flow, especially in elderly clients. Certain antibiotics (e.g., streptomycin) and heavy metals (e.g., mercury) also are nephrotoxic. Acute renal failure can be reversed if identified and promptly treated before kidneys are permanently damaged.

Diagnostic Cluster

▲ Time Frame

Initial diagnosis (postintensive care)
Recurrent acute episodes

▲ Discharge Criteria

Before discharge, the client or family will:

1. Relate an intent to comply with agreed-on restrictions and follow-up
2. State signs and symptoms that must be reported to a health care professional
3. Identify how to reduce the risk of infection

Collaborative Problems

Potential Complications:
Fluid Overload
Metabolic Acidosis
Electrolyte Imbalances

Nursing Diagnoses

Potential for Infection related to invasive procedure
Altered Nutrition: Less Than Body Requirements related to anorexia, nausea, vomiting, loss of taste, loss of smell, stomatitis, and unpalatable diet

Related Care Plans

Hemodialysis or Peritoneal Dialysis
Chronic Renal Failure

Refer to:

Chronic Renal Failure

Collaborative Problems

▲ Nursing Goal

The nurse will manage and minimize complications of acute renal failure.

Potential Complication: Fluid overload
Potential Complication: Metabolic acidosis
Potential Complication: Electrolyte imbalances

Interventions

1. Monitor for signs of fluid overload:
   a. Weight gain
   b. Increased blood pressure and pulse rate, neck vein distention
   c. Dependent edema (periorbital, pedal, pretibial, sacral)
   d. Adventitious breath sounds (e.g., wheezes, crackles)
   e. Urine specific gravity < 1.010.
2. Weigh the client daily or more often, if indicated. Assure accuracy by weighing at the same time every day, on the same scale, and with the client wearing the same amount of clothing.

Rationale

1. The oliguric phase of acute renal failure usually lasts from 5 to 15 days and often is associated with fluid volume excess. Functionally, the changes result in decreased glomerular filtration, decreased tubular transport of substances, decreased urine formation, and decreased renal clearance.

2. Daily weights can help determine fluid balance and appropriate fluid intake.

Interventions

3. Maintain strict intake and output records; determine the net fluid balance and compare with daily weight loss or gain for correlation.
4. Inform the client about fluid management goals.
5. Adjust the client's fluid intake so it approximates fluid loss plus 300 to 500 mL/day.
6. Distribute fluid intake fairly evenly throughout the entire day and night.

7. Encourage the client to express feelings and frustrations; give positive feedback.
8. Consult with a dietitian regarding the fluid plan and overall diet.

9. Administer oral medications with meals whenever possible. If medications must be administered between meals, give with the smallest amount of fluid necessary.
10. Avoid continuous IV fluid infusion whenever possible. Dilute all necessary IV drugs in the smallest amount of fluid that is safe for IV administration.
11. Monitor for signs and symptoms of metabolic acidosis:
    a. Rapid, shallow respirations
    b. Headache
    c. Nausea and vomiting
    d. Negative base excess
    e. Behavior changes, drowsiness

12. Limit fat and protein intake. Assure caloric intake (consult dietitian for appropriate diet).

13. Assess for signs and symptoms of hypocalcemia, hypokalemia, and alkalosis as acidosis is corrected.
14. Consult with the physician to initiate bicarbonate/acetate dialysis if above measures do not correct metabolic acidosis.
    a. Bicarbonate dialysis for severe acidosis:
       Dialysate $-$ $NaHCO_3$ = 100 mEQ/L
    b. Bicarbonate dialysis for moderate acidosis:
       Dialysate $-$ $NaHCO_3$ = 60 mEQ/L
15. Monitor for signs and symptoms of hypernatremia with fluid overload:
    a. Thirst
    b. CNS effects ranging from agitation to convulsions
16. Maintain sodium restriction.

Rationale

3. A 1-kg weight gain should correlate with excess intake of 1 liter (1 liter of fluid weighs 1 kg, or 2.2 lb).
4. The client's understanding can help gain his or her cooperation.
5. Fluid overload can be prevented with careful replacement.
6. Toxins can accumulate with decreased fluid and cause nausea and sensorium changes. It may be necessary to match fluid intake with loss every 8 hours or even every hour if the client is critically imbalanced.
7. Fluid and diet restrictions can be extremely frustrating.
8. The fluid content of nonliquid food, amount and type of liquids, liquid preferences, and sodium content are all important in fluid management.
9. This prevents the fluid allowance from being used up unnecessarily.

10. Small IV bags, Buretrol, or an infusion pump is preferred to avoid accidental infusion of a large volume of fluid.

11. Acidosis results from the kidney's inability to excrete hydrogen ions, phosphates, sulfates, and ketone bodies. Bicarbonate loss results when the kidney reduces its reabsorption. Metabolic acidosis is aggravated by hyperkalemia, hyperphosphatemia, and decreased bicarbonate levels. Excessive ketone bodies cause headaches, nausea, vomiting, and abdominal pain. Respiratory rate and depth increase to increase CO_2 excretion and reduce acidosis. Acidosis affects the CNS and can increase neuromuscular irritability because of the cellular exchange of hydrogen and potassium.
12. Fats and protein are not used as main energy sources, so acidic end-products do not accumulate.
13. Rapid correction of acidosis may cause rapid excretion of calcium and potassium and rebound alkalosis.
14. The acetate anion converted by the liver to bicarbonate is used in dialysate to combat metabolic acidosis. Use of bicarbonate dialysis is indicated for clients with liver impairment, lactic acidosis, or severe acid–base imbalance.

15. Hypernatremia results from excessive sodium intake or increased aldosterone output. Water is pulled from the cells, causing cellular dehydration and producing CNS symptoms. Thirst is a compensatory response to dilute sodium.
16. Hypernatremia must be corrected slowly to minimize CNS deterioration.

Interventions

17. Monitor for signs and symptoms of hyponatremia:
    a. CNS effects ranging from lethargy to coma
    b. Weakness
    c. Abdominal pain
    d. Muscle twitching or convulsions
18. Monitor for signs and symptoms of hyperkalemia:
    a. Weakness to paralysis
    b. Muscle irritability
    c. Paresthesias
    d. Nausea, abdominal cramping, or diarrhea
    e. Irregular pulse
    f. ECG changes: high T wave, dysrhythmias, wide QRS complex, and flat P wave
19. Intervene for hyperkalemia:
    a. Restrict potassium-rich foods and fluids.
    b. Maintain rapid inflow and outflow during peritoneal dialysis.
20. Monitor for signs and symptoms of hypokalemia:
    a. Weakness or paralysis
    b. Decreased or absent deep tendon reflexes
    c. Hypoventilation
    d. Polyuria
    e. Hypotension
    f. Paralytic ileus
    g. ECG changes: U wave, flat T wave, dysrhythmias, and prolonged Q-T interval.

21. Intervene for hypokalemia: Encourage increased intake of potassium-rich foods.
22. Monitor for signs and symptoms of hypocalcemia:
    a. Altered mental status
    b. Numbness or tingling in fingers and toes
    c. Muscle cramps
    d. Seizures
    e. ECG changes: prolonged Q-T interval, prolonged ST segment, and dysrhythmias.

23. Intervene for hypocalcemia: Administer a high-calcium, low-phosphorus diet.
24. Monitor for signs and symptoms of hypermagnesemia:
    a. Weakness
    b. Hypoventilation
    c. Hypotension
    d. Flushing
    e. Behavioral changes
25. Monitor for signs and symptoms of hyperphosphatemia:
    a. Tetany
    b. Numbness or tingling in fingers and toes
    c. Soft tissue calcification

26. For a hyperphosphatemic client, administer phosphorus-binding antacids, calcium supple-

Rationale

17. Hyponatremia results from sodium loss through vomiting, diarrhea, or diuretic therapy; excessive fluid intake; or insufficient dietary sodium. Cellular edema, caused by osmosis, produces cerebral edema, weakness, and muscle cramps.
18. Hyperkalemia results from the kidney's decreased ability to excrete potassium, or from excess intake of potassium. Acidosis increases the release of potassium from cells. Fluctuations in potassium affect neuromuscular transmission, producing cardiac dysrhythmias, reducing action of GI smooth muscle, and impairing electrical conduction.

19. High potassium levels necessitate a reduction in potassium intake. Prolonged dwell time during dialysis increases potassium excretion.

20. Hypokalemia results from losses associated with vomiting, diarrhea, or diuretic therapy, or from insufficient potassium intake. Hypokalemia impairs neuromuscular transmission and reduces the efficiency of respiratory muscles. Kidneys are less sensitive to antidiuretic hormone (ADH) and thus excrete large quantities of dilute urine. Gastrointestinal smooth muscle action also is reduced. Abnormally low potassium levels also impair electrical conduction of the heart.
21. An increase in dietary potassium intake helps ensure potassium replacement.
22. Hypocalcemia results from the kidneys' inability to metabolize vitamin D (needed for calcium absorption); retention of phosphorus causes a reciprocal drop in serum calcium level. Low serum calcium levels produce increased neural excitability resulting in muscle spasms (cardiac, facial, extremities) and CNS irritability (seizures). It also causes cardiac muscle hyperactivity, as evidenced by ECG changes.
23. Elevated phosphate levels lower serum calcium level, necessitating dietary replacement.
24. Hypermagnesemia results from the kidneys' decreased ability to excrete magnesium. Its effects include CNS depression, respiratory depression, and peripheral vasodilatation.

25. Hyperphosphatemia results from the kidneys' decreased ability to excrete phosphorus. Elevated phosphorus does not cause symptoms in itself but contributes to tetany and other neuromuscular symptoms in the short term, and to soft-tissue calcification in the long term.
26. Supplements are needed to overcome vitamin D deficiency and to compensate for a calcium-

▲ **Documentation**

Flow records
  Vital signs
  Respiratory assessment
  Weight
  Edema (sites, amount)
  Specific gravity
  Intake and output
  Complaints of nausea, vomiting, or muscle cramps
  Treatments
Progress notes
  Changes in behavior and sensorium
  EKG changes

Interventions

ments, or vitamin D, and restrict phosphorus-rich foods.

Rationale

poor diet. High phosphate decreases calcium, which increases parathyroid hormone (PTH). PTH is ineffective in removing phosphates due to renal failure, but causes calcium reabsorption from bone and decreases tubular reabsorption of phosphate.

27. Monitor bone x-ray films for signs of osteodystrophy.

27. Osteodystrophy may result from disrupted calcium/phosphorus metabolism.

Related Physician-Prescribed Interventions

Medications

Diuretics
Antihypertensives
Electrolyte inhibitors or replacements; e.g., calcium gluconate, aluminum hydroxide gels

Vitamin and mineral supplements

Intravenous Therapy

Fluid and electrolyte replacement

Laboratory Studies

Urine pH, osmolality, creatinine clearance, specific gravity, sodium, HCO_3, casts, protein, RBCs)
Hemoglobin, RBCs
Serum pH

Blood urea nitrogen, creatinine
Serum osmolarity
Serum protein
Serum glucose
Electrolytes

Diagnostic Studies

ECG
X-ray film (kidney–ureter–bladder [KUB])

Retrograde pyelogram
Renal arteriogram, ultrasound
Voiding cystourethrogram

Therapies

Dialysis
Indwelling catheter
Fluid restrictions

Dietary restrictions dependent on laboratory findings

Nursing Diagnoses

▲ *Outcome Criteria*

The client will:

1. Describe the reasons for increased susceptibility
2. Relate precautions to prevent infection

Potential for Infection related to invasive procedure

Focus Assessment Criteria

1. IV lines (peripheral and subclavian), arterial catheters, central venous lines, venipuncture sites, and dialysis accesses for signs of infection:
   a. Redness
   b. Swelling
   c. Drainage
   d. Warmth
2. Cloudy or odorous urine, dysuria

Clinical Significance

1,2. Prompt recognition of signs of infection and immediate institution of appropriate treatment can help prevent systemic infection.

Interventions

1. Instruct the client about his or her increased susceptibility to infection and responsibility in prevention.

Rationale

1. Infections are a leading cause of death in acute renal failure; urinary tract infection is a major type. A client with acute renal failure has altered immunity, altered nutritional status, disruptive biochemical status, poor healing potential, edema, and decreased activity, all of which predispose him or her to infection. Therefore, implementation of preventive measures is mandated.

Interventions

2. Use an indwelling bladder catheter only when necessary, for the shortest time possible, and with diligent care.
3. Avoid other invasive procedures as much as possible:
   a. Repeated venous punctures
   b. IV lines
   c. Central venous lines
   d. Arterial catheters
4. Whenever possible, avoid placing the client with a roommate who has an indwelling catheter, urinary tract infection, or upper respiratory infections.
5. Use aseptic technique with all invasive procedures and when caring for lines, catheters, dressing changes, suctioning, and dialysis accesses. Do not use access catheters for blood sampling.
6. Teach the client to avoid contacting people with any infection, especially an upper respiratory tract infection.
7. Use written signs to alert visitors to wash hands before and after contacting the client.

Rationale

2,3. Avoiding catheters and invasive procedures helps prevent introducing microorganisms into the body.

4. Selected isolation can decrease the risk of cross-contamination and possible spread of infection.

5. Microorganisms are introduced with each disruption of invasive lines. Aseptic technique reduces the quantity of microorganisms introduced.

6. Selected isolation can help protect against contacting an infection.

7. Handwashing reduces the risk of cross-contamination.

▲ **Documentation**

Flow records
  Urine color and other characteristics
Progress notes
  Redness, swelling, drainage, or warmth at sites

References/Bibliography

Gutch, C.F., & Stoner, M.H. (1983). *Review of hemodialysis for nurses and dialysis personnel* (4th ed.). St. Louis: C.V. Mosby.

Kee, J.L. (1982). *Fluids and electrolytes and clinical applications: A programmed approach* (3rd ed.). New York: John Wiley & Sons.

Lancaster, L.E. (1987). *The patient with end stage renal disease.* New York: John Wiley & Sons.

Lancaster, L.E. (1987). *Core curriculum for nephrology nursing, American Nephrology Nurses Association.* Pitman, NJ: Anthony J. Jannette.

Larsen, E., Lindbloom, L., & Davis, K.B. (1986). *Development of the clinical nephrology practitioner: A focus on independent learning.* Seattle: University of Washington Hospital.

Levine, D.Z. (1984). *Care of the renal patient.* Philadelphia: W.B. Saunders.

Massry, S.G., & Sellers, A.L. (1979). *Clinical aspects of uremia and dialysis.* Springfield, IL: Charles C Thomas.

Norris, M.K.G. (1989). Acute tubular necrosis: Preventing complications. *Dimensions in Critical Care Nursing, 8*(1), 16–26.

Price, S., & Wilson, L. (1986). *Pathophysiology: Clinical concepts of disease process.* New York: McGraw-Hill.

Richard, C.J. (1986). *Comprehensive nephrology nursing.* Boston: Bozeman, Little, Bunn and Co.

Snyder, T.E. (1989). An exercise program for dialysis patients. *American Journal of Nursing, 89*(3), 362–364.

Staff. (1987). Outcome criteria and nursing diagnosis in ESRD patient care planning, Section 1, Constructive management. *ANNA, 14,* 36–39.

Chronic Renal Failure

Chronic renal failure, or end-stage renal disease, involves progressive, irreversible reduction in functioning renal tissue. The body is unable to maintain metabolic, fluid, and electrolyte balance, resulting in uremia. A reduced glomerular filtration rate is the source of the renal dysfunction. Causes of chronic renal failure include chronic glomerulonephritis; pyelonephritis; systemic diseases such as diabetes mellitus, hypertension, and systemic lupus erythematosus; and irreversible acute renal failure.

Diagnostic Cluster

▲ Time Frame
Acute exacerbations

▲ Discharge Criteria
Before discharge, the client or family will:

1. Describe dietary restrictions, medications, and treatment plan
2. Maintain contact and follow-up with health care providers
3. Keep complete daily records as instructed
4. Verbalize community resources available
5. Relate an intent to comply with agreed-on restrictions and follow-up
6. State the signs and symptoms that must be reported to a health care professional
7. Relate the importance of an outlet for feelings and concerns

---

Collaborative Problems

Potential Complications:
GI Bleeding
Hyperparathyroidism
Pathological Fractures
Anemia
Polyneuropathy
Hypoalbuminemia
Congestive Heart Failure
Metabolic Acidosis
Pleural Effusion
Pericarditis, Cardiac Tamponade
Fluid/Electrolyte Imbalance
Fluid Overload

Refer to:

Acute Renal Failure
Acute Renal Failure

Nursing Diagnoses

Altered Nutrition: Less Than Body Requirements related to anorexia, nausea, vomiting, loss of taste, smell, stomatitis, and unpalatable diet
Altered Sexuality Patterns related to decreased libido, impotence, amenorrhea, or sterility
Powerlessness related to progressive disabling nature of illness
Potential Altered Health Maintenance related to insufficient knowledge of condition, dietary restriction, daily recording, pharmacological therapy, signs and symptoms of complications, follow-up visits, and community resources
Potential for Infection related to invasive procedures
Pruritus related to calcium phosphate or urate crystals on skin

Acute Renal Failure
Cirrhosis

Related Care Plan

Hemodialysis

Collaborative Problems

▲ Nursing Goal
The nurse will manage and minimize complications of chronic renal failure.

Potential Complication: **GI bleeding**
Potential Complication: **Hyperparathyroidism**
Potential Complication: **Pathological Fractures**
Potential Complication: **Anemia**
Potential Complication: **Polyneuropathy**
Potential Complication: **Hypoalbuminemia**
Potential Complication: **Congestive Heart Failure**
Potential Complication: **Metabolic Acidosis**
Potential Complication: **Pleural Effusion**
Potential Complication: **Pericarditis, Cardiac Tamponade**

Interventions

1. Monitor for manifestations of GI bleeding:
   a. Nausea
   b. Hemoptysis
   c. Blood in stool
   d. Drop in hematocrit
   e. Hypotension
   f. Diarrhea or constipation
   g. Anorexia

2. Examine stools and vomitus.

3. Monitor vital signs frequently, particularly blood pressure and pulse.
4. Monitor hematocrit each treatment.
5. Administer bulk-forming laxatives or stool softeners if the client is constipated. Avoid magnesium-containing laxatives.

6. Consult with the physician to use mini-heparin dose during dialysis, if signs and symptoms of GI bleeding are present.
7. Monitor for manifestations of hyperparathyroidism:
   a. Low serum calcium (< 9 mg/100 mL)
   b. Elevated serum phosphate (> 4.5 mg/100 mL)
   c. Elevated alkaline phosphatase (> 90 IU/L)
   d. Limited mobility
   e. Muscle pain
   f. Itching
   g. Deposits of calcium in joints, arteries and arterioles, soft tissue, and other sites
   h. Demineralization of bones, causing osteodystrophy (seen on x-ray film and bone scan)
8. Inspect the client's gait, range of motion of joints, and muscle strength. Palpate joints for enlargement, swelling, and tenderness.
9. As indicated, develop a plan of weight-bearing exercise, e.g., walking. Avoid immobilization if possible.

10. Question the client about signs and symptoms of hypocalcemia:
    a. Tetany
    b. Carpopedal spasms
    c. Seizures
    d. Confusion
    e. Numbness and tingling of fingertips and toes

11. Monitor the ECG for prolonged Q-T interval, irritable dysrhythmias, and A–V conduction defects.
12. Monitor for manifestations of pathological fractures:
    a. Evidence of bone degeneration on x-ray film
    b. Incidence of pathological fractures
    c. Elevated serum phosphate level

Rationale

1. Bleeding may be aggravated by the poor platelet aggregation and capillary fragility associated with high serum levels of nitrogenous wastes. Heparinization required during dialysis in the presence of gastric ulcer disease may precipitate GI bleeding. Constipation is a common symptom in renal failure, owing to restricted fluid intake and phosphate-binding medications.
2. Gross and occult blood can be detected by visual examination.
3. Circulating volume must be monitored with renal failure to prevent severe hypervolemia.
4. Blood loss can result from treatments.
5. Certain laxatives elevate serum magnesium levels. Clients with renal failure already have difficulty excreting usual intake of magnesium in foods.
6. Low heparin dose reduces the risk of bleeding.

7. Phosphate clearance ceases when the glomerular filtration rate (GFR) falls below 10%. Despite a high level of parathormone, and as reabsorption of calcium and phosphate from bone takes place, the plasma phosphate level also rises. This additional phosphate cannot be disposed of through the renal route, preventing an increase in serum calcium concentration and stimulating increased parathyroid secretion. A secondary hyperparathyroidism develops, contributing to bone degeneration.

8. Identification of mobility problems points to the need for a structured exercise program.

9. Exercise helps maintain strength and mobility and decrease calcium reabsorption. Immobilization increases protein catabolism and bone demineralization.
10. Chronic renal failure causes decreased absorption of calcium caused by the kidney's inability to metabolize vitamin D and by loss of calcium with phosphorus retention.

11. Calcium imbalances can cause cardiac muscle hyperactivity.

12. Pathological fractures are related to calcium–phosphate imbalance, decreased calcium intake, calcium malabsorption, hyperphosphatemia, inefficient dialysis, or low calcium concentration in the dialysis.

Interventions

   d. Bone pain
   e. Limited mobility
   f. Swelling of surrounding tissues and skin
13. Request a dietary consultation regarding calcium intake.
14. Review medication dosage and the importance of taking phosphate binders (Basaljel, Amphojel, etc.)
15. Increase the calcium level in the dialysate, if indicated.
16. Monitor for manifestations of anemia:

   a. Dyspnea
   b. Fatigue

   c. Tachycardia
   d. Palpitations

   e. Pallor of nail beds and mucous membranes
   f. Low hemoglobin and hematocrit
   g. Bruising
17. Avoid unnecessary collection of blood specimens.
18. Instruct the client to use a soft toothbrush and avoid vigorous nose blowing, constipation, and contact sports.
19. Demonstrate the pressure method to control bleeding should it occur.
20. Monitor for manifestations of polyneuropathy (peripheral neuropathy):
   a. Decreased sensation in feet
   b. Numbness and burning of feet
   c. Muscle cramps
   d. Restlessness of legs: creeping, crawling, prickling, and itching sensations
   e. Loss of muscle strength
   f. Footdrop
   g. Decreased vibratory perception
   h. Abnormal deep tendon reflexes

21. Caution the client to check for skin pressure sores and to eliminate hazards, such as prolonged pressure, ill-fitting shoes, and thermal or friction burns.
22. Provide for movement and mobility: range of motion exercises, as indicated.
23. Monitor for manifestations of decreased albumin levels:
   a. Serum albumin < 3.5 g/dL and proteinuria (< 100–150 mg protein/24 hours)
   b. Edema formation: pedal, facial, sacral
   c. Hypovolemia, increased hematocrit/hemoglobin
   d. Signs and symptoms of negative nitrogen balance:
     • Decreased serum cholesterol
     • Decreased caloric intake (< 45 Kcal/kg)
     • Decreased protein intake (< 0.75 g/kg)

Rationale

13. A consultation is necessary to evaluate the need for increased calcium in the diet.
14. These medications reduce phosphate loss.

15. Supplemental calcium may be required to maintain calcium balance.
16. Causes of anemia in chronic renal failure include these:
   a. Decreased RBC production
   b. Decreased RBC survival time, owing to elevated uremic toxins
   c. Loss of blood through GI bleeding
   d. Blood loss during hemodialysis from membrane rupture, hemolysis, and residual dialyzer blood loss
   e. Dilution caused by volume overload.

17. Blood loss occurs with every blood collection.

18. Trauma should be avoided to reduce the risk of bleeding and infection.

19. Direct, constant pressure prevents excess blood loss.
20. Peripheral neuropathy results from demyelination of large muscle fibers and axonal degeneration secondary to uremia and decreased GFR. Symptoms of peripheral neuropathy usually do not occur until GFR is below 1 mL/min. Other possible etiologies include: pyridoxine deficiencies, especially during isoniazid (INH) or hydralazine use; biotin deficiencies; vitamin B$_{12}$ deficiencies; and acid–base and electrolyte imbalances. Neuropathy usually is bilateral and distal and occurs in lower extremities first.
21. Peripheral neuropathies can cause loss of sensation and temperature perception.

22. Relief of pain from neuropathies often is obtained from movement.
23. When albumin is lost through urinary excretion or peritoneal dialysis, the liver responds by increasing production of plasma proteins. However, when the loss is great, the liver cannot compensate, and hypoalbuminemia results. Edema formation results from decreased plasma proteins and consequent decreased plasma oncotic pressure, which causes a fluid shift from the vascular to the interstitial compartment. Hypovolemia can result from fluid loss, which leads to hemoconcentration and a consequent increase in hemoglobin and hema-

Interventions

- Delayed wound healing
- Muscle wasting

24. Administer intravenous salt-free albumin per physician's order. Avoid diuretics.

25. Hold a dietary consultation for nutritional assessment and to provide for the following:
    a. Fluid restrictions (with massive edema)
    b. Low-sodium diet
    c. Adequate calorie and protein intake
    d. Low protein diet with high biological protein included

26. Evaluate daily:
    a. Weight
    b. Fluid intake and output records
    c. Circumference of the edematous part(s)
    d. Laboratory data: hematocrit, serum sodium, and plasma protein in specific serum albumin
27. Monitor for signs and symptoms of congestive heart failure and decreased cardiac output:
    a. Gradual increase in heart rate
    b. Increased shortness of breath
    c. Diminished breath sounds, rales
    d. Decreased systolic BP
    e. Presence of or increase in S3 and/or S4
    f. Gallop
    g. Peripheral edema
    h. Distended neck veins
28. Encourage adherence to strict fluid restrictions: 800–1000 mL/24 hours, or 24-hour urine output plus 500 mL.

Rationale

tocrit. If the volume loss becomes great, shock occurs.

A negative nitrogen balance results from protein and caloric malnutrition, leading to an oxygen and nutrient deficit, which causes cellular catabolism, cell breakdown, and nitrogen loss. Humoral defenses to infection are depressed owing to protein loss, and general protein reserves are depleted, resulting in slowed healing.

24. Parenteral administration of albumin-containing solutions results only in a transient increase in serum albumin concentrations; however, it is helpful to circumvent life-threatening hypotension. Diuretics are contraindicated if the plasma volume is low, and in low output renal failure.

25. With chronic renal failure (on dialysis), protein is usually restricted to 0.75–1.25 g/kg, with emphasis on high biological value protein (HBV). HBV proteins (dairy products, eggs, meat) supply the essential amino acids necessary for cell growth and repair. Calories should be generous (35–45 Kcal/kg) to allow use of the minerals in protein for tissue maintenance. (*Note:* Because of the greater permeability of the peritoneal membrane, protein loss is larger in chronic peritoneal dialysis than in hemodialysis; therefore, more protein may be needed in the diet to offset hypoalbuminemia.)

A low-sodium diet may be beneficial to prevent additional fluid retention. The client should not become totally edema-free, however, because of the dangers of hypovolemia and hypotension.
26. As GFR decreases and the functioning nephron mass continues to diminish, the kidneys lose the ability to concentrate urine and to excrete sodium and water, resulting in hypervolemia.

27. Congestive heart failure can occur from increased cardiac output, hypervolemia, dysrhythmias, and hypertension, resulting in reduced ability of the left ventricle to eject blood and consequent decreased cardiac output and increased pulmonary vascular congestion. This causes fluid to enter pulmonary tissue, causing the symptoms of respiratory distress and signs of rales, productive cough, and cyanosis.
28. A client who presents with evidence of fluid overload requires fluid restriction based on urine output. In an anuric client, restriction generally is 800 mL/day, which accounts for insensible losses from metabolism, the GI tract, perspiration, and respiration.

Interventions

29. Reevaluate and reestablish the client's optimal "dry" weight—that weight at which the client is free of any signs or symptoms of overload and maintains a normal blood pressure.

30. Collaborate with physician or dietitian in planning an appropriate diet. Encourage adherence to a low-sodium diet (2–4 g/24 hr).

31. Monitor for manifestations of pleural effusion:
    a. Variable dyspnea
    b. Pleuritic pain
    c. Diminished and delayed chest movement on involved side
    d. Bulging of intercostal spaces (in massive effusion)
    e. Decreased breath sounds over site of pleural effusion
    f. Decreased vocal and tactile fremitus
    g. Increased rate and depth of respirations

32. Monitor for manifestations of pericarditis:
    a. Pericardial friction rub
    b. Elevated temperature
    c. Elevated WBC count
    d. Substernal or precordial pain increasing during inspiration

33. Explain the cause of the pain to the client.

34. Monitor for signs and symptoms of cardiac tamponade:
    a. Rapid decrease in blood pressure
    b. Narrowed pulse pressure
    c. Muffled heart sounds
    d. Distended neck veins
    e. Decreased blood pressure during hemodialysis with intolerance to ultrafiltration

35. Discuss with the physician changing to peritoneal dialysis until pericarditis resolves.

Rationale

29. A client with chronic renal failure is prone to fluctuations in weight, necessitating frequent re-evaluation for optimal fluid balance. Accepted interdialytic weight gain is 1 to 2 lb per 24 hours.

30. Sodium restrictions should be adjusted based on urine sodium excretion.

31. Pleural effusion is a collection of fluid, either transudates or exudates, in the pleural cavity. Transudates are seen in chronic renal failure and result from a rise in pulmonary venous pressure secondary to fluid overload. This transudation also may occur owing to the hypoproteinemia often seen in chronic renal failure.

32. Pericarditis results from irritation by accumulated serum nitrogenous wastes.

33. The client may fear that chest pain is signaling a heart attack.

34. Exaggerated signs and symptoms of effusion implicate worsening pericarditis, pericardial effusion, and slowly developing cardiac tamponade. It can develop at any time in a client with uremic pericarditis.

35. Heparin infusion exacerbates the bloody effusions of pericarditis and increases the risk of cardiac tamponade.

▲ **Documentation**

Flow records
    Weight (actual, dry)
    Vital signs
    Laboratory values
    Intake and output
    Evidence of bleeding, e.g., blood in stool, bruises
    Status of edema
Progress notes
    Chest complaints

Related Physician-Prescribed Interventions

Medications
    Diuretics
    Antihypertensives
    Electrolyte inhibitors or replacements, e.g., calcium gluconate, aluminum hydroxide gels
    Vitamins and minerals

Intravenous Therapy
    Fluid or electrolyte replacement

Laboratory Studies
    Urine (pH, osmolality, creatinine clearance, specific gravity, sodium HCO_3, casts, protein, RBC)
    Hemoglobin, RBC count
    Serum pH
    Serum osmolality
    Serum protein
    Blood urea nitrogen (BUN), creatinine
    Electrolytes
    Serum glucose

Diagnostic Studies
    ECG
    X-ray films (kidney–ureter–bladder [KUB])
    Retrograde pyelogram
    Renal arteriogram, ultrasound
    Renal biopsy
    X-ray film (feet, hands, spine)

Therapies
    Hemodialysis
    Indwelling catheter
    Fluid restrictions
    Dietary restrictions dependent on laboratory findings

Nursing Diagnoses

Altered Nutrition: Less Than Body Requirements related to anorexia, nausea and vomiting, loss of taste, loss of smell, stomatitis, and unpalatable diet

Focus Assessment Criteria

1. Appetite, senses of taste and smell
2. Weight
3. Condition of mouth and lips
4. Complaints of diarrhea, constipation, nausea, or vomiting
5. Laboratory values: electrolytes, BUN, serum proteins
6. Diet history
7. Knowledge of nutritional requirements and restrictions

Clinical Significance

1–7. A uremic client has particular nutritional needs in order to avoid negative nitrogen imbalance, long periods of fasting to avoid endogenous protein breakdown, and dehydration. Another problem involves high levels of ammonia caused by breakdown of salivary urea by bacterial urease. Establishing the client's ideal weight—considering actual weight (versus fluid), nutritional requirements of activity, and stressors of chronic illness—provides a goal for treatment. A uremic client often has dental problems related to altered calcium and phosphorus metabolism and bleeding of soft tissues. Inflammation and ulcerations in the mouth contribute to unpleasant taste. Appetite may be diminished owing to dry mucous membranes, sour or metallic taste in mouth, or painful chewing and swallowing.

Interventions

1. Consult a dietitian for assistance with nutritional assessment, identifying nutritional needs, prescribing diet modifications, and providing nutritional instruction to the client.
2. Reinforce dietary instructions and provide written materials for verbal instructions.

3. Encourage the client to verbalize his or her feelings and frustrations about diet modifications.

4. Provide for and encourage good oral hygiene before and after meals.
5. Administer antiemetics, as ordered, on a timely basis before meals.
6. Provide a pleasant environment during mealtimes and assist as indicated.
7. Administer vitamins and phosphate binders as ordered.
8. Check meal trays for proper content and encourage the client to eat.
9. Document all fluid and food intake.

10. Evaluate the client's nutritional status and the diet's effectiveness with the dietitian and physician.
11. Explain the need for the client to eat the maximum protein allowed on the diet.
12. Prepare for and administer total parenteral nutrition (TPN) as ordered. (Refer to the Total

Rationale

1. A properly prescribed diet is essential in the management of chronic renal failure.

2. Empathy and reinforcement of dietary instructions can increase compliance with diet restrictions.
3. The client should be given as much control as possible over his or her diet—for example, have the patient make a list of food and fluid preferences and dislikes and try to incorporate these into the prescribed diet.
4. Proper oral hygiene reduces microorganisms and helps prevent stomatitis.
5. Control of nausea and vomiting stimulates appetite and increases intake.
6. Appetite is stimulated in a relaxed, pleasant setting.
7. Supplements control plasma phosphate levels and help maintain nutritional status.
8. Positive feedback for dietary adherence can promote compliance.
9. Accurate documentation is essential to assessment of nutritional status.
10. Continued evaluation enables alteration of the diet according to the client's specific nutritional needs.
11. Adequate protein is needed to prevent protein catabolism and muscle wasting.
12. For a client unable to maintain nutritional status through the GI route, TPN can provide

▲ Documentation

Flow records
  Daily weights
  Intake (specify food types
    and amounts)
  Output
  Mouth assessment
Discharge summary records
  Client teaching
  Referrals

▲ Outcome Criteria

The client will:

1. Relate the causes of decreased libido and impaired sexual functioning
2. Discuss own feelings and partner's concerns regarding sexual functioning
3. Verbalize an intention to discuss concerns with partner

Interventions

  Parenteral Nutrition Care Plan, page 613, for more information.)

13. Prepare for dialysis, as indicated, and monitor for potential complications. (Refer to the Hemodialysis and Peritoneal Dialysis Care Plans for more information.)
14. Work with the client to develop a plan to incorporate the diet prescription successfully into his or her daily life.

Rationale

  amino acids necessary for healing, especially renal tissue, and for preventing a catabolic state.

13. Dialysis is indicated for rising BUN that cannot be controlled through dietary management. It also may be necessary to remove excess fluid administered with TPN.
14. Collaboration provides opportunities for the client to exert control, which tends to increase compliance.

Potential Altered Sexuality Patterns related to fatigue, decreased libido, impotence, amenorrhea, or sterility

Focus Assessment Criteria	*Clinical Significance*
1. Knowledge of the effects of condition on sexual function 2. Sexual function: 　a. Pattern 　b. Satisfaction 　c. Libido 　d. Erectile problems 3. Menstrual pattern	1,2. Chronic renal failure has a profound impact on the client's life. As the disorder progresses, the client experiences a narrowing of existence; mobility decreases, and pain, discomfort, and fatigue commonly increase. These all contribute to decreased libido. In a male client, impotence may result from neuropathy and possibly from antihypertensive medications. 3. Amenorrhea may result from malnourishment, anemia, or chronic debilitation.

Interventions

1. Explore the client's patterns of sexual functioning, encouraging him or her to share concerns. Assume that all clients have had some sexual experience, and convey a willingness to discuss feelings and concerns.
2. Explain the possible effects of chronic renal failure on sexual functioning and sexuality.

3. Reaffirm the need for frank discussion between sexual partners.

4. Explain how the client and partner can use role-playing to discuss concerns about sex.

5. Reaffirm the need for closeness and expressions of caring through touching, massage, and other means.
6. Suggest that sexual activity need not always culminate in vaginal intercourse but that the partner can reach orgasm through noncoital manual or oral stimulation.
7. Explain the function of a penile prosthesis; point out that both semirigid and inflatable penile prostheses have a high rate of success.
8. Refer the client to a certified sex or mental health professional, if desired.

Rationale

1. Many clients are reluctant to discuss sexuality issues. The proper approach can encourage the client to share feelings and concerns.

2. Explaining that impaired sexual functioning has a physiological basis can reduce feelings of inadequacy and decreased self-esteem, which actually may help improve sexual function.
3. Both partners probably have concerns about sexual activity. Repressing these feelings negatively influences the relationship.
4. Role-playing helps a person gain insight by placing himself or herself in another's position, and allows more spontaneous sharing of fears and concerns.
5. Sexual pleasure and gratification is not limited to intercourse. Other expressions of caring may prove more meaningful.
6. Sexual gratification is an individual matter. It is not limited to intercourse, but includes closeness, touching, and giving pleasure to others.

7. Explaining penile prostheses can give an impaired client hope for renewed sexual function.

8. Certain sexual problems require continuing therapy and the advanced knowledge of specialists.

▲ Documentation

Progress notes
  Dialogues
  Client teaching

▲ **Outcome Criteria**

The client will:

1. Identify personal strengths
2. Identify factors that he or she can control

▲ **Documentation**

Progress Notes
    Dialogues

▲ **Outcome Criteria**

The outcome criteria for this diagnosis represent those associated with discharge planning. Refer to the discharge criteria.

Powerlessness related to feeling of loss of control and life style restrictions

Focus Assessment Criteria

1. Understanding of disease process
2. Perception of control
3. Effects on life style
4. Participation in care and decision making

Clinical Significance

1–4. A client's response to loss of control depends on the meaning of the loss, individual coping patterns, personal characteristics, and response to others.

Interventions

1. Explore with the client the disorder's effects on the following:
   a. Occupation
   b. Role responsibilities
   c. Relationships
2. Determine the client's usual response to problems, i.e., whether the client usually seeks to change his or her own behaviors to control problems or whether he or she expects others or external factors to control problems.
3. Help the client identify personal strengths and assets.

4. Help the client identify energy patterns; explain the need to schedule activities around these patterns. Encourage the client to identify those activities that are personally important and schedule them when energy usually is high.
5. Explain the need to accept help from others and to delegate some tasks.
6. Provide opportunities for the client to make decisions about goals.

7. Assist the client in seeking support from other sources, e.g., self-help groups, support groups.

Rationale

1. Chronic renal failure typically has a negative impact on a client's concept of self, the ability to achieve goals, and relationships.

2. Identifying the client's usual response to problems can help the nurse plan appropriate and effective interventions.

3. Identifying personal strengths helps to discourage the client from focusing only on limitations.

4,5. Adequate rest and pacing of activities is essential to prevent exhaustion and hypoxia. Feelings of self-worth and dignity will be fostered if the client can continue personally important activities.

6. Having mutually agreed-upon goals can improve the client's sense of self-worth and control.
7. Opportunities to share experiences and problem-solving strategies with others in a similar situation can help both the client and his family gain a sense of control over the disorder and their lives.

Potential Altered Health Maintenance related to insufficient knowledge of condition, dietary restrictions, daily recording, pharmacological therapy, signs/symptoms of complications, follow-up visits, and community resources

Focus Assessment Criteria

1. Knowledge of the disease, therapeutic regimen, and future treatment alternatives
2. Ability and readiness to learn, considering level of literacy
3. Barriers to learning (e.g., pain, fatigue, stress)
4. Past experiences influencing current health status
5. Nature of concerns and fears

Clinical Significance

1–5. Effective client teaching involves guided interaction between the nurse and client that results in a change in client behavior. A warm, accepting environment helps ensure learning success. The timing and content of teaching are crucial to the client's understanding, acceptance, and compliance with the plan of care.

Interventions

1. Develop and implement a teaching plan, using teaching techniques and tools appropriate to the client's understanding; this includes but is not necessarily limited to the following:

Rationale

1. Presenting relevant and useful information in an understandable format greatly reduces learning frustration and enhances teaching efforts. Some factors specific to a client with

Interventions

    a. Current condition

    b. Diet and fluid restrictions

    c. Medication therapy (purpose, dosage, route, side effects, precautions)

    d. Daily recordings (intake, output, and weight)

    e. Signs and symptoms of complications

    f. Need for follow-up visits

    g. Available community resources

2. Encourage the client to verbalize anxiety, fears, and questions.
3. Identify factors that may help predict noncompliance:
   a. Lack of knowledge
   b. Noncompliance in the hospital
   c. Failure to perceive the seriousness or chronicity of the disorder
   d. Belief that the condition will "go away" on its own
   e. Belief that the condition is hopeless
4. Include significant others in teaching sessions. Encourage them to provide support without acting as "police."

5. Emphasize to the client that ultimately it is his or her choice and responsibility to comply with the therapeutic regimen.
6. If the cost of medications is a financial burden for the client, consult with social services.
7. Assist the client to identify his or her ideal or desired weight.
8. Teach the client to record weight and urinary output daily.

9. Explain the signs and symptoms of electrolyte imbalances, and the need to watch for and report them. (See Collaborative Problems in this entry for more information.)
10. Teach the client measures to reduce the risk of urinary tract infection:
    a. Perform proper hygiene after toileting, to prevent fecal contamination of the urinary tract.
    b. Drink the maximum amount of fluids allowed, to prevent urinary stasis.
11. Reinforce the need to comply with diet and fluid restrictions and follow-up care.
12. Teach the client who has fluid restrictions to relieve thirst by other means:
    a. Sucking on a lemon wedge, a piece of hard candy, a frozen juice pop, or an ice cube
    b. Spacing fluid allotment over 24 hours
13. Encourage the client to express feelings and frustrations; give positive feedback for adherence to fluid restrictions.
14. Consult with a dietitian regarding the fluid plan and overall diet.

Rationale

chronic renal failure influence the teaching–learning process:

- Depressed mentation, which necessitates repeating information
- Short attention span, which may limit teaching sessions to 10 to 15 minutes
- Altered perceptions, which necessitate frequent clarification and reassurance
- Sensory alterations, causing a better response to ideas presented using varied audiovisual formats

2. Recognition of the client's fear of failure to learn is vital to successful teaching.
3. Openly addressing barriers to compliance may help minimize or eliminate these barriers.

4. Significant others must be aware of the treatment plan so they can support the client. "Policing" the client can disrupt positive relationships.
5. The client must understand that he has control over his choices and that his choices can improve or impair his health.
6. A referral for financial support can prevent discontinuation due to financial reasons.
7. Establishing an achievable goal may help improve compliance.
8. Daily weight and urine output measurements allow the client to monitor his or her own fluid status and limit fluid intake accordingly.
9. Early detection of electrolyte imbalance enables prompt intervention to prevent serious complications.

10. Repetitive infections can cause further renal damage.

11. Compliance reduces the risk of complications.

12. Strategies to reduce thirst without significant fluid intake reduce the risk of fluid overload.

13. Fluid and diet restrictions can be extremely frustrating; positive feedback and reassurance can contribute to continued compliance.

14. Consultation may be required for specific instructions.

Interventions	*Rationale*
15. Teach the client to take oral medications with meals whenever possible. If medications must be administered between meals, give with the smallest amount of fluid possible.	15. Planning can reduce unnecessary fluid intake and conserve fluid allowance.
16. Encourage the client to maintain his or her usual level of activity and continue activities of daily living to the extent possible.	16. Regular activity helps maintain strength and endurance and promotes overall well-being.
17. Teach the client and family to watch for and report the following:	17. Early reporting of complications enables prompt intervention to prevent worsening.
a. Weight gain greater than 2 lb or weight loss	a. Weight gain greater than 2 lb may indicate fluid retention; weight loss may point to insufficient intake.
b. Shortness of breath	b. Shortness of breath may be an early sign of pulmonary edema.
c. Increasing fatigue or weakness	c. Increasing fatigue or weakness may indicate increasing uremia.
d. Confusion, change in mentation	d. Confusion or other changes in mentation may point to acidosis or fluid and electrolyte imbalances.
e. Palpitations	e. Palpitations may indicate electrolyte imbalances (K, Ca).
f. Excessive bruising; excessive menses; excessive bleeding from gums, nose, or cut; or blood in urine, stool, or vomitus	f. Excessive bruising, excessive menses, and abnormal bleeding may indicate reduced prothrombin, clotting factors III and VIII, and platelets.
g. Increasing oral pain or oral lesions	g. Oral pain or lesions can result as excessive salivary urea is converted to ammonia in the mouth, which is irritating to the oral mucosa.
18. Discuss with the client and family any anticipated disease-related stressors:	18. Discussing the nonphysiological effects of chronic renal failure can help the client and family identify effective coping strategies.
a. Financial difficulties	
b. Reversal of role responsibilities	
c. Dependency (Refer to Chapter 3, The Ill Adult: Issues and Responses, for information regarding the effects of chronic illness on families.)	
19. Provide information about or initiate referrals to community resources (e.g., American Kidney Association, counseling, self-help groups).	19. Assistance with home management and in dealing with the potential destructive effects on the client and family may be needed.

▲ **Documentation**

Discharge summary record
Client teaching
Outcome achievement or status
Referrals, if indicated

References/Bibliography

Refer to Acute Renal Failure

Urolithiasis (Renal Calculi)

Urolithiasis refers to the presence of calculi (stones) in the urinary tract—in the kidneys, ureters, or bladder. Composed of crystalline substances such as calcium oxalate, urate calcium phosphate, uric acid, and magnesium, calculi can cause obstruction, infection, or edema in the urinary tract. About 75% of all stones are composed of calcium.

Risk factors for renal calculi include urinary stasis, urinary tract infection, hyperthyroidism, inflammatory bowel disease, gout, excessive intake of calcium and vitamin D, prolonged immobility, and dehydration. Treatment involves promoting stone passage, dissolving the stones, or crushing the stones using ultrasonic waves or electrical discharge. Surgical removal is indicated if these measures prove unsuccessful. In about 25% of cases, calculi recur.

Diagnostic Cluster

▲ Time Frame

Initial diagnosis
Recurrent acute episode

▲ Discharge Criteria

Before discharge, the client or family will:

1. Explain the factors that contribute to calculi formation
2. Demonstrate the ability to test urine pH
3. Describe daily fluid requirement
4. State dietary restrictions
5. Relate signs and symptoms that must be reported to a health care professional
6. Relate an intent to alter the life style to help prevent recurrence

Collaborative Problems

Potential Complications:
Pyelonephritis
Renal Insufficiency

Nursing Diagnoses

Altered Comfort: Pain, Nausea, Vomiting, Diarrhea related to inflammation secondary to irritation of calculi and spasms of the smooth muscles of enteric tract and adjacent structures secondary to renointestinal reflexes

Potential Altered Health Maintenance related to prevention of recurrence, dietary restrictions, and fluid requirements

Collaborative Problems

▲ Nursing Goal

The nurse will manage and minimize renal complications.

Potential Complication: Pyelonephritis
Potential Complication: Renal Insufficiency

Interventions	*Rationale*

1. Monitor for signs and symptoms of pyelonephritis:
  a. Chills, fever
	1. Urinary tract infections can be caused by urinary stasis or irritation of tissue by calculi.
	  a. Bacteria can act as pyrogen by raising the hypothalamic thermostat through the production of endogenous pyrogen, which may mediate through prostaglandins. Chills can occur when the temperature set-point of the hypothalamus changes rapidly.

b. Costovertebral angle (CVA) pain (a dull, constant backache below the 12th rib)	b. CVA pain results from distention of the renal capsule.
c. Leukocytosis	c. Leukocytosis reflects an increase in WBCs to fight infection through phagocytosis.
d. Bacteria and pus in urine	d. Bacteria and pus in the urine indicate a urinary tract infection.
e. Dysuria, frequency	e. Bacteria irritates bladder tissue, causing spasms and frequency.

Interventions

2. Monitor for early signs and symptoms of renal insufficiency:
   a. Sustained elevated urine specific gravity
   b. Elevated urine sodium levels

   c. Sustained insufficient urine output (< 30 mL/hr)
   d. Elevated blood pressure

▲ **Documentation**

Flow records
  Intake and output
  Urine specific gravity

   e. Elevated blood urea nitrogen (BUN), serum creatinine, potassium, phosphorus, and ammonia, and decreased creatinine clearance

Rationale

2. Early detection enables prompt treatment to prevent serious renal dysfunction.
   a,b. Decreased ability of renal tubules to reabsorb electrolytes causes increased urine sodium levels and increased specific gravity.
   c,d. Decreased glomerular filtration rate eventually causes insufficient urine output and stimulates renin production, resulting in elevated blood pressure in an attempt to increase blood flow to the kidney.
   e. Decreased excretion of urea and creatinine in the urine elevates BUN and creatinine levels.

Related Physician-Prescribed Interventions

Medications
  Analgesics
  Antiemetics
  Antibiotics

Antispasmodics
Corticosteroids

Intravenous Therapy
  Fluid replacement

Laboratory Studies
  Urinalysis
  24-hour urine
  Nitroprusside urine test
  Uric acid
  Phosphates
  Urine culture

Serum calcium, protein
Electrolytes
BUN
Creatinine
WBC count

Diagnostic Studies
  Kidney, ureters, bladder (KUB) x-ray film
  Intravenous pyelography

Cystoscopy
Computed tomography

Therapies
  Indwelling catheter
  Diet as indicated by stone composition, e.g., low purine, low calcium, low oxylate, low calcium/phosphate

Nursing Diagnoses

▲ *Outcome Criteria*

The client will:

1. Describe causes of symptoms
2. Relate progressive relief of symptoms after pain-relief measures

Altered Comfort: Pain, Nausea, Vomiting, Diarrhea related to inflammation secondary to irritation of calculi and spasms of the smooth muscles of enteric tract and adjacent structures secondary to renointestinal reflexes

Focus Assessment Criteria

1. Location of pain

2. Severity of pain based on a pain scale of 0 to 10 (0 = absence of pain; 10 = worst pain), rated as follows:
   a. At its best
   b. At its worst
   c. After each pain relief measure

Clinical Significance

1. Documentation of the pain location can help evaluate progress of calculi movement.
2. A rating scale provides a good method for a client to relate the subjective sensations of pain.

Focus Assessment Criteria	*Clinical Significance*
3. Complaints of nausea, vomiting, diarrhea, abdominal pain	3. Afferent stimuli in the renal capsule may cause pylorospasm of the smooth muscle of the enteric tract and adjacent structures. Increased ureteral pressure may cause extravasation of urine into perirenal spaces, causing abdominal pain and predisposing to infection.

Interventions

1. Collaborate with the client to identify methods to reduce pain intensity

2. Relate to the client your acceptance of his response to pain
   a. Acknowledge the presence of his pain
   b. Listen attentively to his descriptions of the pain
   c. Convey that you are assessing his pain because you want to understand its nature better
3. Take steps to reduce fear and correct misinformation:
   a. Explain causes of the pain, nausea, vomiting, and diarrhea.
   b. Relate how long the pain will last, if known.
   c. If indicated, provide accurate information to reduce fear of addiction to pain medications.
4. Provide the client with privacy for his or her pain experience.

5. Provide optimal pain relief with prescribed analgesics.
   a. Use a preventive approach; instruct the client to request pain medication as needed before the pain becomes severe.

   b. After administering a pain relief medication, return in ½ hour to ask the client to rate the severity of his pain. Compare this rating with the rating before medication administration to assess pain relief.
   c. Consult with the physician for antispasmodics, as necessary.
6. As necessary, take steps to decrease nausea and vomiting:
   a. Reduce unpleasant sights and odors.
   b. Provide good mouth care after vomiting.
   c. Teach the client to practice deep breathing and voluntary swallowing to suppress the vomiting reflex.
   d. Instruct him to sit after eating but not to lie down.
   e. Encourage him to eat smaller meals and eat slowly.

Rationale

1. The client has the most intimate knowledge of his pain and can provide valuable insight into its management.
2. If a client must try to convince health care providers that he has pain, he experiences increased anxiety, which in turn may increase the pain.

3. A client who is prepared for pain through explanations of the actual sensations that he will feel tends to experience less stress than a client who receives vague or no explanations. Addiction is a psychological phenomenon involving the regular use of narcotics for emotional, not medical, reasons.
4. The client's embarrassment at having others observe his response to pain can increase anxiety and heighten pain.
5. Optimal pain relief decreases anxiety related to pain recurrence.
   a. The preventive approach—as compared to the p.r.n. approach—may reduce the total 24-hour dose; it provides a constant blood level of the drug, reduces craving for the drug, and reduces the anxiety of having to ask and wait for relief.
   b. This assessment helps evaluate the effectiveness of the pain relief regimen.

   c. Antispasmodics decrease the spasms that cause the pain of renal colic.
6. Unpleasant sights and odors (food, oral, environmental) and overdistention or compression of the stomach serve as noxious stimuli to the vomiting center.

Interventions

   f. Tell him to restrict liquids with meals to avoid overdistending the stomach; also avoid fluids 1 hour before and after meals.

   g. Caution him to avoid the smell of food preparation, if possible.

   h. Suggest that he try eating cold foods, which have less odor.

   i. Encourage him to loosen clothing and eat in fresh air.

   j. Instruct him to avoid lying down flat for at least 2 hours after eating. (If he must rest, he should sit or recline with his head at least 4 inches higher than his feet.)

7. Provide cool, clear liquids and bland foods as tolerated.

Rationale

7. These dietary restrictions reduce digestive activity, which allows the GI tract to rest.

▲ **Documentation**

Medication administration record
  Type, route, dosage of all
    medications
Progress notes
  Location and status of pain
  Unsatisfactory relief from
    pain-relief measures
  Complaints of nausea, vomit-
    ing, diarrhea

▲ **Outcome Criteria**

The outcome criteria for this diagnosis represent those associated with discharge planning. Refer to the discharge criteria.

Potential Altered Health Maintenance related to prevention of recurrence, dietary restrictions, and fluid requirements

Focus Assessment Criteria	*Clinical Significance*
1. Readiness and ability to learn and retain information	1. A client or family that does not achieve goals for learning requires a referral for assistance postdischarge.

Interventions

1. Explain the relationship of dehydration, urinary stasis, acidic urine, and diet to calculi formation.
2. Stress the importance of adequate hydration (especially during periods of excessive perspiration):
  a. 8 oz every hour
  b. 16 oz before retiring
  c. 8 to 16 oz in the midsleep cycle if he awakens to void
3. Teach the client to avoid extended periods of immobility (sitting, driving, or lying down).
4. Teach the client about dietary modifications needed to prevent future stone formation:
  a. If the stone is composed of calcium phosphate or calcium, the client must do the following:
    • Limit foods/fluids high in calcium or phosphorus (e.g., milk, cheese, organ meats, beans, legumes, whole grains, cocoa, carbonated drinks, nuts, chocolate)
    • Maintain an acidic urine pH
  b. If the stone is composed of oxalate, uric acid, or cystine, the following must be done:
    • Avoid tea, cocoa, instant coffee, cola, beer, rhubarb, beans, spinach, apples, cranberries, grape and citrus fruits
    • Maintain an alkaline urine pH
5. If indicated, teach the client how to self-test urine pH.

Rationale

1. Inaccurate perceptions of health status and the nature of the condition can increase the client's susceptibility to complications or recurrence.
2. Stones form more readily in concentrated urine. Adequate hydration dilutes urine.

3. Inactivity contributes to urinary stasis, altered calcium metabolism, and stone formation.
4. If the composition of the stone is known, certain dietary changes can help to prevent future stone formation by reducing intake and changing the pH of the urine to one incompatible with the stone constituents.

5. Urine pH testing provides the data to determine whether the diet is maintaining the pH as prescribed (acid or alkaline).

Interventions

6. If indicated, teach the client how to strain urine to obtain a stone sample.
7. Teach the client to watch for and report the following:
    a. Decreased urine output
    b. Inability to maintain urine pH
    c. Abdominal pain, distention
    d. Sediment in urine
    e. Recurrent flank pain
    f. Blood in urine
8. Instruct the client to consult with a pharmacist before using any over-the-counter (OTC) drugs.

Rationale

6. Acquiring a stone sample confirms stone formation and enables analysis of stone constituents.
7. Prompt reporting of the signs and symptoms of recurrent calculi enables interventions to reduce their severity.

8. Many OTC drugs contain contraindicated ingredients, e.g., calcium, phosphorus.

▲ **Documentation**

Discharge summary record
  Client teaching
  Outcome achievement
  Referrals, if indicated

References/Bibliography

Connor, P.A., Neskey, K. (1988). Nursing implications of renal pelvis irrigations for chemolysis. *Journal of Urological Nursing, 7*(1), 350–356.

Cuber, A.J., & Whalen-Myers, M.A. (1985). Ureteroscopy. *AORN Journal, 42*(6), 853–858.

McConnell, E.A., & Zimmerman, M.I. (1983). *Care of patients with urologic problems.* Philadelphia: J.B. Lippincott.

Parker-Cohen, P.D. (1988). Extracorporeal shock-wave lithotripsy treatment for kidney stones. *Nurse Practitioner, 13*(3), 32–42.

Staff. (1985). Percutaneous lithotripsy for urinary calculi. *American Journal of Nursing, 85*(7), 772–773.

Neurological Disorders

Cerebrovascular Accident (Stroke)

Cerebrovascular accident, or stroke, involves a sudden onset of neurological deficits due to insufficient blood supply to a part of the brain. Insufficient blood supply is caused by a thrombus, usually secondary to atherosclerosis, to embolism originating elsewhere in the body, or to hemorrhage from a ruptured artery (aneurysm). Stroke is the third leading cause of death in the United States. Predisposing factors include arteriosclerosis, heart disease, pulmonary infections, hypertension, brain tumors, and cerebral atherosclerosis.

Diagnostic Cluster

▲ Time Frame

Initial diagnosis
Recurrent episodes

▲ Discharge Criteria

Before discharge, the client and/ or family will:

1. Describe measures for reducing or eliminating selected risk factors
2. Relate an intent to discuss fears and concerns with family members after discharge
3. Identify methods for management, e.g., of dysphagia, incontinence
4. Demonstrate or relate techniques to increase mobility
5. State signs and symptoms that must be reported to a health care professional
6. Relate community resources that can provide assistance with management at home

Collaborative Problems

Potential Complications:
Increased Intracranial Pressure
Pneumonia, Atelectasis

Refer to:

Nursing Diagnoses

Impaired Communication related to dysarthria or aphasia

Potential for Injury related to visual field, motor or perception deficits

Impaired Physical Mobility related to decreased motor function of (specify) secondary to damage to upper motor neurons

Functional Incontinence related to inability or difficulty in reaching toilet secondary to decreased mobility or motivation

Unilateral Neglect related to (specify site) secondary to right hemispheric brain damage

Impaired Swallowing related to muscle paralysis or paresis secondary to damage to upper motor neurons

Potential Impaired Home Maintenance Management related to altered ability to maintain self at home secondary to sensory/motor/cognitive deficits and lack of knowledge of caregivers of home care, reality orientation, bowel/bladder program, skin care and signs and symptoms of complications, and community resources

Total Incontinence related to loss of bladder tone, loss of sphincter control, or inability to perceive bladder cues — Neurogenic Bladder

Self-Care Deficit related to impaired physical mobility or confusion — Immobility or Unconsciousness

Potential Colonic Constipation related to prolonged periods of immobility, inadequate fluid intake, and inadequate nutritional intake — Immobility or Unconsciousness

Potential Impaired Skin Integrity related to immobility, incontinence, sensory deficits, or motor deficits — Immobility or Unconsciousness

Grieving (individual, family) related to loss of function and inability to meet role responsibilities — Radical Vulvectomy

Potential Impaired Social Interactions related to difficulty communicating and embarrassment regarding disabilities — Enucleation

Potential Fluid Volume Deficit related to dysphagia, difficulty in obtaining fluids secondary to weakness or motor deficits — Immobility or Unconsciousness

Potential Self-Concept Disturbance related to effects of prolonged debilitating condition on achieving developmental tasks and life style — Multiple Sclerosis

Related Care Plan

Immobility or Unconsciousness

202

Collaborative Problems

▲ *Nursing Goal*

The nurse will manage and minimize complications of cerebral vascular accident.

Potential Complication: Increased Intracranial Pressure
Potential Complication: Pneumonia, Atelectasis

Interventions

1. Monitor for signs and symptoms of increased intracranial pressure (ICP).

   a. Assess the following:
  - Best eye opening response: spontaneously, to auditory stimuli, to painful stimuli, or no response
  - Best motor response: obeys verbal commands, localizes pain, flexion-withdrawal, flexion-decorticate, extension-decerebrate, or no response
  - Best verbal response: oriented to person, place, and time; confused conversation, inappropriate speech, incomprehensible sounds, or no response

   b. Assess for changes in vital signs:

  - Pulse changes: slowing rate to 60 or below or increasing rate to 100 or above

  - Respiratory irregularities: slowing of rate with lengthening periods of apnea

  - Rising blood pressure or widening pulse pressure

   c. Assess pupillary responses:

  - Inspect the pupils with a flashlight to evaluate size, configuration, and reaction to light. Compare both eyes for similarities and differences.
  - Evaluate gaze to determine whether it is conjugate (paired, working together) or if eye movements are abnormal.
  - Evaluate ability of the eyes to adduct and abduct.

   d. Note the presence of the following:
  - Vomiting

Rationale

1. Cerebral tissue is compromised by deficiencies of cerebral blood supply caused by hemorrhage, hematoma, cerebral edema, thrombus, or emboli. Monitoring ICP serves as an indicator of cerebral perfusion.

   a. These responses evaluate the client's ability to integrate commands with conscious and involuntary movement. Cortical function can be assessed by evaluating eye opening and motor response. No response may indicate damage to the midbrain.

   b. These vital sign changes may reflect increasing ICP.
  - Changes in pulse may indicate brainstem pressure, slowed at first, then increasing to compensate for hypoxia.
  - Respiratory patterns vary with impairments at various sites. Cheyne-Stokes breathing (a gradual increase followed by a gradual decrease, then a period of apnea) points to damage in both cerebral hemispheres, midbrain, and upper pons. Ataxic breathing (irregular with random sequence of deep and shallow breaths) indicates medullar dysfunction.
  - Blood pressure and pulse pressure changes are late signs indicating severe hypoxia.

   c. Pupillary changes indicate pressure on oculomotor or optic nerves.
  - Pupil reactions are regulated by the oculomotor nerve (cranial nerve III) in the brain stem.

  - Conjugate eye movements are regulated from parts of the cortex and brain stem.

  - Cranial nerve VI, or the abducent nerve, regulates abduction and adduction of the eyes. Cranial nerve IV, or the trochlear nerve, also regulates eye movement.

   d.
  - Vomiting results from pressure on the medulla, which stimulates the brain's vomiting center.

Interventions

- Headache (constant, increasing in intensity, or aggravated by movement or straining)
- Subtle changes, e.g., lethargy, restlessness, forced breathing, purposeless movements, and changes in mentation

2. Elevate the head of the bed 15 to 30 degrees unless contraindicated. Avoid changing position rapidly.
3. Avoid the following:

   a. Carotid massage

   b. Neck flexion or extreme rotation

   c. Digital anal stimulation
   d. Breath holding, straining
   e. Extreme flexion of hips and knees

4. Consult with the physician for stool softeners, if needed.
5. Maintain a quiet, calm, softly lit environment. Plan activities to minimize ICP.

6. Monitor for signs and symptoms of pneumonia:

   a. Increased respiratory rate

   b. Fever, chills (sudden or insidious)

   c. Productive cough

   d. Diminished or absent breath sounds

   e. Pleuritic pain

7. Monitor for signs and symptoms of atelectasis:

   a. Pleuritic pain

   b. Diminished or absent breath sounds
   c. Dull percussion sounds over area

   d. Tachycardia
   e. Increased respiratory rate
   f. Elevated temperature

   g. Marked dyspnea

Rationale

- Compression of neural tissue movement increases ICP and increases pain.

- These changes may be early indicators of ICP changes.

2. Slight head elevation can aid venous drainage to reduce cerebrovascular congestion.
3. These situations or maneuvers can increase ICP.
   a. Carotid massage slows heart rate and reduces systemic circulation, which is followed by a sudden increase in circulation.
   b. Neck flexion or extreme rotation disrupts circulation to the brain.
   c,d,e. These activities initiate Valsalva's maneuver, which impairs venous return by constricting the jugular veins and increases ICP.
4. Stool softeners prevent constipation and straining, which initiate Valsalva's maneuver.
5. These measures promote rest and decrease stimulation, helping decrease ICP. Suctioning, position changes, and neck flexion in succession will markedly increase cranial pressure.
6. Inactivity causes shallow respirations, which can cause pooling of secretions.
   a. Increased respiratory rate is a compensatory mechanism for hypoxia.
   b. Bacteria can act as pyrogen by raising the hypothalamic thermostat through the production of endogenous pyrogen, which may mediate through prostaglandins. Chills can occur when the temperature set-point of the hypothalamus rapidly changes.
   c. Productive cough indicates increased mucus production in response to irritant (bacteria).
   d. Airflow through the tracheobronchial tree is affected or obstructed by the presence of fluid or mucus.
   e. Pleuritic pain results from the rubbing together of inflamed pleural surfaces during respiration.
7. Inactivity can cause retained secretions, leading to obstruction or infection.
   a. Pleuritic pain results from the rubbing together of inflamed pleural surfaces during respiration.
   b,c. Changes in breath and percussion sounds represent increased density of lung tissue secondary to fluid accumulation.
   d,e. Tachycardia and tachypnea are compensatory mechanisms for hypoxia.
   f. Bacteria can act as pyrogen by raising the hypothalamic thermostat through the production of endogenous pyrogen, which may mediate through prostaglandins.
   g. Dyspnea points to hypoxia.

Interventions	Rationale
h. Cyanosis	h. Cyanosis indicates vasoconstriction in response to hypoxia.

8. Monitor hydration status by evaluating the following:
  a. Oral intake
  b. Parenteral therapy
  c. Intake and output
  d. Urine specific gravity
	8. A balance must be maintained to ensure hydration to liquefy secretions while at the same time preventing hypervolemia, which increases ICP.

9. Monitor the effectiveness of airway clearance by evaluating these things:
  a. Effectiveness of cough effort
  b. The need for tracheobronchial suctioning
	9. Immobility increases the pooling of pulmonary secretions.

▲ **Documentation**

Flow records
  Neurological assessment
  Vital signs
  Complaints of vomiting or
    headache
  Changes in status
  Respiratory assessment

Related Physician-Prescribed Interventions

Medications
  Antihypertensives   Stool softeners
  Peripheral vasodilators   Corticosteroids
  Anticoagulants

Intravenous Therapy
  Fluid/electrolyte replacements

Laboratory Studies
  Complete blood count   Prothrombin time
  Chemistry profile   Urinalysis

Diagnostic Studies
  Computed tomography (CT) scan of head   Lumbar puncture
  Cerebral angiography   Magnetic resonance imaging (MRI)
  Positron emission   Tomography scan
  Brain scan   Doppler ultrasonography
  Electroencephalography (EEG)   Skull x-ray film

Therapies
  Antiembolism stockings   Speech therapy
  Physical therapy

Nursing Diagnoses

▲ **Outcome Criteria**

The client will:

1. Be able to communicate basic needs
2. Demonstrate improved ability to express self and understand others
3. Report decreased frustration during communication efforts

Impaired Communication related to dysarthria or aphasia

Focus Assessment Criteria	Clinical Significance
1. Ability to comprehend simple commands and complex ideas	1. Injury to Wernicke's area, located in the temporal lobe, disrupts communication between the auditory and visual fields and interferes with interpretation of the sounds of speech.

2. Ability to speak:
  a. Clear
  b. Slurred
  c. Stuttering
  d. Appropriate use of words
	2. Damaged cells in the frontal lobe near the motor cortex control the movement of the lips, jaw, tongue, soft palate, and vocal cords.

3. Ability to read and write	3. Injury to Wernicke's area also disrupts the ability to read and write.
4. Ability to hear and the functioning of hearing aids, if applicable	4,5. Hearing or vision impairment calls for specific interventions.
5. Ability to see and the correctness of glasses, if applicable	

Interventions

1. Provide an atmosphere of acceptance and privacy:
   a. Do not rush.
   b. Speak in a normal tone and slowly.
   c. Decrease external noise and distractions.
   d. Encourage the client to share his frustrations; validate his nonverbal expressions.
   e. Provide the client with opportunities to make decisions about his care, when appropriate.
2. Make every effort to understand the client's communication efforts:
   a. Listen attentively.
   b. Repeat the client's message back to him to ensure understanding.
   c. Ignore inappropriate word usage; do not correct mistakes.
   d. Do not pretend you understand if you do not, ask the client to repeat.
3. Teach the client techniques to improve speech:
   a. Instruct him to speak slowly and in short phrases.
   b. Initially, ask questions that he can answer with a "yes" or "no."
   c. With improvement, allow person to complete some phrases, e.g., "This is a _____."
   d. As the client is able, encourage him to share feelings and concerns.
4. Use strategies to improve the client's comprehension:
   a. Gain the client's attention before speaking to him.
   b. Practice consistent speech patterns:
      • Speak slowly.
      • Use common words and use the same words consistently for a task.
      • Repeat or rephrase when indicated.
   c. Add other methods of communication in addition to verbal:
      • Point or use flash cards for basic needs.
      • Use pantomime.
      • Display at the client's bedside which methods are most effective.
5. Refer to the Parkinson's disease care plan for further strategies to manage dysarthria.

Rationale

1. Communication is the core of all human relations. Impaired ability to communicate spontaneously is frustrating and embarrassing. Nursing actions should focus on decreasing the tension and conveying an understanding of how difficult the situation must be for the client.

2. The nurse should make every attempt to understand the client. Each success, regardless of how minor, decreases frustration and increases motivation.

3. Deliberate actions can be taken to improve speech. As speech improves, confidence will increase and more attempts at speaking will be made.

4. Improving the client's comprehension can help decrease frustration.

▲ **Documentation**

Progress notes
  Dialogues
  Method to use (care plan)

▲ **Outcome Criteria**

The client will:

1. Identify factors that increase the risk for injury
2. Demonstrate safety measures to prevent injury
3. Request assistance when needed

Potential for Injury related to visual field, motor, or perception deficits

Focus Assessment Criteria	*Clinical Significance*

1. Acuity:
  a. Vision
  b. Bearing
  c. Thermal and tactile perception
2. Mental status
	1,2. This assessment helps determine whether the client can detect environmental hazards.

3. Mobility for ambulation and for self-care activities	3. This assessment determines whether the client needs assistance or assistive devices.
4. Gait	4. A client with unstable gait needs assistance with ambulation.

Interventions

1. Take steps to reduce environmental hazards:
   a. Orient the client to his surroundings.
   b. Instruct him to use a call bell to summon assistance.
   c. Keep the bed in a low position with all side rails up.
   d. Keep paths to the bathroom obstacle-free.
   e. Provide adequate lighting in all areas.
   f. Provide a night light.
   g. Ensure that a light switch is accessible next to the bed.
2. If decreased tactile sensitivity is a problem, teach the client to do the following:
   a. Carefully assess temperature of bathwater and heating pads prior to use, using a thermometer if possible
   b. Assess extremities daily for undetected injuries
   c. Keep feet warm and dry and skin softened with emollient lotion (e.g., lanolin, mineral oil).
3. Take steps to reduce risks associated with assistive devices:
   a. Assess for the proper use of devices.
   b. Assess devices for fit and condition.
   c. Consult with a physical therapist for gait training.
   d. Instruct the client to wear shoes with non-skid soles.
4. Teach the client and family to maximize safety at home:
   a. Eliminate throw rugs, clutter and litter, and highly polished floors.
   b. Provide nonslip surfaces in the bathtub or shower by applying commercially available traction tapes.
   c. Provide hand grips in the bathroom.
   d. Provide railings in hallways and on stairs.
   e. Remove protruding objects (e.g., coat hooks, shelves, light fixtures) from stairway walls.

Rationale

1. Emphasizing safety can help reduce injuries.

2. Post-CVA sensory impairment can interfere with the client's perception of temperature and injuries.

3. Improper use or fit of assistive devices can cause straining or falls.

4. A client with mobility problems needs such safety devices installed and hazards eliminated to aid in activities of daily living.

▲ **Documentation**

Discharge summary record
Client teaching

▲ **Outcome Criteria**

The client will demonstrate measures to increase mobility.

Impaired Physical Mobility related to decreased motor function of (specify) secondary to damage to upper motor neurons

Focus Assessment Criteria	*Clinical Significance*
1. Dominant hand	1. If the client's dominant hand is impaired, he requires more assistance.
2. Motor function, range of motion, and strength in hands, arms, and legs	2,3. These assessments provide baseline data to determine the assistance needed and to evaluate progress.
3. Mobility: ability to turn, sit, stand, transfer, and ambulate	

Interventions

1. Teach the client to perform active range-of-motion (ROM) exercises on unaffected limbs at least four times a day, if possible.

Rationale

1. Active ROM increases muscle mass, tone, and strength and improves cardiac and respiratory functioning.

Interventions

2. Perform passive ROM on affected limbs. Do the exercises slowly to allow the muscles time to relax, and support the extremity above and below the joint to prevent strain on joints and tissues.
3. When the client is in bed, take steps to maintain alignment:

   a. Use a foot board.
   b. Avoid prolonged periods of sitting or lying in the same position.
   c. Change position of the shoulder joints every 2 to 4 hours.
   d. Use a small pillow or no pillow when in Fowler's position.
   e. Support the hand and wrist in natural alignment.
   f. If the client is supine or prone, place a rolled towel or small pillow under the lumbar curvature or under the end of the rib cage.
   g. Place a trochanter roll or sand bags alongside the hips and upper thighs.
   h. If the client is in the lateral position, place pillow(s) to support the leg from groin to foot, and a pillow to flex the shoulder and elbow slightly; if needed, support the lower foot in dorsal flexion with a sandbag.
   i. Use hand-wrist splints.

4. Provide progressive mobilization:
   a. Assist the client slowly from the lying to the sitting position.
   b. Allow the client to dangle his legs over the side of the bed for a few minutes before he stands up.
   c. Initially limit the time out of bed to 15 minutes, three times a day.
   d. Increase time out of bed by 15-minute increments, as tolerated.
   e. Progress to ambulation with or without assistive devices.
   f. If the client cannot walk, assist him out of bed to a wheelchair or chair.
   g. Encourage short, frequent walks (at least three times daily), with assistance if unsteady.
   h. Increase the length of walks each day.
5. Gradually help the client progress from active ROM to functional activities, as indicated.

Rationale

2. Passive ROM improves joint mobility and circulation.

3. Prolonged immobility and impaired neurosensory function can cause permanent contractures.
   a. This measure helps prevent foot drop.
   b. This measure prevents hip flexion contractures.
   c. This measure prevents shoulder contractures.
   d. This measure prevents flexion contracture of the neck.
   e. This measure prevents dependent edema and flexion contracture of the wrist.
   f. This measure prevents flexion or hyperflexion of lumbar curvature.

   g. This measure prevents external rotation of femurs and hip.
   h. These measures prevent internal rotation and adduction of the femurs and hip, internal rotation and adduction of the shoulder, and foot drop.

   i. These splints prevent flexion or extension contractures of fingers and abduction of the thumb.
4. Prolonged bed rest or decreased blood volume can cause a sudden drop in blood pressure (orthostatic hypotension) as blood returns to peripheral circulation. Gradual progression to increased activity reduces fatigue and increases endurance.

5. Exercise increases independence. Incorporating ROM exercises into the client's daily routine encourages their regular performance.

▲ **Documentation**

Flow records
   Range of motion exercises
   Progress in activities, ambulation

▲ **Outcome Criteria**

The client will:
1. Describe causative factors for incontinence
2. Eliminate or reduce incontinent episodes

Functional Incontinence related to inability or difficulty in reaching toilet secondary to decreased mobility or motivation

Focus Assessment Criteria	*Clinical Significance*
1. Mobility, desire to be continent	1. Specific assessments are needed to evaluate self-care ability.
2. Ability to delay urination after urge	2. A small bladder capacity interferes with retraining.
3. Perception of need to void	3. The client's ability to recognize bladder cues is necessary to enable participation in bladder retraining.
4. Incontinence episodes	4. A baseline assessment provides a means for evaluating progress.

Interventions

1. Assess the environment for barriers to the client's access to the bathroom.

2. Provide grab rails and a raised toilet seat, if necessary.
3. If the client requires assistance, provide ready access to a call bell and respond promptly when summoned.
4. Encourage the client to wear pajamas or ordinary clothes.

5. For a client with cognitive deficits, do the following:
   a. Offer toileting reminders every 2 hours after meals and before bedtime.
   b. Provide verbal instruction for toileting activities.
   c. Praise success and good attempts.
6. Maintain optimal hydration (2000 to 2500 mL/ day, unless contraindicated). Space fluids every 2 hours.

7. Minimize intake of coffee, tea, colas, and grapefruit juice.

Rationale

1. Barriers can delay access to the toilet and cause incontinence if the client cannot delay urination.

2. These devices can promote independence and reduce toileting difficulties.
3. A few seconds' delay in reaching the bathroom can make the difference between continence and incontinence.
4. Wearing normal clothing or nightwear helps simulate the home environment, where incontinence may not occur. A hospital gown may reinforce incontinence.
5. A client with a cognitive deficit needs constant verbal cues and reminders to establish a routine and reduce incontinence.

6. Dehydration can prevent the sensation of a full bladder and can contribute to loss of bladder tone. Spacing fluids help promote regular bladder filling and emptying.
7. These beverages act as diuretics, which can cause urgency.

▲ **Documentation**

Flow records
  Intake and output
  Incontinent episodes

▲ **Outcome Criteria**

The client will:

1. Demonstrate an ability to scan the visual field to compensate for loss of function or sensation in affected limb(s)
2. Describe the deficit and the rationale for treatments

Unilateral Neglect related to (specify site) secondary to right hemispheric brain damage

Focus Assessment Criteria	*Clinical Significance*
1. Cuts in visual acuity and visual field	1. Loss of vision may occur on the side contralateral to the brain injury.
2. Sensory losses	2. Perceptual deficits result from right hemispheric brain damage.
3. Presence of neglect in one side of the body or face or in one limb	3. This assessment identifies what areas are neglected.

Interventions

1. Initially adapt the client's environment:
   a. Place the call light, telephone, and bedside stand on the unaffected side.
   b. Always approach the client from the unaffected side.
2. Orient the client to the environment, and teach him to recognize the forgotten field (e.g., place the telephone out of his visual field).

Rationale

1. Environmental adaptations enhance security and safety.

2. These reminders can help the client adapt to the environment.

Interventions

3. Teach the client to:
   a. Stroke the affected side
   b. Watch the body part as he strokes
   c. Vary tactile stimulation (e.g., warm, cold, rough, soft)
4. Teach the client to scan the entire environment, turning the head to compensate for visual field cuts. Remind him to scan when ambulating.
5. Teach the client to:
   a. Wear an arm sling when upright
   b. Position the arm on a lapboard
   c. Use a Plexiglass lapboard so he can view the affected leg
   d. Recognize the danger of sources of cold and heat and moving machinery to the affected limb(s).
6. For self-care, instruct the client to:
   a. Attend to the affected side first
   b. Use adaptive equipment as needed
   c. Always check the affected limb(s) during activities of daily living (ADLs).

Rationale

3. Tactile stimulation of the affected parts promotes their integration into the whole body.

4. Scanning can help prevent injury.

5. Decreased sensation or motor function increases the vulnerability to injury.

6. The client may need specific reminders to prevent him from ignoring nonfunctioning body parts.

▲ **Documentation**

Progress notes
    Presence of neglect
Discharge summary record
    Client teaching
    Response to teaching

▲ **Outcome Criteria**

The client will:
1. Verbalize feelings and concerns related to impaired swallowing
2. Demonstrate effective swallowing
3. Avoid complications of impaired swallowing

Impaired Swallowing related to muscle paralysis or paresis secondary to damage to upper motor neurons

Focus Assessment Criteria	*Clinical Significance*
1. Ability to swallow food and liquid	1. Post-CVA paresis or paralysis can interfere with the ability to chew and swallow.
2. Gag and swallowing reflexes	2. Impaired reflexes increase the risk of aspiration.

Interventions

1. Position the head of the bed in semi- or high Fowler's position, with the neck flexed forward slightly.
2. Plan meals when client is well rested; ensure that reliable suction equipment is on hand during meals.
3. Instruct the client to attempt swallowing in a stepwise fashion. Cue him to follow these steps:
   a. Place food on the tongue.
   b. Move food over to the teeth on the unaffected side using the tongue.
   c. Chew food completely.
   d. Hold breath.
   e. Swallow.
4. Assist with meals, as necessary:
   a. Give solids and liquids separately; begin with solids.
   b. Provide small amounts.
   c. Instruct the client to hold breath while swallowing.
   d. Check the mouth for emptying after he swallows.
5. For a client with cognitive deficits, do the following:

Rationale

1. This position uses the force of gravity to aid downward motion of food.

2. Fatigue can increase the risk of aspiration.

3. The client may require verbal cues to complete the eating and swallowing process.

4. The client may be unable to eat unassisted.
   a. Solids stimulate the muscles needed for swallowing and closure of the epiglottis.
   b. Small portions prevent overloading.
   c. Breath-holding during swallowing prevents aspiration by closing the epiglottis.
   d. Checking the mouth determines whether swallowing has occurred.
5. A confused client needs repetitive, simple instructions.

Interventions

    a. Divide eating tasks into the smallest steps possible.

    b. Provide a verbal command for each step.

    c. Progress slowly.

    d. Continue verbal assistance at each meal as needed.

    e. Provide a written checklist as appropriate.

6. Collaborate with a speech pathologist if the client does not progress adequately.

Rationale

6. Expert consultation for swallowing problems may be needed.

▲ **Documentation**

Flow records
    Intake of foods and fluids
Progress notes
    Swallowing difficulties

▲ **Outcome Criteria**

The outcome criteria for this diagnosis represent those associated with discharge planning.

Potential Impaired Home Maintenance Management related to altered ability to maintain self at home secondary to sensory/motor/cognitive deficits and lack of knowledge of caregivers of home care, reality orientation, bowel/bladder program, skin care and signs and symptoms of complications, and community resources

Focus Assessment Criteria	*Clinical Significance*
1. Readiness and ability to learn and retain information	1. A client and/or family that does not achieve goals for learning requires a referral for assistance postdischarge.

Interventions

1. Teach about the condition, its cause, and treatments.

2. Identify risk factors that can be controlled:

    a. Hypertension

    b. Smoking

    c. Obesity

    d. High-fat diet

    e. High-sodium diet

3. Explain signs and symptoms of complications, and stress the need for prompt reporting:

    a. Development of or increase in weakness, lethargy, dysphagia, aphasia, vision problems, confusion

    b. Seizures

4. Discuss with family the anticipated stressors associated with CVA and its treatment:

    a. Financial

    b. Changes in role responsibilities

    c. Dependency

    (Refer to Chapter 3, the Ill Adult: Issues and Responses, for information regarding the effects of chronic illness on families.)

5. Provide information about or initiate referrals to community resources, e.g., counselors, home health agencies, American Heart Association.

Rationale

1. Understanding can reinforce the need to comply with the treatment regimen.

2. Focusing on factors that can be controlled can improve compliance, increase self-esteem, and reduce feelings of helplessness.

    a. Hypertension with increased peripheral resistance damages the intima of blood vessels, contributing to arteriosclerosis.

    b. Smoking produces tachycardia, raises blood pressure, and constricts blood vessels.

    c. Obesity increases cardiac workload.

    d. A high-fat diet may increase arteriosclerosis and plaque formation.

    e. Sodium controls water distribution throughout the body. A gain in sodium causes a gain in water, thus increasing the circulating volume.

3. These signs and symptoms may indicate increasing ICP or cerebral tissue hypoxia.

4. Serious illness of a family member can cause disruption of family functioning.

5. Such resources can provide needed assistance with home management and help minimize the potentially destructive effects on the client and family.

▲ **Documentation**

Discharge summary record
    Client teaching
    Outcome achievement or status
    Referrals, if indicated

References/Bibliography

Burgener, S. (1989). Sexuality concerns of the post-stroke patient. *Rehabilitation Nursing, 14*(4), 178–181.

Carr, E.K. (1988). Lip function and eating after a stroke: A nursing perspective. *Journal of Advanced Nursing, 13*(4), 447–451.

Kernich, C.A. (1988). Development of a stroke family support and education program. *Journal of Neuroscience Nursing 20*(3), 193–197.

Novack, T.A. (1987). Prediction of stroke rehabilitation outcome from psychologic screening. *Archives of Physical Medical Rehabilitation 68*(10), 729–734.

Tanner, D.C. (1989). Guidelines for treatment of chronic depression in the aphasic patient. *Rehabilitation Nursing 14*(2), 77–80.

Multiple Sclerosis

Multiple sclerosis (MS) is a chronic degenerative disease involving destruction of myelin (fatty and protein material of the nerve sheath). This demyelination slows or blocks transmission of nerve impulses, producing neuromuscular deficits. The etiology of MS is unclear; however, it may be linked to a virus that triggers an abnormal immune response. Characterized by periodic remissions and exacerbations, MS produces varying signs and symptoms depending on the location of the lesions.

Diagnostic Cluster

▲ **Time Frame**

Initial diagnosis
Recurrent acute exacerbations

Collaborative Problems

Potential Complications:
Urinary Tract Infection
Renal Insufficiency
Pneumonia

Refer to:

Cerebrovascular Accident
(Stroke)

Nursing Diagnoses

Potential Self-Concept Disturbance related to the effects of prolonged debilitating condition on life style and on achieving developmental tasks

Altered Family Processes related to nature of disorder, role disturbances, and uncertain future

Potential Altered Health Maintenance related to lack of knowledge of condition, treatments, prevention of infection, stress management, aggravating factors, signs and symptoms of complications, and community resources

Potential for Injury related to unsteady gait, visual disturbances, weakness, or uncontrolled movement

Cerebrovascular Accident (Stroke)

Impaired Swallowing related to cerebellar lesions

Cerebrovascular Accident (Stroke)

Impaired Verbal Communication related to dysarthria secondary to ataxia of muscles of speech

Parkinson's Disease

Fatigue related to extremity weakness, spasticity, fear of injury, and stressors

Inflammatory Joint Disease

Urinary Retention related to sensorimotor deficits

Neurogenic Bladder

Incontinence (specify) related to poor sphincter control and spastic bladder

Neurogenic Bladder

Powerlessness related to the unpredictable nature of condition (remissions/exacerbation)

Chronic Obstructive Pulmonary Disease

Related Care Plans

Immobility or Unconsciousness
Corticosteroid Therapy

▲ **Discharge Criteria**

Before discharge, the client and/or family will:

1. Relate an intent to share concerns with other family members or trusted friend(s)
2. Identify one strategy to increase independence
3. Describe actions that can reduce the risk of exacerbation
4. Identify signs and symptoms that must be reported to a health care professional

Collaborative Problems

▲ **Nursing Goal**

The nurse will manage and minimize urinary and renal complications.

Potential Complication: Urinary Tract Infections
Potential Complication: Renal Insufficiency

Interventions

1. Monitor for signs and symptoms of urinary tract infection:

Rationale

1. MS can cause urinary retention owing to lesions of afferent pathways from the bladder. Re-

Interventions

Rationale

sulting urine stasis contributes to microorganism growth. Also, corticosteroid therapy reduces the effectiveness of WBCs against infection.

a. Chills, fever

a. Bacteria can act as a pyrogen by raising the hypothalamic thermostat through the production of endogenous pyrogen, which may mediate through prostaglandins. Chills can occur when the temperature set-point of the hypothalamus rapidly changes.

b. Costovertebral angle (CVA) pain (a dull, constant backache below the 12th rib)

b. CVA pain results from distention of the renal capsule.

c. Leukocytosis

c. Leukocytosis reflects an increase in WBCs to fight infection through phagocytosis.

d. Foul odor or pus in urine

d. Bacteria changes the odor and pH of urine.

e. Dysuria, frequency

e. Bacteria irritates bladder tissue, causing spasms and frequency.

2. Monitor for early signs and symptoms of renal insufficiency:

2. Repeated infections can alter renal function.

a. Sustained elevated urine specific gravity
b. Elevated urine sodium levels

a,b. Decreased ability of the renal tubules to reabsorb electrolytes causes increased urine sodium levels and increased specific gravity.

c. Sustained insufficient urine output (30 mL/hr)
d. Elevated blood pressure

c,d. Decreased glomerular filtration rate eventually causes insufficient urine output and stimulates renin production, which raises blood pressure in an attempt to increase blood flow to the kidneys.

e. Increasing blood urea nitrogen (BUN) and pressure serum creatinine, potassium, phosphorus, and ammonia, and decreased creatinine clearance

e. Decreased excretion of urea potassium, and creatinine in the urine results in elevated BUN potassium, and creatinine levels. The kidneys' inability to excrete hydrogen ions, phosphates, sulfates, and ketone bodies causes increased levels of acidosis.

▲ **Documentation**

Flow records
　Intake and output
　Urine specific gravity

Related Physician-Prescribed Treatments
Medications
　Muscle relaxants
　Corticosteroids
　　　　　Vitamin B
　　　　　Immunosuppressives
Intravenous Therapy
　Adrenocorticotropic hormone (ACTH)
Laboratory Studies
　Electrophoresis gammaglobulin level
Diagnostic Studies
　Electroencephalography (EEG)
　Computed tomography (CT) scan of the brain
　　　　　Magnetic resonance imaging (MRI)
　　　　　Lumbar puncture
Therapies
　Dependent on deficits, e.g., urinary, motor

Nursing Diagnoses

▲ *Outcome Criteria*

The client will:
1. Acknowledge changes in body structure and function
2. Communicate feelings about disability
3. Participate in self-care

Potential Self-Concept Disturbance related to the effects of prolonged debilitating condition on life style and on achieving developmental tasks

Focus Assessment Criteria

1. Previous exposure to persons with MS
2. Ability to express feelings about condition
3. Ability to share feelings with family members or significant others

Clinical Significance

1–4. This information helps the nurse detect patterns of response due to adaptation. It may be helpful to note how the client's support persons view the client's self-con-

Focus Assessment Criteria	*Clinical Significance*
4. Evidence of or others' reports of negative self-concept	cept; they can provide insight into factors that may have had a negative impact on self-concept, and tend to be sensitive to subtle changes.
5. Participation in self-care 6. Evidence of adapting life style to disabilities	5,6. Participation in self-care and adapting goals to the disability indicate attempts to cope with the changes.

Interventions

1. Contact the client frequently and treat him with warm, positive regard.

2. Encourage the client to express feelings and thoughts about the following:
   a. Condition
   b. Progress
   c. Prognosis
   d. Effects on life style
   e. Support system
   f. Treatments

3. Provide reliable information and clarify any misconceptions.

4. Help the client to identify positive attributes and possible new opportunities.

5. Assist with hygiene and grooming, as needed.

6. Encourage visitors.

7. Help the client identify strategies to increase independence and maintain role responsibilities, such as the following:
   a. Prioritizing activities
   b. Getting assistance with less valued or most fatiguing activities, e.g., shopping, housekeeping
   c. Using energy conservation techniques (Refer to the nursing diagnosis Fatigue in the Inflammatory Joint Disease care plan, page 297, for specific strategies.)
   d. Using mobility aids and assistive devices, as needed

8. Discuss ways that the client can provide support to support persons:
   a. Actively listening to their problems
   b. Attempting to decrease the focus on disabilities (Refer to Chapter 3, the Ill Adult: Issues and Responses, for more information.)

9. Allow the client's support persons to share their feelings regarding the diagnoses and actual or anticipated effects.

Rationale

1. Frequent contact by the caregiver indicates acceptance and may facilitate trust. The client may be hesitant to approach the staff because of negative self-concept.

2. Encouraging the client to share feelings can provide a safe outlet for fears and frustrations and can increase self-awareness.

3. Misconceptions can needlessly increase anxiety and damage self-concept.

4. The client may tend to focus only on the change in self-image and not on the positive characteristics that contribute to the whole concept of self. The nurse must reinforce these positive aspects and encourage the client to reincorporate them into his new self-concept.

5. Participation in self-care and planning can aid positive coping.

6. Frequent visits by support persons can help the client feel that he is still a worthwhile, acceptable person, which should promote a positive self-concept.

7. A strong component of self-concept is the ability to perform functions expected of one's role, thus decreasing dependency and reducing the need for others' involvement.

8. The nurse can help the client learn how to balance relationships and preserve the family system.

9. Degenerative chronic disease can negatively affect support persons financially, socially, and emotionally.

Interventions

10. Assess for signs of negative response to changes in appearance:
    a. Refusal to discuss loss
    b. Denial of changes
    c. Decreased self-care ability
    d. Social isolation
    e. Refusal to discuss the future
11. Refer an at-risk client for professional counseling.

Rationale

10. These signs may indicate that the client is at high risk for unsuccessful adjustment.

11. Follow-up therapy may be indicated to assist with adjustment.

▲ **Documentation**

Progress notes
  Present emotional status
  Interventions
  Response to interventions

▲ **Outcome Criteria**

The client and family will:
1. Verbalize feelings regarding the diagnosis and disabilities
2. Identify signs of family dysfunction
3. Identify appropriate resources to seek when needed

Altered Family Processes related to the nature of the disorder, role disturbances, and uncertain future

Focus Assessment Criteria	*Clinical Significance*
1. Understanding of condition 2. Family coping patterns 3. Current response 4. Available resources	1–4. The family unit is a system based on interdependency between members and patterns that provide structure and support. Chronic illness in one family member disrupts these relationships and patterns.

Interventions

1. Convey an understanding of the situation and its impact on the family.

2. Explore family members' perceptions of the situation. Encourage verbalization of feelings such as guilt, anger, and blame.
3. Determine whether present coping mechanisms are effective.

4. Take steps to promote family strengths:
   a. Acknowledge the assistance of family members.
   b. Involve the family in the client's care.
   c. Encourage time away from caregiving to prevent burnout.
   d. Encourage humor.
   (Refer to Chapter 3, The Ill Adult: Issues and Responses, for more information.)
5. Assist to reorganize roles at home, set new priorities, and redistribute responsibilities.
6. Prepare the family for signs of depression, anxiety, anger, and dependency in the client and other family members.
7. Encourage the family to call on its social network (e.g., friends, relatives, church members) for emotional and other support.
8. Identify dysfunctional coping mechanisms:
   a. Substance abuse
   b. Continued denial
   c. Exploitation of one or more family members
   d. Separation or avoidance (Friedman, 1981)
   Refer for counseling as necessary.
9. Direct to community agencies and other sources of assistance (e.g., financial, housekeeping, direct care), as needed.

Rationale

1. Communicating understanding and a sense of caring and concern facilitates trust and strengthens the nurse's relationship with the client and family.
2. Verbalization can provide opportunities for clarification and validation of feelings and concerns, contributing to family unity.
3. Illness of a family member may cause great changes, putting the family at high risk for maladaptation.
4. This can help maintain the existing family structure and its function as a supportive unit.

5. Planning and prioritizing can help maintain family integrity and reduce stress.
6. Anticipatory guidance can alert members to potential problems before they occur, enabling prompt intervention at early signs.
7. Outside assistance may help reduce the perception that the family must "go it alone."

8. A family with a history of unsuccessful coping may need additional resources. A family with unresolved conflicts prior to diagnosis is at high risk.

9. The family may need assistance to help with management at home.

▲ **Documentation**

Progress notes
  Present family functioning
  Interventions
  Family's response to interventions
Discharge summary record
  Referrals, if indicated

▲ **Outcome Criteria**

The outcome criteria for this diagnosis represent those associated with discharge planning. Refer to the discharge criteria.

Potential Altered Health Maintenance related to lack of knowledge of condition, treatments, prevention of infection, stress management, aggravating factors, signs and symptoms of complications, and community resources.

Focus Assessment Criteria	*Clinical Significance*
1. Readiness and ability to learn and retain information	1. A client or family that does not achieve goals for learning requires a referral for assistance postdischarge.

Interventions

1. Assist in formulating and accepting realistic short- and long-term goals.
2. Teach about the diagnosis and management techniques.
3. Discuss the importance of strengthening and stretching exercises for the arms, legs, and facial and respiratory muscles. Consult with a physical therapist.
4. Discuss the factors known to trigger exacerbation (Hickey, 1986):
   a. Undue fatigue or excessive exertion
   b. Overheating or excessive chilling or cold exposure
   c. Infections
   d. Hot baths
   e. Fever
   f. Emotional stress
   g. Pregnancy
5. Teach energy conservation techniques. (Refer to the nursing diagnosis Fatigue in the Inflammatory Joint Disease care plan, page 297, for more information.)
6. Instruct a pregnant client or a client contemplating pregnancy to consult with a physician to discuss the problems associated with pregnancy.
7. Explain the hazards of infection and ways to reduce the risk:
   a. Avoid contact with infected persons.

   b. Receive immunization against influenza and streptococcal pneumonia, if advised.
   c. Cleanse all equipment and utensils well.

   d. Eat a well-balanced diet and get sufficient rest.

   e. Drink 2000 mL of fluids daily unless contraindicated by renal insufficiency.
8. Teach the importance of constructive stress management and reduction; explain measures such as the following:
   a. Progressive relaxation techniques
   b. Self-coaching
   c. Thought-stopping
   d. Assertiveness techniques
   e. Guided imagery
   If possible, refer to community resources for specific courses or assistance.

Rationale

1. Mutual goal-setting reinforces the client's role in improving his own quality of life.
2. Understanding can help improve compliance and reduce exacerbations.
3. Exercise can prevent underused muscles from becoming weak. Facial and respiratory muscle exercises can improve speech deficits.

4. This information gives the client insight into aspects of the condition that can be controlled, which may promote a sense of control and encourage compliance.

5. Energy conservation can prevent fatigue.

6. Pregnancy is associated with onset and exacerbations of MS.

7. Minor infections can cause serious problems in a client with MS.
   a. This precaution reduces the risk of cross-infection.
   b. Immunization confers protection against these infections.
   c. Proper cleansing removes microorganisms and secretions that are a medium for microorganism growth.
   d. Adequate nutrition and rest promote overall good health and increase the resistance to infection.
   e. Adequate hydration prevents concentrated urine with high levels of bacteria.
8. Stress management minimizes external and internal demands and conflicts (Lazarus and Folkman, 1984), releasing energy for more positive functioning.

Interventions

9. Teach the effects of MS on bowel function and the techniques to prevent constipation or incontinence. (Refer to the appropriate nursing diagnoses in the Immobility or Unconsciousness care plan, page 243, for specific interventions.)
10. Explore with the client and partner problems that may interfere with sexual activity:
    a. Low self-esteem
    b. Fatigue
    c. Ejaculatory disorders
    d. Thigh muscle spasms
    e. Fear of bowel or bladder incontinence
11. Refer to a counselor for continued therapy.
12. Explain the signs and symptoms that must be reported to a health care professional:
    a. Worsening of symptoms (e.g., weakness, spasticity, visual disturbances)
    b. Temperature elevation
    c. Change in urination patterns or cloudy, foul-smelling urine
    d. Productive cough with cloudy greenish sputum
    e. Cessation of menses

13. Provide information and materials to assist the client and family to maintain goals and manage at home, from sources such as the following:
    a. Multiple Sclerosis Society
    b. Home health agencies
    c. American Red Cross
    d. Individual/family counselors

Rationale

9. Constipation results from decreased paralysis due to immobility and decreased fluid and fiber intake. Bowel incontinence is caused by lesions of the efferent pathways of the corticospinal tract, resulting in loss of sphincter control.
10. Libido is negatively influenced by stress, fatigue, and low self-esteem. Ejaculatory disorders result from lesions in the pyramidal tracts of the spinal cord.

11. The client may need follow-up therapy.
12. Early detection enables prompt intervention to minimize complications.
    a. Worsening symptoms may herald an exacerbation.
    b,c,d These symptoms may indicate infection (urinary tract or pulmonary).

    e. Cessation of menses may indicate pregnancy, which can exacerbate MS.
13. A client who feels well-supported can cope more effectively with the multiple stressors associated with chronic debilitating disease.

▲ **Documentation**

Discharge summary record
    Client teaching
    Outcome achievement or status
    Referrals, if indicated

References/Bibliography

Burr, B., Good, B.J., & Good, M.D. (1978). The impact of illness on the family. In R.B. Taylor (Ed.). *Family medicine: Principles and practice.* New York: Springer-Verlag.

Christensen, K.E. (1979). Family epidemiology: An approach to assessment and intervention. In D.P. Hymovich & M.V. Barnard (Eds.). *Family health care* (2nd ed.). New York: McGraw-Hill.

Dewis M.D., & Thornton, N.G. (1989). Sexual dysfunction in multiple sclerosis. *Journal of Neuroscience Nursing, 21*(3), 175–180.

Fife, B.L. (1985). A model for predicting the adaptation of families to medical crisis: An analysis of role integration. *Image: The Journal of Nursing Scholarship, 18*(4), 108–112.

Friedman, M. (1981). *Family nursing: Theory and assessment.* New York: Appleton-Century-Crofts.

Henderson, J.S. (1988). A pubococcygeal exercise program for simple urinary stress incontinence; Applicability to the female client with multiple sclerosis. *Journal of Neuroscience Nursing, 20*(3), 185–188.

Hickey, J. (1986). *The clinical practice of neurological and neurosurgical nursing* (2nd ed.). Philadelphia: J.B. Lippincott.

Lazarus, R.S., & Folkman, R. (1984). *Stress, appraisal, and coping.* New York: Springer-Verlag Publishing.

Miller, S., & Winstead-Fry, P. (1982). *Family systems theory in nursing practice.* Reston, VA: Reston Publishing.

Minuchin, A. (1974). *Families and family therapy.* Cambridge, MA: Harvard University Press.

Morgante, L., Madonna, M., & Pokoluk, R. (1989). Research and treatment in multiple sclerosis: Implications for nursing practice. *Journal of Neuroscience Nursing, 21*(5), 285–289.

Samonds, R.J., & Cammermeyer, M. (1989). Perceptions of body image in subjects with multiple sclerosis: A pilot study. *Journal of Neuroscience Nursing, 21*(3), 190–195.

Parkinson's Disease

Parkinson's disease is a chronic degenerative disorder of the basal ganglia causing impairment of extrapyramidal tracts, semiautomatic functions, and coordinated movements. Initial symptoms typically develop after age 60. Onset is insidious, and a diagnosis may not be made for years.

Diagnostic Cluster

▲ Time Frame

Secondary diagnosis (hospitalization not usual)

▲ Discharge Criteria

Before discharge, the client and/or family will:

1. Relate an intent to share concerns with another family member or a trusted friend
2. Identify one strategy to increase independence
3. Describe measures that can reduce the risk of exacerbation
4. Identify signs and symptoms that must be reported to a health care professional

Nursing Diagnoses

Impaired Verbal Communication related to dysarthria secondary to ataxia of muscles of speech

Impaired Physical Mobility related to effects of muscle rigidity, tremors, and slowness of movement on activities of daily living

Related Care Plans

Immobility or Unconsciousness
Multiple Sclerosis

Nursing Diagnoses

▲ Outcome Criteria

The client will:

1. Demonstrate techniques and exercises to improve speech and strengthen muscles
2. Demonstrate improved ability for self-expression

Impaired Communication related to dysarthria secondary to ataxia of muscles of speech

Focus Assessment Criteria

1. Speech:
   a. Volume
   b. Intonation (monotone)
   c. Quality (breathy, hoarse)
   d. Fate
   e. Rhythm (hesitation)
2. Articulation
3. Hearing

Clinical Significance

1,2. Speech is a motor activity involving complex coordination of intrinsic and extrinsic muscles of the larynx with those of the pharynx, soft palate, lips, and tongue. Parkinson's disease causes neuromuscular incoordination of these muscles.

3. Communication problems are complicated by hearing impairments.

Interventions

1. Explain the effects of the disorder on speech.

2. Explain the benefits of daily speech improvement exercises.

3. Teach the client measures recommended by the American Parkinson's Disease Association:
   a. Practice in front of a mirror.

   b. Do exercises to improve voice loudness:
      • Place hands on abdomen, inhale slowly, and exhale slowly. Repeat several times.

Rationale

1. Understanding may promote compliance with speech improvement exercises.

2. Daily exercises help improve the efficiency of speech musculature and increase rate, volume, and articulation.

3. These exercises improve muscle tone and control and speech clarity.
   a. Practicing in front of a mirror allows the client to see and evaluate his lip and tongue movements.

   b. These exercises increase air intake and improve control over air intake and exhalation during speech.

Interventions   *Rationale*

- Breathe in and then pronounce tones as
  you breathe out. Hold sound only as long
  as your voice is strong, as follows:
      Breathe in, say "Ah," and rest.
      Breathe in, say "Oh," and rest.
      Breathe in, say "Aw," and rest.
      Breathe in, say "Oo," and rest.
- Count from one to ten and take a breath
  between each number. Forcefully push
  out each number. Progress to two or
  three sets of numbers, as below:
      Breathe in, say "One."
      Breathe in, say "Two, three."

c. Do exercises to improve voice variation: c. These exercises enhance speech intelligibil-
- Practice regulating voice from soft to   ity.
  loud. Breathe in each time you start an
  exercise and stop when voice fades:
      "I will" (softly)
      "I will" (a little louder)
      "I will" (much louder)
- Say a sentence several times and stress a
  word. Change the word each time. For example, use the following sentence:
      I don't want that blue hat.
      I *don't* want that blue hat.
      I don't *want* that blue hat.
      I don't want *that* blue hat.
      I don't want that *blue* hat.
      I don't want that blue *hat.*
- Practice asking questions and giving answers. Raise the voice after a question,
  lower it with an answer, as below:
      "Are you cold?" (raise voice)
      "No, I am not." (lower voice)
      "Can I help you?" (raise voice)
      "Yes, you can." (lower voice)

d. Practice tongue exercises several times: d. These exercises strengthen the tongue and
- Stick tongue out as far as you can, hold,   increase its range of motion, to improve
  relax.   articulation.
- Stick tongue out and move slowly from
  corner to corner.
- Stretch tongue to chin and then to nose.
- Stick tongue out and put it back as fast
  as you can.
- Move tongue in a circle as quickly as you
  can around lips.
- Practice words with final consonant
  sounds *k* or *g*:
      Luck   Egg
      Back   Dog
      Lake   Pig
      Sick   Frog
- Practice words that end with the following
  consonant sounds:
      t—cat   s—face
      d—paid   z—hose
      n—seen   sh—fish
      l—mail   dz—cage

Interventions

Rationale

- Practice words that end with these consonant sounds:

p—top	f—safe
b—job	v—love
m—him	

e. Practice lip and jaw exercises; repeat several times:
  - Open and close mouth slowly, close lips completely. Do another set but as fast as you can.
  - Close lips and press together tightly for a few seconds.
  - Stretch lips into a wide smile—hold—relax.
  - Pucker lips—hold—relax.
  - Pucker—hold—smile—hold.
  - Say "ma-ma-ma-ma" as fast as you can.
  - Breathe in and talk, overexaggerating the pronunciation of these words:

    Map—mad—mug
    Bob—bat—bag
    Pipe—pool—park
    Game—goat—gang
    Warm—wool—wig

f. Do exercises to slow the rate of speaking:
  - Say words in syllables:

    Pos-si-bil-i-ty
    pa-ci-fic
    hor-ri-ble
  - Say phrases in syllables:

    when-ever pos-si-ble
    fam-i-ly bus-i-ness

g. Practice varying facial expression: Using a mirror, make faces (e.g., smile, frown, laugh, grin, whistle, puff out cheeks).

h. Read the newspaper out loud. Determine how many words you can speak in one breath before the volume decreases.

4. Refer the client to a speech therapist and reference material from:

   American Parkinson's Disease Association
   116 John St.
   New York, NY 10038
   1-800-223-2732

e. These exercises strengthen and increase the range of lip movements for the formation of speech sounds.

f. These exercises help improve deliberate word-by-word pronunciation.

g. Parkinson's disease causes limited movement of facial muscles, producing a mask-like facies; these exercises help overcome this effect.

h. This helps the client learn to maintain volume for each syllable and final consonant sounds.

4. The client requires additional instruction and follow-up monitoring.

▲ **Documentation**

Discharge summary record
    Assessment of speech
    Exercises taught
    Outcome achievement or status
    Referrals, if indicated

▲ **Outcome Criteria**

The client will:

1. Demonstrate exercises to improve mobility
2. Demonstrate a wide base gait with arm swinging
3. Identify one strategy to increase independence
4. Relate an intent to exercise at home

Impaired Physical Mobility related to effects of muscle rigidity, tremors, and slowness of movement on activities of daily living

Focus Assessment Criteria	*Clinical Significance*
1. Gait, balance 2. Range of motion 3. Presence of tremors, akinesia (no movement), bradykinesia (slowed movements) 4. Muscle rigidity (trunk, facial, intercostal)	1–3. Parkinson's disease disrupts the extrapyramidal motor system, which is responsible for control of posture, semiautomatic actions, muscle tone, and coordination of movements. 4. Affected muscles include two-joint flexor muscles (e.g., trunk) and striated muscles (e.g., face, intercostal).

Interventions	*Rationale*
1. Explain the cause of symptoms.	1. The client's understanding may help promote compliance with an exercise program at home.
2. Teach the client to walk erect, looking at the horizon, with the feet separated and arms swinging normally.	2. Conscious efforts to simulate a normal gait and position can improve mobility and reduce loss of balance.
3. Instruct the client to exercise three to five times a week, at least 30 minutes each session.	3. Regular exercise can prevent deconditioning of muscles, which results from inactivity or slowed movements. Specific benefits include the following: a. Increased muscle strength b. Improved coordination and dexterity c. Reduced rigidity d. Help preventing contractures e. Improved flexibility f. Enhanced peristalsis g. Improved cardiovascular endurance h. Increased ability to tolerate stress i. A sense of control, which reduces feelings of powerlessness
4. Teach that an exercise program should include the following: a. Warm-up for 10 minutes b. Cool-down for 10 minutes c. Lower body, torso, upper body, and head exercises d. Relaxation exercises	4. a. Warm-up stretches muscles to help prevent injury. b. Cool-down promotes excretion of body wastes from exercise and reduces heart rate slowly. c. A range of exercises ensures that all the affected muscle areas are exercised. d. Relaxation exercises provide some control over the anxiety associated with fear of "freezing" or falling.
5. Stress to the client that compliance with the exercise program is ultimately his or her choice.	5. Promoting the client's feelings of control and self-determination may improve compliance with the exercise program.
6. Include family members or significant others in teaching sessions; stress that they are not to "police" the client's compliance.	6. Support from family members or significant others can encourage the client to comply with the exercise program.
7. Refer to a physical therapist or reference material for specific exercise guidelines, e.g., material from the American Parkinson's Disease Association.	7. The client may require additional instructions and follow-up monitoring.

▲ **Documentation**

Discharge summary record
   Assessment of mobility
   Exercises taught
   Outcome achievement or status
   Referrals, if indicated

References/Bibliography

Calne, S. (1989). Parkinson's disease problems in nursing management related to medication. *Axon, 9*(4), 55–58.

Delgado, J.M., et al. (1988). Care of the patient with Parkinson's disease: Surgical and nursing interventions. *Journal of Neuroscience Nursing, 20*(3), 142–150.

Duvoisin, R. (1984). *Parkinson's disease: A guide for patient and family.* New York: Raven Press.

Hurwitz, A. (1989). The benefit of a home exercise regimen for ambulatory Parkinson's disease patients. *Journal of Neuroscience Nursing, 21*(3), 180–184.

Mitchell, P.H., Merts, M.A., & Catanzaro, M. (1987). Group exercise: A nursing therapy in Parkinson's disease. *Rehabilitation Nursing, 12*(5), 34–38.

Pitzele, S.K. (1985). *We are not alone: To live with chronic illness.* Minneapolis: Thompson & Co., Inc.

Stern, M.B., & Hurtig, H.I. (1988). *The comprehensive management of Parkinson's disease.* Great Neck, N.Y.: PMA Publishing Corp.

Strauss, A. (1984). *Chronic illness and the quality of life.* St. Louis: C.V. Mosby.

The Parkinson's Disease Foundation. (1986). *The Parkinson patient at home.* New York: Parkinson's Disease Foundation.

Vernon, G. (1989). Parkinson's disease. *Journal of Neuroscience Nursing, 21*(5), 273–281.

Seizure Disorders

Seizure disorders constitute a chronic syndrome in which a neurological dysfunction in cerebral tissue produces seizures—disturbances of behavior, mood, sensation, perception, movement, and muscle tone. The disorder is thought to be an electrical disturbance in cerebral nerve cells that causes them to produce abnormal, repetitive electrical charges. Seizures can be partial (involving one part of the brain) or generalized (involving the entire brain).

Diagnostic Cluster

▲ Time Frame

Initial diagnosis
Recurrent acute episodes

▲ Discharge Criteria

Before discharge, the client or family will:

1. State an intent to wear medical identification
2. Relate activities to be avoided
3. Relate the importance of complying with the prescribed medication regimen
4. Relate the side effects of prescribed medications
5. State situations that increase the possibility of a seizure
6. State signs and symptoms that must be reported to a health care professional

Nursing Diagnoses

Potential Ineffective Airway Clearance related to relaxation of tongue and gag reflexes secondary to disruption in muscle innervation

Potential Social Isolation related to fear of embarrassment secondary to having a seizure in public

Potential Altered Health Maintenance related to insufficient knowledge of condition, medication, care during seizures, environmental hazards, and community resources

Nursing Diagnoses

▲ Outcome Criteria

1. The client will demonstrate continued airway patency.
2. The family will describe interventions to maintain a patent airway during seizures.

Potential Ineffective Airway Clearance related to relaxation of tongue and gag reflexes secondary to disruption in muscle innervation

Focus Assessment Criteria

1. History of seizure activity
2. Respiratory status during seizure activity

Clinical Significance

1,2. The tonic/clonic movements during a seizure can cause the tongue to drop backward and obstruct the airway.

Interventions

1. During a seizure, do the following:
   a. Provide privacy, if possible.
   b. Ease the client to the floor, if possible.
   c. Place him in a side-lying position.
   d. Loosen clothing around the neck.
   e. If unable to position the client on his side, lift his chin up and forward with his head tilted back, to help open the airway.
2. Observe the seizure and document its characteristics:
   a. Onset and duration
   b. Preseizure events (e.g., visual, auditory, olfactory, or tactile stimuli)

Rationale

1. These measures can help reduce injury and embarrassment.

2. This information gives clues to the location of the epileptogenic focus in the brain and is useful in guiding treatment.

Interventions

    c. Part of body where the seizure started, initial movement
    d. Eyes: open or closed, pupil size
    e. Body parts involved, type of movements
    f. Involuntary motor activities (e.g., lip smacking, repeated swallowing)
    g. Incontinence (fecal or urinary)
    h. Loss of consciousness
    i. Postseizure: ability to speak, sleeping, confusion, weakness, paralysis (Brunner and Suddarth, 1989).

3. If the client reports an aura, have him lie down.

4. Teach family members or significant others how to respond to the client during a seizure.

Rationale

3. A recumbent position can prevent injuries from a fall.

4. Others can be taught measures to prevent airway obstruction and injury.

▲ **Documentation**

Progress notes
    Description of seizures
Discharge summary record
    Client teaching

▲ **Outcome Criteria**

The client will identify appropriate diversional activities.

Potential Social Isolation related to fear of embarrassment secondary to having a seizure in public

Focus Assessment Criteria	*Clinical Significance*

1. Usual socialization patterns:
  a. Hobbies
  b. Other interests
  c. Church
  d. Work
  e. Neighborhood
  f. School
	1. An at-risk client must be assessed carefully, because the suffering associated with social isolation is not always readily apparent.

2. Concerns regarding socialization	2. Feelings of rejection and embarrassment are common.

Interventions

1. Help the client recognize the need for socialization.

2. Provide support and validate that his or her concerns are normal.

3. Assist the client in identifying activities that are pleasurable and nonhazardous.
4. Stress the importance of adhering to the treatment plan.
5. Discuss sharing the diagnosis with family members, friends, coworkers, and social contacts.

6. Discuss situations through which the client can meet others in a similar situation:
    a. Support groups
    b. Epilepsy Foundation of America

Rationale

1. A client prone to seizures may separate himself or herself from family, friends, and other social contacts.
2. The nurse must be sensitive to the impact of seizures on the client's body image, resulting self-concept, and interest in social activities.
3. Fear of injury may contribute to isolation.

4. Adherence to the medication regimen can help prevent or reduce seizure episodes.
5. Open dialogue with others forewarns them of possible seizures, which can reduce the shock of witnessing a seizure and possibly enable assistive action.
6. Sharing with others in a similar situation may give the client a more realistic view of seizure disorder and societal perception of it.

▲ **Documentation**

Progress notes
    Client's concerns
    Interaction with client

▲ **Outcome Criteria**

The outcome criteria for this diagnosis represent those associated with discharge planning. Refer to the discharge criteria.

Potential Altered Health Maintenance related to insufficient knowledge of condition, medications, care during seizures, environmental hazards, and community resources

Focus Assessment Criteria

1. Current knowledge of seizures and their management
2. Contributing factors, including the following:
   a. Anxiety
   b. New diagnosis
   c. Lack of previous instruction
3. Resources, e.g., family, financial, community
4. Attitudes, feelings, and concerns related to seizure disorders
5. Readiness and ability to learn

Clinical Significance

1–5. Assessment helps identify any factors that may interfere with learning. A client or family that does not achieve goals for learning requires a referral for assistance postdischarge.

Interventions

1. Teach about seizure disorders and treatment; correct misconceptions.

2. If the client is on medication therapy, teach the following information
   a. Never to discontinue a drug abruptly

   b. Side effects and signs of toxicity

   c. The need to have drug blood levels monitored
   d. The need for periodic complete blood counts, if indicated

   e. The effects of diphenylhydantoin (Dilantin), if ordered, on gingival tissue and the need for regular dental examinations
3. Provide information regarding situations that increase the risk of seizure:
   a. Alcohol ingestion
   b. Excessive caffeine intake
   c. Excessive fatigue or stress
   d. Febrile illness
   e. Poorly adjusted TV screen
   f. Sedentary activity level (Hickey, 1986)
4. Discuss why certain activities are hazardous and should be avoided:
   a. Swimming alone
   b. Driving alone (unless seizure-free for 5 years)
   c. Operating potentially hazardous machinery
   d. Mountain climbing
5. Provide opportunities for the client and significant others to express their feelings alone and with each other.

6. Refer the client and family to community resources and reference material for assistance with management (e.g., Epilepsy Foundation of America, counseling, occupational rehabilitation).

Rationale

1. The client's and family's understanding of seizure disorder and the prescribed treatment regimen strongly influence compliance with the regimen.
2. Certain precautions must be emphasized to ensure safe, effective drug therapy.
   a. Abrupt discontinuation can precipitate status epilepticus.
   b. Early identification of problems enables prompt intervention to prevent serious complications.
   c. Drug blood levels provide a guide for adjusting drug dosage.
   d. Long-term use of some anticonvulsive drugs, such as hydantoins (e.g., Dilantin) can cause blood dyscrasias.
   e. Long-term phenytoin (Dilantin) therapy can cause gingival hyperplasia.

3. Certain situations have been identified as increasing seizure episodes, although the actual mechanisms behind them are unknown.

4. Generally, a client prone to seizures should avoid any activity that could place him or others in danger should a seizure occur.

5. Witnessing a seizure is terrifying for others and embarrassing for the client prone to them. This shame and humiliation contribute to anxiety, depression, hostility, and secrecy. Family members also may experience these feelings. Frank discussions may reduce feelings of shame and isolation.
6. Such resources may provide additional information and support.

▲ Documentation

Discharge summary record
  Client teaching
  Outcome achievement or status
  Referrals, if indicated

References/Bibliography

Barry, K., & Teixeira, S. (1983). The role of the nurse in the diagnostic classification and management of epileptic seizures. *Journal of Neurosurgical Nursing, 15*(4), 243–249.

Brunner, L., & Suddarth, D. (1988). *Textbook of medical–surgical nursing* (6th ed.). Philadelphia: J.B. Lippincott.

Hickey, J. (1986). *The clinical practice of neurological and neurosurgical nursing* (2nd ed.). Philadelphia: J.B. Lippincott.

Spinal Cord Injury

Spinal cord injuries can be caused by four major mechanisms: acceleration/deceleration, deformation, vertical loading, and penetration wounds. Acceleration/deceleration–caused injuries (e.g., rear-end collisions) produce hyperextension and hyperflexion. Deformation-caused injuries involve tissues and other structures that support the spinal cord. In vertical loading–caused injuries (e.g., diving accidents), damage results from compression of the spinal column. Penetration wounds are commonly caused by knives or other sharp objects. The consequences of spinal cord injury depend on the location and extent of cord injury.

Diagnostic Cluster

▲ **Time Frame**

Initial acute episode (post–intensive care)
Secondary diagnosis

Collaborative Problems

Potential Complications: *Refer to:*
Fracture Dislocation
Cardiovascular
Hypoxemia
Paralytic Ileus
Urinary Retention
Pyelonephritis
Renal Insufficiency
Gastrointestinal (GI) Bleeding
Hemorrhage   Fractures
Electrolyte Imbalance   Acute Renal Failure
Thrombophlebitis   Fractures

Nursing Diagnoses

Anxiety related to perceived effects of injury on life style and unknown future
Grieving related to loss of body function and its effects on life style
Potential Self-Concept Disturbance related to effects of disability on achieving developmental tasks and life style
Bowel Incontinence: Reflexic related to lack of voluntary sphincter control secondary to spinal cord injury above the eleventh thoracic vertebra (T11)
Bowel Incontinence: Areflexic related to lack of voluntary sphincter secondary to spinal cord injury involving sacral reflex arc (S2–S4)
Potential Dysreflexia related to reflex stimulation of sympathetic nervous system secondary to loss of autonomic control
Altered Family Processes related to adjustment requirements, role disturbances, and uncertain future
Potential Altered Sexuality Pattern related to physiological, sensory, and psychological effects of disability on sexuality or function
Potential Impaired Home Maintenance Management related to insufficient knowledge of the effects of altered skin, bowel, bladder, respiratory, thermoregulation, and sexual function and their management; signs and symptoms of complications; follow-up care; and community resources
Self-Care Deficit related to sensorimotor deficits secondary to   Immobility or Unconsciousness
level of spinal cord injury

Related Care Plans

Immobility or Unconsciousness
Neurogenic Bladder
Tracheostomy

▲ **Discharge Planning**

Before discharge, the client and/ or family will:

1. Describe the effects of injury on functioning and methods of home management
2. Express feelings regarding the effects of injury on life style
3. Relate an intent to share feelings with significant others after discharge
4. State signs and symptoms that must be reported to a health care professional
5. Identify a plan for rehabilitation and follow-up care
6. Identify available community resources

Collaborative Problems

▲ **Nursing Goal**

The nurse will manage and minimize complications of spinal cord injury.

Potential Complication: Fracture Dislocation
Potential Complication: Cardiovascular
Potential Complication: Hypoxemia
Potential Complication: Hemorrhage
Potential Complication: Electrolyte Imbalance
Potential Complication: Paralytic Ileus
Potential Complication: Urinary Retention
Potential Complication: Pyelonephritis
Potential Complication: Renal Insufficiency
Potential Complication: Gastrointestinal (GI) Bleeding

Interventions	*Rationale*
1. Maintain immobilization with skeletal traction (e.g., tongs, calipers, halo vest); ensure that ropes and weights hang freely.	1. Skeletal traction stabilizes the vertebral column to prevent further spinal cord injury and to allow reduction of the vertebral column into correct alignment by constant traction force.
2. Use the triple log-rolling technique with a fourth person to stabilize weights during turning.	2. Log-rolling helps maintain spinal alignment during turning.
3. If traction disconnects or fails, stabilize the head, neck, and shoulders with a cervical collar, hands, or sand bags.	3. Stabilization of the injured area is vital to prevent misalignment and further damage.

4. Monitor for cardiovascular complications:
  a. Bradycardia
	4.
	  a. Cardiac function is altered because of the vagal stimulation, which has no sympathetic control (unopposed parasympathetic response).

b. Hypotension, decreased cardiac output	b. Sympathetic blockage causes vasodilatation, with resulting decreased venous return.
5. Monitor for signs of hypoxemia:	5. Spinal cord injuries can impair the muscles of respiration depending on the level of injury, e.g., diaphragm (C3,C4,C5), intercostals (T1–T7), accessory muscles (C2–C7), and abdominal muscles (T6–T12).
a. Abnormal arterial blood gases (ABGs) (pH < 7.35 and $pCO_2 > 46$ mmg)	a. ABG analysis helps evaluate gas exchange in the lungs.
b. Increased and irregular heart rate c. Increased respiratory rate followed by decreased rate	b,c. Respiratory acidosis results from excessive CO_2 retention. A client with respiratory acidosis initially exhibits increased heart rate and respirations in an attempt to correct decreased circulating oxygen, then begins to breathe more slowly and with prolonged expiration.
d. Changes in mentation	d. Altered mentation may indicate cerebral tissue hypoxia.
e. Decreased urine output (< 30 mL/hr) f. Cool, pale, or cyanotic skin	e,f. The compensatory response to decreased circulating oxygen is to increase heart and respiratory rates and to decrease circulation to the kidneys (resulting in decreased urine output) and to the extremities (resulting in diminished pulses and skin changes).
6. Administer low-flow (2 L/min) oxygen as needed through a cannula.	6. Supplemental oxygen therapy increases circulating oxygen. Higher flow rates increase CO_2 retention. Use of a nasal cannula rather than a mask minimizes feelings of suffocation.

Interventions	*Rationale*
7. Assess ability to cough and use of accessory muscles. Suction as needed.	7. Lost innervation of intercostal muscles (T1–T7) and abdominal muscles (T6–T12) destroys the ability to cough and deep breathe effectively.
8. Auscultate lung fields regularly.	8. Auscultation can detect accumulation of retained secretions and asymmetric breath sounds.

9. Monitor for signs of paralytic ileus:
  a. Decreased or absent bowel sounds
  b. Abdominal distention
	9. Gastric dilatation and ileus can result from depressed reflexes and hypoxia.

10. Monitor for signs of urinary retention:
  a. Bladder distention
  b. Decreased urine output
	10. Urinary retention is caused by bladder atony and contraction of the urinary sphincter during spinal shock. Bladder distention can lead to urinary reflux, pyelonephritis, stone formation, and renal insufficiency.

11. Monitor for signs and symptoms of pyelonephritis:
  a. Fever, chills
	11. Urinary tract infections can be caused by urinary stasis. •
	  a. Bacteria can act as a pyrogen by raising the hypothalamic thermostat through the production of endogenous pyrogen, which may mediate through prostaglandins. Chills can occur when the temperature setpoint of the hypothalamus rapidly changes.

b. Costovertebral angle (CVA) pain if sensation is intact at this level; otherwise vague, referred pain
  c. Leukocytosis
 	
  d. Bacteria and pus in urine
  e. Dysuria, frequency
	b. CVA pain results from distention of the renal capsule.
	
	  c. Leukocytosis reflects an increase in WBCs to fight infection through phagocytosis.
	  d. Bacteria changes the odor and *p*H of urine.
	  e. Bacteria irritates bladder tissue, causing spasms and frequency.

12. Monitor for early signs and symptoms of renal insufficiency:
  a. Sustained elevated urine specific gravity
  b. Elevated urine sodium level
 	
  c. Sustained insufficient urine output (< 30 mL/hr)
  d. Elevated blood pressure
	12. Repeated infections can alter renal function.
	
	  a,b. Decreased ability of the renal tubules to reabsorb electrolytes causes increased urine sodium levels and increased specific gravity.
	  c,d. Decreased glomerular filtration rate eventually causes insufficient urine output and stimulates renin production, which raises blood pressure in an attempt to increase blood flow to the kidneys.

e. Elevated blood urea nitrogen (BUN); serum creatinine, potassium, phosphorus, and ammonia; and creatinine clearance	**e.** Decreased excretion of urea and creatinine in the urine results in elevated BUN and creatinine levels.
13. Monitor intake and output.	13. Intake and output measurements help evaluate hydration status.

14. Monitor for signs and symptoms of GI bleeding:
  a. Shoulder pain (referred pain)
  b. Frank or occult blood in stool
  c. Hemoptysis
  d. Nausea and vomiting.
	14. GI bleeding can result from irritation of gastric mucosa as a side effect of corticosteroids or from a stress ulcer caused by vagal stimulation, which produces gastric hyperacidity.

15. Assess vital signs frequently, especially blood pressure and pulse.	15. Vital signs assessment evaluates circulatory status and monitors for shock.

▲ **Documentation**

Flow records
  Vital signs
  Intake and output
  Respiratory assessment
  Abdominal assessment
    (bowel sounds, distention)
  Stool and emesis assessment
    (blood)
  Traction (type, weights)
Progress notes
  Change in status
  Interventions
  Response to interventions

Related Physician-Prescribed Interventions

Medications
  Muscle relaxants   Stool softeners, laxatives, suppositories

Related Physician-Prescribed Interventions (Continued)

Intravenous Therapy
 Not indicated
Laboratory Studies
 Renal function studies
Diagnostic Studies
 Spinal x-ray films   Magnetic resonance imaging (MRI)
 Computed tomography (CT) scan   Pulmonary function studies
Therapies
 Immobilization devices   Physical therapy
 Alternating pressure beds   Indwelling catheterization
 Antiembolic stockings

Nursing Diagnoses

▲ **Outcome Criteria**

The client will:

1. Share feelings and fears
2. Discuss feelings with significant others

Anxiety related to perceived effects of injury on life style and unknown future

Focus Assessment Criteria	*Clinical Significance*
1. Understanding of injury 2. Knowledge of structure and function of affected organs	1,2. The client's understanding of the disorder can affect his anxiety level. The client may be influenced, either positively or negatively, by information from others. Assessing his knowledge level also helps the nurse plan teaching strategies.
3. Life style, strengths, coping mechanisms, available support systems	3. This helps identify the client's resources for managing stress and anxiety.

Interventions

1. Provide opportunities for the client to share his feelings and concerns. Maintain a calm, relaxed atmosphere, convey a nonjudgmental attitude, and listen attentively. Identify the client's support systems and coping mechanisms, and suggest alternatives as necessary.
2. Explain the following:
   a. The need for frequent assessments
   b. Diagnostic tests
   c. The consequences of spinal shock (flaccid paralysis and absent reflexes)
   d. Treatment
3. Attempt to provide consistency with staff assignments.
4. Provide opportunities for family members or significant others to share their concerns.

5. Identify a client at risk for unsuccessful adjustment; look for the following characteristics:
   a. Poor ego strength
   b. Ineffective problem-solving strategies
   c. Lack of motivation
   d. External focus of control
   e. Poor health
   f. Unsatisfactory preinjury sex life
   g. Lack of positive support systems
   h. Unstable economic status
   i. Rejection of counseling

Rationale

1. Sharing feelings openly facilitates trust and helps reduce anxiety.

2. Accurate descriptions of expected sensations and procedures help ease anxiety and fear.

3. Familiarity may increase opportunities for sharing and provide stability and security.
4. Exploration gives the nurse the opportunity to correct misinformation and validate the situation as difficult and frightening.

5. A client's successful adjustment is influenced by such factors as previous coping success, achievement of developmental tasks before the injury, the extent to which the disability interferes with goal-directed activity, sense of control, and realistic perception of situation by himself and support persons.

▲ **Documentation**

Progress notes
 Present emotional status
 Interventions
 Client's and/or family's response to interventions

▲ *Outcome Criteria*

The client will:

1. Express grief
2. Describe the meaning of loss
3. Report an intent to discuss feelings with significant others

Grieving related to loss of body function and its effects on life style

Focus Assessment Criteria	*Clinical Significance*
1. Signs and symptoms of grief reaction, e.g., crying, withdrawal, anxiety, fear, restlessness, decreased appetite, decreased interest, and participation in activities	1. The client is experiencing losses related to sexual identity, function, and independence. The grief response may be profound or subtle.

Interventions

1. Provide opportunities for the client and family members to ventilate feelings, discuss the loss openly, and explore the personal meaning of the loss. Explain that grief is a common and healthy reaction.
2. Encourage use of positive coping strategies that have proven successful in the past.
3. Encourage the client to express positive self-attributes.
4. Implement measures to support the family and promote cohesiveness:
   a. Help them acknowledge and accept losses.
   b. Explain the grieving process.
   c. Encourage verbalization of feelings.
   d. Allow family members to participate in client care.
5. Promote grief work with each response:
   a. Denial:
      - Encourage acceptance of the situation; do not reinforce denial by giving false reassurance.
      - Promote hope through assurances of care, comfort, and support.
      - Explain the use of denial by one family member to other members.
      - Do not push a person to move past denial until he is emotionally ready.
   b. Isolation:
      - Convey acceptance by encouraging expressions of grief.
      - Promote open, honest communication to encourage sharing.
      - Reinforce the client's self-worth by providing for privacy, when desired.
      - Encourage socialization as feasible (e.g., support groups, church activities).
   c. Depression:
      - Reinforce the client's self-esteem.
      - Employ empathetic sharing and acknowledge grief.
      - Identify the degree of depression and develop appropriate strategies.
   d. Anger:
      - Explain to other family members that anger represents an attempt to control the environment, stemming from frustration at the inability to control the disease.
      - Encourage verbalization of anger.
   e. Guilt:
      - Acknowledge the person's expressed self-image.

Rationale

1. Loss may give rise to feelings of powerlessness, anger, profound sadness, and other grief responses. Open, honest discussions can help the client and family members accept and cope with the situation and their response to it.
2. Positive coping strategies aid acceptance and problem-solving.
3. Focusing on positive attributes increases self-acceptance and acceptance of the loss.
4. Family cohesiveness is important to client support.

5. Grieving involves profound emotional responses; interventions depend on the particular response.

Interventions

   - Encourage identification of the relationship's positive aspects.
   - Avoid arguing and participating in the person's system of thinking, "I should have . . ." and, "I shouldn't have. . . ."
f. Fear:
   - Focus on the present and maintain a safe and secure environment.
   - Help the person explore reasons for and meanings of the fears.
g. Rejection:
   - Provide reassurance by explaining what is happening.
   - Explain this response to other family members.
h. Hysteria:
   - Reduce environmental stressors (e.g., limit personnel).
   - Provide a safe, private area in which to express grief.

Rationale

▲ *Documentation*

Progress notes
   Present emotional status
   Interventions
   Response to nursing interventions

Potential Self-Concept Disturbance related to the effects of disability on achieving developmental tasks and life style

▲ *Outcome Criteria*

The client will:

1. Acknowledge changes in body structure and function
2. Communicate feelings about disability
3. Participate in self-care

Focus Assessment Criteria	*Clinical Significance*
1. Previous exposure to persons with spinal cord injury	1–4. This information helps the nurse detect patterns of response due to adaptation. It may be helpful to note how the client's support persons view the client's self-concept; they can provide insight into factors that may have had a negative impact on self-concept, and they tend to be sensitive to subtle changes.
2. Ability to express feelings about condition	
3. Ability to share feelings with family members or significant others	
4. Evidence of or others' reports of negative self-concept	
5. Participation in self-care	5,6. Participation in self-care and adaptation of goals to disability indicate attempts to cope with the changes (Hamburg, 1983).
6. Evidence of adapting life style to disabilities	

Interventions

1. Contact the client frequently and treat him with warm, positive regard.

2. Encourage the client to express feelings and thoughts about the following:
   a. Condition
   b. Progress
   c. Prognosis
   d. Effects on life style
   e. Support system
   f. Treatments
3. Provide reliable information and clarify any misconceptions.
4. Help the client to identify positive attributes and possible new opportunities.

Rationale

1. Frequent contact by the caregiver indicates acceptance and may facilitate trust. The client may be hesitant to approach the staff because of negative self-concept.
2. Encouraging the client to share feelings can provide a safe outlet for fears and frustrations and can increase self-awareness.

3. Misconceptions can needlessly increase anxiety and damage self-concept.
4. The client may tend to focus only on the change in self-image and not on the positive characteristics that contribute to the whole concept of self. The nurse must reinforce these positive aspects and encourage the client to reincorporate them into his new self-concept.

Interventions

5. Assist with hygiene and grooming, as needed.

6. Encourage visitors.

7. Help the client identify strategies to increase independence and maintain role responsibilities:
   a. Prioritizing activities
   b. Using mobility aids and assistive devices, as needed.
8. Discuss ways that the client can provide support to support persons:
   a. Actively listening to their problems
   b. Attempting to decrease the focus on disabilities.
   (Refer to Chapter 3, The Ill Adult: Issues and Responses, for more information.)
9. Allow the client's support persons to share their feelings regarding the diagnoses and actual or anticipated effects.
10. Assess for signs of negative response to changes in appearance:
    a. Refusal to discuss loss
    b. Denial of changes
    c. Decreased self-care ability
    d. Social isolation
    e. Refusal to discuss future
11. Refer an at-risk client for professional counseling.

Rationale

5. Participation in self-care and planning can aid positive coping.

6. Frequent visits by support persons can help the client feel that he is still a worthwhile, acceptable person, which should promote a positive self-concept.

7. A strong component of self-concept is the ability to perform functions expected of one's role, thus decreasing dependency and reducing the need for others' involvement.

8. The nurse can help the client learn how to balance relationships and preserve the family system.

9. Spinal cord injury can negatively affect support persons financially, socially, and emotionally.

10. These signs may indicate that the client is at high risk for unsuccessful adjustment.

11. Follow-up therapy may be indicated to assist with adjustment.

▲ **Documentation**

Progress notes
  Present emotional status
  Interventions
  Response to interventions

Potential Dysreflexia related to reflex stimulation of sympathetic nervous system below the level of cord injury secondary to loss of autonomic control

Focus Assessment Criteria

1. History of dysreflexia:
   a. Triggered by:
      • Bladder distention
      • Bowel distention
      • Tactile stimulation
      • Skin lesion(s)
      • Sexual activity
      • Menstruation
      • Urinary tract infection
   b. Initial symptoms:
      • Headache
      • Sweating above the level of injury
      • Chills
      • Metallic taste
      • Nasal congestion
      • Blurred vision
      • Numbness
      • "Goose bumps" above the level of injury
      • Others
   c. Medications used; any recent changes in use

Clinical Significance

1. With spinal cord injury (T7 or above), the cord activity below the injury is deprived of the controlling effects from the higher centers, which results in poorly controlled responses (Hickey, 1986). The uninhibited responses are life-threatening if not reversed. A baseline of history, triggering activities, initial symptoms, and medication use enables the nurse to make subsequent assessments of dysreflexic activity.

▲ **Outcome Criteria**

The client will:
1. State factors that cause dysreflexia
2. Describe the treatment for dysreflexia
3. Relate when emergency treatment is indicated

Focus Assessment Criteria

2. Bladder program: type, problems, any recent changes
3. Bowel program: type, problems, any recent changes
4. Knowledge of dysreflexia

Clinical Significance

2,3. A distended bowel or bladder can trigger dysreflexia.

4. The client and family can be taught how to prevent and treat dysreflexia.

Interventions

1. Monitor for signs and symptoms of dysreflexia:
   a. Paroxysmal hypertension (sudden periodic elevated blood pressure: systolic pressure > 140 mm Hg, diastolic > 90 mm Hg)
   b. Bradycardia or tachycardia
   c. Diaphoresis
   d. Red splotches on skin above the level of injury
   e. Pallor below the level of injury
   f. Headache
2. If signs of dysreflexia occur, raise the head of the bed and remove the noxious stimuli, as follows:
   a. Bladder distention:
      • Check for distended bladder
      • If catheterized, check the catheter for kinks or compression; irrigate with only 30 mL of saline solution, instilled very slowly; replace the catheter if it will not drain.
      • If not catheterized, insert a catheter using dibucaine hydrochloride ointment (Nupercaine). Then, remove the 500 mL clamp for 15 minutes; repeat until the bladder is drained.
   b. Fecal impaction:
      • First, apply Nupercaine to the anus and about 1 inch into the rectum.
      • Gently check the rectum with a well-lubricated gloved finger.
      • Insert a rectal suppository or gently remove the impaction.
   c. Skin stimulation: Spray the skin lesion triggering dysreflexia with a topical anesthetic agent.
3. Continue to monitor blood pressure every 3 to 5 minutes.

4. Immediately consult the physician for pharmacological treatment if symptoms or noxious stimuli are not eliminated.

5. Initiate health teaching and referrals, as indicated:
   a. Teach signs and symptoms and treatment of dysreflexia.

Rationale

1. Spasms of pelvic viscera and arterioles cause vasoconstriction below the level of injury, producing hypertension and pallor. Afferent impulses triggered by high blood pressure cause vagal stimulation, resulting in bradycardia. Baroreceptors in the aortic arch and carotid sinus respond to the hypertension, triggering superficial vasodilatation, flushing, diaphoresis, and headache (above the level of cord injury).

2. These interventions aim to reduce cerebral hypertension.

   a. Bladder distention can trigger dysreflexia by stimulating sensory receptors. Nupercaine ointment reduces tissue stimulation. Too rapid removal of urine can result in compensatory hypotension.

   b. Fecal impaction prevents stimulation of sensory receptors.

   c. Dysreflexia can be triggered by stimulation (e.g., of the glans penis or skin lesions).

3. Failure to reverse severe hypertension can result in status epilepticus, cerebrovascular accident, and death.
4. Intravenous pharmacological intervention may be warranted if the noxious stimuli cannot be removed or hypertension reduced. Medications used may include diazoxide (Hyperstat), hydralazine (Apresoline), sodium nitroprusside (Nipride), and ganglionic blocking agents such as phenoxybenzamine (Dibenzyline) and guanethidine sulfate (Ismelin).
5. Good teaching can help the client and family successfully prevent or treat dysreflexia at home.

Interventions

b. Teach when immediate medical intervention is warranted.

c. Explain what situations can trigger dysreflexia (e.g., menstrual cycle, sexual activity, bladder or bowel routines).

d. Teach to watch for early signs and to intervene immediately.

e. Teach to observe for early signs of bladder infections and skin lesions (e.g., pressure ulcers, ingrown toenails).

f. Advise to consult with the physician for long-term pharmacological management if the client is very vulnerable to dysreflexia.

Rationale:

▲ **Documentation**

Progress notes
    Episodes of dysreflexia (cause, treatment, response)
Discharge summary record
    Client teaching

▲ **Outcome Criteria**

The client and/or family members will:

1. Verbalize feelings regarding the situation
2. Identify signs of family dysfunction
3. Identify appropriate resources to seek when needed

Altered Family Processes related to the adjustment requirements, role disturbance, and uncertain future

Focus Assessment Criteria	*Clinical Significance*
1. Understanding of condition	1–4. The family unit is a system based on interdependence among members and patterns that provide structure and support. Chronic disability disrupts these relationships and patterns.
2. Family coping patterns	
3. Current response	
4. Available resources	

Interventions

1. Convey an understanding of the situation and its impact on the family.

2. Explore family members' perceptions of the situation. Encourage verbalization of feelings such as guilt, anger, and blame.

3. Determine whether present coping mechanisms are effective.

4. Take steps to promote family strengths:
   a. Acknowledge the assistance of family members.
   b. Involve them in the client's care.
   c. Encourage time away from caregiving to prevent burnout.
   d. Encourage humor.
   (Refer to Chapter 3, The Ill Adult: Issues and Responses, for more information.)

5. Assist to reorganize roles at home, set new priorities, and redistribute responsibilities.

6. Prepare the family for signs of depression, anxiety, anger, and dependency in the client and other family members.

7. Encourage the family to call on its social network (e.g., friends, relatives, church members) for emotional and other support.

8. Identify dysfunctional coping mechanisms, such as the following:
   a. Substance abuse
   b. Continued denial
   c. Exploitation of one or more family members
   d. Separation or avoidance
   Refer for counseling as necessary.

Rationale:

1. Communicating understanding and a sense of caring and concern facilitates trust and strengthens the nurse's relationship with the client and family.

2. Verbalization can provide opportunities for clarification and validation of feelings and concerns, contributing to family unity.

3. Illness of a family member may cause great changes, putting the family at high risk for maladaptation.

4. This can help maintain the existing family structure and its function as a supportive unit.

5. Planning and prioritizing can help maintain family integrity and reduce stress.

6. Anticipatory guidance can alert members to potential problems before they occur, enabling prompt intervention at early signs.

7. Outside assistance may help reduce the perception that the family must "go it alone."

8. A family with a history of unsuccessful coping may need additional resources. A family with unresolved conflicts prior to diagnosis is at high risk.

▲ **Documentation**

Progress notes
    Present family functioning
    Interventions
    Family's response to interventions
Discharge summary record
    Referrals, if indicated

Interventions

9. Direct to community agencies and other sources of assistance (e.g., financial, housekeeping, direct care), as needed.

Rationale

9. The family may need assistance to help with management at home.

Potential Altered Sexuality Pattern related to physiological, sensory, and psychological effects of disability on sexual functioning and self-concept

▲ *Outcome Criteria*

The client will:

1. Discuss own feelings and partner's concerns regarding sexual functioning
2. Verbalize intention to discuss concerns with partner before discharge.

Focus Assessment Criteria	*Clinical Significance*
1. Previous sexual patterns 2. Partner availability 3. Upper extremity muscle strength 4. Presence of catheters	1–4. Loss of sensory and motor function can cause erectile problems in men and libido problems in both genders. Sexual options available to the spinal cord-injured client are influenced (Woods, 1979) by sexual value system, previous sexual function, upper-extremity muscle strength, presence of hip flexors and extensors, presence of appliances (e.g., casts, catheters), and availability of a caring partner.
5. Family planning decisions	5. Cord injuries usually do not affect fertility. Paraplegic females can become pregnant and deliver vaginally.

Interventions

1. Initiate a discussion regarding concerns associated with sexuality and sexual function.

2. Provide accurate information on the effect of the cord injury on sexual functioning.
3. Reaffirm the need for frank discussion between sexual partners.

4. Explain how the client and partner can use role-playing to bring concerns about sex out in the open.

5. Discuss alternate means for sexual satisfaction for self and partner (e.g., vibrators, touching, oral–genital techniques, body massage); consider past sexual experiences before suggesting specific techniques.
6. Encourage the client to consult with others with spinal cord injuries for an exchange of information; refer him to pertinent literature and organizations.
7. Refer the client and partner to certified sex or mental health professional, if desired.

Rationale

1. Many clients are reluctant to discuss sexual matters; initiating discussions demonstrates your empathy and concern.
2. Accurate information can prevent false hope or give real hope, as appropriate.
3. Both partners have fears and concerns about sexual activity. Repressing these feelings negatively influences the relationship.
4. Role-playing helps a person gain insight by placing himself in the position of another and allows more spontaneous sharing of fears and concerns.
5. The client and partner can experience sexual satisfaction and gratification through various alternatives to intercourse.

6. Interacting with others in a similar situation can help reduce feelings of isolation, provide information on alternative sexual practices, and allow frank sharing of problems and concerns.
7. Certain sexual problems require continuing therapy and the advanced knowledge of therapists.

▲ *Documentation*

Progress notes
    Dialogues
Discharge summary record
    Referrals, if indicated

Bowel Incontinence: Reflexic related to lack of voluntary sphincter control secondary to spinal cord injury above T11

▲ *Outcome Criteria*

The client will evacuate a soft formed stool every other day or every third day.

Focus Assessment Criteria	*Clinical Significance*
1. Understanding of injury 2. Previous and current bowel patterns 3. Control of rectal sphincter, presence of anal wink and bulbocavernosus reflex	1–4. Complete central nervous system lesions or trauma occurring above sacral cord segments (S2, S3, S4) (T12-L1-L2 vertebral level) result in a reflexic neurogenic

Focus Assessment Criteria

4. Awareness of bowel cues

Clinical Significance

bowel. The ascending sensory signals between the sacral reflex center and the brain are interrupted, resulting in the inability to feel the urge to defecate. Descending motor signals from the brain are also interrupted, causing loss of voluntary control over the anal sphincter. Once spinal shock has abated, the bulbocavernosus reflex usually returns. Because the sacral reflex center is preserved, it is possible to develop a stimulation–response bowel evacuation program using digital stimulation or digital stimulation devices. Fecal incontinence may occur through sacral arc reflex action, although this occurs less frequently than in areflexic bowel owing to the fact that in a reflexic bowel, the external anal sphincter usually remains in the contracted state until stimulated to relax.

Interventions

1. Assess previous bowel elimination patterns, diet, and life style.

2. Determine present neurological and physiological status and functional level.

3. Plan a consistent, appropriate time for elimination. Institute a daily bowel program for 5 days or until a pattern develops, then an alternate-day program (morning or evening).

4. Provide privacy and a nonstressful environment.

5. Position in an upright or sitting position if functionally able. If not functionally able (quadriplegic), position in left side-lying position, use digital stimulation—gloves, lubricant, or index finger (adults).

6. For a functionally able client, use assistive devices, e.g., dil stick, digital stimulator, raised commode seat, and lubricant and gloves, as appropriate.

7. For a client with upper extremity mobility and abdominal musculature innervation, teach bowel elimination facilitation techniques as appropriate:
   a. Valsalva's maneuver
   b. Forward bends
   c. Sitting push-ups
   d. Abdominal massage

8. Assist with or provide equipment needed for hygiene measures, as necessary.

9. Maintain an elimination record or a flow sheet of the bowel schedule that includes time, stool characteristics, assistive method(s) used, and number of involuntary stools, if any.

Rationale

1. This assessment enables the nurse to plan a bowel program to meet the client's habits and needs.

2. Establishing an appropriate bowel program in accordance with the client's functional level and ability helps reduce frustration.

3. A routine evacuation schedule decreases or eliminates the chance of involuntary stool passage.

4. Privacy decreases anxiety and promotes self-image and esteem.

5. Upright positioning facilitates movement of stool by enlisting the aid of gravity and by aiding emptying of the transverse colon into the descending colon.

6. A dil stick and digital stimulator stimulate the rectal sphincter and lower colon, initiating peristalsis for movement of fecal material.

7. These techniques increase intra-abdominal pressure to facilitate passage of stool at evacuation time.

8. Good hygiene helps prevent skin breakdown.

9. Ongoing documentation of elimination schedule and results provides data helpful to bowel program management.

Interventions	*Rationale*
10. Provide reassurance and protection from embarrassment while establishing the bowel program.	10. Reassurance decreases anxiety and promotes self-esteem.
11. Initiate a nutritional consultation; provide a diet high in fluid and fiber content. Monitor fluid intake and output.	11. Frequency and consistency of stool are related to fluid and food intake. Fiber increases fecal bulk and enhances absorption of water into the stool. Adequate dietary fiber and fluid intake promote firm but soft, well-formed stools and decrease the risk of hard, dry constipated stools.
12. Provide physical activity and exercise appropriate to the client's functional ability and endurance.	12. Physical activity promotes peristalsis, aids digestion, and facilitates elimination.
13. Teach appropriate use of stool softeners, laxatives, and suppositories, and explain the hazards of enemas.	13. Laxatives upset a bowel program, because they cause much of the bowel to empty and can cause unscheduled bowel movements. With constant use, the colon loses tone and bowel retraining becomes difficult. Chronic use of bowel aids can lead to inconsistent stool consistency, which interferes with the scheduled bowel program and bowel management. Stool softeners may not be necessary if diet and fluid intake are adequate. Enemas lead to overstretching of the bowel and loss of bowel tone, contributing to further constipation.
14. Explain the signs and symptoms of fecal impaction and constipation.	14. Fecal impaction and constipation may lead to autonomic dysreflexia in a client with injury at T7 or higher, owing to bowel overdistention. Chronic constipation can lead to overdistention of the bowel, with further loss of bowel tone. Unrelieved constipation may result in fecal impaction. Early intervention in diet and fluid intake, bowel evacuation methods, and schedules helps prevent constipation, further loss of bowel tone, and fecal impaction.
15. Initiate teaching of a bowel program before discharge. If the client is functionally able, encourage independence with the bowel program; if client is quadriplegic with limited hand function, incorporate assistive devices or attendant care, as needed.	15. Teaching bowel management techniques, bowel complications, and the impact of diet, fluids, and exercise on elimination can help promote independent functioning or help the client to instruct others in specific care measures, promoting adequate elimination and preventing complications.

▲ **Documentation**

Flow records
  Stool results (time, method used, involuntary stools)
Discharge summary record
  Client teaching
  Outcome achievement or status

▲ **Outcome Criteria**

The client will evacuate a firm, formed stool every day or every other day.

Bowel Incontinence: Areflexic related to lack of voluntary sphincter secondary to spinal cord injury involving sacral reflex arc (S2–S4)

Focus Assessment Criteria	*Clinical Significance*
1. Understanding of injury	1. Complete spinal cord injury, spinal cord lesions, neurological disease, or congenital defects causing an interruption of the sacral reflex arc (at the sacral segments S2, S3, S4) result in an areflexic (autonomous) or flaccid bowel. Flaccid paralysis at this level, known as an LMN lesion, results in loss of the defecation reflex, loss of sphincter control (flaccid anal sphincter), and absence of the bulbocavernosus reflex.

Focus Assessment Criteria	*Clinical Significance*
2. Previous and present bowel patterns 3. Dietary patterns: food and fluid intake	2,3. Because of an interrupted sacral reflex arc and a flaccid anal sphincter, bowel incontinence can occur without rectal stimulation whenever stool is present in the rectal vault. The stool may leak out if too soft or remain (if not extracted), predisposing the client to fecal impaction or constipation. Some intrinsic contractile abilities of the colon remain, but peristalsis is sluggish, leading to stool retention with contents present in the rectal vault.
4. Awareness of bowel cues	4. Interruption of the sensory and motor pathways to the brain usually results in loss of cerebral awareness and control of elimination.

Interventions

1. Assess previous bowel elimination patterns, diet, and life style.

2. Determine present neurological and physiological status and functional level.

3. Plan a consistent, appropriate time for elimination. Institute a daily bowel program for 5 days or until a pattern develops, then an alternate-day program (morning or evening).

4. Provide privacy and a nonstressful environment.

5. Position in an upright or sitting position if functionally able. If not functionally able (quadriplegic), position in left side-lying position, use digital stimulation—gloves, lubricant, or index finger (adults).

6. For a functionally able client, use assistive devices, e.g., dil stick, digital stimulator, raised commode seat, and lubricant and gloves, as appropriate.

7. For a client with upper extremity mobility and abdominal musculature innervation, teach bowel elimination facilitation techniques as appropriate:
   a. Valsalva's maneuver
   b. Forward bends
   c. Sitting push-ups
   d. Abdominal massage

8. Assist with or provide equipment needed for hygiene measures, as necessary.

9. Maintain an elimination record or a flow sheet of the bowel schedule that includes time, stool characteristics, assistive method(s) used, and number of involuntary stools, if any.

10. Provide reassurance and protection from embarrassment while establishing the bowel program.

11. Initiate a nutritional consultation; provide a diet high in fluid and fiber content. Monitor fluid intake and output.

Rationale

1. This assessment enables the nurse to plan a bowel program to meet the client's habits and needs.

2. Establishing an appropriate bowel program in accordance with the client's functional level and ability helps reduce frustration.

3. A routine evacuation schedule decreases or eliminates the chance of involuntary stool passage.

4. Privacy decreases anxiety and promotes self-image and esteem.

5. Upright positioning facilitates movement of stool by enlisting the aid of gravity and by aiding emptying of the transverse colon into the descending colon.

6. A dil stick and digital stimulator stimulate the rectal sphincter and lower colon, initiating peristalsis for movement of fecal material.

7. These techniques increase intra-abdominal pressure to facilitate passage of stool at evacuation time.

8. Good hygiene helps prevent skin breakdown.

9. Ongoing documentation of elimination schedule and results provides data helpful to bowel program management.

10. Reassurance decreases anxiety and promotes self-esteem.

11. Frequency and consistency of stool are related to fluid and food intake. Fiber increases fecal bulk and enhances absorption of water into

Interventions

12. Provide physical activity and exercise appropriate to the client's functional ability and endurance.
13. Teach appropriate use of stool softeners, laxatives, and suppositories and explain the hazards of enemas.

14. Explain the signs and symptoms of fecal impaction and constipation.

15. Initiate teaching of a bowel program before discharge. If the client is functionally able, encourage independence with the bowel program; if not, incorporate assistive devices or attendant care, as needed.

Rationale

the stool. Adequate dietary fiber and fluid intake promote firm but soft, well-formed stools and decrease the risk of hard, dry constipated stools.
12. Physical activity promotes peristalsis, aids digestion, and facilitates elimination.
13. Laxatives upset a bowel program, because they cause much of the bowel to empty and can cause unscheduled bowel movements. With constant use, the colon loses tone and bowel retraining becomes difficult. Chronic use of bowel aids can lead to inconsistent stool consistency, which interferes with the scheduled bowel program and bowel management. Stool softeners may not be necessary if diet and fluid intake are adequate. Enemas lead to overstretching of the bowel and loss of bowel tone, contributing to further constipation.
14. Bowel motility is decreased in LMN cord damage; decreased movement of stool through the colon can result in increased fluid absorption from stool, resulting in hard, dry stools and constipation. Unrelieved constipation may result in fecal impaction. Early intervention in diet and fluid intake, bowel evacuation methods, and schedules help prevent constipation, further loss of bowel tone, and fecal impaction.
15. Teaching bowel management techniques, bowel complications, and the impact of diet, fluids, and exercise on elimination can help promote independent functioning or help the client to instruct others in specific care measures, promoting adequate elimination and preventing complications.

▲ **Documentation**

Flow records
    Consistency of stool
    Amount of stool
    Time of evacuation
    Time and number of involuntary stools, if any
    Any leakage of stool from rectum
    Bowel sounds
    Intake and output
    Assistive devices, if any
Progress notes
    Unsatisfactory results/toleration of procedure
    Evidence of hemorrhoids, bleeding, abnormal sacral skin appearance
Discharge summary record
    Client teaching

▲ **Outcome Criteria**

The outcome criteria for this diagnosis represent those associated with discharge planning. Refer to the discharge criteria.

Potential Impaired Home Maintenance Management related to insufficient knowledge of the effects of altered skin, bowel, bladder, respiratory, thermoregulatory, and sexual function and their management; signs and symptoms of complications; follow-up care; and community resources

Focus Assessment Criteria	*Clinical Significance*
1. Readiness and ability to learn and retain information	1. A client or family that fails to achieve learning goals requires a referral for assistance postdischarge.

Interventions

1. Reinforce the effects of injury on bowel, bladder, thermoregulation, respiratory system, and integumentary function.
2. Assist in formulating and accepting realistic short- and long-term goals.
3. Evaluate the client's and family member's or significant other's ability to perform the following:

Rationale

1. This information may encourage the client and family to comply with the therapeutic regimen.
2. Mutual goal-setting reinforces the client's sense of control over his life.
3. These skills are essential to an effective home management program.

Interventions

   a. Skin care and assessment
   b. Bowel program
   c. Bladder program
   d. Proper positioning
   e. Transfer techniques
   f. Application of abdominal binder, antiembolic hose, splints, and protectors
   g. Range-of-motion exercises (active and passive).

4. Reinforce the teaching about dysreflexia and its treatment.
5. Explain the reasons for temperature fluctuation and the risks of hypothermia and hyperthermia.

6. Explain the importance of a well-balanced diet with caloric intake appropriate for activity level.

7. Instruct to report the following:
   a. Cloudy, foul-smelling urine
   b. Unresolved signs of dysreflexia
   c. Fever, chills
   d. Green, purulent, or rust-colored sputum
   e. Nausea and vomiting
   f. Persistent skin lesion or irritation
   g. Swelling and redness of lower extremities
   h. Increased restriction of movement
   i. Unsatisfactory bowel or bladder results
8. Emphasize the need to participate in the scheduled rehabilitation plan.

9. Initiate a referral for assistance with home care, e.g., community nurses, social service.

10. Provide information on self-help sessions and hand out printed material, such as the following:

   National Spinal Cord Injury Association
   369 Elliot St.
   Newton Upper Falls, MA 02164

Rationale

4. Reinforcement promotes feelings of competency and confidence.
5. Interruption in the sympathetic system disrupts the vasoconstriction or vasodilatation response to temperature changes. Also, diaphoresis is absent below the level of cord injury. As a result, the client's body assumes the temperature of the environment (poikilothermia).
6. A well-balanced diet is needed to maintain tissue integrity, prevent complications (e.g., skin problems, infection, osteoporosis), and prevent weight gain.

7. Early detection of complications enables prompt interventions to prevent debilitating results. Complications can include infections (urinary tract, respiratory, or GI), thrombophlebitis, pressure ulcers, contractures, and dysreflexia.

8. With training and assistance, most spinal cord-injured clients can attain some degree of independence in activities of daily living.
9. Regardless of the success experienced in the hospital, the client and family need assistance with adjustment postdischarge.
10. Specialized organizations can provide timely information on a variety of related issues or problems.

▲ **Documentation**

Discharge summary record
   Client teaching
   Outcome achievement or status
   Referrals, if indicated

References/Bibliography

Adams, G. (1976). The sexual history as an integral part of the patient history. *Maternal–Child Nursing Journal, 1*(3), 170–175.

Annon, J.S. (1976). The PLISS T model: A proposed conceptual scheme for the behavioral treatment of sexual problems. *Journal of Sexual Education and Therapy, 2*, 211–215.

Baxter, R. (1978). Sex counseling and the spinal cord injured patient. *Nursing, 8*(9), 46–52.

Bertino, L. (1989). Stress management with SCI clients. *Rehabilitation Nursing, 14*(3), 127–129.

Calderone, M., & Johnson, E. (1981). *Family book about sexuality.* New York: Harper and Row.

Comfort, A. (1978). *Sexual consequences of disability.* Philadelphia: G.F. Stickley.

Decker, S., Schultz, R., & Wood, D. (1989). Determinants of well-being in primary caregivers of spinal cord injured persons. *Rehabilitation Nursing, 14*(1), 6–8.

Evans, R., Halar, E.M., DiFreece, A.B., et al. (1976). Multidisciplinary approach to sex education of spinal cord injured patients. *Physical Therapy, 56*, 541–545.

Hamburg, D.A., Adams, J.E. (1983). A perspective on coping behaviors. *Archives of General Psychiatry, 17*(3), 1–20.

Hickey, J. (1986). *The clinical practice of neurological and neurosurgical nursing* (2nd ed.). Philadelphia: J. B. Lippincott.

Hogan, R. (1980). *Human sexuality: A nursing perspective.* New York: Appleton-Century-Crofts.

Kolodney, R.C., Masters, W.H., Johnson, V.E., et al. (1979). *Textbook of human sexuality for nurses.* Boston: Little, Brown.

Krozy, R. (1978). Becoming comfortable with sexual assessment. *American Journal of Nursing, 78,* 1036–1038.

Lion, E. (1982). *Human sexuality in the nursing process.* New York: John Wiley & Sons.

Macrae, I., & Henderson, M. (1975). Sexuality and irreversible health limitations. *Nursing Clinics of North America, 10*(3), 587–597.

Mitchell, P., Hodges, L., Mawaswes, M., & Walleck, C. (1988). *AANN's neuroscience nursing.* Norwalk, CT: Appleton and Lange.

Mooney, T. (1975). *Sexual options for paraplegics and quadriplegics.* Boston: Little, Brown.

Rudy, E. (1984). *Advanced neurological and neurosurgical nursing.* St. Louis: C.V. Mosby Co.

Schiller, P. (1977). The nurse's role as sex counselor. *Nursing Care, 10,* 10–13.

Siemens, S., & Brandzel, R. (1982). *Sexuality: Nursing assessment and intervention.* Philadelphia: J.B. Lippincott.

Woods, N.F. (1979). *Human sexuality in health and illness* (2nd ed.). St. Louis: C.V. Mosby.

Immobility or Unconsciousness

This care plan addresses the needs of clients who are either unconscious or conscious but immobile. In addition to the following diagnostic cluster, refer to the specific coexisting medical disease or condition, e.g., renal failure, cancer.

Diagnostic Cluster

▲ **Time Frame**

Variable

Collaborative Problems

Potential Complications:	Refer to:
Pneumonia, Atelectasis	Cerebrovascular Accident (Stroke)
Fluid/Electrolyte Imbalance	General Surgery
Negative Nitrogen Balance	Chronic Renal Failure
Sepsis	Urolithiasis
Thrombophlebitis	General Surgery
Renal Calculi	Chronic Renal Failure
Urinary Tract Infection	Chronic Renal Failure

Nursing Diagnoses

Potential for Disuse Syndrome related to effects of immobility on body systems	
Self-Care Deficit (specify) related to immobility	
Powerlessness related to feelings of loss of control and the restrictions that are placed on life style	
Potential Ineffective Airway Clearance related to stasis of secretions secondary to inadequate cough and decreased mobility	Chronic Obstructive Pulmonary Disease
Total Incontinence related to unconscious state	Neurogenic Bladder
Potential Altered Oral Mucous Membrane related to immobility to perform own mouth care and pooling of secretions	Pneumonia

▲ **Discharge Criteria**

Before discharge, the client and/or family will:

1. Relate ways to prevent complications of immobility
2. State signs and symptoms that must be reported to a health care professional
3. Identify community services available for assistance

Nursing Diagnoses

▲ **Outcome Criteria**

The client will:

1. Demonstrate intact skin and tissue integrity
2. Demonstrate maximum pulmonary function
3. Demonstrate maximum peripheral blood flow
4. Demonstrate full range of motion
5. Demonstrate adequate bowel, bladder, and renal function
6. Make use of social contacts and activities when possible
7. Explain rationale for treatments
8. Make decisions regarding care when possible
9. Share feelings regarding immobile state

Potential for Disuse Syndrome related to effects of immobility on body systems

Focus Assessment Criteria

1. Level of consciousness
2. Motor function in arms and legs
3. Mobility: ability to turn self, sit, stand, transfer, ambulate
4. Restrictive devices (e.g., casts, ventilator, Foley catheter, IV lines)
5. Range of motion: full or limited
6. Elimination pattern
7. Respiratory status
8. Circulatory status, skin condition
9. Intake and output

Clinical Significance

1–9. Musculoskeletal inactivity has adverse effects on all body systems. The nurse must assess the client's functional ability in order to determine the type and frequency of interventions required.

Interventions

1. Explain the effects of immobility on body systems and the reason for interventions, as indicated.

Rationale

1. Understanding may help elicit cooperation in reducing immobility.

Interventions

2. Take steps to promote optimal respiratory function:
   a. Vary bed position, unless contraindicated, to change the horizontal and vertical position of the thorax gradually.
   b. Assist with repositioning, turning from side to side every hour if possible.
   c. Encourage deep breathing and controlled coughing exercises five times an hour.
   d. Teach to use a blow bottle or incentive spirometer every hour when awake. (A client with severe neuromuscular impairment may have to be awakened during the night as well.)
   e. For a child, try using colored water in the blow bottle; also have him blow up balloons, blow soap bubbles, blow cotton balls with a straw, and other "fun" breathing exercises.
   f. Auscultate lung fields every 8 hours or less, if altered breath sounds occur.
   g. Encourage small, frequent feedings.
3. Encourage increased oral fluid intake, as indicated.

4. Explain the effects of daily activity on elimination. Assist with ambulation when possible.

5. Promote factors that contribute to optimal elimination:
   a. Balanced diet:
      • Review a list of foods high in bulk, e.g., fresh fruits with skins, bran, nuts and seeds, whole grain breads and cereals, cooked fruits and vegetables, and fruit juices.
      • Discuss dietary preferences.
      • Encourage intake of approximately 800 g of fruits and vegetables (about four pieces of fresh fruit and a large salad) for normal daily bowel movement.
   b. Adequate fluid intake:
      • Encourage intake of at least 8 to 10 glasses (about 2000 mL) daily, unless contraindicated.
      • Discuss fluid preferences.
      • Set up a regular schedule for fluid intake.
   c. Regular time for defecation:
      • Identify normal defecation pattern before onset of constipation.
      • Review daily routine.
      • Include time for defecation as part of the regular daily routine.
      • Discuss a suitable time, based on responsibilities, availability of facilities, etc.
      • Suggest that the client attempt defecation about an hour following a meal and

Rationale

2. Immobility contributes to stasis of secretions and possible pneumonia or atelectasis. These measures help increase lung expansion and the ability to expel secretions.

3. Optimal hydration liquefies secretions for easier expectoration and prevents stasis of secretions that provide a medium for microorganism growth.
4. Activity influences bowel elimination by improving muscle tone and stimulating appetite and peristalsis.
5.

   a. A well-balanced diet high in fiber content stimulates peristalsis.

   b. Sufficient fluid intake is necessary to maintain bowel patterns and promote proper stool consistency.

   c. Taking advantage of circadian rhythms may aid in establishing a regular defecation schedule.

Interventions	*Rationale*

remain in the bathroom a suitable length of time.

d. Simulation of the home environment:
- Have the client use the bathroom instead of a bedpan, if possible; offer a bedpan or a bedside commode if the client cannot use the bathroom.
- Assist into position on the toilet, commode, or bedpan if necessary.
- Provide privacy, e.g., close the door, draw curtains around the bed, play a TV or radio to mask sounds, make room deodorizer available.
- Provide for comfort (e.g., provide reading materials as a diversion) and safety (e.g., make a call bell readily available).

e. Proper positioning:
- Assist the client to a normal semisquatting position on the toilet or commode, if possible.
- Assist onto a bedpan if necessary, elevating the head of the bed to high Fowler's position or to the elevation permitted.
- Stress the need to avoid straining during defecation efforts.

6. Institute measures to prevent pressure ulcers. (Refer to the Pressure Ulcers care plan, page 266, for specific interventions.)

7. Promote optimum circulation when the client is sitting:
   a. Limit sitting time for a client at high risk for ulcer development.
   b. Instruct the client to lift himself every 10 minutes, using the chair arms, if possible, or assist him with this maneuver.

8. With each position change, inspect areas at risk for developing ulcers:
   a. Ears
   b. Elbows
   c. Occiput
   d. Trochanter
   e. Heels
   f. Ischia
   g. Sacrum
   h. Scapula
   i. Scrotum

9. Observe for erythema and blanching, palpate for warmth and tissue sponginess, and massage vulnerable areas lightly with each position change.

10. Teach the client to do the following:
    a. Elevate the legs above the level of the heart. (*Note,* this may be contraindicated if severe cardiac or respiratory disease is present.)
    b. Avoid standing or sitting with legs dependent for long periods

Rationale

d. Privacy and a sense of normalcy can promote relaxation, which can enhance defecation.

e. Proper positioning uses the abdominal muscles and the force of gravity to aid defecation.

6. The immobile client is at risk for pressure ulcers—localized areas of cellular necrosis that tend to occur when soft tissue is compressed between a bony prominence and a firm surface for a prolonged period. Avoiding prolonged pressure can prevent pressure ulcer formation.

7. Capillary flow is increased if pressure is relieved and redistributed. Prolonged compromised capillary flow leads to tissue hypoxia and necrosis.

8. Certain areas over bony prominences are more prone to cellular compression.

9. Erythema and blanching are early signs of tissue hypoxia. Deep massage can injure capillaries, but light massage stimulates local circulation.

10.

a,b. Immobility reduces venous return and increases intravascular pressure, which contributes to venous stasis and thrombophlebitis.

Interventions

    c. Consider using Ace bandages or below-knee elastic stockings

    d. Avoid using pillows behind the knees or a gatch on the bed elevated at the knees

    e. Avoid leg crossing

    f. Change positions, move extremities, or wiggle fingers and toes every hour

    g. Avoid garters and tight elastic stockings above the knees

    h. Perform leg exercises every hour when advisable

11. Measure baseline circumference of calves and thighs daily if the client is at risk for deep venous thrombosis, or if it is suspected.

12. Institute measures to increase limb mobility:
    a. Perform range-of-motion (ROM) exercises as frequently as the client's condition warrants.
    b. Support limbs with pillows to prevent or reduce swelling.
    c. Encourage the client to perform exercise regimens for specific joints, as prescribed by the physician or physical therapist.

13. Take steps to maintain proper body alignment:

    a. Use a footboard.
    b. Avoid prolonged periods of sitting or lying in the same position.
    c. Change position of the shoulder joints every 2 to 4 hours.
    d. Use a small pillow or no pillow when the client is in Fowler's position.
    e. Support the hand and wrist in natural alignment.
    f. If the client is supine or prone, place a rolled towel or small pillow under the lumbar curvature or under the end of the rib cage.
    g. Place a trochanter roll or sandbags alongside the hips and upper thighs.
    h. If the client is in the lateral position, place pillow(s) to support the leg from groin to foot, and a pillow to flex the shoulder and elbow slightly; if needed, support the lower foot in dorsal flexion with a sandbag.
    i. Use hand–wrist splints.

14. Monitor for and take steps to reduce bone demineralization:
    a. Monitor for signs and symptoms of hypercalcemia, e.g., elevated serum calcium level, nausea and vomiting, polydipsia, polyuria, lethargy.
    b. Provide weightbearing whenever possible; use a tilt table, if indicated.

Rationale

    c. Elastic stockings reduce venous pooling by exerting even pressure over the leg and increase flow to deeper veins by reducing the caliber of the superficial veins.

    d–g. External venous compression impedes venous flow.

    h. Leg exercises promote the muscle pumping effect on the deep veins.

11. Thrombophlebitis causes edema, which increases leg measurements.

12. Joints without range of motion exercise develop contractures in 3 to 7 days because flexor muscles are stronger than extensor muscles.

13. Prolonged immobility and impaired neurosensory function can cause permanent contractures.
    a. This measure prevents foot drop.
    b. This measure prevents hip flexion contractures.
    c. This measure can help prevent shoulder contractures.
    d. This measure prevents flexion contracture of the neck.
    e. This measure can help prevent dependent edema and flexion contracture of wrist.
    f. This measure prevents flexion or hyperflexion of lumbar curvature.

    g. This prevents external rotation of the femurs and hips.
    h. These measures prevent internal rotation and adduction of the femur and shoulder, and prevent foot drop.

    i. Splints prevent flexion or extension contractures of fingers and abduction of the thumbs.

14. Lack of motion and weightbearing results in bone destruction, which releases calcium into the bloodstream, resulting in hypercalcemia.

Interventions

15. Take measures to prevent urinary stasis and calculi formation:

   a. Provide a daily intake of fluid of 2000 mL or greater a day (unless contraindicated).

   b. Maintain urine pH below 6.0 (acidic) with acid ash foods (e.g., cereals, meats, poultry, fish, cranberry juice, apple juice).

   c. Teach the client to avoid these foods:
- Milk, milk products, cheese
- Bran cereals
- Cranberries, plums, raspberries, gooseberries, olives
- Asparagus, rhubarb, spinach, kale, Swiss chard, turnip greens, mustard greens, broccoli, beet greens
- Legumes, whole grain rice
- Sardines, shrimp, oysters
- Chocolate
- Peanut butter

16. Maintain vigorous hydration unless contraindicated:
   a. Adult: 2000 mL/day
   b. Adolescent: 3000 to 4000 mL/day

Rationale

15. The peristaltic contractions of the ureters are insufficient when in a reclining position, resulting in urine stasis in the renal pelvis.
   a. Stones form more readily in concentrated urine.
   b. These measures reduce the formation of calcium calculi.

   c. These foods are high in calcium and oxalate and can contribute to stone formation.

16. Optimal hydration reduces the blood coagulability, liquefies secretions, inhibits stone formation, and promotes glomerular filtration of body wastes.

▲ **Documentation**

Flow records
   Exercise
   Turning
   Assessment results (circulatory, respiratory, skin)
Discharge summary record
   Client teaching

▲ **Outcome Criteria**

The client will:

1. Perform self-care activities (specify feeding, toileting, dressing, grooming, or bathing)
2. Demonstrate use of adaptive devices (specify), if necessary
3. Demonstrate optimal hygiene after care is provided

Self-Care Deficit (specify) related to immobility

Focus Assessment Criteria	Clinical Significance
1. Self-feeding abilities	1–6. A baseline is needed to assess improvement in self-care activities.
2. Self-bathing abilities	
3. Self-dressing abilities	
4. Self-toileting abilities	
5. Motivation	
6. Endurance	

Interventions

1. Promote the client's maximum involvement in feeding activities:

   a. Ascertain from the client or family members what foods he likes and dislikes.

   b. Have the client eat all meals in the same setting—pleasant surroundings that are not too distracting.

   c. Provide good oral hygiene before and after meals.

   d. Encourage the client to wear dentures and eyeglasses, as necessary.

   e. Place the client in the most normal eating position suited to his physical disability (best is sitting in a chair at a table).

   f. Provide social contact during meals.

   g. Encourage eating of "finger foods" (e.g., bread, bacon, fruit, hot dogs) to promote independence.

   h. To enhance independence, provide necessary adaptive devices (e.g., plate guard to avoid pushing food off plate, suction device under plate or bowl for stabilization, padded handles on utensils for a more secure grip, wrist

Rationale

1. Eating has physiological, psychological, social, and cultural implications. Providing control over meals promotes overall well-being.

Interventions

or hand splints with clamp to hold eating utensils, special drinking cup, rocker knife for cutting).

  i. Assist with set-up, if needed, e.g., opening containers, napkins, and condiment packages; cutting meat; buttering bread.

  j. Arrange food so the client has adequate amount of space to perform the task of eating.

2. Promote the client's maximum involvement in bathing activities:

  a. Bathing time and routine should be consistent to encourage greatest amount of independence.

  b. Encourage the client to wear prescribed corrective lenses or hearing aid.

  c. Keep bathroom temperature warm; ascertain the client's preferred water temperature.

  d. Provide for privacy during the bathing routine.

  e. Provide for adaptive equipment as needed (e.g., bath board for transferring to tub chair or stool, washing mitts with pocket for soap, adapted toothbrushes, shaver holders, hand-held shower spray).

  f. Place bathing equipment in the location most suitable to the client.

  g. Keep a call bell within reach if the client is to bathe alone.

3. Promote the client's maximum involvement in toileting activities:

  a. Observe his ability to obtain equipment or get to the toilet unassisted.

  b. Provide only the amount of supervision and assistance necessary.

  c. Provide the necessary adaptive devices to enhance independence and safety (e.g., commode chairs, spill-proof urinals, fracture bedpans, raised toilet seats, support side rails for toilets).

  d. Avoid the use of bedpans and urinals whenever possible; provide a normal atmosphere of elimination in the bathroom, and use the same toilet to promote familiarity.

4. Promote or provide assistance with grooming and dressing:

  a. Deodorant application daily

  b. Cosmetics of choice

  c. Hair care (shampoo, styling)

  d. Facial hair

  e. Nail and foot care

Rationale

2. Inability for self-care produces feelings of dependency and poor self-concept. With increased ability for self-care, self-esteem increases.

3. These measures can reduce the embarrassment associated with assistance with toileting.

4. Optimal personal grooming promotes psychological well-being.

▲ **Documentation**

Progress notes
  Involvement in self-care

Powerlessness related to loss of control and disorder-related life style restrictions

Focus Assessment Criteria	Clinical Significance
1. Understanding of activity restrictions 2. Perception of control 3. Effects on life style	1–3. A client's response to loss of control depends on the personal meaning of the loss, individual coping patterns, personal characteristics, and response of others.

Interventions	*Rationale*
1. Encourage the client to share his or her feelings and fears regarding restricted movement.	1. Open dialogue promotes sharing and a sense of well-being.
2. Determine the client's usual response to problems.	2. To plan effective care, the nurse must determine whether the client usually seeks to change his or her own behaviors to control problems or expects others or external factors to control problems.
3. Encourage the client to wear clothes rather than pajamas and to wear desired personal adornments, e.g., baseball cap, colorful socks.	3. Street clothes allow the client to express his or her individuality, which promotes self-esteem and reduces feelings of powerlessness.
4. Plan strategies to reduce the monotony of immobility: a. Vary the daily routine when possible. b. Have the client participate in daily planning when possible. c. Try to make the routine as normal as possible, e.g., have the client dress in street clothes during the day if feasible. d. Encourage visitors. e. Alter the physical environment when possible, e.g., update bulletin boards, change pictures on the walls, rearrange furniture. f. Maintain a pleasant, cheerful environment. Position the client near a window if possible. If appropriate, provide a goldfish bowl for visual variety. g. Provide a variety of reading materials (or "books on tape" if impairment hinders reading ability), and a television and radio. h. Discourage excessive TV watching. i. Plan some "special" activity daily to give the client something to look forward to each day. j. Consider enlisting a volunteer to read to the client or help with activities, if necessary. k. Encourage the client to devise his own strategies to combat boredom.	4. These measures may help reduce the monotony of immobility and compensate for psychological effects of immobility (e.g., decreased attention span, decreased motivation).
5. Provide opportunities for the client to make decisions regarding his surroundings, activities and routines, and short- and long-term goals, as appropriate.	5. Mobility enables a client to actualize his or her decisions (e.g., when to eat, where to go, what to do. Loss of mobility can impact autonomy and control.
6. Encourage family members to request the client's opinions when making family decisions.	6. The family can provide opportunities for the client to maintain role responsibilities, which can help minimize feelings of powerlessness.

▲ **Documentation**
Progress notes
   Interactions
   Response

References/Bibliography

Milde, F.K. (1988). Impaired physical mobility. *Journal of Gerontological Nursing, 14*(3), 20–40.
Rubin, M. (1988). The physiology of bed rest. *American Journal of Nursing, 88*(1), 50–58.

Neurogenic Bladder

Resulting from impaired neurological control of micturition, neurogenic bladder may be classified as autonomous, reflexive, atonic, and uninhibited. Classification depends on the level of central nervous system disruption:

☐ *Autonomous* neurogenic bladder results from destruction of the bladder center in the sacral spinal cord. The client feels no conscious sensation to void and has no micturition reflex, and the bladder empties irregularly.

☐ In *reflexive* neurogenic bladder, occurring from spinal cord damage between the sacral spinal cord and the cerebral cortex, the client has no sensation to void and no ability to inhibit reflex contractions of the bladder.

☐ *Atonic* neurogenic bladder results from damage to the posterior nerve roots. The client retains voluntary control but loses the sensation of bladder distention. Overflow incontinence occurs when the bladder contains a high volume of urine.

☐ In *uninhibited* neurogenic bladder, resulting from damage to the bladder center in the cerebral cortex, the client has limited sensation of bladder distention but no ability to inhibit urination. Urgency results from the short time between limited sensation to void and the uninhibited bladder contraction.

Diagnostic Cluster

▲ Time Frame

Secondary diagnosis (hospitalization not usual for neurogenic bladder)

▲ Discharge Criteria

Before discharge, the client or family will:

1. Identify measures to reduce incontinence
2. Relate an intent to discuss fears and concerns with family after discharge
3. Relate signs and symptoms that must be reported to a health care professional
4. Demonstrate correct self-catheterization technique
5. Relate an intent to continue exercises and fluid intake program at home

---

Collaborative Problems

Potential Complication:
Renal Calculi

Refer to:

Nursing Diagnoses

Urinary Retention related to chronically overfilled bladder with loss of sensation of bladder distention

Reflex Incontinence related to absence of sensation to void and loss of ability to inhibit bladder contraction

Potential for Infection related to retention of urine or introduction of urinary catheter

Urge Incontinence related to disruption of the inhibitory efferent impulses secondary to brain or spinal cord dysfunction

Potential Social Isolation related to embarrassment from wetting self in front of others and fear of odor from urine

Potential Altered Health Maintenance related to insufficient knowledge of etiology of incontinence, management, bladder retraining programs, signs and symptoms of complications, and community resources

Potential Dysreflexia related to reflex stimulation of sympathetic nervous system secondary to loss of autonomic control   Spinal Cord Injury

Potential Impaired Skin Integrity related to constant irritation from urine   Pressure Ulcers

---

Collaborative Problems

▲ Nursing Goal

The nurse will manage and minimize episodes of renal calculi.

Potential Complication: Renal Calculi

Interventions

1. Monitor for signs and symptoms of renal calculi:

Rationale

1. Urinary stasis and infection increase the risk of renal calculi because of increased precipitants in the urine.

▲ Documentation

Flow records
    Urine output and characteristics
Progress notes
    Complaints of pain, nausea, vomiting

Interventions

  a. Acute flank pain
  b. Costovertebral angle (CVA) pain (a dull, constant backache below the 12th rib)
  c. Hematuria

  d. Nausea and vomiting

Rationale

  a,b. Stones can cause severe pain owing to obstruction and ureter spasms or CVA pain due to distention of the renal capsule.
  c. The abrasive action of the stone can sever small blood vessels.
  d. Afferent stimuli in the renal capsule may cause pylorospasm of the smooth muscle of the GI tract.

Related Physician-Prescribed Interventions
None applicable

Nursing Diagnoses

▲ Outcome Criteria

The client will not be wet from urine.

Urinary Retention related to chronically overfilled bladder with loss of sensation of bladder distention

Focus Assessment Criteria	*Clinical Significance*
1. Perception of need to void 2. Complaints of incontinence or dribbling 3. Reports of relief after voiding 4. Urine characteristics 5. Bladder distention and capacity	1–5. Although the client has voluntary control over urination, an atonic detrusor muscle prevents him from feeling when the bladder is full. When sufficient urine collects in the bladder to stretch the detrusor muscle, bladder pressure exceeds urethral pressure, resulting in overflow incontinence or dribbling.

Interventions

1. Instruct the client in appropriate measures to minimize urine dribbling:

  a. Stop smoking.

  b. Reduce weight.

  c. Eat a high-fiber diet.

  d. Practice Kegel exercises (start and stop urine flow three times at each voiding).
2. Teach measures to help reduce detrusor activity:
  a. Resist voiding for as long as possible.
  b. Drink sufficient fluid to distend the bladder.
  c. Time fluid intake so that detrusor activity is restricted to waking hours.

3. Reduce any impediments to voiding routine by providing the following:
  a. Velcro straps on clothes, if necessary
  b. Handrails or mobility aids to bathroom if necessary
  c. Bedside commode, if necessary
  d. Urinal, if necessary
4. Teach the client methods to empty the bladder.
  a. Credé's maneuver:
    • Place the hands (either flat or in fists) just

Rationale

1. Dribbling of urine often can be reduced by reducing the pressure in the bladder and abdomen and strengthening the periurethral tissue.
  a. Coughing associated with smoking increases intra-abdominal pressure.
  b. Obesity increases pressure on the pelvic floor and sphincter.
  c. A high-fiber diet can help prevent constipation with associated straining, which decreases sphincter tone.
  d. Kegel exercises strengthen and tone muscles of the pelvic floor.
2. To increase comfort associated with voiding, the client must condition the voiding reflex by ingesting adequate fluids and inhibiting bladder contractions. Frequent toileting causes chronic low-volume voiding and increases detrusor activity. Resisting the urge to void may increase voiding intervals and reduce detrusor muscle activity.
3. These measures ensure the ability to self-toilet before incontinence occurs. Often, little time exists between onset of the sensation to void and the bladder contraction.

4.
  a. In many clients, Credé's maneuver can help empty the bladder. This maneuver is inap-

Interventions

below the umbilical area, one hand on top of the other.
- Firmly press down and in toward the pelvic arch.
- Repeat six or seven times until no more urine is expelled.
- Wait several minutes, then repeat again to ensure complete emptying.

b. Cutaneous triggering by suprapubic tapping:
- Assume a half-sitting position.
- Using the fingers of one hand, aim tapping directly at the bladder wall; tap at a rate of 7 or 8 times every 5 seconds, for a total of 50 taps.
- Shift the site of tapping over the bladder to find the most effective site.
- Continue stimulation until a good stream starts.
- Wait about 1 minute, then repeat stimulation until bladder is empty. (One or two series of stimulations without urination indicates bladder emptying.)
- If tapping is ineffective, perform each of the following for 2 to 3 minutes each:
  Stroke the glans penis.
  Lightly punch the abdomen above the inguinal ligaments.
  Stroke the inner thigh.

c. Valsalva's maneuver (bearing down):
- Lean forward on thighs.
- Contract abdominal muscles, if possible, and strain or bear down, holding the breath while doing so.
- Hold until urine flow stops; wait 1 minute, then repeat.
- Continue until no more urine is expelled.

d. The anal stretch maneuver:
- Sit on the commode or toilet, leaning forward on the thighs.
- Insert one or two lubricated fingers into the anus to the anal sphincter.
- Spread fingers apart or pull in the posterior direction to stretch the anal sphincter.
- Bear down and void, performing Valsalva's maneuver.
- Relax, then repeat the procedure until the bladder is empty.

e. Clean intermittent self-catheterization (CISC), used alone or in combination with the above methods. (Refer to the nursing diagnosis Altered Health Maintenance in this care plan for specific teaching points.)

5. Consult with the physician to restrict certain medications (e.g., diuretics, hypnotics, diazepam, phenothiazines, and ganglion-blocking agents) to reduce iatrogenic incontinence.

Rationale

propriate, however, if the urinary sphincters are chronically contracted. In this case, pressing the bladder can force urine up the ureters as well as through the urethra. Reflux of urine into the renal pelvis may result in renal infection.

b. External cutaneous stimulation can stimulate the voiding reflex.

c. Valsalva's maneuver contracts the abdominal muscles, which manually compresses the bladder.

d. Anal sphincter stimulation can stimulate the voiding reflex.

e. CISC prevents overdistention, helps maintain detrusor muscle tone, and ensures complete bladder emptying. CISC may be used initially to determine residual urine following Credé's maneuver or tapping. As residual urine decreases, catheterization may be tapered. CISC may recondition the voiding reflex in some clients.

5. These drugs induce incontinence—particularly in elderly clients—by increasing urinary output, causing sedation, altering conscious inhibition, and impairing recognition of bladder cues.

Documentation

Flow records
  Fluid intake
  Voiding patterns (amount, time, method used)
Discharge summary record
  Client teaching
  Outcome achievement or status

Outcome Criteria

The client will not be wet from urine.

Interventions

6. If other measures fail, plan for managing incontinence:
   a. Incontinent males can manage fairly easily by using an external condom drainage system and leg bag or pubic pressure urinal.
   b. Incontinent females have a more difficult problem. Incontinence pads are frequently used; new external collection devices are being marketed but are not yet perfected.

Rationale

6. If bladder emptying techniques are unsuccessful, other methods of managing incontinence are necessary.

Reflex Incontinence related to absence of sensation to void and loss of ability to inhibit bladder contraction

Focus Assessment Criteria	Clinical Significance
1. Level of cord injury 2. Perception of need to void 3. Relief after voiding 4. Voiding pattern 5. Reflexes (anal, bulbocavernosus) 6. Bladder distention, residual urine (amount) 7. Fluid intake pattern 8. Urine characteristics 9. Use of external stimuli (triggering)	1–9. Reflex incontinence entails partial or complete loss of the sensation of bladder distention, resulting in repeated involuntary reflexes that produce spontaneous voiding. Data collection is indicated to determine the extent of bladder control and identify appropriate interventions.

Interventions

1. Ensure adequate fluid intake (at least 2000 mL/day, unless contraindicated).

2. Consult with the physician about prescribing medication to relax the bladder (e.g., anticholinergics).
3. Teach techniques to trigger reflex voiding. (See the nursing diagnosis Urinary Retention in this care plan for details.)

Rationale

1. Adequate fluid intake prevents concentrated urine, which can irritate the bladder and cause increased bladder instability.
2. Anticholinergic medications can eliminate hyperirritable and uninhibited bladder contractions and allow successful bladder retraining.
3.
   a,b. Stimulating the reflex arc relaxes the internal sphincter of the bladder, allowing urination. The reflex arc can be triggered by stimulating the bladder wall or cutaneous sites (e.g., suprapubic, pubic).
   c. Regular voiding prevents distention, stasis, and infection.
   d. Contraction of abdominal muscles compresses the bladder to empty it.

Documentation

Flow records
  Fluid intake
  Voiding patterns (amount, time, method used)
Discharge summary record
  Client teaching
  Outcome achievement or status

Outcome Criteria

The client will be free of bladder infection.

4. Encourage the client to void or trigger at least every 3 hours.
5. Manage incontinence with clean intermittent self-catheterization (CISC) or external urine collection devices, and incontinence products, whichever are most appropriate for the client and caregiver.

4. A regular voiding pattern can prevent incontinent episodes.
5. Loss of both the sensation to void and the ability to inhibit contractions makes bladder retraining impossible. CISC, often in conjunction with medications, is then the procedure of choice for managing incontinence.

Potential for Infection related to retention of urine or introduction of urinary catheter

Focus Assessment Criteria	Clinical Significance
1. Urine color, odor, volume 2. Temperature 3. Urethral orifice condition	1–3. The catheter, as a foreign body in the urethra, irritates mucosa and can introduce bacteria into the urinary tract, increasing the risk of infection.
4. Presence of urinary retention	4. Stagnant urine provides a good medium for bacterial growth.

Interventions

1. Ensure adequate fluid intake (at least 2000 mL/day, unless contraindicated).
2. Eliminate residual urine by aiding urine outflow through methods such as these:
   a. Credé's maneuver
   b. Suprapubic tapping
   c. Multiple voiding
   d. Valsalva's maneuver
   e. Intermittent catheterization
3. Consult with the physician for medication to relieve detrusor/sphincter dyssynergia (DSD).
4. As ordered, administer vitamin C and methenamine mandelate (Mandelamine) to acidify urine.
5. Monitor residual urine (should be no more than 50 mL).

6. Test an uncontaminated urine sample for bacteria.
7. Maintain sterile technique for intermittent catheterization while the client is hospitalized.

8. Avoid using an indwelling catheter.

Rationale

1. Dilute urine helps prevent infection and bladder irritation.
2. Bacteria multiply rapidly in stagnant urine retained in the bladder. Moreover, overdistention hinders blood flow to the bladder wall, increasing the susceptibility to infection from bacterial growth. Regular, complete bladder emptying greatly reduces the risk of infection.

3. DSD is associated with large amounts of residual urine.
4. Acidic urine deters the growth of most bacteria implicated in cystitis.
5. Careful monitoring detects problems early, enabling prompt intervention to prevent urine stasis.
6. A bacteria count over 10^5/mL of urine indicates infection.
7. The most common cause of infection is bacteria introduced by a caregiver who did not wash his or her hands adequately between clients.
8. Indwelling catheters are associated with urinary tract infection related to the catheter sliding in and out of the urethra, which introduces pathogens.

▲ *Documentation*

Flow records
   Urine characteristics
   Temperature
   Elimination pattern (amount, time)
   Urine retention > 50 mL

▲ *Outcome Criteria*

The client will report a decrease in or an elimination of incontinence.

Urge Incontinence related to disruption of the inhibitory efferent impulses secondary to brain or spinal cord dysfunction

Focus Assessment Criteria

1. Incontinence history (onset, pattern, complaints of frequency or urgency)

2. History of cerebrovascular accident, brain tumor, spinal cord injury or tumor, or demyelinating disease, e.g., multiple sclerosis
3. Bladder sensation, bulbocavernosus reflex

Clinical Significance

1. Descriptions of the incontinence can help distinguish urge incontinence from other types.
2. Defects in corticoregulatory pathways (cerebral, spinal cord) can cause urgency, frequency, and decreased bladder capacity.
3. If bladder sensation and bulbocavernosus reflex remain intact, stimulated voiding is possible.

Interventions

1. Assess voiding patterns and develop a schedule of frequent timed voiding.
2. If indicated, restrict fluid intake during the evening.
3. If needed, teach trigger voiding, external manual compression, or abdominal straining. (Refer to the nursing diagnosis Urinary Retention in this care plan for specific teaching points.)
4. If incontinence occurs, decrease the time between planned voidings.

5. Reinforce the need for optimal hydration (at least 2000 mL/day, unless contraindicated).

Rationale

1. Frequent timed voiding can reduce urgency from bladder overdistention.
2. Evening fluid restrictions may help prevent enuresis.
3. A client with an intact reflex arc may be taught parasympathetic stimulation of the detrusor muscle, which will initiate and sustain bladder contractions to aid bladder emptying.
4. Bladder capacity may be insufficient to accommodate the urine volume, necessitating more frequent voiding.
5. Optimal hydration is needed to prevent urinary tract infection and renal calculi.

▲ *Documentation*

Flow records
   Intake
   Voidings (amount, time)
   Method used
   Incontinent episodes
Discharge summary record
   Client teaching

▲ Outcome Criteria

The client will:

1. Express a willingness to socialize
2. State an intent to reestablish or increase socialization pattern

Potential Social Isolation related to embarrassment from wetting self in front of others and fear of odor from urine

Focus Assessment Criteria	*Clinical Significance*
1. Socialization history 2. Anticipated or actual decrease in social contacts	1,2. Feelings of embarrassment, rejection, and low self-esteem may contribute to isolation. An at-risk client must be assessed carefully, as the suffering associated with social isolation is not always readily apparent.

Interventions	*Rationale*
1. Acknowledge the client's frustration with incontinence.	1. To the client, incontinence may seem like a reversion to an infantile state in which he has no control over his body functions and feels ostracized by others. Acknowledging the difficulty of the situation can help reduce his feelings of frustration.
2. Determine the client's eligibility for bladder training, CISC, or other methods to manage incontinence.	2. These measures can increase control and reduce fear of accidents.
3. Teach the client ways to control wetness and odor. Many products make wetting manageable by providing reliable leakage protection and masking odors.	3. Helping the client manage incontinence encourages socialization.
4. Encourage the client to venture out socially for short periods initially, then increase the length of social contacts as success at managing incontinence increases.	4. Short trips help the client gradually gain confidence and reduce his or her fears.

▲ Documentation

Progress notes
  Significant dialogue
  Discharge summary record
Client teaching

▲ Outcome Criteria

The outcome criteria for this diagnosis represent those associated with discharge planning. Refer to the discharge criteria.

Potential Altered Health Maintenance related to insufficient knowledge of etiology of incontinence, management, bladder retraining programs, signs and symptoms of complications, and community resources

Focus Assessment Criteria	*Clinical Significance*
1. Readiness and ability to learn and retain information	1. A client or family failing to achieve learning goals requires a referral for assistance postdischarge.

Interventions	*Rationale*
1. Teach about the condition, its cause, and management.	1. Understanding can encourage compliance with and participation in the treatment regimen.

2. If the client has voluntary control, institute a bladder training program.
   a. Document fluid intake, incontinence episodes, periods of continence, and client behavior on a voiding chart, to provide reinforcement for the client.
   b. Have the patient void "by the clock" rather than from an urge.
   c. Ensure that the client assumes an anatomically correct position for voiding attempts.
   d. Ensure privacy.
   e. Encourage use of the toilet 30 minutes before any usual incontinent episodes.
   f. Increase the scheduled time between voidings as the client remains continent for longer periods.
	2. Bladder training, an acceptable treatment for urge incontinence, can help increase bladder volume and extend the length of time between voidings.

Interventions	*Rationale*
3. Encourage an obese client to lose weight.	3. Obesity places excessive intra-abdominal pressure on the bladder, which can aggravate incontinence.
4. Teach pelvic floor exercises (Kegel exercises) to help restore bladder control, if the client is a candidate: a. Obtain an audio cassette tape and exercise booklet from Help for Incontinent People (HIP), P.O. Box 544, Union, SC 29379. b. Help the client identify the muscles that start and stop urination. c. Instruct the client to try the exercises for 3 to 4 months to strengthen periurethral tissue.	4. Useful for some clients with stress incontinence, Kegel exercises strengthen the pelvic floor muscles, which in turn may increase urinary sphincter competence.
5. Teach biofeedback if the client is a candidate. (He must be alert and have a good memory.) He may be able to learn to control the sphincter and prevent uninhibited bladder contractions by watching information on a screen as the bladder fills during cystometry or by hearing the activity of the sphincter muscles in action.	5. Effective for some clients with urge incontinence, biofeedback uses behavior modification to habituate the client to recognize and control unwanted bladder spasms.
6. Teach the client about any drugs prescribed for managing incontinence: a. Anticholinergics decrease uninhibited bladder contractions. b. Smooth muscle relaxants increase bladder capacity. c. Alpha-adrenergic agents stimulate the urethral sphincter. d. Alpha blocking agents decrease neural sphincter resistance and help reduce overflow incontinence.	6. Understanding the actions of medications may encourage compliance with the therapeutic regimen.
7. Explain possible surgical options, as appropriate: a. Artificial urinary sphincters are increasing in popularity for clients with a malfunctioning sphincter or those who have undergone prostatectomy. b. Prostate resection often can eliminate overflow incontinence. c. Subarachnoid block, sacral rhizotomy, sacral nerve dissection, sphincterectomy, and urinary diversions may benefit spinal cord-injured clients with severe spasticity. The client must have a complete neurological and urodynamic evaluation to identify the appropriate surgical or medical treatment.	7. The client may be a candidate for surgery to control or cure incontinence.
8. If indicated, teach clean intermittent self-catheterization (CISC) to the client or caregiver. a. In women follow this procedure: • Wash hands thoroughly. • Hold the catheter 1½ inches from the tip. With the other hand, separate the labia, using the second and fourth fingers, and locate the urethral meatus with the middle finger. Use this finger as a guide for insertion.	8. Intermittent self-catheterization is appropriate for children and adults who are motivated and physically able to perform the procedure. Often, a caregiver may be taught to catheterize the client. CISC stimulates normal voiding, prevents infection, and maintains integrity of the ureterovesical junction. In the hospital, aseptic technique is used because of increased microorganisms in the hospital environment. At home, clean technique is used. CISC entails

Interventions

- Gently insert the catheter into the urethral meatus by slipping the catheter tip just under the middle finger. Advance the catheter in an upward direction.
- Guide the catheter into the bladder, about 1 inch past the point at which urine begins to flow.
- Drain the bladder of urine. When urine stops flowing, slowly begin removing the catheter. If urine flow begins again during removal, hold the catheter in position and wait until flow stops.
- After removal, cleanse the outer surface of the catheter with water and the same soap used to wash hands, then rinse the inside and outside with clear water.
- Dry and store it in its container. Remember to discard a catheter that becomes too stiff or soft.

b. In men use the following procedure:
- Wash hands and prepare the catheter. Generously apply water-soluble lubricant to the catheter tip.
- Hold the catheter about 1½ inches from the tip. With the other hand, hold the penis straight out from the body.
- Insert the catheter into the urinary meatus until slight resistance is felt. Then, using gentle but firm pressure, advance the catheter to the bladder, 1 inch past the point at which urine begins to flow.
- Drain the bladder of urine. When urine stops flowing, slowly begin removing the catheter. If urine flow begins again during removal, hold the catheter in position and wait until flow stops.
- After removal, cleanse the outer surface of the catheter with water and the same soap used to wash hands, then rinse the inside and outside with clear water.
- Dry and store it in its container. Remember to discard a catheter that becomes too stiff or soft.

9. Teach the client to keep a record of catheterization times, amount of fluid intake and urine output, and any incontinent periods.
10. Teach the client to notify the physician of the following:
   a. Bleeding from urethral opening

   b. Reactions from medications
   c. Difficulty inserting catheter

   d. Dark, bloody, cloudy, or strong-smelling urine
   e. Pain in the abdomen or back
   f. Elevated temperature

Rationale

fewer complications than an indwelling catheter. However, it is not the procedure of choice for clients who are unable to empty the bladder completely.

9. Accurate record-keeping aids in evaluating status.

10. Early reporting enables prompt treatment to prevent serious problems.
   a. Bleeding may indicate trauma or renal calculi.
   b. Drug reactions may indicate overdose.
   c. Difficult catheter insertion may indicate a stricture.
   d. These urine changes may point to infection.
   e. Pain may indicate renal calculi.
   f. Fever may be the first sign of urinary tract infection.

▲ **Documentation**

Discharge summary record
   Client teaching
   Outcome achievement or status

Interventions	Rationale
11. Explain available community resources, e.g., Help for Incontinent People (see References).	11. The client and family may need assistance or more information for home care.

References/Bibliography

Alterescu, V. (1986). Theoretical foundation for an approach to urinary incontinence. *Journal of Enterostomal Therapy, 13*(3), 105–107.

Creason, N.S. (1989). Prompted voiding therapy for urinary incontinence in aged female nursing home residents. *Journal of Advanced Nursing, 14*(2), 120–126.

DeRosa, S. (1985). Urinary incontinence. In M.M. Jacobs & W. Geels (Eds.). *Signs and symptoms in nursing interpretation and management.* Philadelphia: J.B. Lippincott.

Henderson, J.S. (1989). Intermittent clean self-catheterization in clients with neurogenic bladder resulting from multiple sclerosis. *Journal of Neuroscience Nursing, 21*(3), 160–164.

Holland, N.J., Wiesel-Levison, P., & Schwedelson, E. (1981). Surgery of neurogenic bladder in multiple sclerosis. *Journal of Neurosurgical Nursing, 13*(6), 337–341.

Irrgang, S.J. (1988). Classification of urinary incontinence. *Journal of Enterostomal Therapy, 13*(2), 62–65.

Jones, R., Young, P., & Marosszeky, J. (1987). Treatment of infection in the presence of an indwelling urethral catheter. *British Journal of Urology, 54,* 316–319.

Maklebust, J.A. (1987). Pressure ulcers: Etiology and prevention. *Nursing Clinics of North America, 22,* 359–377.

Malvern, J. (1986). The mechanism of continence. In Stanton, S. & Tanagho, J. (Eds.). *Surgery of female incontinence.* New York: Springer.

Mandelstom, D. (1980). Strengthening pelvic floor muscles. *Geriatric Nursing, 1,* 251–252.

McConnell, E.A., & Zimmerman, M.F. (1983). *Care of patients with urological problems.* Philadelphia: J.B. Lippincott.

McCormick, K.A. (1988). Urinary incontinence in the elderly. *Nursing Clinics of North America, 23*(1), 135–137.

McCormick, K.A., et al. (1988). Nursing management of urinary incontinence in geriatric inpatients. *Nursing Clinics of North America, 23*(1), 231–264.

Newman, D.K. (1989). The treatment of urinary incontinence in adults. *The Nurse Practitioner, 14*(6), 21–34.

Ruff, C.C., & Reaves, E.L. (1989). Diagnosing urinary incontinence in adults. *The Nurse Practitioner, 14*(6), 8–20.

Weigel, J.W. (1988). Urinary incontinence. *Journal of Enterostomal Therapy, 15*(1), 24–29.

Wells, T., & Brink, C. (1981). Urinary incontinence: Assessment and management. In I. Burnside (Ed.). *Nursing and the aged.* New York: McGraw-Hill.

Sensory Disorders

Glaucoma

Glaucoma involves intraocular pressure increase due to pathological changes at the iridocorneal angle that prevent the normal outflow of aqueous humor. This increased pressure causes progressive structural or functional damage to the eye, eventually leading to blindness.

Diagnostic Cluster

▲ **Time Frame**

Secondary diagnosis

▲ **Discharge Criteria**

Before discharge, the client or family will:

1. Describe the causes and effects of glaucoma
2. Identify present visual impairments, if any
3. Describe the need for daily medications and regular follow-up
4. State the signs and symptoms that must be reported to a health care professional

Collaborative Problems

Potential Complication:
Increased Intraocular Pressure

Refer to:

Nursing Diagnoses

Anxiety related to actual or potential vision loss and perceived impact of chronic illness on life style

Potential Noncompliance related to negative side effects of prescribed therapy versus the belief that no treatment is needed without the presence of symptoms

Potential Altered Health Maintenance related to insufficient knowledge of disease process, current clinical status, and treatment plan

Potential for Injury related to visual limitations — Enucleation

Potential Social Isolation related to reduced peripheral vision and altered visual acuity — Enucleation

Potential Self-Concept Disturbance related to effects of visual limitations — Enucleation

Collaborative Problems

▲ **Nursing Goal**

The nurse will manage and minimize changes in intraocular pressure.

Potential Complication: Increased Intraocular Pressure

Interventions

1. Teach the client to report the following:
   a. Difficulty perceiving changes in colors
   b. Blurred vision
   c. Persistent aching in eyes
   d. Intense eye pain
   e. Sudden decrease in or loss of vision
   f. Halos around lights (blue, violet, yellow, red)

Rationale

1. If aqueous humor production exceeds its outflow into the Schlemm's canal to the venous system, increased intraocular pressure will result. If untreated, this can lead to compression of nerve fibers and blood vessels in the optic disc, with possible permanent damage.

Related Physician-Prescribed Interventions

Medications
Miotics
Beta-adrenergic receptor blockers
Carbonic anhydrase inhibitors
Anticholinesterases

Intravenous Therapy
Not indicated

Laboratory Studies
Not indicated

Diagnostic Studies
Tonometry
Electronic tonometry
Gonioscopy

▲ **Documentation**

Progress notes
Complaints of visual or eye problems

Therapies
Laser trabeculoplasty

Nursing Diagnoses

▲ *Outcome Criteria*

The client will verbalize his or her concerns and fears.

Anxiety related to actual or potential vision loss and perceived impact of chronic illness on lifestyle

Focus Assessment Criteria:	*Clinical Significance*
1. Verbal and nonverbal indicators of anxiety 2. Perception of illness 3. Understanding of information presented 4. Available support systems 5. Coping mechanisms	1–5. The client diagnosed with glaucoma frequently experiences anxiety and fear. Many people associate glaucoma with blindness, fear of dependence on others, and lifestyle changes. Because few symptoms are associated with the more common forms of the disease, some vision loss may already have occurred by the time of diagnosis. The client may express concerns regarding vision loss and how well the treatment regimen is maintaining intraocular pressure within an acceptable range.

Interventions

1. Explore the client's perception of the condition and its effects on his or her life style and self-concept.

2. Provide accurate information and correct any misconceptions.

3. Assist the client to identify and use past successful coping mechanisms and support systems.

4. Discuss strategies for socialization and role development:
   a. Continued involvement in prehospitalization activities
   b. Investigating possible new roles and activities

5. Refer to outside agencies, as appropriate:
   a. Glaucoma Research Foundation
   b. Sight Center/Services for Visually Impaired
   c. Support groups

Rationale

1. Because each person manifests anxiety or fear in a unique manner, the nurse must be alert to subtle changes in the client's behavior. In addition, clients view their disease differently. A client with declining vision may focus only on negative aspects, especially if glaucoma threatens his or her self-concept. For example, to a pilot the diagnosis may mean loss of his work role, but a retired gardener may perceive the diagnosis as less threatening to his role. The nurse should attempt to move the client from this phase toward a broadening view of self, one that incorporates positive role aspects.

2. Common misconceptions, such as "all people with glaucoma go blind," "increased intraocular pressure is like high blood pressure," and "the side effects of the medications are worse than the disease," can create or intensify anxiety. Accurate information on disease progression, treatments, and necessary lifestyle changes usually reduces client anxiety.

3. Examining past coping mechanisms and support systems provides the nurse with insight into previous behaviors and a source of data from which to guide future development of coping skills.

4. Increased socialization can promote self-esteem and reduce anxiety.

5. Referrals to outside agencies may decrease client anxiety by providing other sources of information and support and by enabling the client to interact with others experiencing similar problems.

▲ **Documentation**

Progress notes
    Verbal and nonverbal indicators of anxiety
    Interventions
    Client response to interventions
Discharge summary record
    Referrals, if indicated

▲ *Outcome Criteria*

The client will:

1. Verbalize an intent to comply with the prescribed treatment after discharge
2. Identify source(s) of support for assisting with compliance
3. Verbalize potential complications of noncompliance

Potential Noncompliance related to negative side effects of prescribed therapy versus the belief that treatment is not needed without the presence of symptoms

Focus Assessment Criteria	*Clinical Significance*
1. Perception and understanding of glaucoma	1. Assessing the client's perception of glaucoma and its seriousness can help predict compliance or noncompliance.

Interventions

1. Identify factors that may predict noncompliance:
   a. Lack of knowledge
   b. Noncompliance in the hospital
   c. Failure to perceive the seriousness or chronicity of glaucoma
   d. Belief that the condition resolves itself
2. Stress the importance of adhering to the treatment regimen and of notifying a health care professional if unable to do so.

3. Point out that elevated intraocular pressure may produce no symptoms.
4. Discuss the effects of the client's vision loss or blindness on family members and significant others.

5. Include family members and/or significant others in teaching sessions, as appropriate.

6. Discuss strategies to improve compliance with the treatment regimen. If noncompliance is related to financial concerns, do the following:
   a. Explore available funding sources (e.g., Lions Club, other civic organizations, social service agencies).
   b. Refer for governmental assistance as appropriate.
   c. Compare costs of medications at various pharmacies, and encourage patronizing the one with the lowest prices.
   d. If noncompliance is related to memory impairment, do the following:
      • Explore mechanisms for cueing (e.g., calendar, notes, reminder calls from family, associating administration with other events).
      • Develop a set time schedule for administration.
      • Simplify the regimen as much as possible.
      • Provide written instructions.

Rationale

1. Openly addressing the barriers to compliance may reduce noncompliance.

2. The client may require frequent motivation to adhere to a sometimes complex routine. If some vision loss has occurred, he may question the need for continued treatment that does not seem effective. The nurse should reinforce the medication as a mechanism for saving sight, even though it cannot restore sight that has already been lost. Conversely, a client with no symptoms also may not perceive the point of medication therapy. The nurse must explain that medication still is important to prevent vision loss.
3. The lack of symptoms often encourages noncompliance.
4. Emphasizing the potential impact of vision loss on the client's support persons (e.g., loss of family income, role changes, possible family dysfunction) may encourage compliance.
5. Family members and significant others who understand the disorder and the treatment regimen may help the client achieve compliance. (They should not be charged with "policing" the client, however.)
6. In order for a regimen to be effective, it must meet the client's individual needs. Involving the client in planning the regimen can help ensure compliance.

Interventions

e. If noncompliance is related to side effects of medication, do the following:
- Discuss side effects with the physician, who may change the prescription.
- Help the client minimize side effects if the prescription cannot be changed; for example, drops may be administered at times when their adverse effect on vision is minimized, such as before bedtime.

7. Emphasize that ultimately it is the client's choice and responsibility to adhere to the treatment plan.

Rationale

7. Stressing the client's decision-making ability and responsibility can strengthen feelings of control and self-determination, which can promote compliance.

▲ **Documentation**

Progress notes
    Noncompliant behavior
Discharge summary record
    Client teaching
    Response to teaching

▲ **Outcome Criteria**

The outcome criteria for this diagnosis represent those associated with discharge planning. Refer to the discharge criteria.

Potential Altered Health Maintenance related to insufficient knowledge of disease process, current clinical status, and treatment plan

Focus Assessment Criteria	Clinical Significance
1. Knowledge of disease at time of diagnosis and at periodic intervals thereafter	**1.** Validating the client's knowledge of the disease process enables the nurse to determine the appropriate information to present. A newly diagnosed client may have little information about the disease; a client with long-standing glaucoma should be evaluated and updated periodically about new information generated by ongoing research.
2. Readiness and ability to learn and retain information	**2.** In a recently diagnosed client, anxiety and denial may impair his or her ability to process information. If such symptoms are noted, reschedule another time to discuss this information.
3. Details and amount of information desired	**3.** Clients differ in the amount of information they find helpful. Detailed instruction may be overwhelming to one, yet allay the anxieties of another.

Interventions

1. Present information necessary for self-care using a variety of instructional aids and teaching methods:
  a. Pamphlets

  b. Audiovisual programs

  c. Demonstrations

2. Discuss the client's current clinical status.

3. Describe the dosage schedule, route of administration, and possible side effects of all prescribed medications.

Rationale

1.

  a. Pamphlets provide material to review later and are of great benefit if the client is experiencing anxiety and a resulting decreased learning retention.

  b. Audiovisual programs enable the client to stop the presentation at any time and to review the material at a later time or with family.

  c. Demonstration provides both visual and verbal reinforcement.

2. Advising the client of the latest assessment data provides him with information on which to base decisions. It also indicates how well self-care activities are reducing or maintaining intraocular pressure.

3. A client is more likely to comply with a medication regimen when he understands it and its importance. If not advised otherwise, the client

Interventions

4. Reiterate plans for follow-up care and testing.

5. Reinforce the need to carry an identification card that specifies the client's diagnosis of glaucoma (crucial in cases of angle closure glaucoma).

6. If peripheral visual losses have occurred, teach the client to scan the environment.
7. Explore with the client and family members or significant others whether vision losses are interfering with activities (e.g., driving, socializing, self-care).

▲ **Documentation**

Discharge summary record
  Material presented
  Teaching methods used
  Response to teaching

8. Provide information on community resources for visually impaired persons, if indicated (e.g., Visually Impaired Society, Bureau of Visually Impaired).

Rationale

may view side effects of glaucoma medications as normal and may not report them.
4. Follow-up care enables evaluation of the efficacy of treatment. These evaluations can only be performed in the physician's office.
5. In a medical emergency, such as cardiac arrest, health care providers need to recognize a client with glaucoma to avoid administering atropine or similar-acting agents, which can cause a dangerous elevation in intraocular pressure.

6. Accommodating for peripheral vision losses can prevent injury.
7. Owing to the nature of the disease, the glaucoma client may lose peripheral vision over time. Side effects of glaucoma medications may further reduce visual ability, especially in poorly illuminated environments. As vision declines, the client may become uneasy in social situations. Rather than risk detection of reduced acuity, he or she may choose to withdraw from social situations.
8. Such resources can provide needed assistance with home management and self-care.

References/Bibliography

Boyd-Monk, H., & Starita, R.J. (1985). Surgical intervention to stop glaucoma. *Journal of Ophthalmic Nursing and Technology, 4*(3), 12–15.

Carpenito, L.J. (1989). *Nursing diagnosis: Application to clinical practice* (3rd ed.). Philadelphia: J.B. Lippincott.

Doenges, M., Jeffries, M., & Moorehouse, M. (1985). *Nursing care plans—Nursing diagnoses in planning patient care.* Philadelphia: F.A. Davis.

Epstein, D. L. (Ed.) (1986). *Chandler and Grantis glaucoma.* Philadelphia: Lea and Febiger.

Miller, J.F. (1983). *Coping with chronic illness: Overcoming powerlessness.* Philadelphia: F.A. Davis.

Schultz, P.J. (1986). Preserving sight in glaucoma patients. *Ophthalmic Nursing Forum, 2*(1), 1–7.

Smith, J., & Nachacl, D. (1980). *Ophthalmic nursing.* Boston: Little, Brown.

Van Buskirk, E.M. (1987). The compliance factor. *American Journal of Ophthalmology, 101*(5), 609–610.

Integumentary Disorders

Pressure Ulcers

Pressure ulcers are localized areas of cellular necrosis that tend to occur from prolonged compression of soft tissue between a bony prominence and a firm surface—most commonly as a result of immobility. Extrinsic factors that exert mechanical force on soft tissue include pressure, shear, friction, and maceration. Intrinsic factors that determine susceptibility to tissue breakdown include malnutrition, anemia, loss of sensation, impaired mobility, advanced age, decreased mental status, incontinence, and infection. Extrinsic and intrinsic factors interact to produce ischemia and necrosis of soft tissue in susceptible persons (Maklebust, 1987).

Diagnostic Cluster

▲ **Time Frame**

Secondary diagnosis

▲ **Discharge Criteria**

Before discharge, the client or family will:
1. Identify factors that contribute to ulcer development
2. Demonstrate the ability to perform skills necessary to prevent and treat pressure ulcers
3. State an intent to continue prevention strategies at home (e.g., activity, nutrition)

Collaborative Problems

Potential Complication:
Septicemia

Nursing Diagnoses

Impaired Tissue Integrity related to mechanical destruction of tissue secondary to pressure, shear, and friction

Impaired Physical Mobility related to imposed restrictions, deconditioned status, loss of motor control, or altered mental status

Altered Nutrition: Less Than Body Requirements related to anorexia

Potential for Infection related to exposure of ulcer base to fecal/urinary drainage

Potential Altered Health Maintenance related to insufficient knowledge of etiology, prevention, treatment, and home care

Related Nursing Care Plan

Immobility or Unconsciousness

Collaborative Problems

▲ **Nursing Goal**

The nurse will manage and minimize septicemic events.

▲ **Documentation**

Flow records
  Vital signs

Potential Complication: Septicemia

Interventions

1. Monitor for signs and symptoms of septicemia:
   a. Temperature > 101° F or < 98.6° F
   b. Tachycardia and tachypnea
   c. Pale, cool skin
   d. Decreased urine output
   e. WBCs and bacteria in urine
   f. Positive blood culture

Rationale

1. Gram-positive and gram-negative organisms can invade the open wounds; debilitated clients are more vulnerable. Response to sepsis results in massive vasodilatation with hypovolemia, resulting in tissue hypoxia and decreased renal function and cardiac output. This in turn triggers a compensatory response of increased heart rate and respirations to correct hypoxia and acidosis. Bacteria in urine or blood indicates infection.

Related Physician-Prescribed Interventions
Medications
  Topical antibiotics   Proteolytic enzymes
Intravenous Therapy
  Not indicated

Related Physician-Prescribed Interventions (Continued)

Laboratory Studies
  Wound cultures

Diagnostic Studies
  Not indicated

Therapies
  Topical skin barriers   Wound care
  Pressure relief systems (air-   Ulcer care
    fluidized bed, low-air-loss
    bed, kinetic bed)

Nursing Diagnoses

Impaired Tissue Integrity related to mechanical destruction of tissue secondary to pressure, shear, and friction

▲ Outcome Criteria

The client will:

1. Identify causative factors for pressure ulcers
2. Identify rationale for prevention and treatment
3. Participate in the prescribed treatment plan to promote wound healing
4. Demonstrate progressive healing of dermal ulcer

Focus Assessment Criteria

1. Skin condition (lesions, circulation)
2. Systemic disorders (e.g., diabetes mellitus)
3. Chemical irritants (e.g., incontinence)
4. Mechanical irritants (e.g., casts)
5. Nutritional or fluid deficits
6. Level of consciousness
7. Ability to move in bed and out of bed

Clinical Significance

1–7. Contributing factors to tissue destruction can be intrinsic (e.g., vulnerable skin, systemic disorders) or extrinsic (e.g., mechanical, chemical). The more factors present, the more vulnerable the client.

Interventions

1. Apply pressure ulcer prevention principles:

    a. Encourage range-of-motion (ROM) exercise and weight-bearing mobility when possible.
    b. Promote optimal mobility. (Refer to the Impaired Mobility care plan, page 269, for more information.)
    c. Keep the bed as flat as possible and support feet with a foot board.

    d. Avoid using a knee gatch.

    e. Use foam blocks or pillows to provide a bridging effect to support the body above and below the high-risk or ulcerated area, preventing the affected area from touching the bed surface. Do not use foam donuts or inflatable rings.
    f. Alternate or reduce the pressure on the skin surface with devices such as these:
        • Air mattresses
        • Low-air-loss beds
        • Air-fluidized beds
        • Vascular boots to suspend heels

Rationale

1. Principles of pressure ulcer prevention include reducing or rotating pressure on soft tissue. If pressure on soft tissue exceeds intracapillary pressure (approximately 32 mm Hg), capillary occlusion and resulting hypoxia cause tissue damage.

    a,b. Exercise and mobility increase blood flow to all areas.

    c. These measures help prevent shear, the pressure created when two adjacent tissue layers move in opposition. If a bony prominence slides across the subcutaneous tissue, the subepidermal capillaries may become bent and pinched, resulting in decreased tissue perfusion.
    d. A knee gatch may promote pooling of blood and decrease circulation in the lower extremities.
    e. This measure helps distribute pressure to a larger area.

    f. Foam mattresses (e.g., egg-crate type) are for comfort; generally, they do not provide adequate pressure relief. Special air mattresses and air beds redistribute the body weight evenly across the surface.

Interventions

Rationale

g. Use sufficient personnel to lift the client up in bed or a chair without sliding or pulling the skin surface. Use Heelbo protectors to reduce friction on elbows and heels.

g. Proper transfer technique reduces friction forces that can rub away or abride the skin.

h. Instruct a sitting client to lift himself using the chair arms every 10 minutes, if possible, or assist him in rising up off the chair every 10 to 20 minutes, depending on risk factors present.

h. This measure allows periodic reperfusion of ischemic areas.

i. Do not elevate legs unless calves are supported.

i. Supporting the calves reduces pressure over the ischial tuberosities.

j. Pad the chair with a pressure-relieving device.

j. Ischial tuberosities are prime areas for pressure ulcer development. Air cushions provide better pressure relief than foam cushions.

k. Inspect other areas at risk of developing ulcers with each position change:
- Ears
- Elbows
- Occiput
- Trochanter
- Heels
- Ischia
- Sacrum
- Scapula
- Scrotum

k. A client with one pressure ulcer is at increased risk to develop others.

l. Observe for erythema and blanching, and palpate surrounding area for warmth and tissue sponginess with each position change.

l. Warmth and sponginess are signs of tissue damage.

m. Massage non-reddened vulnerable areas gently with each position change.

m. Gentle massage stimulates circulation.

2. Compensate for sensory deficits:

2.

a. Inspect the skin every 2 hours for signs of injury.

a. An immobilized client may have impaired sensation, interfering with the ability to perceive pain from skin damage.

b. Teach the client and family members to inspect the skin frequently. Show the client how to use a mirror to inspect hard-to-see areas.

b. Regular skin inspection enables early detection of damage. The client's involvement promotes responsibility for self-care.

3. Identify the stage of pressure ulcer development:

3. Each stage involves different nursing interventions.

a. Stage I: nonblanchable erythema or ulceration limited to epidermis

b. Stage II: ulceration of dermis not involving underlying subcutaneous fat

c. Stage III: ulceration involving subcutaneous fat

d. Stage IV: extensive ulceration penetrating muscle and bone

4. Reduce or eliminate factors that contribute to extension of existing pressure ulcers:

4.

a. Wash area surrounding ulcer gently with a mild soap, rinse area thoroughly to remove soap, and pat dry.

a. Soap is an irritant and dries skin.

b. Gently massage healthy skin around the ulcer to stimulate circulation; do not massage any reddened areas.

b. Gentle massage may stimulate circulation. Vigorous massage angulates and tears the vessels. Massaging over reddened areas may cause breaking of capillaries and traumatize skin.

c. Institute one or a combination of the following:
- Apply a thin coat of liquid copolymer skin sealant.

c. Healthy skin should be protected.

Interventions

- Cover area with a moisture-permeable film dressing.
- Cover area with a hydroactive wafer barrier and secure with strips of 1 inch microscope tape; leave in place for 4 to 5 days.

5. Devise a plan for pressure ulcers using moist wound healing principles, as follows:

   a. Avoid breaking blisters.

   b. Flush ulcer base with sterile saline solution. If it is infected, use forceful irrigation.

   c. Avoid using wound cleaners and topical antiseptics.
   d. Consult with a surgeon or wound specialist to debride necrotic tissue mechanically or surgically.
   e. Cover pressure ulcers with a sterile dressing that maintains a moist environment over the ulcer base (e.g., film dressing, hydrocolloid wafer dressing, absorption dressing, moist gauze dressing).
   f. Avoid drying agents (e.g., heat lamps, Maalox, Milk of Magnesia).

6. Consult with a nurse specialist or physician for treatment of deep or infected pressure ulcers.

Rationale

5. When wounds are semi-occluded and the surface of the wound remains moist, epidermal cells migrate more rapidly over the surface.

   a. Blisters indicate stage II pressure ulcers; the fluid contained in the blister provides an environment for formation of granulation tissue.
   b. Irrigation with normal saline solution may aid in removing dead cells and reducing the bacterial count. Forceful irrigation should not be used in the presence of granulation tissue and new epithelium.
   c. These products may be cytotoxic to tissue.

   d. A necrotic ulcer does not heal until the necrotic tissue is removed.

   e. Moist wounds heal faster.

   f. Heat creates an increase in oxygen demand. Heat lamps are contraindicated in pressure ulcers, as they increase the oxygen demand to tissue that is already stressed.

6. Expert consultation may be needed for more specific interventions.

▲ **Documentation**

Flow records
  Size of ulcer base (length, width, depth)
  Ulcer characteristics: granulation, epithelialization, necrotic tissue, undermined areas, sinus tracts, drainage, surrounding erythema, induration
  Treatment
  Unsatisfactory response

▲ **Outcome Criteria**

The client will:
1. Have body weight shifted at least every 2 hours
2. Demonstrate reduced interface pressure over the ulcer to less than 32 mm Hg

Impaired Physical Mobility related to imposed restrictions, deconditioned status, loss of motor control, altered mental status

Focus Assessment Criteria	*Clinical Significance*
1. Ability to move within the environment, e.g., in bed, transfer from bed to chair	1,2. Impaired physical mobility forces the client to maintain the same body posture for long periods. Constant unrelieved pressure causes ischemia in compressed tissue, the primary cause of soft tissue ulceration.
2. Ability of the primary caregiver to move and turn the client in bed, transfer him from bed to chair, etc.	

Interventions

1. Encourage the highest level of mobility. Provide devices such as an overhead or partial side rails, if possible, to facilitate independent movement.
2. Promote optimal circulation while in bed.
   a. If the client cannot turn himself, reposition him every 2 hours. Use a "turn clock" to indicate the appropriate position for each full body turn.
   b. Make minor shifts in body position between full turns.

Rationale

1. Regular movement relieves constant pressure over a bony prominence.

2.
   a. Intermittent pressure relief lets blood reenter capillaries that compression had deprived of blood and oxygen.

   b. Minor shifts in body weight aid reperfusion of compressed areas.

Interventions

Rationale

c. Examine bony prominences with each repositioning. If reddened areas do not fade within 30 minutes after repositioning, turn the client more frequently.

c. Reactive hyperemia may be insufficient to compensate for local ischemia.

d. Position the client in a 30-degree, laterally inclined position. Do *not* use high Fowler's position.

d. This position relieves pressure over the trochanter and sacrum simultaneously. High Fowler's position increases sacral shear.

e. Use a pressure-relief device to augment the turning schedule.

e. Pressure-reducing devices may increase the time intervals between necessary repositioning.

f. Do not use foam donuts or rubber rings.

f. These devices compress the surrounding vasculature, increasing the area of ischemia.

g. Pay particular attention to the heels.

g. Studies demonstrate that the heels are extremely vulnerable to breakdown because of the high concentration of body weight over their relatively small surface.

h. *Gently* massage around bony prominences. *Do not* massage reddened areas.

h. Vigorous massage can angulate and break capillaires.

▲ **Documentation**

Flow record
    Degree of mobility
    Frequency of repositioning
    Actual body position (e.g., left side, supine, right side, prone, 30 degree laterally inclined on left or right)
    Pressure relief devices used
Progress notes
    Abnormal local tissue response to repositioning

▲ **Outcome Criteria**

The client will:

1. Be in positive nitrogen balance
2. Demonstrate increase in body weight and muscle mass
3. Demonstrate decreasing wound size

Altered Nutrition: Less Than Body Requirements related to anorexia

Focus Assessment Criteria

1. Dietary history
2. Present nutritional status
    a. Weight
    b. Nutritional intake (e.g., ability to eat, dentition, nausea/vomiting)
    c. Laboratory values: hemoglobin, serum albumin, serum transferrin

3. Loss of nitrogen from wound drainage

Clinical Significance

1,2. Poor general nutrition commonly leads to weight loss and muscle atrophy. Reduction of subcutaneous fat and muscle tissue eliminates some of the padding between the skin and underlying bony prominences, increasing the susceptibility to pressure ulcers. Poor nutrition also decreases resistance to infection and interferes with wound healing.

    Adequate hemoglobin is required to transport oxygen to cells. Hemoglobin and serum albumin levels often provide good clues to overall nutritional status. Decreased albumin levels may result from inadequate protein intake or protein loss from a draining ulcer. (Protein is essential to new tissue synthesis.) Studies show a threefold increase in pressure ulcer incidence with every 1-g decrease in serum albumin level. Serum transferrin also evaluates protein levels, but is a more costly procedure.

3. Daily drainage from wounds may contain up to 100 g of protein. Replacement therapy may be necessary.

▲ **Documentation**

Flow records
    Actual nutritional intake
    Twice-weekly weights
    Status of wounds
    Amount of wound drainage
    Serum albumin levels

Interventions

1. Refer to the nursing diagnosis Altered Nutrition: Less than Body Requirements in the Thermal Injury care plan, page 280, for specific interventions and rationales.

▲ Outcome Criteria

The client will not become infected from exposure to fecal/urinary drainage.

Potential for Infection related to exposure of ulcer base to fecal/urinary drainage

Focus Assessment Criteria	*Clinical Significance*
1. Skin and ulcer base for exposure to urine or feces	1. Infection can penetrate all skin layers, exacerbating ulcers. The proximity of pelvic pressure ulcers to fecal and urinary drainage increases the risk of infection in these areas.

Interventions	*Rationale*
1. Teach the importance of good skin hygiene. Use emollients if skin is dry, but do not leave skin "wet" from too much lotion or cream.	1. Dry skin is susceptible to cracking and infection. Excessive emollient use can lead to maceration.
2. Protect the skin from exposure to urine/feces: a. Cleanse the skin thoroughly after each incontinent episode, using a liquid soap that does not alter skin pH. b. Collect feces and urine in an appropriate containment device (e.g., condom catheter, fecal incontinence pouch, polymer-filled incontinent pads), or apply a skin sealant, cream, or emollient to act as a barrier to urine and feces.	2. Contact with urine and stool can cause skin maceration. Feces may be more ulcerogenic than urine, owing to bacteria and toxins in stool.
3. Consider using occlusive dressings on clean superficial ulcers, but never on deep ulcers.	3. Occlusive dressings protect superficial wounds from urine and feces, but can trap bacteria in deep wounds.
4. Ensure meticulous handwashing to prevent infection transmission.	4. Improper handwashing by caregivers is the primary source of infection transmission in hospitalized clients.
5. Use sterile technique during all dressing changes.	5. Sterile technique reduces the entry of pathogenic organisms into the wound.
6. Flush the ulcer base with sterile saline solution.	6. Infection produces necrotic debris with secretions that provide an excellent medium for microorganism growth. Flushing helps remove necrotic debris and dilutes the bacterial count. An infected partial-thickness wound may progress to wound sepsis with increasing necrosis, then eventually to a full-thickness lesion.
7. Use new sterile gloves for each dressing change on a client with multiple pressure ulcers.	7. Each ulcer may be contaminated with different organisms; this measure helps prevent cross-infection.
8. Monitor for signs of local wound infection, e.g., purulent drainage, cellulitis.	8. Infected ulcers require additional interventions.

▲ Documentation

Flow records
  Skin condition (e.g., redness, maceration, denuded areas)
  Amount and frequency of incontinence
  Skin care and hygiene measures
  Containment devices used
Progress notes
  Change in skin condition

▲ Outcome Criteria

The outcome criteria for this diagnosis represent those associated with discharge planning. Refer to the discharge criteria.

Potential Altered Health Maintenance related to insufficient knowledge of etiology, prevention, treatment, and home care

Focus Assessment Criteria	*Clinical Significance*
1. Ability of the client or family members to perform necessary turning, lifting, bathing, food purchase and preparation, and other necessary care activities 2. Available support systems for sharing caretaking responsibilities 3. Readiness and ability to learn pressure ulcer prevention and care techniques	1–3. An assessment of client and family learning needs allows the nurse to plan appropriate teaching strategies. About 80% of healed pressure ulcers recur, many because of failure to maintain a regimen for ulcer prevention.

Interventions	*Rationale*

1. Teach measures to prevent pressure ulcers:
  a. Adequate nutrition
  b. Mobility
  c. Turning and pressure relief
  d. Small shifts in body weight
  e. Active and passive range of motion
  f. Skin care
  g. Skin protection from urine and feces
  h. Recognition of tissue damage
	1. Preventing pressure ulcers is much easier than treating them.

2. Teach methods of treating pressure ulcers:
  a. Use of pressure ulcer prevention principles
  b. Wound care specific to each ulcer
  c. How to evaluate effectiveness of current treatment
	2. These specific instructions help the client and family learn to promote healing and prevent infection.

3. Ask family members to determine the amount of assistance they need in caring for the client.	3. This assessment is required to determine if the family can provide necessary care and assistance.
4. Determine equipment and supply needs (e.g., pressure relief devices, wheelchair cushion, dressings). Consult with social services, if necessary, for assistance in obtaining needed equipment and supplies.	4. Equipment and supplies should be arranged for before discharge.
5. If appropriate, refer the client and family to a home health agency for ongoing assessment and evaluation of complex care.	5. Ongoing assessment and teaching may be necessary to sustain the complex level of care.
6. Encourage available caregivers to share the chores of client care.	6. Role fatigue and burnout may occur when one person devotes an inordinate amount of time to caregiving. Periodic relief or assistance can help prevent this situation.
7. Stress the need to continue wound care and maintain adequate nutrition at home. (Refer to the nursing diagnoses Impaired Tissue Integrity and Altered Nutrition in this care plan for specific information.)	7. Strategies must be continued at home for complete healing to occur.

▲ **Documentation**

Discharge summary record
  Client teaching
  Outcome achievement or status
  Referrals, if indicated

References/Bibliography

Abruzzese, R.S. (1985). Early assessment and prevention of pressure sores. In B.Y. Lee (Ed.). *Chronic ulcers of the skin.* New York: McGraw-Hill.

Agarwal, N., DelGuercio, L.R.M., & Lee, B. (1985). The role of nutrition in the management of pressure sores. In B.Y. Lee (Ed.). *Chronic ulcers of the skin.* New York: McGraw-Hill.

Allman R.M., Laprade C.A., Noel L.B., et al. (1986). Pressure sores among hospitalized patients, *Annals of Internal Medicine, 105*(3), 337.

Andberg, M.N., Rudolph, A., & Anderson, T.P. (1983). Improving skin care through patient and family training. *Topics in Clinical Nursing,* July, 45–54.

Barbenel, J.C., Ferguson-Pell, M.W., & Beale, A.Q. (1985). Monitoring the mobility of patients in bed. *Medical and Biological Engineering and Computing, 23*(5), 466–468.

Bennett, L., & Lee, B.Y. (1985). Pressure versus shear in pressure sore causation. In B. Y. Lee (Ed.). *Chronic ulcers of the skin.* New York: McGraw-Hill.

Bergstrom, N., Branden, B., Laquzza, A., & Holman, V. (1985). The Bradan Scale for predicting pressure sore risk: Reliability studies. *Nursing Research, 34*(6), 383.

Bobel, L.M. (1987) Nutritional implications in the patient with pressure sores. *Nursing Clinics of North America, 22*(2), 379–390.

Carpenito, L.J. (1987). *Nursing diagnosis: Application to clinical practice* (2nd ed.). Philadelphia: J.B. Lippincott.

Delisa, J.A., & Mikulic, M.A. (1985). Pressure ulcers—What to do if prevention fails. *Postgraduate Medicine, 77*(6), 209–220.

Fowler, E. (1987). Equipment and products used in management and treatment of pressure ulcers. *Nursing Clinics of North America, 22*(2), 449–461.

Gosnell, D.J. (1973). An assessment tool to identify pressure sores. *Nursing Research, 22*(1), 55–59.

Horsley, J.A. (1981). *Preventing decubitus ulcers: CURN Project.* New York: Grune & Stratton.

Krouskop, T.A., Williams, R., Krebs, M., Herszkowicz, I., & Garber, S. (1985). Effectiveness of mattress overlays in reducing interface pressure during recumbency. *Journal of Rehabilitation Research and Development, 22*(3), 7–10.

Kynes, P. (1986). A new perspective on pressure sore prevention. *Journal of Enterostomal Therapy, 13*(2), 42–43.

Lehman, K.B. (1983). Administrator's role in prevention and care of decubitus ulcers. *The Journal of Long-Term Care Administration, 11*(1), 21–25.

Maklebust, J. (1987). Pressure ulcers: Etiology and prevention. *Nursing Clinics of North America, 22*(2), 359–377.

Maklebust, J., Mondoux, L., & Sieggreen, M. (1986). Pressure relief characteristics of various support surfaces used in prevention and treatment of pressure ulcers. *Journal of Enterostomal Therapy, 14*(3), 85–89.

Maklebust, J., Sieggreen, M., Mondoux, L., LaPlante, J., Lenk, D., Singer, D., & Cameron, O. (1987). *Pressure ulcers: Nursing diagnoses and management* (2nd ed.) Detroit: Harper-Grace Hospitals.

Maklebust, J., Sieggreen, M., Mondoux, L., LaPlante, J., Lenk, D., & Singer, D. (in press). Capabilities: A comparison of the Sof.Care bed cushion and the Clinitron bed. *Decubitus: A Compendium of Prevention and Treatment of Pressure Ulcers.* New York: SN Publications.

Natow, A. (1983). Nutrition in prevention and treatment of pressure sores. *Topics in Clinical Nursing,* July, 39–44.

Shea, D.J. (1975). Pressure sores: Classification and management. *Clinical Orthopedics, 112,* 89–100.

Sieggreen, M. (1987). Healing of physical wounds. *Nursing Clinics of North America, 22*(2), 439–447.

Stotts, N.A. (1985). Nutritional parameters as predictors of pressure sores in surgical patients. *Nursing Research, 34*(6), 383.

Zacharkow, D. (1985). Effect of posture and distribution of pressure in the prevention of pressure sores. In B.Y. Lee (Ed.). *Chronic ulcers of the skin.* New York: McGraw-Hill.

Thermal Injuries

Thermal injuries, or burns, are classified according to cause as thermal (e.g., fire, steam, hot liquids), chemical (e.g., acid, oven cleaners), electrical, or radiation (e.g., sun, x-rays). They also are classified according to the depth of tissue injury, as first degree (epidermis only), second degree (epidermis and part of the dermis), and third degree (complete epidermis and dermis). First- and second-degree burns are also known as partial-thickness burns; third-degree burns, as full-thickness burns. This care plan focuses on the period of hospitalization after emergency treatment on admission and before admission to a rehabilitation unit.

Diagnostic Cluster

▲ Time Frame
Acute episode (nonintensive care)

Collaborative Problems

Potential Complications:
Hypovolemic Shock
Hypervolemia
Electrolyte Imbalance
Metabolic Acidosis
Respiratory
Septicemia
Negative Nitrogen Balance
Thromboembolism
Renal Insufficiency
Curling's Ulcer
Adrenal Insufficiency
Paralytic Ileus
Graft Rejection/Infection

Refer to:

Nursing Diagnoses

Anxiety related to sudden injury, treatments, uncertainty of outcome, and pain

Altered Comfort related to thermal injury treatments and immobility

Altered Nutrition: Less Than Body Requirements related to increased caloric requirement secondary to thermal injury and inability to ingest sufficient quantities to meet increased requirements.

Potential Self-Concept Disturbance related to effects of burn on appearance, increased dependence on others, and disruption of life style and role responsibilities

Diversional Activity Deficit related to prolonged hospitalization, physical limitations, and monotony of confinement

Potential Altered Health Maintenance related to insufficient knowledge of exercise program, wound care, nutritional requirements, pain management, signs and symptoms of complications, and burn prevention and follow-up care

Potential Disuse Syndrome related to effects of immobility and pain on muscle and joint function

Immobility or Unconsciousness

Self-Care Deficit (specify) related to impaired range-of-motion ability secondary to pain

Immobility or Unconsciousness

Potential for Infection related to loss of protective layer secondary to thermal injury

Pressure Ulcers

Grieving (Family, Individual) related to actual or perceived impact of injury on appearance, relationships, and life style

Radical Vulvectomy

Related Care Plan

Immobility or Unconsciousness

▲ Discharge Criteria
Before discharge, the client or family will:

1. Relate an intent to discuss feelings and concerns with significant others after discharge
2. Relate the need to comply with the prescribed dietary and daily exercise program and the consequences of noncompliance
3. Demonstrate correct wound care
4. Describe methods to decrease the risk of infection
5. State the signs and symptoms that must be reported to a health care professional
6. Relate an intent to adhere to the follow-up schedule
7. Describe community resources available for assistance at home

Collaborative Problems

▲ *Nursing Goal*

The nurse will detect, manage, and minimize complications of thermal injuries.

Potential Complication: **Hypovolemic Shock**
Potential Complication: **Hypervolemia**
Potential Complication: **Electrolyte Imbalance**
Potential Complication: **Metabolic Acidosis**
Potential Complication: **Respiratory Complication**
Potential Complication: **Septicemia**
Potential Complication: **Negative Nitrogen Balance**
Potential Complication: **Thromboembolism**
Potential Complication: **Renal Insufficiency**
Potential Complication: **Curling's Ulcer**
Potential Complication: **Adrenal Insufficiency**
Potential Complication: **Paralytic Ileus**
Potential Complication: **Graft Rejection/Infection**

Interventions	*Rationale*

1. Monitor for signs and symptoms of hypovolemia/shock:
  a. Increasing pulse rate with normal or slightly decreased blood pressure
  b. Urine output < 30 mL/hr
  c. Restlessness, agitation, change in mentation
  d. Increasing respiratory rate
  e. Diminished peripheral pulses
  f. Cool, pale, or cyanotic skin
  g. Thirst
	1. In the immediate period after the burn, the body releases large amounts of vasoactive substances, which increases capillary permeability. Serum, proteins, and electrolytes leak into damaged and normal tissue, resulting in severe hypovolemia the first 48 hours postburn (a phenomenon known as third-space fluid shift, or just third-spacing). The compensatory response to decreased circulatory volume is to increase blood oxygen by increasing heart and respiratory rates and decreasing circulation to extremities (manifested by decreased pulses and cool skin). Diminished cerebral oxygenation can cause changes in mentation.

2. Monitor fluid status:
  a. Intake (parenteral, oral)
  b. Output and loss (urinary, nasogastric tube drainage, vomiting)
	2. Fluid shifts can occur postburn. Stress can produce sodium and water retention.

3. Monitor laboratory study results: electrolytes, glucose, arterial blood gases (ABGs), blood urea nitrogen (BUN), serum creatinine, serum albumin, protein, hematocrit, hemoglobin, red blood cell (RBC) count, and leukocytes.	3. A major burn affects all body systems either through direct burn damage or through compensatory mechanisms that attempt to maintain homeostasis. All body system functioning must be assessed frequently for status and response to treatment.

4. Monitor for signs and symptoms of hypervolemia:
 	
  a. Rapid weight gain
  b. Increased pulse rate and blood pressure, neck vein distention
  c. Dependent edema (preorbital, pedal, pretibial, sacral)
  d. Adventitious breath sounds (e.g., wheezing, rales)
  e. Urine specific gravity < 1.010
	4. Within 36 to 48 hours after a major burn, capillary permeability returns to normal. Fluids in body tissues reenter vascular spaces and blood volume increases, resulting in profound diuresis. Circulatory overload can result if cardiac or renal function is compromised.
	  a,b. Hypervolemia causes weight gain, neck vein distention, and pulse and blood pressure increase.
	  c. Edema may occur in various sites depending on the client's body positioning.
	  d. Adventitious breath sounds indicate pulmonary congestions.
	  e. Decreased urine specific gravity indicates impaired renal function.

5. Weigh the client daily or more often if indicated. Ensure accuracy by using the same scale and weighing at the same time of day with the client wearing the same amount of clothing.	5. Daily weights provide data on which to base fluid intake recommendations.

Interventions

6. Adjust fluid intake so it approximates fluid loss plus 300 to 500 mL/day.

7. Monitor for signs and symptoms of electrolyte imbalances:
   a. Hyperkalemia (serum potassium > 5.5 mEq/L):
      • Weakness or paralysis
      • Muscle irritability
      • Paresthesias
      • Nausea, abdominal cramps, diarrhea
      • Irregular pulse

   b. Hyponatremia (serum sodium < 135 mEq/L):
      • Lethargy, coma
      • Weakness
      • Abdominal pain
      • Muscle twitching, convulsions

8. Monitor for signs and symptoms of metabolic acidosis:
   a. Rapid, shallow respirations
   b. Headache
   c. Nausea and vomiting
   d. Negative base excess
   e. Behavioral changes, drowsiness

9. Monitor respiratory function: breath sounds, ABGs.

10. Monitor for signs and symptoms of septicemia:
    a. Temperature > 101° F or < 98.6° F
    b. Decreased urine output
    c. Tachycardia and tachypnea
    d. Pale, cool skin
    e. WBCs and bacteria in urine
    f. Positive blood culture

11. Monitor for signs of negative nitrogen imbalance:
    a. Weight loss
    b. 24-Hour urine nitrogen balance below zero

12. Consult with the physician on the need for hyperalimentation.

13. Monitor for signs and symptoms of thromboembolism:

    a. Positive Homans' sign (dorsiflexion of the foot causes pain)
    b. Calf tenderness, unusual warmth, redness

Rationale

6. This measure is necessary to prevent dehydration. Normal daily fluid loss is 300 to 500 mL; a client with fever or pulmonary complications may lose more.

7.
   a. Damaged cells release potassium into the circulation. If renal insufficiency is present, serum potassium levels rise. Acidosis increases the release of potassium from cells. Fluctuations in potassium affect neuromuscular transmission and can cause such complications as cardiac dysrhythmias, reduced action of GI smooth muscles, and impaired electrical conduction.
   b. Sodium losses result from denuded skin areas and the shift into interstitial spaces during periods of increased capillary permeability. Cellular edema, caused by osmosis, produces changes in sensorium, weakness, and muscle cramps.

8. Metabolic acidosis can result from fixed acids released from damaged cells, hyperkalemia, or reduced renal tubular function. Excessive ketone bodies cause headaches, nausea, vomiting, and abdominal pain. Respiratory rate and depth increase in an attempt to increase excretion of CO_2 and reduce acidosis. Acidosis affects the CNS and can increase neuromuscular irritability.

9. Pulmonary damage can occur from inhalation of smoke, superheated gases, or chemical irritants and from carbon monoxide intoxication.

10. Gram-positive and gram-negative organisms can invade open wounds; a debilitated client is most vulnerable. Bacteria in urine or blood indicates infection. Sepsis results in massive vasodilatation with hypovolemia, leading to tissue hypoxia and resulting decreased renal function and decreased cardiac output. The compensatory response of increased heart rate and respiration attempts to correct hypoxia and acidosis.

11. Protein losses occur from the burn exudate and the kidneys. Catabolism occurs, resulting in negative nitrogen balance. Wound healing is slowed if nutritional status deteriorates.

12. Hyperalimentation may be needed if the client's oral intake is insufficient to overcome negative nitrogen balance.

13. Hypovolemia increases blood viscosity because of hemoconcentration. Immobility reduces vasomotor tone, resulting in decreased venous return with peripheral blood pooling.
    a. Positive Homans' sign indicates insufficient circulation
    b. These signs and symptoms point to inflammation.

Interventions

14. Monitor for early signs and symptoms of renal insufficiency:

    a. Sustained elevated urine specific gravity
    b. Elevated urine sodium

    c. Sustained insufficient urine output (<30 mL/hr)
    d. Elevated blood pressure

    e. Elevated BUN, serum creatinine, potassium, phosphorus, and ammonia, and decreased creatinine clearance

15. Monitor for signs of Curling's ulcer: GI bleeding (manifested by blood in stool or emesis).

16. Monitor for signs of adrenal insufficiency:
    a. Hyponatremia
    b. Hypotension
    c. Hyperkalemia
    d. Blood glucose fluctuations

17. Monitor for signs and symptoms of paralytic ileus:
    a. Decreased or absent bowel sounds
    b. Abdominal distention
    c. Abdominal discomfort

18. Monitor for signs of graft rejection or infection:

    a. Sloughing, darkened edges
    b. Continued pale white-yellow appearance
    c. Increased redness, warmth, swelling, and foul-smelling drainage

19. Teach the client to do the following:
    a. Avoid movement or pressure on the graft

    b. Elevate the involved body part

Rationale

14. Decreased renal blood flow results from hypotension and secretion of antidiuretic hormone (ADH) and aldosterone. Nephrons can be blocked by free hemoglobin increased by red blood cell destruction.
    a,b. Decreased ability of the renal tubules to reabsorb electrolytes results in increased urine sodium levels and urine specific gravity.
    c,d. Decreased glomerular filtration rate eventually leads to insufficient urine output and increased renin production, resulting in elevated blood pressure in an attempt to increase renal blood flow.
    e. These changes result from decreased excretion of urea and creatinine in urine.

15. Ulcers can develop a few days after burn injury. Profound stimulation of the vagus nerve causes hypersecretion of gastric juices, which can erode gastric mucosa.

16. Adrenal insufficiency results from increased demands on the adrenal glands to secrete steroids and catecholamines. Decreased mineralocorticoids leads to decreased sodium reabsorption, potassium excretion, and water reabsorption; decrease in glucocorticoids interferes with blood glucose stability.

17. Paralytic ileus can result from hypoxia secondary to hypovolemia, which reduces peristalsis.

18. Skin grafts are used for deep dermal burns to provide protection from infection and to hasten healing.
    a,b. These signs indicate failure of graft revascularization.
    c. These signs indicate wound infection.

19.
    a. Pressure on graft can disrupt revascularization.
    b. Elevation facilitates venous return.

▲ **Documentation**

Flow records
  Vital signs
  Respiratory assessment
  Weight
  Edema (sites, amount)
  Urine specific gravity
  Intake and output (calories, amounts)
  Occult blood tests
  Bowel sounds
Progress notes
  Complaints of nausea, vomiting, muscle cramps
  Changes in behavior or sensorium
  Treatments
  Condition of graft and donor sites

Related Physician-Prescribed Interventions

Medications
  Antacids   Analgesics
  Antibiotics   Topical agents
  Histamine inhibitors

Intravenous Therapy
  Hyperalimentation   Replacement therapy (fluids, electrolytes, plasma, albumin)

Laboratory Studies
  Complete blood count   Serum electrolytes
  Serum glucose   BUN
  WBC count   Alkaline phosphatase
  Serum albumin   Wound cultures

Related Physician-Prescribed Interventions (Continued)

Diagnostic Studies
  Serial chest x-ray films
Therapies
  Pressure relief beds   Wound care

Nursing Diagnoses

▲ Outcome Criteria

The client will:

1. Effectively communicate feelings regarding injuries
2. Report reduced anxiety to a mild-moderate level

Anxiety related to sudden injury, treatment, uncertainty of outcome, and pain

Focus Assessment Criteria	*Clinical Significance*

1. Anxiety level:
  a. Mild: broad perceptual field, relaxed facial expression, lack of muscle tension, learning ability intact
  b. Moderate: narrowed perceptual field, increased respiratory and pulse rate, visible nervousness, problem-solving ability intact
  c. Severe: distorted sense of time, inattentiveness, greatly reduced perception, hyperventilation, complaints of headache and dizziness
  d. Panic: distorted perception: profound confusion; possible incoherence, vomiting, and violence; learning impossible
	1. Anxiety level varies depending on the client's perception of burn severity and on successful or unsuccessful coping.

2. Personal stressors 3. Specific concerns and fears	2,3. A seriously burned client may have many legitimate fears, such as pain, death, abandonment, dependency, and disfigurement. Recognizing and expressing fears may help reduce anxiety.
4. Available support systems	4. The client needs much support during the acute and rehabilitative periods.

Interventions

1. Help the client reduce anxiety:
   a. Provide constant comfort and reassurance.
   b. Stay with him as much as possible.
   c. Speak in a calm, soothing voice.
   d. Identify and support effective coping mechanisms.
   e. Convey your understanding and empathy.
   f. Encourage the client to verbalize fears and concerns.
2. If anxiety is mild to moderate, take the opportunity to provide client teaching about procedures.
3. Encourage family and friends to verbalize their fears and concerns to staff. Prepare them for initial visit by discussing the client's appearance and any invasive lines or other care measures they may see.
4. Encourage the use of relaxation techniques.

5. Notify the physician immediately if anxiety reaches the severe or panic level.

Rationale

1. An anxious client has a narrowed perceptual field and a diminished ability to learn. He may experience muscle tension, pain, and sleep disturbances, and tend to overreact to situations. Anxiety tends to feed on itself, and can catch the client in a widening spiral of tension and physical and emotional pain; thus, anxiety reduction is essential to effective client care.

2. Accurate information about what to expect may help reduce anxiety associated with the unknown.
3. Discussions help clarify misconceptions and allow sharing. Descriptions of what to expect help to prevent a shocked response, which may trigger anxiety in the client.

4. Relaxation exercises provide control over the body's response to stress and can help reduce anxiety.
5. Severe to panic anxiety can lead to injury or other problems, and makes learning and compliance with treatment impossible.

▲ Documentation

Progress notes
  Present emotional status
  Response to nursing interventions

Altered Comfort related to thermal injury, treatment, and immobility

Focus Assessment Criteria

1. Source of pain:
   a. Burn area
   b. Donor site
   c. Invasive lines
   d. Pressure ulcer
   e. Abdomen
   f. Muscle
2. Client's perception of pain severity, based on a scale of 0 to 10 (0 = no pain; 10 = most severe pain), rated as follows:
   a. At its best
   b. At its worst
   c. After each pain relief intervention
3. Physical signs of pain, e.g., increased pulse rate and respirations, elevated blood pressure, restlessness, facial grimacing, guarding

Clinical Significance

1. Burn pain stems from nerve and tissue destruction; other pain may develop from complications (e.g., ileus, electrolyte imbalance, thrombus) or from treatment. Distinguishing the source of pain guides pain relief interventions.

2. This scale provides a good method of evaluating the subjective experience of pain.

3. In some clients objective signs may be more reliable indicators of pain; for whatever reason, some clients are reluctant to express pain or request pain relief medications.

Interventions

1. Collaborate with the client to identify effective pain relief measures.
2. Convey that you acknowledge and accept his pain.

3. Provide accurate information:
   a. Explain the cause of the pain, if known.
   b. Explain how long the pain should last, if known.
   c. If indicated, reassure the client that narcotic addiction is not likely to develop from the pain relief regimen.
4. Provide privacy for the client during acute pain episodes.
5. Provide optimal pain relief with prescribed analgesics.
   a. Determine the preferred route of administration; consult with the physician.

   b. Assess vital signs, especially respiratory rate, before and after administration.
   c. Consult with a pharmacist for possible adverse interactions with other medications the client is taking, such as muscle relaxants and tranquilizers.
   d. Use a preventive approach to pain medication; administer before treatment procedures or activity, and instruct the client to request p.r.n. pain medications before pain becomes severe.
   e. About ½ hour after administration, assess pain relief.
6. Explain and assist with noninvasive pain relief measures, such as these:
   a. Splinting
   b. Positioning

Rationale

1. The client can provide valuable insight into the pain and its relief.
2. A client who feels that he must convince skeptical caregivers of the seriousness of his pain experiences increased anxiety, which can increase pain.
3. A client who understands and is prepared for pain by detailed explanations tends to experience less stress—and, consequently, less pain—than a client who receives vague or no explanations.

4. Privacy reduces embarrassment and anxiety and enables more effective coping.
5.

   a. If frequent injections are necessary, the IV route is preferred because it is not painful and absorption is guaranteed.
   b. Narcotics depress the brain's respiratory center.
   c. Some medications potentiate the effects of narcotics.

   d. The preventive approach may reduce the total 24-hour drug dose as compared to the p.r.n. approach, and it may reduce the client's anxiety associated with having to ask for and wait for p.r.n. medications.
   e. Response to analgesics can vary with stress levels, fatigue, and pain intensity.
6. Certain measures can relieve pain by preventing painful stimuli from reaching higher brain centers. They also may improve the client's sense of control over pain.

Interventions

    c. Distraction

    d. Massage

    e. Relaxation techniques

7. Explain the prescribed burn wound care, and its advantages and disadvantages.

    a. Open method: no dressings with frequent reapplication of ointment. Advantages: no dressings, hastened eschar separation reduces infection. Disadvantages: requires frequent reapplication, increased heat loss.

    b. Semiclosed method: dressings with antimicrobials changed once or twice a day. Advantages: dressing removal debrides wounds, heat loss is reduced, wounds are not always visible. Disadvantages: dressing changes are required, débridement is painful.

    c. Closed method: occlusive dressings not changed for up to 72 hours. Advantages: fewer dressing changes, others the same as semiclosed. Disadvantages: wounds cannot be inspected daily, dressings can be too tight or too loose.

8. Explain that dressings must not be removed dry.

9. Take steps to reduce pain during dressing changes:

    a. Apply ointment to dressing rather than directly to skin.

    b. Administer analgesics ½ hour before treatment.

    c. Use a bed cradle.

10. Keep the room as warm as possible with a humidity of 40% to 50%, and reduce exposure time during treatments and baths.

Rationale

7. Explaining the method and its advantages and disadvantages can help the client recognize and report any problems or complications.

8. Removing dry dressings causes the removal of burned skin or eschar, which interferes with healing or grafting.

9. Dressing changes are painful because of the associated débridement.

    a. Ointment reduces pain from pressure.

    b. Early administration allows full drug effects during the dressing change.

    c. A bed cradle relieves pressure on wounds.

10. Loss of insulating skin surface increases heat loss. High humidity prevents eschar from drying or cracking prematurely.

▲ **Documentation**

Medication administration record
    Type, dosage schedule, and route of all medications administered
Progress notes
    Pain relief measures
    Unsatisfactory pain relief from these measures

▲ **Outcome Criteria**

The client will resume ingesting the daily nutritional requirements, which include the following:

1. Selections from the basic four food groups
2. 2000 to 3000 mL of fluids/day
3. Adequate vitamins, fiber, and minerals

Potential Altered Nutrition: Less Than Body Requirements related to increased protein/vitamin requirements for wound healing and decreased intake secondary to pain, nausea, and vomiting

Focus Assessment Criteria	*Clinical Significance*
1. Intake (caloric count, types of foods)	1. Wound healing requires increased protein and carbohydrate intake.
2. Daily weight, laboratory values: serum albumin, protein, urine nitrogen (24 hours)	2. Daily weights and laboratory studies enable early detection of negative nitrogen balance.

3. Presence of the following:
  a. Bowel sounds
  b. Nausea
  c. Vomiting
  d. Flatus
	3. Medications and immobility can disrupt GI function.

Interventions

1. Explain the need for increased consumption of carbohydrates, fats, protein, vitamins, minerals, and fluids.

Rationale

1. Wound healing requires increased intake of nutrients to prevent negative nitrogen balance.

Interventions

2. Consult with a nutritionist to establish daily caloric and food type requirements.
3. Explain the causes of anorexia and nausea.

4. Teach the client to rest before meals.

5. Offer frequent small feedings (six per day plus snacks) rather than infrequent large meals.
6. Restrict liquids with meals and 1 hour before and after meals.
7. Maintain good oral hygiene before and after meals.

8. Arrange to have foods with the highest protein and calorie content served at the times when the client usually feels most like eating.
9. Prevent pain from interfering with eating:
   a. Plan care so that painful procedures are not done immediately before meals.
   b. Provide pain medication ½ hour before meals, as ordered.
10. Take steps to prevent nausea and vomiting:

    a. Frequently provide small amounts of ice chips or cool clear liquid (e.g., dilute tea, Jello water, flat ginger ale, or cola), unless vomiting persists.
    b. Eliminate unpleasant sights and odors.

    c. Provide good oral care after vomiting.
    d. Encourage deep breathing.

    e. Restrict liquids before meals.

    f. Avoid having the client lie down for at least 2 hours after meals. (A client who must rest should sit or recline so the head is at least 4 inches higher than the feet.)
    g. Administer antiemetics before meals if indicated.
11. Encourage the client to try commercial supplements available in many forms (liquids, powder, pudding); keep switching brands until some are found that are acceptable to the individual in taste and consistency.
12. Teach techniques to enhance nutritional content of food:
    a. Add powdered milk or egg to milkshakes, gravies, sauces, puddings, cereals, etc., to increase protein and calorie content.
    b. Add blenderized or baby foods to meat juices or soups.
    c. Use fortified milk—1 cup nonfat dry milk added to 1 quart fresh milk.
    d. Use milk, half-and-half, or soy milk instead of water when making soups and sauces.
    e. Add cheese or diced meat to foods whenever able.

Rationale

2. Meeting a burn client's special nutritional needs requires expert consultation.
3. Pain, fatigue, analgesics, and immobility can contribute to anorexia and nausea. Explanations can reduce the anxiety associated with the unknown.
4. Fatigue further diminishes a decreased desire to eat.
5. Distributing the caloric intake over the day helps increase total intake.
6. Overdistending the stomach decreases appetite and intake.
7. Accumulation of food particles can contribute to foul odors and taste, which diminish appetite.
8. This measure may improve protein and calorie intake.

9. Pain causes fatigue, which can reduce appetite.

10. Control of nausea and vomiting improves nutritional status.
    a. Frequent intake of small amounts of fluid helps prevent overdistension.

    b. This diminishes visual and olfactory stimulation of the vomiting center.
    c. Good oral hygiene can reduce nausea.
    d. Deep breathing can suppress the vomiting reflex.
    e. Restricting liquids can prevent overdistension.
    f. Sitting reduces gastric pressure.

    g. Antiemetics prior to meals can prevent nausea and vomiting.
11. These supplements can substantially increase caloric intake without the need to consume large quantities of food.

12. Simple food additives can increase calorie, protein, carbohydrate, and fat intake.

Interventions

    f. Spread cream cheese or peanut butter on toast, crackers, celery sticks.
    g. Add extra butter or margarine to foods.
    h. Use mayonnaise instead of salad dressing.
    i. Add raisins, dates, nuts, and brown sugar to hot and cold cereals.
    j. Keep snacks readily available.
13. If the client still has insufficient nutritional intake, consult with the physician for alternate strategies.

Rationale

13. The client may require high-protein supplements, tube feedings, or total parenteral nutrition.

▲ **Documentation**

Flow records
    Weight
    Intake (type, amount)

▲ **Outcome Criteria**

The client will:

1. Communicate his or her feelings about the burns
2. Participate in self-care

Potential Self-Concept Disturbance related to the effects of burns on appearance, increased dependence on others, and disruption of life style and role responsibilities

Focus Assessment Criteria

1. Experience with or previous exposure to persons with burns
2. Ability to visualize burned area
3. Ability to express feelings about appearance
4. Ability to share feelings about appearance with family members and significant others
5. Participation in self-care activities

Clinical Significance

1–5. This information helps the nurse evaluate the client's understanding of the burn injury, emotional response to the injury and body changes, and coping ability.

Interventions

1. Contact the client often, and treat him with warm, positive regard.

2. Incorporate emotional support into technical self-care sessions. Encourage narration, visualization, participation, and exploration.

3. Encourage the client to look at burned areas.

4. Encourage the client to verbalize feelings and perceptions of life style effects. Validate his perceptions and assure him that his responses are normal and appropriate.
5. Have the client participate in care as much as possible. Provide feedback on progress and reinforce positive behavior and proper techniques.

Rationale

1. Frequent client contact indicates acceptance and may facilitate trust. The client may be hesitant to approach staff because of a poor self-concept.
2. These activities promote exploration of feelings and resolution of emotional conflicts during acquisition of technical skills. Four stages of psychological adjustment have been identified:
    a. Narration: The person recounts his injury experience and reveals his understanding of how and why he is in this situation.
    b. Visualization and verbalization: The person looks at and expresses feelings about the injury.
    c. Participation: The person progresses from observer to assistant and then to independent practitioner of the mechanical aspects of wound care.
    d. Exploration: The person begins to explore methods of incorporating appearance changes into his life style.
3. The client begins the adaptation process by acknowledging the injury and loss.
4. Validating the client's feelings and perceptions increases self-awareness and boosts self-concept.

5. Participation in care can improve the client's self-esteem and sense of control; feedback and reinforcement encourage continued participation.

Interventions

6. Have the client demonstrate wound care and teach procedure independently to a support person.
7. Involve family members and/or significant other(s) in learning wound care.

8. Encourage the client to verbalize positive self-attributes.

9. Encourage contact with others on the unit.

10. Identify a client at risk for unsuccessful adjustment; look for these characteristics:

    a. Poor ego strength
    b. Ineffective problem-solving ability

    c. Learning difficulty

    d. Lack of motivation
    e. External focus of control

    f. Poor health
    g. Unsatisfactory preinjury sex life
    h. Lack of positive support systems
    i. Rejection of counseling
11. Refer an at-risk client for professional counseling.

Rationale

6. Evaluation of a return demonstration helps the nurse identify the need for further teaching and supervision.
7. The acceptance of support persons is one of the most important factors in the client's acceptance of body image changes.
8. Evidence that the client will pursue his goals and maintain his life style reflects positive adjustment.
9. Such contacts give the client the opportunity to test the response of others to his injuries and possible altered appearance.
10. Successful adjustment to changes in appearance are influenced by factors such as the following:
    a. Previous successful coping
    b. Achievement of developmental tasks preinjury
    c. The extent to which injury interferes with goal-directed activity
    d. Sense of control
    e. Realistic self-perception and realistic perception from support persons

11. The client may need follow-up therapy to aid in successful adjustment.

▲ **Documentation**

Progress notes
    Present emotional status
    Interventions
    Client's or family's response
      to nursing interventions

Diversional Activity Deficit related to prolonged hospitalization, physical limitations, and monotony of confinement

▲ **Outcome Criteria**

The client will:

1. Relate feelings of boredom and discuss methods of finding diversional activities
2. Relate methods of coping with feelings of anger or depression caused by boredom
3. Engage in a diversional activity

Focus Assessment Criteria	*Clinical Significance*
1. Current activity level 2. Past activity pattern 3. Motivation	1–3. Previous activity levels and motivation influence the client's response to reduced activity levels.

Interventions

1. Validate the client's boredom.

2. Explore the client's likes and dislikes.

3. Vary the client's routine, when possible.
4. Encourage visitors

5. Use various strategies to vary the physical environment and the daily routine to reduce boredom:
   a. Update bulletin boards, change pictures on the walls, rearrange furniture.
   b. Maintain a pleasant, cheerful environment. Position the client near a window if possible. If appropriate, provide a goldfish bowl for visual variety.
   c. Provide a variety of reading materials (or "books on tape" if impairment hinders reading ability), and a TV and radio.

Rationale

1. Acknowledgment may increase motivation to increase stimulation.
2. Exploration may help to identify possible recreational activities.
3. Monotony contributes to boredom.
4. Visitors provide social interaction and mental stimulation.
5. Creative strategies to vary the environment and daily routine can reduce boredom.

Interventions

    d. Discourage excessive TV watching.
    e. Plan some "special" activity daily to give the client something to look forward to each day.
    f. Consider enlisting a volunteer to read to the client or help with activities, if necessary.
    g. Encourage the client to devise his own strategies to combat boredom.
6. If feasible, enlist the client to assist with clerical work for inservice or the public relations department, e.g., addressing envelopes.
7. Encourage staff and visitors to discuss experiences, trips, and issues of interest or controversy with the client.

Rationale

6. Such work provides opportunities to assist others and reduces feelings of dependency and isolation.
7. Initiating such discussions validates that the client has interests and opinions and also involves him in subjects outside of personal concerns.

▲ **Documentation**

Progress notes
    Activities
    Participation in self-care
        activities

▲ **Outcome Criteria**

The outcome criteria for this diagnosis represent those associated with discharge planning. Refer to the discharge criteria.

Potential Altered Health Maintenance related to insufficient knowledge of exercise program, wound care, nutritional requirements, pain management, signs and symptoms of complications, and burn prevention and follow-up care

Focus Assessment Criteria	*Clinical Significance*
1. Readiness and ability to learn and retain information	**1.** A client or family failing to meet learning goals requires a referral for assistance post-discharge.

Interventions

1. Explain the healing process, eschar formation, and débridement.

2. Explain the need to maintain adequate nutrition after discharge. (Refer to the nursing diagnosis Altered Nutrition in this care plan for specific instructions.)
3. Explain the importance of continuing range-of-motion exercises at home.

4. Describe the action of pressure garments (e.g., Jobst) and the need to wear them 23 hours a day (1 hour to launder).
5. Discuss skin care measures:
    a. Apply lubricant frequently (e.g., cocoa butter) to healed and unaffected skin.

    b. Avoid sun on burned areas for 1 year.

    c. Wear cotton garments next to skin.

    d. Avoid harsh soaps and hot water.
6. Instruct the client and family to watch for and report the following:
    a. Change in healed areas

    b. Change in wound drainage or color
    c. Fever, chills
    d. Weight loss

Rationale

1. Explanations are needed to prepare for changes in the burn area and to verify the need for débridement.
2. Burn healing requires increased protein and carbohydrate intake.

3. As the burn heals, hypertrophic scar tissue formation causes some shortening or contraction. Daily exercise can help reduce severity.
4. Constant pressure on the wound throughout scar maturation (usually 1 year) can retard scar growth.
5. Healing skin is more vulnerable to injury.
    a. Lubricants relieve pruritus of dry skin. (Grafted skin areas do not contain sweat or oil glands.)
    b. Burned and grafted skin tans unevenly, and burned skin is more vulnerable to skin cancer.
    c. Cotton garments reduce itching and abrasion.
    d. Healed burned skin may be hypersensitive.
6. Healing burns are prone to infection and require optimal nutrition.
    a. Changes may point to infection or graft rejection.
    b,c. These signs may indicate infection.

    d. Weight loss indicates that intake is insufficient to meet metabolic needs.

▲ **Documentation**

Discharge summary record
    Client teaching
    Outcome achievement or
        status
    Referrals, if indicated

Interventions	**Rationale**
7. Describe available community resources (e.g., home care, vocational rehabilitation, financial assistance).	7. Such resources may assist in recovery.

References/Bibliography

Cooper, S., et al. (1988). An effective method of positioning the burn patient. *Journal of Burn Care Rehabilitation, 9*(3), 288–289.

Duncan, C.E. (1988). Use of a pillow in exercises for burn patients. *Journal of Burn Care Rehabilitation, 9*(3), 293.

Kneish, C., & Ames, S. (1986). *Adult health nursing.* Reading, MA: Addison-Wesley.

Ninnemann, J.L. (1987). Trauma, sepsis and the immune response. *Journal of Burn Care Rehabilitation, 8*(6), 462–468.

Quested, K.A., et al. (1988). Relating mental health and physical function at discharge to rehabilitation status at three months postburn. *Journal of Burn Care Rehabilitation, 9*(1), 87–89.

Sutherland, S. (1988). Burned adolescents' descriptions of their coping strategies. *Heart & Lung, 17*(2), 150–157.

Watkins, P.N., et al. (1988). Psychological stages in adaptation following burn injury: A method for facilitating psychological recovery of burn victims. *Journal of Burn Care Rehabilitation, 9*(4), 376–384.

Musculoskeletal and Connective-Tissue Disorders

Fractures

Breaks in the continuity of bone, fractures result from external pressure greater than the bone can absorb. When the fracture displaces the bone, surrounding structures (muscles, tendons, nerves, and blood vessels) are also damaged. Traumatic injuries cause most fractures. Pathological fractures occur without trauma in bones weakened from excessive demineralization.

Diagnostic Cluster

▲ **Time Frame**

Initial diagnosis

Collaborative Problems

Potential Complications: *Refer to:*
Neurovascular Compromise
Fat Embolism
Hemorrhage/Hematoma Formation
Thromboemboli

Nursing Diagnoses

Impaired Physical Mobility related to tissue trauma secondary
to fracture
Potential Altered Health Maintenance related to insufficient
knowledge of condition, signs and symptoms of complications,
activity restrictions
Self-Care Deficit (specify) related to limitation of movement   Casts
secondary to fracture
Potential Altered Respiratory Function related to immobility   Immobility or
secondary to traction or fixation devices   Unconsciousness

Related Care Plan

Casts

▲ **Discharge Criteria**

Before discharge, the client or family will:

1. Describe necessary precautions during activity
2. State signs and symptoms that must be reported to a health care professional
3. Demonstrate the ability to provide self-care or report available assistance at home

Collaborative Problems

▲ **Nursing Goal**

The nurse will detect, manage, and minimize complications of fractures.

Potential Complication: **Neurovascular Compromise**
Potential Complication: **Fat Embolism**
Potential Complication: **Hemorrhage/Hematoma Formation**
Potential Complication: **Thromboembolism**

Interventions

1. Monitor for signs and symptoms of neurovascular compromise, comparing findings on affected limb to other limb:
   a. Diminished or absent pedal pulses
   b. Numbness or tingling
   c. Capillary refill time exceeding 3 seconds
   d. Pallor, blanching, cyanosis, coolness
   e. Inability to flex or extend extremity
2. Monitor for signs and symptoms of fat embolism:
   a. Tachypnea
   b. Sudden onset of chest pain or dyspnea
   c. Restlessness, apprehension
   d. Confusion
   e. Elevated temperature
   f. Increased pulse rate

Rationale

1. Trauma causes tissue edema and blood loss, which reduce tissue perfusion. Inadequate circulation and edema damage peripheral nerves, resulting in decrease in sensation, movement, and circulation.

2. A fracture can release bone marrow into the bloodstream, where it forms an embolism that can obstruct circulation (distal, cerebral, or pulmonary). Symptoms depend on the site of obstruction.

Interventions

3. Minimize movement of a fractured extremity for the first 3 days after the injury.
4. Monitor for signs and symptoms of hemorrhage/shock:
    a. Increasing pulse rate with normal or slightly decreased blood pressure
    b. Urine output < 30 mL/hr
    c. Restlessness, agitation, change in mentation
    d. Increasing respiratory rate
    e. Diminished peripheral pulses
    f. Cool, pale, or cyanotic skin
    g. Thirst
5. Monitor for signs and symptoms of thrombophlebitis:
    a. Positive Homans' sign. (Dorsiflexion of the foot causes pain from insufficient circulation.)
    b. Calf tenderness, unusual warmth, redness
6. In leg fracture, encourage exercises of the unaffected leg. Discourage placing pillows under the knees, using a knee gatch, crossing the legs, and prolonged sitting.

Rationale

3. Immobilization minimizes further tissue trauma and reduces the risk of embolism dislodgement.
4. Bone is very vascular; blood loss can be substantial, especially with multiple fractures and fractures of the pelvis and femur. The compensatory response to decreased circulatory volume involves increasing blood oxygen by raising heart and respiratory rates and decreasing circulation to the extremities (marked by decreased pulses, cool skin). Diminished cerebral oxygenation can cause altered mentation.

5. Immobility reduces vasomotor tone, resulting in decreased venous return with peripheral blood pooling and an increased risk of thrombophlebitis.

6. Leg exercises help increase venous return; avoiding external pressure helps prevent venous stasis.

▲ **Documentation**

Flow records
    Vital signs
    Pulses, color, warmth, sensation, movement of distal areas
    Intake and output
Progress notes
    Unusual complaints

Related Physician-Prescribed Interventions

Medications
    Analgesics   Muscle relaxants

Intravenous Therapy
    Not indicated

Laboratory Studies
    Complete blood count   Blood chemistry studies

Diagnostic Studies
    X-ray examinations   Tomograms
    Bone scans

Therapies
    Casts   Wound care
    Traction (skin, skeletal)

Nursing Diagnoses

▲ **Outcome Criteria**

The client will report progressive reduction of pain and relief after pain relief measures.

Impaired Physical Mobility related to tissue trauma secondary to fracture

Focus Assessment Criteria

1. Source of pain:
    a. Fracture
    b. Edema
    c. Poor alignment
    d. Splint or traction
    e. Cast

2. Client's perception of pain severity, based on a pain scale of 0 to 10 (0 = absence of pain; 10 = worst pain), rated as follows:
    a. At its best
    b. At its worst
    c. After each pain relief measure
3. Physical signs of pain: increased heart rate, respirations, and blood pressure; restlessness; facial grimacing; guarding

Clinical Significance

1. Postfracture pain can result from destruction of nerves and tissue by trauma, tissue edema during healing, poor alignment, and poorly fitted splints, traction devices, or casts. The nurse should assess the client carefully to differentiate fracture pain from the other possible causes.
2. Such a rating scale enables the nurse to assess the subjective experience of pain.

3. Objective data may be a more reliable indicator of pain in certain clients. Some clients are reluctant to admit the extent of pain or to request pain medications.

Interventions

1. Refer to the General Surgery care plan, Appendix II, for general pain relief interventions.
2. Immobilize the injured part as much as possible, using splints when indicated.
3. Teach the client to change position slowly.
4. Elevate an injured extremity unless contraindicated.
5. Investigate pain not relieved by pain medications or other relief measures.

Rationale

1. Rationale is self-evident.
2. Immobilization reduces pain and displacement.
3. Slow movements decrease muscle spasms.
4. Elevation reduces edema and the resulting pain from compression.
5. Unrelenting pain can indicate neurovascular compression from embolism, edema, or bleeding.

▲ **Documentation**

Medication administration record
  Type, dosage, route of all
    medications administered
Progress notes
  Unrelieved pain and actions
    taken

▲ **Outcome Criteria**

The outcome criteria for this diagnosis represent those associated with discharge planning. Refer to the discharge criteria.

Potential Altered Health Maintenance related to insufficient knowledge of condition, signs and symptoms of complications, and activity restrictions

Focus Assessment Criteria	Clinical Significance
1. Readiness and ability to learn and retain information	1. A client or family failing to achieve learning goals requires a referral for assistance post-discharge.

Interventions

1. Teach to watch for and report the following immediately:
   a. Severe pain
   b. Tingling, numbness
   c. Skin discoloration
   d. Cool extremities
2. Explain the risks of infection and signs of osteomyelitis:
   a. Chills, high fever
   b. Rapid pulse
   c. Malaise
   d. Painful, tender extremity
3. Explain activity restrictions.
4. Instruct on proper ambulation techniques, as appropriate.

Rationale

1. These signs may indicate neurovascular compression, a condition requiring immediate medical intervention.

2. Bone infections can occur during the first 3 months after fracture.

3. Resting the affected limb promotes healing.
4. Improper use of assistive devices can cause injuries.

▲ **Documentation**

Discharge summary record
  Client teaching
  Outcome achievement or
    status

References/Bibliography

Callahan, J. (1985). Compartmental syndrome. *Orthopedic Nursing, 4*(14), 11–15.

Farrel, J. (1986). *Illustrated guide to orthopedic nursing* (3rd ed.). Philadelphia: J.B. Lippincott.

Gillie, G. (1985). Patient care not injury care: Fracture and tissue injuries. *Emergency, 17*(3), 36–39.

Gameron, R. (1988). Taking the pressure out of compartmental syndrome. *American Journal of Nursing, 88*(8), 1076.

Laughlin, R.M., & Clancy, G.J. (1982). Musculoskeletal assessment: Neurovascular examination of the injured extremity. *Orthopedic Nursing, 1*(1), 43–48.

Wittert, D.W., & Barden, R.N. (1985). Deep vein thrombosis, pulmonary emboli, and prophylaxis in the orthopedic patient. *Orthopedic Nursing, 4*(4), 27–32.

Osteoporosis

In osteoporosis, the rate of bone resorption exceeds the rate of bone formation. As a result, the bones become progressively porous and brittle and are prone to fracture from minimal trauma and even normal stress. Small-framed, nonobese Caucasian women are at greatest risk.

Diagnostic Cluster

▲ Time Frame
Secondary diagnosis

▲ Discharge Criteria
Before discharge, the client and/or family will:
1. Relate those risk factors that can be modified or eliminated
2. Describe dietary modifications
3. Relate signs and symptoms that must be reported to a health care professional

---

Collaborative Problems

Potential Complications:
Fractures
Kyphosis
Paralytic Ileus

Nursing Diagnoses

Potential Altered Health Maintenance related to insufficient knowledge of condition, risk factors, nutritional therapy, and prevention

---

Collaborative Problems

▲ Nursing Goal
The nurse will manage and minimize complications of osteoporosis.

Potential Complication: Fractures
Potential Complication: Kyphosis
Potential Complication: Paralytic Ileus

Interventions
1. Monitor for signs and symptoms of fractures (vertebral, hip, or wrist):
   a. Pain in lower back or neck
   b. Localized tenderness
   c. Pain radiating to abdomen and flank
   d. Spasm of paravertebral muscles
2. Monitor for kyphosis of dorsal spine, marked by loss of height. Kyphosis is indicated when the distance between the foot and the symphysis pubis exceeds the distance between the head and the symphysis pubis by more than 1 cm.
3. Monitor for signs and symptoms of paralytic ileus:
   a. Absent bowel sounds
   b. Abdominal discomfort and distention

Rationale
1. Bones with high amounts of trabecular tissue (e.g., hip, vertebrae, wrist) are more affected by progressive osteoporosis.

2. This spinal change can cause height loss of 2.5 to 15 cm.

3. Vertebral collapse involving the tenth to twelfth thoracic vertebrae (T10–T12) can interfere with bowel innervation, resulting in ileus.

▲ Documentation
Progress notes
  Complaints of pain or discomfort
Flow records
  Bowel sounds
  Height

Related Physician-Prescribed Interventions

Medications
Calcium, vitamin D supplements   Estrogen-progesterone replacement

Intravenous Therapy
Not indicated

Laboratory Studies
Serum calcium and phosphate   Urine calcium excretion
Alkaline phosphatase   Hematocrit

Diagnostic Studies
X-ray examinations   Computed tomography (CT) scan

Therapies
Not indicated

Nursing Diagnoses

Potential Altered Health Maintenance related to insufficient knowledge of condition, risk factors, nutritional therapy, and prevention

▲ Outcome Criteria

The outcome criteria for this diagnosis represent those associated with discharge planning. Refer to the discharge criteria.

Focus Assessment Criteria	Clinical Significance
1. Knowledge of or experience with osteoporosis	1. This assessment helps the nurse plan teaching strategies.
2. Readiness and ability to learn and retain information	2. A client or family failing to meet learning goals requires a referral for assistance post-discharge.

Interventions

1. Discuss osteoporosis using teaching aids appropriate to the client's or family's level of understanding (e.g., pictures, slides, models). Explain the following:
   a. Loss of bone density

   b. Increased incidence of vertebral, hip, and wrist fractures

2. Explain risk factors and which ones can be eliminated or modified:
   a. Sedentary life style

   b. Thinness, small body frame

   c. Diet low in calcium and vitamin D and high in phosphorus

   d. Menopause or oophorectomy

   e. Medications

Rationale

1. Various teaching strategies may be necessary to maximize understanding and retention of information.

   a. Bone mass decreases as a result of decreased bone formation or increased bone resorption.
   b. These bones contain large amounts of porous trabecular tissue, making them more susceptible to the effects of osteoporosis. About one half of women experience vertebral fracture due to osteoporosis before age 75. The incidence of osteoporosis-related hip fracture in women doubles every 5 years after age 60.

2. Focusing on those factors that can be modified can help decrease feelings of helplessness.
   a. Inactivity leads to increased rate of bone resorption.
   b. Thin women typically have less bone mass than obese women. Caucasian women with small skeletal frames are at greatest risk. Black and Oriental women tend to have more bone mass and thus are at less risk.
   c. Insufficient dietary calcium and vitamin D can contribute to decreased bone reformation. High phosphate intake, associated with high-protein diets, stimulates parathyroid activity and thus increases bone resorption.
   d. Decreased plasma estrogen level increases bone sensitivity to the resorptive action of parathyroid hormone.
   e. Various medications have been linked to progression of osteoporosis, e.g., some anticonvulsants, aluminum-containing antacids, thyroid supplements, isoniazid, prolonged heparin therapy, tetracycline, furosemide, and corticosteroids (particularly if dosage exceeds 15 mg/day for more than 2 years). Corticosteroids affect calcium absorption by interfering with vitamin D metabolism. Discontinuation of therapy does not result in restoration of lost bone mass; however, it does prevent further disease progression.

Interventions

    f. Alcohol ingestion

    g. Caffeine

    h. Low sodium fluoride levels

    i. Cigarette smoking

3. Refer to community resources such as smoking cessation workshops, Alcoholics Anonymous, and the Arthritis Foundation.
4. Teach to monitor for and report signs and symptoms of fracture:
   a. Sudden severe pain in the lower back, particularly after lifting or bending
   b. Painful paravertebral muscle spasms
   c. Gradual vertebral collapse (assessed by changes in height or measurements indicating kyphosis)
   d. Chronic back pain
   e. Fatigue
   f. Constipation
5. Reinforce explanations for nutritional therapy, consulting with a dietitian when indicated.
   a. Encourage calcium intake of 1000 to 1500 mg/day.

   b. Identify foods high in calcium, e.g., sardines, salmon, tofu, dairy products, and dark green leafy vegetables.
   c. Monitor for signs and symptoms of lactose intolerance, such as diarrhea, flatulence, and bloating.
   d. Recommend vitamin D intake of 100 to 500 IU/day.
   e. Identify food sources of vitamin D, e.g., fortified milk, cereals; egg yolks, liver, and saltwater fish.
   f. Encourage adequate but not excessive protein intake, approximately 44 g/day in most clients.

6. Explain the need for increased physical activity and certain restrictions.
   a. Encourage exercise that results in movement, pull, and stress on the long bones, e.g., walking, stationary bicycling, and rowing.

Rationale

    f. Alcohol impairs calcium absorption in the intestines, increases urinary loss of calcium, and has a possible effect on liver activation of vitamin D.
    g. Early research results provide some evidence that caffeine increases calcium loss in kidneys and intestines.
    h. Sodium fluoride stimulates osteoblastic activity.
    i. On average, smokers are thinner than nonsmokers; moreover, female smokers usually experience menopause earlier than nonsmokers.

3. These resources can provide needed assistance after discharge.

4. Early detection and treatment of fractures can prevent serious tissue damage and disabilities.

5. Nutritional therapy is a critical component of treatment.
   a. Although the recommended calcium requirement for most persons is only 800 mg/day, older women need increased intake to compensate for decreased absorption, and premenopausal women should prepare for expected bone resorption by increasing intake.
   b. Dietary sources provide a good means of increasing calcium intake.

   c. Increased intake of dairy products may lead to development of lactose intolerance, particularly in older clients.
   d,e. Vitamin D is necessary for the use and absorption of available calcium and phosphorus. However, excessive vitamin D intake can result in bone loss.

   f. Protein intake should not exceed normal recommended requirements, as excessive protein can enhance bone loss by causing increased urinary acid and resulting increased calcium excretion.

6. Immobilization results in bone resorption exceeding bone formation.
   a. Weightbearing exercises increase bone mass. Caution should be used in choosing activities that do not carry a high risk of fractures. Activities such as jogging and bicycling over rough roads may increase pressure on weightbearing vertebrae.

Interventions

b. Instruct the client to exercise at least three times a week for 30 to 60 minutes each session, as ability allows.

c. Discourage flexion exercises of the spine and sudden bending, jarring, and strenuous lifting.

d. Plan adequate rest periods, lying in supine position for at least 15 minutes when chronic pain increases or at certain intervals during day.

e. Instruct the client in the use of a back brace, corset, or splint, if necessary.

f. Encourage family members or other caregivers to provide passive range-of-motion exercises for a client immobilized in bed.

7. Explain the importance of safety precautions such as the following:
   a. Supporting the back with a firm mattress, body supports, and good body mechanics
   b. Protecting against accidental falls by wearing walking shoes with low heels; removing environmental hazards such as throw rugs, slippery floors, electrical cords in pathways, and poor lighting; and avoiding alcohol, hypnotics, and tranquilizers.

   c. Using assistive devices as necessary, e.g., a cane or crutches
   d. Avoiding any flexion movement, such as stooping, bending, and lifting. Explain that vertebral compression fractures can result from minimal trauma resulting from opening a window, lifting a child, coughing, or stooping.

8. Explain any prescribed medication therapy, stressing the importance of adhering to the plan and understanding possible side effects. As appropriate, reinforce the following:

   a. Calcium supplement: 1000 to 1500 mg/day, 1500 mg/day after menopause, accompanied by increased fluid intake
   b. Vitamin D supplement: 100 to 500 IU/day. (*Note:* if vitamin D is used in conjunction with calcitriol, plasma calcium levels should be monitored weekly for 4 to 6 weeks and then less frequently.)
   c. Low-dose estrogen therapy: 0.3 to 0.625 mg/day for postmenopausal women, accompanied by monthly self-breast examination and regular pelvic exam with Pap smear to monitor for side effects.
   d. Calcitonin: 100 U/day 3 times a week initially; then, after x-ray films and evaluation of serum calcium, dosage may decrease to 50 U/day at frequency of 3 times/week.

Rationale

b. A consistent exercise program stimulates bone formation and slows bone loss. It also provides a secondary benefit of improved neuromuscular conditioning and decreased likelihood of falls.

c. These maneuvers increase vertical compression force, increasing the risk of vertebral fractures.

d. Fatigue decreases the motivation to exercise.

e. This intervention minimizes the possibility of spontaneous fractures.

f. Many studies have demonstrated that prolonged immobilization causes even young persons to experience bone loss (approximately 1% of bone mass per week).

7. Osteoporosis increases the risk of spontaneous fractures.
   a. Spontaneous fractures occur most often in the mid to lower thoracic and lumbar spine.
   b. Often a fall is caused by a spontaneous fracture of the hip. Falling from a standing position can result in a fracture of the proximal femur; falling on an outstretched hand can cause Colles's fracture. Even though wrist fractures heal easily, they are significant because they are predictors of hip fractures.
   c. Assistive devices can decrease stress on bones.
   d. Any flexion movement should be eliminated to decrease the risk of fracture.

8. Compliance with the medication regimen can slow the progression of osteoporosis. Awareness of possible side effects allows prompt reporting and intervention to minimize adverse effects.
   a. The risk of renal calculi can be diminished with increased fluid intake.

   b. Vitamin D supplements increase utilization of phosphorus and calcium in clients with no exposure to sunlight and with inadequate dietary vitamin intake. Hypercalcemia can result.
   c. Estrogens have been linked to breast and endometrial hyperplasia and cancer. The risks are reduced with low cyclic doses with progesterone (Bellantoni, 1988).

   d. Serum calcium levels should be monitored closely because of an increased risk of hypercalcemia with induced hyperparathyroidism.

▲ *Documentation*

Discharge summary record
    Client teaching
    Outcome achievement or
        status
    Referrals, if indicated

Interventions	*Rationale*
e. Sodium fluoride: usually 60 mg/day at separate time from calcium administration.	e. Taking calcium with fluoride may interfere with fluoride absorption.

References/Bibliography

Bellantoni, M.F., Blackman, M.R. (1988). Osteoporosis: Diagnostic screening and its place in current care. *Geriatrics, 43*(2), 63–70.

Chambers, J.K. (1987). Metabolic bone disorders: Imbalances of calcium and phosphorus. *Nursing Clinics of North America, 22*(4), 861–872.

Circullo, J.A. (1989). Osteoporosis. *Clinical Management Physical Therapy, 9*(1), 14–19.

MacKinnon, J.L. (1988). Osteoporosis: A review. *Physical Therapy, 68*(10), 1533–1540.

Perry, G.R. (1988). Living with osteoporosis: Early awareness and attention to life-style can delay or prevent osteoporosis. *Geriatric Nursing, 9*(3), 174–176.

Inflammatory Joint Disease (Rheumatoid Arthritis, Infectious Arthritis)

Rheumatoid arthritis is a systemic disease characterized primarily by chronic inflammation of the synovial lining of the joint. The etiology is unknown. The joints involved are usually symmetrically affected. Extra-articular involvement of rheumatoid arthritis can include muscle atrophy, anemia, osteoporosis, and skin, ocular, vascular, pulmonary, and cardiac symptoms.

Infectious arthritis is an inflammation of a joint resulting from a viral, bacterial, or fungal organism invading the synovium and synovial fluid. Individuals at risk for this opportunistic disease are those immunocompromised by a chronic disease or medications.

Diagnostic Cluster

▲ **Time Frame**

Initial diagnosis
Secondary diagnosis

▲ **Discharge Criteria**

Before discharge, the client or family will:

1. Identify components of a standard treatment program for inflammatory arthritis
2. Relate proper use of medications and other treatment modalities
3. Identify characteristics common to "quack" cures
4. Identify factors that restrict self-care and home maintenance
5. Relate signs and symptoms that must be reported to a health care professional

Collaborative Problems

Potential Complications:
Septic Arthritis
Sjögren's Syndrome
Neuropathy
Anemia, Leukopenea

Refer to:

Inflammatory Bowel Disease

Nursing Diagnoses

Fatigue related to decreased mobility, stiffness
Potential Altered Oral Mucous Membrane related to effects of medications and/or Sjögren's Syndrome
Sleep Pattern Disturbance related to pain or secondary fibrositis
Potential Social Isolation related to ambulation difficulties and fatigue
(Specify) Self-Care Deficit related to limitations secondary to disease process
Altered Sexuality Patterns related to pain, fatigue, difficulty in assuming positions, and lack of adequate lubrication (female) secondary to disease process
Impaired Physical Mobility related to pain and limited joint motion
Chronic Pain related to inflammation of joints and juxta-articular structures
Potential Altered Health Maintenance related to insufficient knowledge of condition, pharmacological therapy, home care, stress management, and quackery
Altered Family Processes related to difficulty/inability of ill person to assume role responsibilities secondary to fatigue and limited motion

Multiple Sclerosis

Powerlessness related to physical and psychological changes imposed by the disease

Chronic Obstructive Pulmonary Disease

Related Care Plans

Corticosteroid Therapy
Raynaud's Disease

Collaborative Problems

▲ Nursing Goal

The nurse will manage and minimize complications of arthritis.

Potential Complication: Septic Arthritis
Potential Complication: Sjögren's Syndrome
Potential Complication: Neuropathy

Interventions

1. Monitor for septic signs and symptoms of arthritis:
   a. Warm, painful, swollen joints
   b. Decreased range of motion
   c. Fever, chills
2. Explain the need to splint or support and rest the inflamed joint.
3. Monitor for signs and symptoms of Sjögren's syndrome:
   a. Dry mucous membranes (mouth, vagina)
   b. Decreased salivary and lacrimal gland secretions
4. Monitor for symptoms of neuropathy:
   a. Paresthesias
   b. Numbness

Rationale

1. The chronic inflammation of arthritis increases the risk of joints becoming infected from infections in other body parts.

2. Reducing movement can decrease permanent damage to articular cartilage.
3. The etiology of this syndrome is unknown. It is characterized by faulty secretion of lacrimal, salivary, gastric, and sweat glands.

4. Swelling and actual joint changes can cause nerve entrapment.

▲ Documentation

Progress notes
    Changes in range of motion
    Complaints

Related Physician-Prescribed Interventions

Medications
  Acetylsalicylates
  Oral chelating agents
  Nonsteroidal anti-inflammatory agents
  Antimalarials

  Antirheumatic agents
  Immunosuppresives
  Corticosteroids

Intravenous Therapy
  Not indicated

Laboratory Studies
  Latex fixation
  WBC count
  Agglutination reactions

  Immunoglobins
  Sedimentation rate

Diagnostic Studies
  X-ray films
  Direct arthroscopy

  Radionuclide scans
  Synovial fluid aspirate

Therapies
  Physical therapy

Nursing Diagnoses

▲ Outcome Criteria

The client will:
1. Identify daily patterns of fatigue
2. Identify signs and symptoms of increased disease activity that affect activity tolerance
3. Identify principles of energy conservation

Fatigue related to decreased mobility and stiffness

Focus Assessment Criteria	Clinical Significance
1. Fatigue pattern (morning, evening, transient, constant)	1. Inflammation produces joint symptoms such as pain and stiffness, which result in fatigue. Identifying periods of decreased fatigue can assist in scheduling activities.
2. Effects of fatigue on activities of daily living (ADLs), role responsibilities, recreation, relationships	2. Fatigue can negatively influence a client's ability for reciprocity—returning support to one's support persons—which is vital for balanced and healthy relationships.

Interventions

1. Encourage taking a warm bath or shower in the morning.
2. Assist in identifying energy patterns; have the client rate his fatigue on a scale of 0 to 10 (0 = not tired; 10 = total exhaustion), every hour for a 24-hour period.
3. Help the client schedule and coordinate procedures and activities to accommodate energy patterns.
4. Instruct in general principles of energy conservation:
   a. Planning ahead
   b. Setting priorities
   c. Scheduling intermittent rest periods
   d. Resting before difficult tasks and stopping before fatigue occurs
5. Teach specific energy-conservation strategies:
   a. Eating small, frequent meals
   b. Using a taxi or public transportation, if possible
   c. Distributing difficult tasks throughout the week
   d. Dividing activities into parts, and delegating some parts to others
6. Teach the client to identify signs and symptoms that indicate increased disease activity and to decrease activities accordingly:
   a. Fever
   b. Weight loss
   c. Worsening fatigue
   d. Increased joint symptoms

Rationale

1. Warmth relaxes muscles, decreasing stiffness.
2. Identifying times of peak energy and exhaustion can aid in planning activities to maximize energy conservation and productivity.
3,4. The client requires rest periods before or after some activities. Planning can provide for adequate rest and reduce unnecessary energy expenditure.
5. Such strategies can enable continuation of activities, contributing to positive self-esteem.
6. During periods of increased disease activity, rest requirements increase to 10 to 12 hr/day.

▲ **Documentation**

Progress notes
    Fatigue pattern assessment
Discharge summary record
    Client teaching

Potential Altered Oral Mucous Membrane related to effects of medications or Sjögren's syndrome

▲ **Outcome Criteria**

The client will:

1. Identify factors contributing to altered oral mucosa
2. Relate the need to report oral ulcers or stomatitis to a health care provider
3. Identify strategies for maintaining moist oral mucosa
4. Identify community resources for Sjögren's syndrome
5. Relate the need for frequent, regular dental care for Sjögren's syndrome sequelae.

Focus Assessment Criteria	*Clinical Significance*

1. Contributing factors:
  a. Immunosuppressive drugs
  b. Disease-modifying agents
  c. Sjögren's syndrome
 	
2. Knowledge of signs and symptoms of oral ulcers and stomatitis
	1. Medications used in the treatment of inflammatory joint disease can result in oral ulcers or stomatitis. The presence of either or both of these conditions may require the health care provider to hold or reduce the dose.
	2. The client's understanding enables monitoring and early detection of complications.

Interventions

1. Teach the client to inspect the mouth during daily oral hygiene activities, and to report ulcers or stomatitis to a health care provider.
2. Teach to drink adequate amounts of nonsugared liquids.
3. Teach the importance of regular dental care.

4. Refer individual to Sjögren's Syndrome Foundation, 29 Gateway Drive, Great Neck, NY 11201

Rationale

1. Early detection of these problems enables prompt intervention to prevent serious complications.
2. Well-hydrated oral tissue is more resistant to breakdown.
3. Secondary Sjögren's syndrome can result in excessively dry oral mucosa and predispose the client to tooth decay and gum disease.
4. This organization can provide more detailed information on the condition and its management.

▲ **Documentation**

Flow records
    Oral assessments
Discharge summary record
    Client teaching
    Outcome achievement or status

Sleep Pattern Disturbance related to pain or secondary fibrositis

▲ *Outcome Criteria*

The client will:

1. Describe factors that inhibit sleep
2. Identify techniques to facilitate sleep
3. Demonstrate an optimal balance of activity and rest

Focus Assessment Criteria	*Clinical Significance*
1. Usual sleep requirements, pattern, nighttime awakenings	1. The amount of sleep a client needs varies with age and life style. Nighttime awakening can disrupt the sleep cycle. Assessment can help determine individual needs.
2. Presence of pain at night	2. Pain can have a negative impact on sleep.
3. Presence of secondary fibrositis, marked by the following: a. Difficulty maintaining sleep or nonrestorative sleep b. Characteristic locally tender body points	3. A syndrome characterized by difficulty maintaining sleep and the presence of locally tender nonarticular body points, fibrositis is often associated with inflammatory joint disease.

Interventions

1. Discuss sleep patterns and requirements:
   a. Explain that they vary with age, activity level, and other factors.
   b. Discourage comparing sleep habits with others.
   c. Discourage focusing on hours slept; instead, focus on whether he feels rested and restored after sleep.
   d. Encourage alternate activities if sleep is difficult, e.g., reading, needlepoint.
2. Encourage performance of a bedtime ritual, e.g., hygiene activity, reading, a warm drink.
3. Initiate pain relief measures before bedtime, if appropriate. (Refer to the nursing diagnosis Chronic Pain in this care plan for more details.)
4. Encourage proper positioning of joints:
   a. Pillows for limb position
   b. Cervical pillow
5. Encourage a balance of activity and rest.

6. Provide for uninterrupted sleep to enable completion of a sleep cycle, e.g., use a fan on low setting to drown out sounds.

Rationale

1. The amount of sleep a person needs varies with life style, health, and age. Older adults generally require slightly less sleep than younger adults.

2. A bedtime ritual helps promote relaxation and prepare for sleep.
3. A client with inflammatory joint disease often experiences worsening of symptoms at night.

4. Proper positioning may help prevent pain during sleep and awakenings.

5. Regular physical exercise also seems helpful in controlling the symptoms of fibrositis.
6. A sleep cycle has an interval of 70 to 100 minutes. Most persons need to complete 4 to 5 cycles each night to feel rested.

▲ *Documentation*

Progress notes
  Sleep patterns
  Reports of feeling rested in the morning

Potential Social Isolation related to ambulation difficulties and fatigue

▲ *Outcome Criteria*

The client will:

1. Identify factors that contribute to isolation
2. Identify strategies to increase social interaction
3. Identify appropriate diversional activities

Focus Assessment Criteria	*Clinical Significance*
1. Previous and present social patterns 2. Anticipated changes, desire for an increase	1,2. At-risk clients must be assessed carefully, because the suffering associated with social isolation is not always visible. The client's perception of the situation and the need for change help guide interventions.

Interventions

1. Encourage the client to share feelings and to evaluate his or her socialization patterns.

2. Discuss ways to initiate social contacts:
   a. Inviting a neighbor (adult or child) over for coffee or a snack 1 or 2 days a week

Rationale

1. Only the client can determine whether socialization patterns are satisfactory or unsatisfactory. Some persons like to spend much of their time alone; others do not.
2. Preoccupation with one's own life, problems, and responsibilities often prevents a person from socializing regularly with neighbors or

Interventions

b. Calling friends and relatives weekly
c. Participating in social clubs, e.g., book discussion groups
d. Volunteering at the library, hospital, or other organizations
3. Discuss the advantages of using leisure time for personal enrichment, e.g., reading, crafts.
4. Discourage excessive TV watching.

5. Discuss possible options to increase social activities:
   a. Exercise groups, e.g., YWCA/YMCA
   b. Senior centers and church groups
   c. Foster grandparent program
   d. Day care centers for the elderly
   e. Retirement communities
   f. House-sharing
   g. College classes open to older persons
   h. Pets
   i. Telephone contact
6. Identify barriers to social contact:
   a. Lack of transportation
   b. Pain
   c. Decreased mobility

Rationale

relatives. Initiating contacts may be needed to break established patterns of isolation.

3. Diversional activities can make a person more interesting to others.
4. Other than educational documentaries, TV encourages passive participation and usually does not challenge the intellect.
5. Socialization can promote positive self-esteem and coping.

6. Mobility problems commonly hinder socialization, but many associated difficulties can be overcome with planning.

▲ **Documentation**

Progress notes
  Feelings regarding social contacts
Discharge summary record
  Client teaching
  Response to teaching

▲ **Outcome Criteria**

The client will:

1. Identify the highest possible level of functioning in the following activities: bathing, dressing, feeding, and toileting
2. Demonstrate the ability to use assistive devices

(Specify) Self-Care Deficit related to limitations secondary to disease process

Focus Assessment Criteria	*Clinical Significance*
1. Extent of disability in self-care activities	1,2. Inflammatory joint disease can result in temporary or permanent loss of joint function or deformity. This functional loss can impair the client's ability to perform self-care activities.
2. Need for and ability to use assistive devices	

Interventions

1. Refer to occupational therapy for instruction in energy conservation techniques and use of assistive devices.
2. Provide pain relief before the client undertakes self-care activities. (Refer to the nursing diagnosis Chronic Pain in this care plan for more information.)
3. Provide privacy and an environment conducive to performance of each activity.
4. Schedule activities to provide for adequate rest periods.
5. Teach about the variety of assistive devices available for use in the home:
   a. Bathing
      • Grip bars in shower and bath
      • Bath seat
      • Washing mitt
      • Long-handled washing appliances
      • Built-up toothbrush
      • Dental floss holder

Rationale

1. Occupational therapy can provide specific instruction and further assistance.

2. Unrelieved pain can hinder self-care.

3. A comfortable, secure environment can reduce anxiety and enhance self-care abilities.
4. Exhaustion decreases motivation for self-care activities.
5. Assistive devices can improve self-care ability and increase the client's sense of control over his or her life.

Interventions

b. Dressing
- Long-handled zipper device
- Buttoning device
- Stocking/sock device
- Long-handled shoe horns

c. Feeding
- Built-up utensils
- Plate guard
- Straw holder

d. Toileting
- Raised toilet seat
- Grip handle around toilet

6. Explain available self-help reference materials, such as those from the Arthritis Foundation.

7. Discuss with family members and/or significant others the changing family processes resulting from the client's illness.

8. Also discuss the importance of promoting the client's self-care at an appropriate level.

Rationale

6. Promoting self-help promotes self-esteem.

7. Disability associated with inflammatory joint disease can interfere with the client's ability to care for himself, his family, his home, which disrupts family functioning.

8. Maximum self-care promotes positive self-esteem and reduces feelings of powerlessness, which can contribute to effective family functioning.

▲ **Documentation**

Progress notes
 Type of assistance needed

▲ **Outcome Criteria**

The client will:
1. Identify factors that compromise sexual function
2. Identify strategies and techniques to facilitate and enhance sexual pleasures and expression.

Altered Sexuality Patterns related to pain, fatigue, difficulty in assuming position, lack of adequate lubrication (female) secondary to disease process

Focus Assessment Criteria

1. Usual sexual activity pattern
2. Client's perception of problem

3. Signal symptoms of secondary Sjögren's syndrome:
   a. Dry eyes
   b. Dry nasal mucosa
   c. Dry oral mucosa
   d. Dry vagina
   e. Recurrent parotiditis

Clinical Significance

1,2. Sexual expression is essential for complete well-being and should be nurtured in all clients. An assessment to determine patterns and gratification helps guide interventions.

3. Sjögren's syndrome causes a decrease in the body's ability to secrete lubricating fluids; vaginal dryness may inhibit sexual activity.

Interventions

1. Encourage the client or couple to identify alternative sexual behaviors that may be used for sexual expression during periods of increased disease activity, e.g., touching, body massage.
2. Teach the client or couple positions that minimize pain and joint stress during sexual intercourse, e.g., client on bottom, side-lying. Refer them to the Arthritis Foundation pamphlet *Living and Loving* for more information.
3. Identify times when sexual activity may be more painful—most commonly in the early morning—and encourage having sex at other times.
4. Identify products that can be used to replace or supplement natural vaginal lubrication, e.g., water-soluble lubricants (KY jelly, Surgilube).

Rationale

1. Sexual expression is not limited to intercourse but encompasses many means of self-pleasure and giving pleasure to others.

2. Inflammatory joint disease can result in the loss of joint motion, owing to damage to both articular and juxta-articular structures (muscle, tendon, ligaments). Positions that lessen strain on the client's joints can enhance sexual pleasure.
3. Inflammatory joint disease is often associated with prolonged morning stiffness.

4. Inflammatory joint disease is sometimes associated with Sjögren's syndrome, characterized by a decreased ability to secrete lubricating

Interventions

Rationale

▲ **Documentation**

Progress notes
    Client teaching
    Discussions

▲ **Outcome Criteria**

The client will:

1. Describe the rationale for interventions
2. Minimize joint stress and injury
3. Maintain and when possible increase strength and endurance in limbs
4. Demonstrate correct performance of exercises

5. Discuss the need to plan for sexual activity, e.g., schedule it for a certain time of day, take a hot shower or bath prior to activity.

fluids (e.g., tears, saliva, vaginal secretions). Use of a lubricant can decrease pain on intercourse.

5. Planning sexual activity allows the client to prepare beforehand, which can increase pleasure for both client and partner.

Impaired Physical Mobility related to pain and limited joint motion

Focus Assessment Criteria	*Clinical Significance*

1. Presence and degree of pain
2. Function and mobility of joints:
    a. Limitations in range of motion
    b. Presence of deformities
3. Muscle strength
	1–3. The chronic inflammation associated with inflammatory joint disease results in damage to articular and juxta-articular structures, such as bone demineralization, tendon and ligament laxity, and muscle wasting. This damage can result in impaired mobility.

Interventions

1. Provide pain relief as necessary. (Refer to the nursing diagnosis Chronic Pain in this care plan for specific interventions.)
2. Encourage compliance with a prescribed exercise program, which may include the following exercises:
    a. Range of motion (ROM)
    b. Muscle strengthening
    c. Endurance
3. Encourage an amount of exercise consistent with the degree of disease activity.

4. Teach the client to perform all the following steps:
    a. Warm-up: Before exercising, take a warm bath or shower or use warm soaks or a heating pad on affected areas. Then, perform gentle stretching.
    b. Gentle ROM without passive pressure at least once daily
    c. Isometric and strengthening exercises: Contract muscle group for a count of eight, then relax for two counts. Perform ten repetitions, three to four times a day, on the quadriceps, abdominal muscles, gluteals, and deltoids.
    d. Endurance/aerobic exercise: Begin with a 5- to 10-minute period and gradually increase. Appropriate activities include walking, swimming, and light racquet games (badminton, ping-pong). Inappropriate activities include heavy racquet sports (tennis, squash, racquetball), contact sports (football, hockey), and weight-lifting or progressive resistance exercise.

Rationale

1. Pain can contribute to decreased mobility.

2. A regular exercise program including ROM, isometrics, and selected aerobic activities can help maintain integrity of joint function.

3. During periods of acute inflammation, the individual may immobilize the joints in the most comfortable position; this is usually partial flexion. Continued immobilization can result in joint stiffness and muscle weakness (extensor groups) that can quickly lead to contractures and more pain.

4.

    a. A warm-up period of local heat or gentle stretching prior to strengthening and endurance exercises allows muscles to become ready gradually for more intense work.
    b. Gentle ROM prevents injury to joint tissue.

    c. Isometric and other strengthening exercises can improve function.

    d. Exercises that jar or bang joints are contraindicated.

Interventions

e. Cool-down period: For 5 to 10 minutes, progressively slow movements of extremities or slow walking pace.

5. If the client complains of postexercise pain persisting longer than 1½ to 2 hours, instruct him to do as follows:
   a. Decrease repetitions the next day
   b. For severe soreness, the next day attempt ROM at least once after local heat application to affected joints.
6. Refer to physical therapy as necessary.

7. Refer to community-based exercise groups for people with arthritis, e.g., an aquatic exercise program at the YWCA/YMCA.

Rationale

e. A cool-down period after more intense exercise allows muscle waste products to be removed and permits the body to return gradually to its preexercise state.

5. Exhaustion and pain decrease motivation to continue in an exercise program.

6. Assistance may be needed for development of an in-depth instruction in a physical activity program.
7. Such a program can provide exercise and socialization.

▲ **Documentation**

Flow records
    Exercises (type, frequency)

▲ **Outcome Criteria**

The client will:
1. Receive validation that pain exists
2. Practice selected noninvasive pain relief measures to manage pain
3. Relate improvement of pain and, when possible, increase daily activities

Chronic Pain related to inflammation of joints and juxta-articular structures

Focus Assessment Criteria

1. Joints affected and the presence of associated warmth, swelling, and erythema
2. Range of motion in affected joints

Clinical Significance

1,2. Inflammatory joint disease is characterized by an activation of the body's inflammatory response. Stable prostaglandins, thromboxanes, and prostacycline are mediators of inflammation. Experimental data show that although these mediators are themselves incapable of provoking pain directly, they do produce hyperalgesia and act synergistically with other inflammation mediators to augment pain. These substances also act on small blood vessels, producing vasodilation and changes in vascular permeability that result in erythema, warmth, and swelling.

Interventions

1. Apply local heat or cold to affected joints for approximately 20 to 30 minutes three to four times a day. Avoid temperatures likely to cause skin or tissue damage by checking the temperature of warm soaks or covering a cold/ice pack with a towel.
2. Encourage a warm bath or shower the first thing in the morning to reduce morning stiffness.
3. Encourage measures to protect affected joints:
   a. Performing gentle active ROM exercises once daily during periods of active inflammation
   b. Using splints
   c. Obtaining assistance with ADLs if necessary
   d. Maintaining proper body alignment
   e. Avoiding pillows under the knees to prevent knee and hip flexion deformities
   f. Using assistive devices as necessary

Rationale

1,2. Treatment of inflammatory joint pain focuses on the reduction of discomfort and inflammation by the use of local comfort measures, joint rest, and the use of anti-inflammatory or disease-modifying medications.

3. Frequent rest periods take the weight off joints and relieve fatigue. Proper positioning is needed to minimize stress on joints.

▲ *Documentation*

Progress notes
    In affected joints: pain,
       swelling, warmth, erythema
    Pain relief measures
    Response to pain relief mea-
       sures

Interventions

4. Encourage the use of adjunctive pain control measures:
    a. Progressive relaxation
    b. Transcutaneous electrical nerve stimulation (TENS)
    c. Biofeedback
5. Warn against using oral or parenteral narcotics to control chronic pain.

Rationale

4. Pain is a subjective, multifactorial experience that can be modified by the use of cognitive and physical techniques to reduce the intensity or perception of pain.

5. Drug tolerance develops, which necessitates increased dosage and increases the risk of narcotic dependency or addiction. Nonsteroidal anti-inflammatory drugs are safer.

▲ *Outcome Criteria*

The outcome criteria for this diagnosis represent those associated with discharge planning. Refer to the discharge criteria.

Potential Altered Health Maintenance related to insufficient knowledge of condition, pharmacological therapy, home care, stress management, and quackery

Focus Assessment Criteria

1. Knowledge of or experience with arthritic conditions, either personal or from relatives or friends; feelings, concerns, and questions
2. Readiness and ability to learn and retain information

Clinical Significance

1. This assessment guides the nurse in developing teaching strategies.

2. A client or family failing to achieve learning goals requires a referral for assistance postdischarge.

Interventions

1. Explain inflammatory arthritis using teaching aids appropriate to the client's and family member's level of understanding. Explain the following:
    a. The inflammatory process
    b. Joint function and structure
    c. Effects of inflammation on joints and juxta-articular structures
    d. Extra-articular manifestations of the disease process
    e. Chronic nature of disease
    f. Disease course (remission/exacerbation)
    g. Low incidence of significant or total disability
    h. Components of the standard treatment program:
       • Medications (e.g., aspirin, nonsteroidal anti-inflammatory drugs, disease-modifying agents, cytotoxic agents, corticosteroids)
       • Local comfort measures
       • Exercise/rest
       • Joint protection/assistive devices
       • Consultation with other disciplines
       • Adequate nutrition
       • Regular follow-up care
2. Teach the client and family to identify characteristics of quackery:
    a. "Secret" formulas or devices for curing arthritis
    b. Advertisements using "case histories" and "testimonials"
    c. Rejection of standard components of treatment program
    d. Claims of persecution by the "medical establishment"

Rationale

1. Inflammatory joint disease is a chronic illness. Education should emphasize a good understanding of the inflammatory process and the actions the client can take to manage symptoms and minimize their impact on his or her life.

2. An accurate and full understanding of inflammatory joint disease and its treatment decrease the client's susceptibility to quackery.

Interventions

3. Teach the client to take prescribed medications properly and to report symptoms of side effects promptly.

4. Explain the proper use of other treatment modalities:
   a. Local heat or cold application
   b. Assistive devices
   c. Exercises
5. Explain the relationship of stress to inflammatory diseases. Discuss stress management techniques:
   a. Progressive relaxation
   b. Guided imagery
   c. Regular exercise
6. Reinforce the importance of routine follow-up care.
7. Refer to appropriate community resources, such as The Arthritis Foundation, 1314 Spring St N.W., Atlanta, GA 30309.

Rationale

3. Adhering to the schedule may help prevent fluctuating drug blood levels, which can reduce side effects. Prompt reporting of side effects enables intervention to prevent serious problems.
4. Injury can further decrease mobility and motivation to continue therapies.

5. Stressful events may be associated with an increase in disease activity. Effective use of stress management techniques can help minimize the effects of stress on the disease process.

6. Follow-up care can identify complications early and help to reduce disabilities from disuse.
7. Such resources can provide specific additional information to enhance self-care.

▲ **Documentation**

Discharge summary record
  Client and family teaching
  Outcome achievement or
    status
  Referrals, if indicated

References/Bibliography

Brassell, M.P. (1988). Pharmacologic management of rheumatic diseases. *Orthopedic Nursing, 7*(2), 43–51.

Crosby, L.J. (1988). Stress factors, emotional stress and rheumatoid arthritis disease activity. *Journal of Advanced Nursing, 13*(4), 452–461.

Geber, L.H., et al. (1988). Rehabilitation in joint and connective tissue diseases: Comprehensive rehabilitation evaluation. *Archives of Physical Medical Rehabilitation* (Suppl.), *69*(3-S), S97–98.

Gill, K.P. (1987). Cementless total hip arthroplasty. *Canadian Nurse, 83*(10), 18–20.

Henderson, L. (1989). Arthritis in motion: An exercise program for chronic arthritis patients. *Orthopedic Nursing, 8*(3), 41–45.

Hicks, J.E., et al. (1988). Rehabilitation in joint and connective tissue diseases: Specific rheumatic diseases. *Archives of Physical Medical Rehabilitation* (Suppl.), *69*(3-S), S84–96.

Schoen, C.H. (1988). Assessment for arthritis. *Orthopedic Nursing, 7*(2), 31–39.

Infectious and Immunodeficient Disorders

Systemic Lupus Erythematosus

A chronic autoimmune inflammatory disease, systemic lupus erythematosus (SLE) affects the connective tissue of one or more organ systems. The etiology has not been confirmed, but latent viruses, genetic factors, hormones, and medications have been linked to onset. Joints, skin, blood, heart, lung, and glomerular tissue may be involved.

Diagnostic Cluster

▲ **Time Frame**

Initial diagnosis
Secondary diagnosis

Collaborative Problems

Potential Complications:
Polymyositis
Vasculitis
Hematological Problem
Raynaud's Disease

Refer to:

Nursing Diagnoses

Potential for Injury related to increased dermal vulnerability secondary to disease process

Potential Altered Health Maintenance related to insufficient knowledge of condition, rest versus activity requirements, pharmacological therapy, signs and symptoms of complications, risk factors, and community resources

Powerlessness related to unpredictable course of disease

Fatigue related to decreased mobility and effects of chronic inflammation

Potential Self-Concept Disturbance related to inability to achieve developmental tasks secondary to disabling condition and changes in appearance

Diabetes Mellitus
Inflammatory Joint Disease

Multiple Sclerosis

Related Care Plan

Corticosteroid Therapy

▲ **Discharge Criteria**

Before discharge, the client and/or family will:

1. State an intent to share concerns with a trusted friend
2. Identify components of a standard treatment program
3. Relate proper use of medications
4. Describe actions to reduce the risk of exacerbation
5. Identify signs and symptoms that must be reported to a health care professional

Collaborative Problems

▲ **Nursing Goal**

The nurse will manage and minimize complications of lupus.

Potential Complication: Polymyositis
Potential Complication: Vasculitis
Potential Complication: Hematological Problem
Potential Complication: Raynaud's Syndrome

Interventions

1. Monitor for polymyositis:
   a. Tendinitis (pain radiating down an extremity)
   b. Pursitis (pain in the shoulder, knee, elbow, or hip)
   c. Pericarditis (pain beneath the left clavicle and in the neck and left scapular region, aggravated by movement)
2. Monitor for the effects of vasculitis:
   a. Hypertension
   b. Peripheral vascular disease
   c. Pericarditis

Rationale

1. Antibodies are produced that damage the nuclei, e.g., lupus erythematosus (LE) factor, DNA, nucleoprotein, and histones. The resulting inflammation stimulates antigens, which in turn stimulate more antibodies, and the cycle begins anew. Inflammation in skeletal muscle (polymyositis) can cause pericarditis.

2. Inflammation of vessel walls decreases blood supply to major organs, causing necrosis, sclerosis, and dysfunction.

Interventions

    d. Hepatomegaly
    e. Splenomegaly
    f. Gastritis
    g. Pneumonitis
    h. Seizures
    i. Renal failure
3. Monitor for hematological disorders:
    a. Hemolytic anemia
    b. Leukopenia
    c. Lymphopenia
    d. Thrombocytopenia
4. Teach the client to report purpura and ecchymosis.
5. Monitor for Raynaud's syndrome:
    a. Vasospasm of arteries in fingers, resulting in pallor changing to cyanosis and ending in rubor
    b. Numbness, tingling, and pain in affected digits

Rationale

3. SLE alters blood components through unknown mechanisms. White blood cells are less attracted to inflamed sites and thus are less effective in fighting infection.
4. Platelet deficiencies may be manifested by purpura and ecchymosis.
5. In Raynaud's syndrome, inflammation and subsequent damage to connective tissue produces vasospasm of arteries and arterioles of the fingers and hands.

▲ **Documentation**

Flow records
    Vital signs
    Peripheral pulses
Progress notes
    Complaints

Related Physician-Prescribed Interventions

Medications
    Nonsteroidal anti-inflammatory agents   Immunosuppressives
    Antimalarials   Cytotoxic agents
    Corticosteroids

Intravenous Therapy
    Not indicated

Laboratory Studies
    Complete blood count   Renal function studies

Diagnostic Studies
    None indicated

Therapies
    None indicated

Nursing Diagnoses

▲ **Outcome Criteria**

The client will:

1. Identify causative factors that may increase disease activity, e.g., sun exposure
2. Identify measures to reduce damage to skin by the sun
3. Identify strategies to manage skin damage should it occur
4. Identify signs and symptoms of cellulitis

Potential for Injury related to increased dermal vulnerability secondary to disease process

Focus Assessment Criteria

1. Knowledge of need to avoid sun exposure

2. Presence of skin manifestations of SLE

Clinical Significance

1. In SLE, the skin is extremely sensitive to sun exposure.
2. Common skin manifestations of SLE include the characteristic "butterfly" facial rash, discoid skin lesions, and patchy alopecia. Other SLE skin manifestations, such as digital or leg ulcers, result from immune complex deposition vasculitis and generally signal active systemic disease.

Interventions

1. Explain the relationship between sun exposure and disease activity.

Rationale

1. Through an unknown mechanism, exposure to ultraviolet light can precipitate an exacerbation of both skin and systemic disease. The client's understanding of this relationship should encourage him to limit sun exposure.

Interventions

2. Identify strategies to limit sun exposure:
   a. Avoid sun exposure between 10 AM and 2 PM.
   b. Use nondeodorant soaps.
   c. Use sunscreens (15 SPF); reapply after swimming or exercise.
   d. Select lightweight long-sleeved clothing and wide-brimmed hats.
3. Explain the need to avoid fluorescent lighting.

4. Teach the client to keep skin ulcers clean and the skin moist.

5. Teach the client to recognize signs and symptoms of cellulitis at open skin area sites and to report them promptly to a health care professional:
   a. Tenderness
   b. Swelling
   c. Warmth
   d. Redness

Rationale

2. A client with SLE should make every attempt to minimize sun exposure.

3. Like sunlight, fluorescent lighting produces ultraviolet rays.
4. Skin changes associated with SLE increase the vulnerability to injury. Reducing bacteria on the skin reduces the risk of infection. Dry skin is more susceptible to breakdown.
5. Cellulitis can develop in open skin areas, owing to loss of protective skin and decreased circulation secondary to vasculitis. Early recognition enables prompt intervention to prevent further complications.

▲ **Documentation**

Flow record
    Skin assessment
Discharge summary record
    Client teaching
    Response to teaching

▲ **Outcome Criteria**

The outcome criteria for this diagnosis represent those associated with discharge planning. See the discharge criteria.

Potential Altered Health Maintenance related to insufficient knowledge of condition, rest versus activity requirements, pharmacological therapy, signs and symptoms of complications, risk factors, and community resources

Focus Assessment Criteria	*Clinical Significance*
1. Readiness and ability to learn and retain information	1. A client or family failing to achieve learning goals requires a referral for assistance post-discharge.
2. Knowledge of or experience with SLE	2. This assessment helps the nurse plan effective teaching strategies.

Interventions

1. Explain SLE using teaching aids appropriate to the client's and family's level of understanding. Discuss the following:
   a. The inflammatory process
   b. Organ systems at risk of involvement (See Potential Complications in this care plan for more information.)
   c. Chronic nature of disease (remission/exacerbation)
   d. Components of standard treatment program
   e. Medications
   f. Exercise and rest
   g. Regular follow-up care
2. Teach the client to take medications properly and to report symptoms of side effects. Drugs prescribed for SLE may include the following:
   a. Ponsteroidal anti-inflammatory drugs
   b. Corticosteroids (Refer to the Corticosteroid care plan, page 542, for more information.)
   c. Immunosuppressive agents, such as azathioprine (Imuran) and cyclophosphamide (Cytoxan)
   d. Antimalarial agents, such as hydroxychloroquine (Plaquenil)

Rationale

1. Understanding may help improve compliance and reduce exacerbations.

2. Knowledge of and proper adherence to the medication regimen can help reduce complications and detect side effects early.

Interventions	*Rationale*
3. Teach the need to balance activity and rest. (Refer to the Inflammatory Joint Disease care plan, page 296, for specific strategies.)	3. The chronic fatigue associated with SLE necessitates strategies to prevent exhaustion and maintain the highest level of independent functioning.
4. Teach the need for meticulous, gentle mouth care.	4. Vasculitis can increase the risk of mouth lesions and injury.
5. Teach to report signs and symptoms of complications:	5. Early detection of complications enables prompt interventions to prevent serious tissue damage or dysfunction.
a. Chest pain and dyspnea	a. Chest pain and dyspnea may indicate pericarditis or pleural effusion.
b. Fever	b. Fever may point to infection.
c. Ecchymoses	c. Ecchymoses may indicate a clotting disorder.
d. Edema	d. Edema may signal renal or hepatic insufficiency.
e. Decreased urine output, concentrated urine	e. These urine changes may indicate renal insufficiency.
f. Nausea and vomiting	f. Nausea and vomiting can indicate GI dysfunction.
g. Leg cramps	g. Leg cramps may result from peripheral vascular insufficiency.

6. Explain the relationship of stress and autoimmune disorders. Discusss stress management techniques:
   a. Progressive relaxation
   b. Guided imagery
   c. Regular exercise (e.g., walking, swimming)
	6. Stress may be associated with an increase in disease activity. Stress management techniques can reduce the stress and fatigue associated with unmanaged conflicts.

7. Refer to appropriate community resources, e.g., The Lupus Foundation.	7. Additional self-help information may be very useful for self-care.

▲ **Documentation**

Discharge summary record
  Client teaching
  Outcome achievement or
    status
  Referrals, if indicated

References/Bibliography

Joyce, K.M., et al. (1985). The patient with lupus nephritis: A nursing perspective. *Heart & Lung, 14*(1), 75–79.

Regan-Gavin, R. (1988). The war within: A personal account of coping with systemic lupus erythematosus. *Health Social Work, 13*(1), 11–19.

Searle, L. et al. (1985). Honoring the personal side of chronic illness: Systemic lupus erythematosus. *Nursing 85, 15*(11), 52–57.

Zeiger, G.C. (1984). Systemic lupus erythematosus and systemic sclerosis. *Nursing Clinics of North America, 19*(4), 673–695.

Acquired Immunodeficiency Syndrome

An infection caused by the human immunodeficiency virus (HIV), acquired immunodeficiency syndrome (AIDS) was first reported in the United States in 1981. AIDS represents the end-stage of a continuum of HIV infection and its sequelae. Major modes of infection transmission include sexual activity with an infected person and exposure to infected needles, blood, or blood products. A fetus can contract HIV infection from an infected mother perinatally. HIV infects primarily the T_4 cell lymphocytes; this interferes with cell-mediated immunity. The clinical consequences of this progressive, irreversible immune deficit are opportunistic infections and malignancies, which prove fatal in 95% of cases.

Diagnostic Cluster

▲ Time Frame
Initial diagnosis
Recurrent acute episodes

▲ Discharge Criteria
Before discharge, the client and/ or family will:
1. Relate the implications of diagnosis
2. Describe the prescribed medication regimen
3. Identify modes of HIV transmission
4. Identify infection control measures
5. Describe signs and symptoms that must be reported to a health care professional
6. Identify available community resources

Collaborative Problems

	Refer to:
Potential Complications:	
Opportunistic Infections	
Malignancies	
Septicemia	
Myelosuppression	Leukemia

Nursing Diagnoses

Altered Family Processes related to the nature of the AIDS condition, role disturbance, and uncertain future	
Potential for Infection Transmission related to contagious nature of blood and body excretions	
Social Isolation related to fear of rejection or actual rejection of others secondary to fear	
Potential Altered Health Maintenance related to insufficient knowledge of condition, medications, home care, infection control, and community resources	
Powerlessness related to unpredictable nature of condition	Chronic Obstructive Pulmonary Disease Cancer (Initial Diagnosis)
Anxiety related to perceived effects of illness on life style and unknown future	
Grieving related to loss of body function and its effects on life style	Cancer (Initial Diagnosis)
Powerlessness related to change from curative to palliative status	Cancer (Initial Diagnosis)
Potential for Infection related to increased susceptibility secondary to compromised immune system	Leukemia
Fatigue related to effects of disease, stress, chronic infections, and nutritional deficiency	Inflammatory Joint Disease
Potential Altered Oral Mucous Membrane related to compromised immune system	Chemotherapy

Related Care Plans

Cancer (End-Stage)

Collaborative Problems

▲ Nursing Goal
The nurse will manage and minimize complications of AIDS.

Potential Complication: Opportunistic Infections
Potential Complication: Malignancies
Potential Complication: Septicemia

Interventions

1. Monitor for opportunistic infections

    a. Protozoal
        - *Pneumocystis carinii* pneumonia (dry, nonproductive cough, fever, dyspnea)
        - *Toxoplasma gondii* encephalitis (headache, lethargy, seizures)
        - *Cryptosporidium* enteritis (watery diarrhea, malaise, nausea, abdominal cramps)
    b. Viral
        - Herpes simplex perirectal abscesses (severe pain, bleeding, rectal discharge)
        - Cytomegalovirus (CMV) retinitis, colitis, pneumonitis, encephalitis, or other organ disease
        - Progressive multifocal leukoencephalopathy (headache, decreased mentation)
        - Varicella zoster, disseminated (shingles)
    c. Fungal
        - *Candida albicans* stomatitis and esophagitis (exudate, complaints of unusual taste in mouth)
        - *Cryptococcus neoformans* meningitis (fever, headaches, blurred vision, stiff neck, confusion)
    d. Bacterial
        - *Mycobacterium avium intracellulare* disseminated
        - *Mycobacterium tuberculosis* extrapulmonary and pulmonary

2. Emphasize the need to report symptoms early.

3. Explain the need to balance activity and rest, consume a nutritious diet, and practice stress management techniques.

4. Refer to the nursing diagnosis Potential for Infection in the Corticosteroid Therapy care plan, page 545 for specific interventions to reduce risks.

5. Monitor for malignancies:

    a. Kaposi's sarcoma
        - Palpable, purplish lesions frequently on trunk, arms, and head
        - Extracutaneous lesions in GI tract, lymph nodes, and lungs
    b. Lymphoma (non-Hodgkin's, Burkitt's)
        - Painless lymphadenopathy (early site neck, axilla, inguinal area)
        - Pruritus, weight loss

6. Monitor for signs and symptoms of septicemia:
    a. Temperature > 101° F or <98.6° F
    b. Decreased urine output
    c. Tachycardia and tachypnea
    d. Pale, cool skin
    e. WBCs and bacteria in urine

Rationale

1. The progressive, irreversible immune deficit causes secondary diseases of opportunistic infections and malignancies
    a. The most common and serious infection is *Pneumocystis carinii* pneumonia.

    b. Herpes simplex is common and painful. The CMV infections are responsible for significant morbidity, e.g., blindness.

    c. Fungal conditions are chronic with relapses.

    d. Bacterial infections frequently affect the pulmonary system.

2. Early treatment can often prevent serious complications, e.g., septicemia, and increases the chance of a favorable response to treatment.

3. Rest and a nutritious diet provide the person with energy to heal and to increase defense systems. Stress management techniques help decrease anxiety, which is fatiguing.

5. The malignancies that affect AIDS clients are related to immunosuppression (Grady, 1988).
    a. Kaposi's sarcoma is frequently seen in AIDS clients who are homosexuals and rarely in AIDS clients who are not homosexuals.

    b. Non-Hodgkin's lymphomas can progress into the bone marrow, liver, spleen, GI, and nervous system.

6. Gram-positive and gram-negative organisms can invade open wounds, causing septicemia. A debilitated client is at increased risk. Sepsis produces massive vasodilatation, resulting in hypovolemia and subsequent tissue hypoxia. Hypoxia leads to decreased renal function and

▲ **Documentation**

Flow records
 Lesions (number, size, locations)
 Respiratory assessment
 Neurological assessment (mentation, orientation, affect)
 Mouth assessment
Progress notes
 Complaints

Interventions

    f. Positive blood culture

Rationale

cardiac output, triggering a compensatory response of increased respirations and heart rate in an attempt to correct hypoxia and acidosis. Bacteria in urine or blood indicates infection.

Related Physician-Prescribed Interventions

Medications

Antibiotics
Antiemetics
Antifungals
Chemotherapy

Antipyretics
Antiviral agents
Antidiarrheals

Intravenous Therapy

Hyperalimentation

Laboratory Studies

Complete blood count
WBC count
Anergy panel
Serum antibody test
Western blot test
Serum protein
Polymerase chain reaction

Cultures
Immunosorbent assay
    T-lymphocyte cells
    T_4 helper cells
    T_8
    p24 antigen
    Immunoglobin

Diagnostic Studies

Magnetic resonance imaging (MRI)
Biopsies
Chest x-ray film

Endoscopy
Gallium scan

Therapies

Nasogastric feeding

Nursing Diagnoses

▲ Outcome Criteria

The client and family members will:

1. Verbalize feelings regarding the diagnosis and prognosis
2. Identify signs of family dysfunction
3. Identify appropriate resources to seek when needed

Altered Family Processes related to the nature of the AIDS condition, role disturbances, and uncertain future

Focus Assessment Criteria	Clinical Significance
1. Understanding of condition (acute versus chronic)	1. The client and family or significant others must understand the reality of AIDS: it is a chronic, debilitating disease with high mortality. Over two-thirds of those with AIDS are not in the hospital or a hospice, but are being cared for at home (Bennett, 1988).
2. Family coping patterns, awareness of client's life style, current response (family, lover, friends)	2. An AIDS diagnosis evokes a variety of responses from family and significant others according to their relationships, their ability to cope, and their knowledge of the client's life style. Responses include shock, disbelief, guilt, or anger in response to the AIDS diagnosis and to the disclosure of client's risk behavior (sexual, drugs). Lovers and friends are confronted with their own mortality and the fear of transmission.
3. Available resources	3. The stigma associated with AIDS may prohibit the client from seeking usual support systems. Expensive treatment, inadequate health insurance, and the inability to work can create serious financial problems for both the patient and family. These feelings and concerns may affect family communication, function, and support and can alter family processes.

Interventions

1. Create a private and supportive environment for the family.

2. Explore family members' perception of the situation. Encourage verbalization of guilt, anger, blame, etc. If family was unaware of the client's sexual or drug use practices prior to the AIDS diagnosis, encourage them to share their feelings.

3. As appropriate, provide information regarding homosexuality and emphasize that the client is the same person he was before the family knew of his sexual orientation.

4. Emphasize aspects of the client's life other than AIDS or risk behaviors, e.g., hobbies, accomplishments.

5. As appropriate, allow the client's lover and friends to share their concerns and previous experiences with AIDS.

6. Discuss with the client the possible conflicts that may arise between his family and his lover and friends.

7. When appropriate, encourage the client to document preferences regarding designated decision-maker, end-of-life care, finances, and funeral arrangements.

8. Determine whether the family's coping mechanisms are effective.

9. Identify dysfunctional coping mechanisms:
   a. Substance abuse
   b. Continued denial
   c. Exploitation of one or more family members
   d. Separation or avoidance
   Refer for counseling as necessary.

10. Promote family strengths:
    a. Acknowledge their assistance.
    b. Involve them in caring for the client.
    c. Encourage time away from the client to prevent burnout.
    d. Encourage a sense of humor.
    Refer to Chapter 3, the Ill Adult: Issues and Responses, for more information.

11. Assist the family to reorganize roles at home, set priorities, and distribute responsibilities. Allow the client to do as much as possible.

12. Warn the family to prepare for depression, anxiety, anger, and dependence from the client.

13. Assist the family to use their social network (e.g., friends, relatives, church or social groups) for support and assistance with care.

Rationale

1. Attempts to communicate a sense of caring and concern to family members can help reduce their feelings of isolation and embarrassment.

2. Open discussions may help reduce feelings of guilt related to causation or anger toward society, the gay community, or the client's lover.

3. These interventions can help decrease guilt and mobilize family members to support the client (Govoni, 1988).

4. This can help deemphasize and destigmatize AIDS (Govoni, 1988).

5. If lovers and friends are members of high-risk groups (homosexuals, IV drug users), they may have experienced AIDS before or may be HIV-positive. Sharing their experiences may help the client and family better understand and cope with the disorder.

6. Initiating dialogue regarding possible conflicts with lovers/friends related to treatment decisions, finances, and care may help clarify misconceptions about roles and responsibilities.

7. This demonstrates that you respect the client's right of self-determination and can help reduce conflict between survivors with contradictory opinions.

8. Illness of a family member may cause significant role changes, putting family members at risk for maladaptation.

9. Any family demonstrating dysfunctional coping may need outside help and additional resources. A family with unresolved conflicts prior to diagnosis is at greatest risk for dysfunctional coping.

10. These interventions can help maintain the family structure and function as a supportive unit.

11. Strategies are needed to maintain family integrity and to reduce stress, as well as to preserve the client's sense of independence and control.

12. Anticipatory guidance can alert family members to impending problems.

13. Outside assistance can help the family avoid isolation and burnout. Your support can encourage a family that is reluctant to disclose

Interventions

Rationale

▲ **Documentation**

Progress notes
    Family functioning
    Dialogues
Discharge summary record
    Referrals, if indicated

14. Direct the family to community agencies and other sources of financial assistance and emotional support.

this situation to others because of the stigma associated with AIDS.

14. The family may need assistance with home care, which helps to maintain personal and family integrity as compared to hospitalization.

▲ **Outcome Criteria**

The client will:

1. Describe how to prevent transmission of infection
2. Describe low-risk sexual behaviors

Potential for Infection Transmission related to contagious nature of blood and body excretions

Focus Assessment Criteria

1. Knowledge of modes of transmission
2. Knowledge of universal precautions
3. Knowledge of high-risk and low-risk behaviors

Clinical Significance

1–3. Knowledge of modes of transmission and prevention strategies can reduce the risk of transmission and the fears associated with it.

Interventions

1. In the hospital:
    a. Wash hands immediately after contact with client materials that may be infectious.
    b. Use masks and gowns if indicated (disposable or nondisposable).

    c. Use disposable gloves as indicated; do not reuse gloves.
    d. Dispose of wastes in accordance with institutional policy.
    e. Dispose of needles and sharps in puncture-proof containers placed in the area of use. Do not recap, bend, or break used needles.
    f. Use protective eye coverings when in close contact with the client's blood or body fluids or when potential exists for splashing or spraying, such as during invasive procedures, suctioning, tracheostomy care, dental care, or postmortem care.
    g. Have disposable resuscitation equipment readily accessible.

    h. Double-bag contaminated items that cannot be disposed of in other ways and according to local regulations for waste disposal, e.g., diapers.
    i. Clean up blood and body fluid spills using gloves and paper towels to get up the majority of the spill; then disinfect with a 1:10 solution of bleach.
    j. Provide a private room if the client has diarrhea or open draining wounds.
2. In the home, teach the client and family members or significant others to do the following:

Rationale

1.
    a. Handwashing is one of the most important means of preventing the spread of infection.
    b. Masks prevent transmission by aerosolization of infectious agents if oral mucosal lesions are present; gowns prevent soiling of clothes if contact with secretions/excretions is likely.
    c. Gloves provide a barrier from contact with infectious secretions and excretions.
    d. Proper disposal reduces the risk of transmission.
    e. These precautions help prevent accidental needlesticks with contaminated equipment.

    f. Eye coverings protect the eyes from accidental exposure to infectious secretions.

    g. Use of resuscitation equipment prevents exposure to infectious body secretions during emergency procedures.
    h. Double-bagging provides extra protection in case of puncture of the first bag.

    i. Proper cleaning and disinfection of the contaminated area prevents transmission of HIV.

    j. Isolation reduces the risk of HIV transmission.
2. Although to date no evidence of viral transmission to anyone other than sexual partners has

Interventions

    a. Wash hands after contact with body fluids (semen, mucus, blood)

    b. Wash hands before handling food

    c. Avoid sharing eating utensils, towels, wash cloths, toothbrushes, razors, and enema equipment.

3. Instruct those who may have been infected to be tested.

4. Teach the client to avoid high-risk behaviors conducive to HIV transmission:

    a. Sexual contact with multiple partners

    b. Oral contact with penis, vagina, and rectum

    c. Sexual practices that can cause tears in mucosal linings of the rectum, penis, or vagina

    d. Sexual intercourse with prostitutes and others identified to be in high-risk groups

    e. Sharing needles with IV drug users; if using IV drugs, use clean needles and syringes

5. Explain measures to help reduce the risk of HIV transmission from the client to others.

    a. Explain low-risk sexual behaviors, such as mutual masturbation, massage, and vaginal intercourse using a condom.

    b. Explain the risk of contact of ejaculate with broken skin or mucous membranes (oral and anal).

    c. Teach to use condoms of latex rubber, not "natural membrane" condoms; teach appropriate storage to preserve latex.

    d. Explain the need to use water-based lubricants to reduce prophylactic breaks and to avoid petroleum-based lubricants, which dissolve latex.

    e. Explain that a condom with a spermicide may provide additional protection by decreasing the number of viable HIV particles.

6. Teach how to disinfect equipment possibly contaminated with the AIDS virus (e.g., needles, syringes, sexual aids):

    a. Wash under running water.

    b. Fill or wash with household bleach.

    c. Rinse well with water.

7. Provide facts to dispel myths regarding AIDS transmission:

    a. The AIDS virus is not transmitted by skin contact, mosquito bites, swimming pools, clothes, eating utensils, telephones, or toilet seats.

    b. Saliva, sweat, tears, urine, and feces do not transmit the AIDS virus.

    c. AIDS cannot be contracted while donating blood.

    d. Blood for transfusions is tested to reduce substantially the risk of contracting the AIDS virus.

8. Provide the national AIDS hotline number (1-800-342-AIDS).

Rationale

been identified (Friedland, Saltzman, and Rogers, 1987), it still is advisable that family members and others caring for or coming in contact with the client take simple precautions.

3. Testing can predict onset of infection, enabling the person to receive medications prophylactically to slow disease progression.

4. HIV is transmitted by sexual contact, by contact with infected blood and blood products, and perinatally (from mother to fetus).

5. These measures aim to prevent contact of body fluids with mucous membranes.

6. HIV is rapidly inactivated by exposure to disinfecting agents. Household bleach solution (dilute 1:10 with water) is an inexpensive choice.

7. Dispelling myths and correcting misinformation can reduce anxiety and allow others to interact more normally with the client.

8. The hotline provides rapid access to accurate information.

▲ **Documentation**

Progress notes
    Precautions needed
    Client teaching
    Outcome achievement or status

▲ **Outcome Criteria**

The client will:

1. Share feelings regarding rejection by others
2. Identify a support system
3. Identify appropriate diversional activities

Social Isolation related to fear of rejection or actual rejection from others secondary to fear

Focus Assessment Criteria	Clinical Significance
1. Previous and current social patterns	1. This assessment helps determine if there has been a negative change, such as lack of participation in social clubs.
2. Support system (family, friends)	2. The nurse should determine what resources and support systems are available to the client. A homosexual client's family may not know of his sexual orientation; fear of this disclosure increases the client's isolation.
3. Emotional status, desire for more contact	3. The emotional suffering associated with social isolation is not always readily apparent.

Interventions	Rationale
1. Encourage the client to share his feelings about changes in his social life after the AIDS diagnosis.	1. The stigma associated with AIDS is connected to the fear of contact, prejudicial attitudes toward homosexuality, family embarrassment, and fear of discovery.
2. Teach the client about HIV transmission. (See the nursing diagnosis Potential for Infection Transmission in this care plan for more information.)	2. Knowledge of the modes of HIV transmission can reduce the fear of casual contact and the need for isolation.
3. Encourage the client to allow friends and family members to share their feelings and fears.	3. Friends and family may need help to deal with their own anxiety, denial, anger, feelings of helplessness, exhaustion, and survivor guilt (Bennett, 1988). Friends and lovers may have lost others to AIDS and may even be HIV-positive themselves.
4. Spend time with the client when support persons are present.	4. The nurse's presence can help validate the client's worth and provides a role model for others for how to interact with the client.
5. Encourage the client to set priorities for the next several months rather than the next several years.	5. Needs typically change over time. Focusing on the "here and now" can decrease anxiety regarding the future (Govoni, 1988).
6. Suggest that the client make contact with those not likely to reject him, e.g., AIDS volunteers, clergy, counselors.	6. Such contacts give the client opportunities to establish trusting relationships and share feelings.
7. Encourage the client to participate in favorite activities and new activities, as able. Enlist the assistance of an occupational or physical therapist, if indicated.	7. Helping the client discover or rediscover pleasure and meaning in activities can promote a focus on life rather than on impending death.
8. Encourage the client to participate in an AIDS support group, if appropriate.	8. Dialogue with others in a similar situation can decrease isolation and allow open confrontation of issues such as death, isolation, fear, and powerlessness. (On the other hand, however, seeing others in advanced stages of the disease can increase fear.)

▲ **Documentation**

Progress notes
    Present activity patterns
    Dialogues

▲ **Outcome Criteria**

The outcome criteria for this diagnosis represent those associated with discharge planning. Refer to the discharge criteria.

Potential Altered Health Maintenance related to insufficient knowledge of condition, medication therapy, modes of transmission, infection control, and community services

Focus Assessment Criteria	Clinical Significance
1. Knowledge of disease, transmission, treatments, complications	1. Assessing knowledge level guides the nurse in determining learning needs and planning teaching strategies.

Focus Assessment Criteria	*Clinical Significance*
2. Ability to learn and retain information	2. High anxiety levels impair learning. A client or family member who does not achieve learning goals requires a referral for assistance postdischarge.

Interventions

1. Help the client formulate and accept realistic short- and long-term goals.

2. Teach about the diagnosis and management techniques.

3. Discuss the vulnerability to misinformation and the need to consult with a knowledgeable nurse or physician.

4. Explain the hazards of infection and ways to reduce the risk:
   a. Avoid contact with infected persons.

   b. Receive immunization against influenza and streptococcal pneumonia, if advisable.
   c. Cleanse all equipment and utensils well before using.

   d. Eat a well-balanced diet and get sufficient rest.

   e. Drink at least 2000 mL of fluids daily, unless contraindicated.

5. Teach energy conservation. (Refer to the Inflammatory Joint Disease care plan, page 296, for specific strategies.)

6. Explain the importance of constructive stress management and reduction; encourage measures such as the following:
   a. Progressive relaxation techniques
   b. Self-coaching
   c. Thought-stopping
   d. Assertiveness training
   e. Guided imagery
   Refer to community resources for further assistance.

7. Teach the effects of medications, immobility, and inadequate nutrition on bowel function and the techniques to prevent constipation or incontinence. (Refer to the Immobility or Unconsciousness care plan, page 243, for specific interventions.)

8. Explore with the client and his or her sex partner(s) problems that may interfere with sexual activity:
   a. Risk and fear of contagion
   b. Fatigue
   c. Guilt
   d. Fear of rejection
   e. Depression
   f. Skin lesions

Rationale

1. Such planning reinforces the client's sense of control over his or her life, which may promote compliance with the treatment regimen.

2. The client's understanding contributes to improved compliance and reduced risk of complications.

3. A person with an incurable disease is vulnerable to inaccurate claims from quacks and well-meaning but misinformed friends.

4. Minor infections can cause serious problems in a client with AIDS.
   a. Minimizing contact with infected persons reduces the risk of cross-infection.

   b. Immunization conveys protection against these infections.
   c. Cleansing removes microorganisms and secretions that provide a medium for microorganism growth.
   d. Good nutrition and adequate rest promote overall good health and increase infection resistance.
   e. Adequate hydration prevents concentrated urine with high bacteria levels.

5. Stress, nutritional deficiencies, and chronic infections cause fatigue.

6. Stress management minimizes external and internal demands and conflicts (Lazarus, 1984), which releases energy for more positive functioning.

7. Constipation results from decreased peristalsis due to immobility, medications, or insufficient fluid and fiber intake. Bowel incontinence is caused by lesions in the efferent pathways of the corticospinal tract, resulting in loss of sphincter control.

8. Libido is negatively influenced by stress, fatigue, low self-esteem, and neurological effects of HIV infection. Skin lesions and other appearance changes can negatively affect a sexual relationship.

Interventions	*Rationale*
9. Explain the signs and symptoms that must be reported to a health care professional:	9. Early detection and reporting of complications enables prompt intervention, which may reduce their severity.
a. Increase in symptoms (e.g., lesions, swollen glands, pain)	a. Worsening symptoms may indicate disease exacerbation.
b. Fever, chills	b–e. These signs and symptoms point to infection.
c. Frequency and burning on urination	
d. Cloudy, foul-smelling urine	
e. Cough or dyspnea	
f. White patches and ulcerations in mouth	f. Skin and mucous membrane lesions may result from Kaposi's sarcoma or fungal infection.
g. Persistent headache or changes in affect and mentation	g. These symptoms may indicate encephalopathy.
10. Emphasize the importance of following the prescribed medication regimen and the need for regular follow-up examinations.	10. A constant blood level of medication must be maintained to ensure antiviral effects. Careful monitoring of hematological results is needed to detect bone marrow depression.
11. Provide information and materials to assist the client and family to maintain goals and manage at home:	11. A client who feels well-supported can cope better with the great stress associated with AIDS.
a. Local AIDS task force	
b. Home health agencies	
c. Hospice	
d. Individual/family counselors	
12. Refer to the nursing diagnoses Potential for Infection in the Leukemia care plan, page 343, and Potential for Infection Transmission in this care plan for specific infection and transmission prevention strategies.	

▲ **Documentation**

Discharge summary record
    Client and family teaching
    Outcome achievement or status
    Referrals, if indicated

References/Bibliography

Bennett, J. (1988). Helping people with AIDS live well at home. *Nursing Clinics of North America, 23*(4), 731–748.

Brunner, L., & Suddarth, D. (1988). *Textbook of medical-surgical nursing* (6th ed.). Philadelphia: J.B. Lippincott.

Carpenito, L.J. (1989). *Nursing diagnosis: Application to clinical practice* (3rd ed.). Philadelphia: J.B. Lippincott.

Friedland, G.H., Saltzman, B.R., & Rogers, M.F. (1987). Additional evidence for lack of transmission of HIV infection to household contacts of AIDS patients. Paper presented at the Third International Conference on AIDS, Washington, D.C., June 2, 1987.

Govoni, L. (1988). Psychosocial issues of AIDS in the nursing care of homosexual men and their significant other. *Nursing Clinics of North America, 23*(4), 749–765.

Grady, C. (Ed.). (1988). AIDS. *Nursing Clinics of North America, 23*(4), 683–862.

Sepes, C. (1988). The haunting facts, the human care (A skillbook with CEUs). *Nursing Life, 8*(2), 33–41.

Neoplastic Disorders

Cancer (Initial Diagnosis)

Cancer involves a disturbance in normal cell growth in which abnormal cells arise from normal cells, reproduce rapidly, and infiltrate tissues, lymph, and blood vessels. The destruction caused by cancer depends on its site, whether it metastasizes, its obstructive effects, and its effects on the body's defense system (e.g., nutrition, hemopoiesis). Cancer is classified according to the cell of origin; malignant tumors from epithelial tissue are called carcinomas, and those from connective tissue are known as sarcomas. Treatment varies depending on classification, cancer stage, and other factors.

Diagnostic Cluster

▲ Time Frame

Initial diagnosis

▲ Discharge Criteria

Before discharge, the client and/or family will:

1. Relate an intent to share concerns with a trusted confidante
2. Describe early signs of family dysfunction
3. Identify signs and symptoms that must be reported to a health care professional
4. Identify available community resources

Nursing Diagnoses

Anxiety related to unfamiliar hospital environment, uncertainty about outcomes, feelings of helplessness and hopelessness, and insufficient knowledge about cancer and treatment

Potential Self-Concept Disturbance related to changes in life style, role responsibilities, and appearance

Altered Family Processes related to fears associated with recent cancer diagnosis, disruptions associated with treatments, financial problems, and uncertain future

Decisional Conflict related to treatment modality choices

Grieving related to potential loss of body function and the perceived effects of cancer on life style

Potential Social Isolation related to fear of rejection or actual rejection secondary to fear

Potential Spiritual Distress related to conflicts centering on the meaning of life, cancer, spiritual beliefs, and death

Refer to:

Acquired Immunodeficiency Syndrome
Cancer (End-Stage)

Related Care Plans

Chemotherapy
Radiation Therapy

Nursing Diagnoses

▲ Outcome Criteria

The client will share concerns regarding the cancer diagnosis.

Anxiety related to unfamiliar hospital environment, uncertainty about cancer treatment outcomes, feelings of helplessness and hopelessness, and insufficient knowledge about cancer and treatments

Focus Assessment Criteria

1. Level of understanding of condition, past experiences with cancer
2. Familiarity with hospital environment, diagnostic tests, and treatment plan
3. Life style, strengths, coping mechanisms, and available support systems

Clinical Significance

1–3. This assessment helps the nurse identify learning needs and plan appropriate teaching strategies. Health professionals recognize that cancer is a chronic disease that can be cured or controlled with treatment. In the general public, however, the term cancer conjures thoughts of death. Lack of knowledge and negative attitudes about cancer, coupled with the unfamiliarity of medical treatments and the hospital environment, cause most newly diag-

Focus Assessment Criteria	*Clinical Significance*
	nosed clients to respond with anxiety and fear, even when the prognosis is good. The physiological and psychological effects of treatments produce changes in body image, life style, and function, which also can contribute to fear and anxiety.

Interventions	*Rationale*

1. Provide opportunities for the client and family members to share feelings.
   a. Initiate frequent contacts and provide an atmosphere that promotes calm and relaxation.
   b. Convey a nonjudgmental attitude and listen attentively.
   c. Explore feelings about upcoming treatments and resources for coping with anxiety. Identify support systems, other resources, and coping strategies for reducing anxiety, e.g., diversion, relaxation techniques, stress management.
	1. Frequent contact by the caregiver indicates acceptance and may facilitate trust. The client may be hesitant to approach the staff because of negative self-concept. The nurse should not make assumptions about a client's or family member's reaction; validating the person's particular fears and concerns helps increase self-awareness.

2. Encourage an open discussion of cancer, experiences of others, and its potential for cure.	2. The nurse who can talk openly about life after a cancer diagnosis offers encouragement and hope.
3. Explain hospital routines and reinforce the physician's explanations of scheduled tests and the proposed treatment plan. Focus on what the client can expect.	3. Accurate descriptions of sensations and procedures help ease anxiety and fear associated with the unknown.

4. Identify those at risk for unsuccessful adjustment:
   a. Poor ego strength
   b. Ineffective problem-solving ability
   c. Poor motivation
   d. External focus of control
   e. Poor overall health
   f. Lack of positive support systems
   g. Unstable economic status
   h. Rejection of counseling (Shipes, 1987).
	4. A client identified as high-risk may need referrals for counseling. Successful adjustment is influenced by factors such as the following: previous coping success; achievement of developmental tasks presurgery; the extent to which the disorder and treatment interfere with goal-directed activity; sense of self-determination and control; and realistic perception of the disorder.

▲ **Documentation**

Progress notes
   Present emotional status
   Interventions utilized
   Response to interventions

▲ **Outcome Criteria**

The client will:

1. Communicate feelings about changes
2. Participate in self-care

Potential Self-Concept Disturbance related to changes in life style, role responsibilities, and appearance

Focus Assessment Criteria	*Clinical Significance*
1. Previous exposure to persons with cancer 2. Ability to express feelings about condition 3. Ability to share feelings with family members and significant others 4. Self-concept, and others' perceptions of client's self-concept	1–4. This information helps the nurse detect patterns of response due to adaptation. It may be helpful to note how the client's support persons view the client's self-concept; they can provide insight into factors that may have had a negative impact on self-concept, and they tend to be sensitive to subtle changes.
5. Participation in self-care 6. Evidence of adapting life style to accommodate disabilities	5,6. Participation in self-care and adapting goals to disability indicates attempts to cope with the changes (Hamburg, 1953)

Interventions	Rationale
1. Contact the client frequently and treat him with warm, positive regard.	1. Frequent contact by the caregiver indicates acceptance and may facilitate trust. The client may be hesitant to approach the staff because of negative self-concept.

2. Encourage the client to express feelings and thoughts about the following:
  a. Condition
  b. Progress
  c. Prognosis
  d. Effects on life style
  e. Support system
  f. Treatments
	2. Encouraging the client to share feelings can provide a safe outlet for fears and frustrations and can increase self-awareness.

3. Provide reliable information and clarify any misconceptions.	3. Misconceptions can needlessly increase anxiety and damage self-concept.
4. Help the client to identify positive attributes and possible new opportunities.	4. The client may tend to focus only on the change in self-image and not on the positive characteristics that contribute to the whole concept of self. The nurse must reinforce these positive aspects and encourage the client to reincorporate them into his new self-concept.
5. Assist with hygiene and grooming, as needed.	5. Participation in self-care and planning can aid positive coping.
6. Encourage visitors.	6. Frequent visits by support persons can help the client feel that he is still a worthwhile, acceptable person, which should promote a positive self-concept.

7. Help the client identify strategies to increase independence and maintain role responsibilities:
  a. Prioritizing activities
  b. Getting assistance with less valued or most fatiguing activities, e.g., shopping, housekeeping
  c. Using energy conservation techniques (Refer to the nursing diagnosis Fatigue in the Inflammatory Joint Disease care plan, page 297, for specific strategies.)
  d. Using mobility aids and assistive devices, as needed
	7. A strong component of self-concept is the ability to perform functions expected of one's role, thus decreasing dependency and reducing the need for others' involvement.

8. Discuss ways that the client can provide support to support persons:
  a. Actively listening to their problems
  b. Attempting to decrease the focus on disabilities
  (Refer to Chapter 3, The Ill Adult: Issues and Responses, for more information.)
	8. The nurse can help the client learn how to balance relationships and preserve the family system.

9. Help the client identify potential opportunities for self-growth through living with cancer:
  a. Living and getting the most out of each day
  b. Value of relationships
  c. Increase in knowledge, personal strength, and understanding
  d. Spiritual and moral development
	9. Experiences with cancer can provide the client with opportunities to reevaluate his or her life and to focus on personal priorities.

10. Allow the client's support persons to share their feelings regarding the diagnoses and actual or anticipated effects.	10. Cancer can have a negative impact on the client's family financially, socially, and emotionally.

Interventions	*Rationale*

11. Assess for signs of negative response to changes in appearance:
   a. Refusal to discuss loss
   b. Denial of changes
   c. Decreased self-care ability
   d. Social isolation
   e. Refusal to discuss future
	11. A client at high risk for unsuccessful adjustment should be identified for additional interventions or referrals.

12. Assist with management of alopecia, as necessary:
   a. Explain when hair loss occurs (usually within 2 to 3 weeks of initiation of therapy) and when regrowth will begin (usually 4 to 6 weeks after discontinuation of therapy).
   b. Suggest cutting long hair to minimize fallout.
   c. Suggest resources for wigs and hairpieces.
   d. Discuss measures to reduce hair loss in low-dose therapy, e.g., wash hair only twice a week, use a mild shampoo, avoid brushing.
   e. Encourage good grooming, hygiene, and other measures to enhance appearance (e.g., makeup, manicures, new clothes).
	12. Embarrassment from alopecia can contribute to isolation and negative self-concept.

13. Discuss possible emotional reactions—sadness, depression, anger. Encourage verbalization of feelings.	13. Changes in appearance often initiate the grieving process.
14. Discuss the advantages and disadvantages of scalp tourniquets and ice caps to prevent hair loss. The advantages are that they provide some control over hair loss and may reduce hair loss, especially in low-dose chemotherapy or radiation therapy. The disadvantages include possible micrometastasis to scalp not protected by chemotherapy, discomfort, and high cost.	14. Understanding advantages and disadvantages allows the client to make an informed decision regarding these treatments.
15. Refer an at-risk client for professional counseling.	15. Some clients may need follow-up therapy to aid with effective adjustment.

▲ **Documentation**

Progress notes
  Present emotional status
  Interventions
  Response to interventions

▲ **Outcome Criteria**

The client and family members will:

1. Verbalize feelings regarding the diagnosis and prognosis
2. Identify signs of family dysfunction
3. Identify appropriate resources to seek when needed

Altered Family Processes related to fears associated with recent cancer diagnosis, disruptions associated with treatments, financial problems, and uncertain future

Focus Assessment Criteria	*Clinical Significance*

1. Understanding of condition
2. Family coping patterns
3. Current response
4. Available resources
	1–4. The family unit is a system based on interdependence between members and patterns that provide structure and support. Chronic illness in one family member disrupts these relationships and patterns. Cancer and its treatment may be as threatening to the family as it is to the client. Common sources of fear and disruption include the following:
	   a. The mistaken belief that cancer is contagious and can be "caught"
	   b. Concerns about the hereditary nature of cancer
	   c. Guilt
	   d. Anger

Focus Assessment Criteria

Clinical Significance

e. Revulsion at the client's appearance
f. Concerns about caregiving ability
g. Worry about death
h. Financial problems
These feelings and concerns can affect family communication, function, and support, and can alter family processes.

Interventions

1. Convey an understanding of the situation and its impact on the family.

2. Explore family members' perceptions of the situation. Encourage verbalization of feelings such as guilt, anger, and blame.
3. Determine whether present coping mechanisms are effective.

4. Take steps to promote family strengths:
   a. Acknowledge the assistance of family members.
   b. Involve the family in the client's care.
   c. Encourage time away from caregiving to prevent burnout.
   d. Encourage humor.
   (Refer to Chapter 3, The Ill Adult: Issues and Responses, for more information.)
5. Assist to reorganize roles at home, set new priorities, and redistribute responsibilities.
6. Prepare the family for signs of depression, anxiety, anger, and dependency in the client and other family members.
7. Encourage the family to call on its social network (e.g., friends, relatives, church members) for emotional and other support.
8. Identify dysfunctional coping mechanisms:
   a. Substance abuse
   b. Continued denial
   c. Exploitation of one or more family members
   d. Separation or avoidance (Friedman, 1981). Refer for counseling as necessary.
9. Direct to community agencies and other sources of assistance (e.g., financial, housekeeping, direct care), as needed.

Rationale

1. Communicating understanding and a sense of caring and concern facilitates trust and strengthens the nurse's relationship with the client and family.
2. Verbalization can provide an opportunity for clarification and validation of feelings and concerns, contributing to family unity.
3. Illness of a family member may cause great changes, putting the family at high risk for maladaption.
4. This can help maintain the existing family structure and its function as a supportive unit.

5. Planning and prioritizing can help maintain family integrity and reduce stress.
6. Anticipatory guidance can alert members to potential problems before they occur, enabling prompt intervention at early signs.
7. Outside assistance may help reduce the perception that the family must "go it alone."

8. A family with a history of unsuccessful coping may need additional resources. A family with unresolved conflicts prior to diagnosis is at high risk.

9. The family may need assistance to help with management at home.

▲ **Documentation**

Progress notes
    Present family functioning
    Interventions
    Response to interventions
Discharge summary record
    Referrals, if indicated

▲ **Outcome Criteria**

The client and family members will:

1. Relate the advantages and disadvantages of choices
2. Share their fears and concerns regarding a decision
3. Make an informed choice

Decisional Conflict related to treatment modality choices

Focus Assessment Criteria

1. Knowledge of cancer diagnosis, treatment options, and treatment plan
2. Decision-making pattern
3. Other involved parties (e.g., relatives, friends, physician)
4. Possible conflicts (e.g., religion, culture, family)

Clinical Significance

1–4. These assessments provide the nurse with needed information to assist the client and family with informed decision-making.

Interventions

1. Provide, reinforce, and clarify information about the diagnosis, treatment options, and treatment plan.
2. Allow the client and family members opportunities to share feelings and concerns regarding the decision.

3. Ensure that the client and family clearly understand what is involved in each treatment alternative.
4. As appropriate, assure the client that he does not have to abide by decisions that others make, but that he can choose for himself. Discourage family members and others from undermining the client's confidence in his decision-making ability.
5. Provide as much time as possible for decision-making.
6. If indicated, encourage the client to seek a second professional opinion.

Rationale

1. The client and family need specific, accurate information in order to make an informed decision.
2. Conflict is more intense when the decision has potentially negative impacts or conflicting opinions exist. Anxiety and fear have a negative impact on decision-making ability. Providing opportunities to share feelings and concerns can help reduce anxiety.
3. Informed decisions support a person's right to self-determination.
4. Each person has the right to make his or her own decisions and to expect respect from others.

5. Effective and informed decision-making requires time to consider all alternatives thoroughly.
6. A second opinion can confirm information and validate options.

▲ **Documentation**

Progress notes
   Dialogues

▲ **Outcome Criteria**

The client and family members will:

1. Express grief
2. Describe the personal meaning of the loss
3. Report an intent to discuss his or her feelings with significant others

Grieving related to potential loss of body function and the perceived effects on life style

Focus Assessment Criteria

1. Signs and symptoms of grief reaction, e.g., crying, anger, withdrawal
2. Significance of loss, coping mechanisms
3. Personal strengths, support systems

Clinical Significance

1–3. At diagnosis, most clients with cancer experience losses secondary to the disease and its treatment; major losses may include the following:
  a. Loss of functional ability
  b. Change in role
  c. Social isolation
  d. Loss of intimacy
  e. Anticipatory loss of life
These losses, like any, are accompanied by grief feelings. Evaluation of the losses, the client's response, and coping mechanisms, personal strengths, and support systems guides the nurse in planning appropriate interventions.

Interventions

1. Provide opportunities for the client and family members to ventilate feelings, discuss the loss openly, and explore the personal meaning of the loss. Explain that grief is a common and healthy reaction.
2. Encourage use of positive coping strategies that have proven successful in the past.
3. Encourage the client to express positive self-attributes.
4. Implement measures to support the family and promote cohesiveness:

Rationale

1. A cancer diagnosis typically gives rise to feelings of powerlessness, anger, profound sadness, and other grief responses. Open, honest discussions can help the client and family members accept and cope with the situation and their response to it.
2. Positive coping strategies aid acceptance and problem-solving.
3. Focusing on positive attributes increases self-acceptance and acceptance of the diagnosis.
4. Family cohesiveness is important to client support.

Interventions

Rationale

    a. Help family members acknowledge losses.

    b. Explain the grieving process.

    c. Encourage verbalization of feelings with the client.

    d. Allow participation in care to promote comfort.

    e. Encourage discussing the significance of the relationship.

5. Promote grief work with each response:

    a. Denial:

      • Encourage acceptance of the situation; do not reinforce denial by giving false reassurance.

      • Promote hope through assurances of care, comfort, and support.

      • Explain the use of denial by one family member to other members.

      • Do not push a person to move past denial until he is emotionally ready.

    b. Isolation:

      • Convey acceptance by encouraging expressions of grief.

      • Promote open, honest communication to encourage sharing.

      • Reinforce the client's self-worth by providing privacy, when desired.

      • Encourage socialization, as feasible (e.g., support groups, church activities).

    c. Depression:

      • Reinforce the client's self-esteem.

      • Employ empathetic sharing and acknowledge grief.

      • Identify the degree of depression and develop appropriate strategies.

    d. Anger:

      • Explain to other family members that anger represents an attempt to control the environment stemming from frustration at the inability to control the disease.

      • Encourage verbalization of anger.

    e. Guilt:

      • Acknowledge the person's expressed self-image.

      • Encourage identification of the relationship's positive aspects.

      • Avoid arguing and participating in the person's system of "I should have . . ." and "I shouldn't have. . . ."

    f. Fear:

      • Focus on the present and maintain a safe and secure environment.

      • Help the person explore reasons for and meanings of the fears.

    g. Rejection:

      • Provide reassurance by explaining what is happening.

      • Explain this response to other family members.

5. Grieving involves profound emotional responses; interventions depend on the particular response.

▲ Documentation

Progress notes
  Present emotional status
  Interventions
  Response to nursing inter-
   ventions

Interventions

h. Hysteria:
- Reduce environmental stressors (e.g., limit personnel).
- Provide a safe, private area in which to express grief.

Rationale

References/Bibliography

Bouchard, R., & Speese, N. (1981). *Nursing care of the cancer patient.* St. Louis: C.V. Mosby.

Carpenito, L.J. (1989). *Nursing diagnosis: Application to clinical practice* (3rd ed.). Philadelphia: J.B. Lippincott.

Chernecky, C.C., & Ramsey, P.W. (1984). *Critical nursing care of the client with cancer.* Norwalk, CT: Appleton-Century Crofts.

Dickson, A.C., Dodd, M.J., Carrier, V., et al. (1985). Comparison of a cancer-specific locus of control and the multidimensional health locus of control scales in chemotherapy. *Oncology Nursing Forum, 12*(3), 49–54.

Friedman, M. (1981). *Family nursing: Theory and assessment.* New York: Appleton-Century-Crofts.

Hamburg, D. A., & Adams, J. E. (1953). A perspective on coping behaviors. *Archives of General Psychiatry, 17,* 1–20.

Highfield, M.F., & Cason, C. (1983). Spiritual needs of patients. *Cancer Nursing, 6*(3), 187–192.

Mariono, L.B. (1981). *Cancer nursing.* St. Louis: C.V. Mosby.

McNally, J.C., Stair, J.C., & Somerville, E. (1985). *Guidelines for nursing practice.* Orlando, FL: Grune & Stratton.

Shipes, E. (1987). Psychosocial issues: The person with an ostomy. *Nursing Clinics of North America, 22*(2), 291–302.

Simko, L.D. (1987). *Cancer nursing principles and practice.* New York: Jones and Bartlett.

Stupczynski, J.S. (1984). Dealing with life-threatening complications of cancer. *Consultant, 24*(3), 207–223.

Ulrich, C.P., Canale, S.W., & Wendell, S.A. (1986). *Nursing care planning guides: A nursing diagnosis approach.* Philadelphia: W.B. Saunders.

End-Stage Cancer

Approximately 400,000 people in the United States die from cancer each year. Cancer that cannot be controlled by treatment metastasizes to adjacent organs and structures or spreads through the blood and lymphatics to a distant site, such as the liver, brain, or bones. For example, a client with end-stage colon cancer may have a tumor in the colon causing bowel obstruction. Metastasis to the liver causes ascites, edema, and clotting problems; metastasis to the lung promotes respiratory alterations.

End-stage cancer with metastasis can result in many structural and functional problems, depending on the body area(s) or system(s) affected. Potential complications also depend on the affected site; only those specific to end-stage cancer are discussed in this care plan.

Diagnostic Cluster

▲ Time Frame

Terminal stage (care in home, hospital, long-term care facility, or hospice)

▲ Discharge Criteria

Before discharge, the client or family will:

1. Relate an intent to share feelings with a trusted friend
2. Relate strategies to manage discomfort
3. Identify personal strengths
4. Identify community resources available for assistance
5. Describe signs and symptoms of complication that must be reported to a health care professional
6. Identify two sources of spiritual comfort

Collaborative Problems

Potential Complications: *Refer to:*
Hypercalcemia
Negative Nitrogen Balance
Malignant Effusions
Narcotic Toxicity
Pathological Fractures
Spinal Cord Compression
Superior Vena Cava Syndrome
Intracerebral Metastasis   Cerebrovascular Accident
                                                     (Stroke)
Myelosuppression   Chemotherapy

Nursing Diagnoses

Anxiety related to effects of disease process and inadequate relief from pain-relief measures

Grieving related to terminal illness, impending death, functional losses, and withdrawal of or from others

Powerlessness related to change from curative status to palliative status

Hopelessness related to overwhelming functional losses or impending death

Potential Spiritual Distress related to fear of death, overwhelming grief, and belief system crisis

Potential Impaired Home Maintenance Management related to insufficient knowledge of home care, pain management, signs and symptoms of complications, and community resources available

Altered Nutrition: Less Than Body Requirements related to   Chemotherapy
decreased oral intake, increased metabolic demands of tumor, and altered lipid metabolism

Constipation related to decreased dietary fiber intake, decreased   Immobility or
intestinal mobility secondary to narcotic medications and   Unconsciousness
inactivity

Pruritus related to dry skin secondary to dehydration or   Hepatitis (Viral)
accumulation of bile salts secondary to biliary duct obstruction

Nursing Diagnoses, cont'd.

Ineffective Airway Clearance related to decreased ability to expectorate secretions secondary to weakness, increased viscosity, and pain	Pneumonia
Potential for Disuse Syndrome related to pain, weakness, fatigue, and edema	Immobility or Unconsciousness
Potential for Injury related to weakness, fatigue secondary to anemia, electrolyte imbalances, or somnolence secondary to medications or disease process	Cerebrovascular Accident (Stroke)
Self-Care Deficit related to fatigue, weakness, sedation, pain, and decreased sensory-perceptual capacity	Immobility or Unconsciousness
Self-Concept Disturbance related to dependence on others to meet basic needs	Multiple Sclerosis
Altered Family Processes related to change to terminal status, unresolved relationship conflicts, and concerns regarding coping and managing home care	Multiple Sclerosis

Related Care Plans

Specific Surgical Care Plan
Radiation Therapy
Chemotherapy

Collaborative Problems

▲ *Nursing Goal*

The nurse will detect, manage, and minimize complications of cancer.

Potential Complication: Hypercalcemia
Potential Complication: Negative Nitrogen Balance
Potential Complication: Malignant Effusions
Potential Complication: Narcotic Toxicity
Potential Complication: Pathological Fractures
Potential Complication: Spinal Cord Compression
Potential Complication: Superior Vena Cava Syndrome

Interventions

1. Monitor for signs and symptoms of hypercalcemia:
   a. Altered mental status
   b. Dysrhythmias
   c. Numbness or tingling in fingers and toes
   d. Muscle cramps
   e. Seizures
2. Monitor for signs of negative nitrogen balance:
   a. Weight loss
   b. 24-Hour urine nitrogen balance below zero

3. Monitor laboratory values:
   a. Serum calcium
   b. Ionized calcium
   c. Serum albumin
   d. Blood urea nitrogen (BUN)
   e. Creatinine
   f. Electrolytes

Rationale

1. Hypercalcemia (serum calcium > 11 mg/dL) is a common complication of end-stage cancer. It occurs most often in multiple myeloma, breast cancer, and metastatic bone cancer, owing to disturbed calcium reabsorption.

2. A client with advanced cancer has an abnormal sugar tolerance with resistance or decreased sensitivity to insulin, which inhibits cell nourishment. Cachexia results from the increased metabolic demands of the tumor, altered lipid metabolism, and anorexia. Impaired carbohydrate metabolism causes increased metabolism of fats and protein, which—especially in the presence of metabolic acidosis—can lead to negative nitrogen balance.

3. Selected laboratory studies are done to monitor nutritional status and to detect early changes in renal function.

Interventions

4. Monitor for malignant effusions (excessive accumulation of fluid in the pleural space, peritoneal cavity [ascites], or pericardial space).
   a. Pleural effusion:
      • Variable dyspnea
      • Pleuritic pain
      • Diminished and delayed chest movement on the involved side
      • Bulging of intercostal spaces (in a large effusion)
      • Decreased breath sounds auscultated over the effusion
      • Decreased vocal and tactile fremitus
      • Increased respiratory rate and depth
   b. Ascites:
      • Abdominal distention
      • Fluid wave
      • Generalized edema
      • Reduced bladder capacity
      • Indigestion
      • Early satiety
      • Decreased serum albumin and protein values
      • Abnormal clotting factors and electrolyte values
   c. Pericardial effusion:
      • Dyspnea
      • Muffled heart sounds
      • Friction rub
      • Orthopnea
      • Neck vein distention
      • Increased central venous pressure
5. Monitor abdominal girth and weight daily.

6. Monitor for signs of narcotic toxicity:
   a. Increased sedation
   b. Drowsiness
   c. Depressed respiratory rate

7. As necessary, intervene for narcotic toxicity:
   a. Monitor sedation level frequently. Expect peak effects from narcotics 5 to 10 minutes after intravenous injection, 30 minutes after intramuscular (IM) injection, and 90 minutes after subcutaneous (SQ) injection.
   b. Withhold narcotic dose if sedation level increases; assess results.
   c. If respirations fall below 12, monitor patient carefully; below 10, notify the physician.
   d. If respirations continue to fall, consult with the physician for a narcotic antagonist (e.g., Naloxone).
8. Monitor for signs and symptoms of pathological fracture:
   a. Pain in the back, neck, or extremities

Rationale

4. Effusions cause pain and discomfort and inhibit function.

   a. Collections of fluid (either transudates or exudates) in the pleural cavity, pleural effusions are common with lung cancer, breast cancer, and lymphomas. Obstruction of the pulmonary vein by the tumor increases hydrostatic pressure and promotes leakage of fluid into the pleural space.

   b. Accumulation of serous fluid in the peritoneal cavity caused by obstruction in portal circulation, ascites is commonly associated with ovarian, endometrial, breast, colon, stomach, and pancreatic cancer.

   c. Tumors of the lung and breast, leukemia, lymphomas, melanomas, and sarcomas metastasize to the pericardium and promote pericardial effusions. These effusions interfere with cardiac function, reducing cardiac volume during diastole and decreasing cardiac output and venous return.
5. These measurements help detect fluid retention and ascites.
6. Many health professionals are overly concerned about narcotic toxicity and may needlessly withold narcotics from a terminally ill client. A client in severe pain can tolerate very high doses of narcotics without developing excessive sedation and respiratory depression.
7. Narcotic toxicity can occur if excretion is impaired, e.g., in liver dysfunction. Sedation usually precedes respiratory depression; withholding drugs when sedation occurs usually heads off respiratory depression. Narcotic antagonists reduce opioid effects by competing for the same receptor sites.

8. Pathological fractures occur in about 8% of clients with bone metastasis. Bones most susceptible to tumor invasion are those with the

Interventions

     b. Visible bone deformity
     c. Crepitation on movement
     d. Loss of movement or use
     e. Localized soft tissue edema
     f. Skin discoloration

9. Maintain alignment and immobilize the site if fracture is suspected.
10. If a stabilization device is necessary, refer to the Casts care plan, page 518, for specific interventions.
11. Monitor for signs and symptoms of spinal cord compression:
     a. Neck or back pain—gradual onset, relieved by sitting, and aggravated by lying and movement
     b. Motor deficits—weakness, spasticity, paralysis, ataxia, flacidity, atrophy, hyporeflexia or hyper-reflexia
     c. Sensory deficits—loss of pain sensation, loss of temperature sensation, paresthesias
12. Maintain bed rest.

13. Monitor respiratory, bowel, and bladder function.

14. Monitor for signs and symptoms of superior vena cava syndrome (SVCS):
     a. Gradual onset of swelling in the face, trunk, and arms
     b. Periorbital edema
     c. Distended thoracic and neck veins
     d. Horner's syndrome (drooping of one eyelid, pupil constriction, conjunctivitis, anhidrosis)
     e. Tachypnea
     f. Tachycardia
     g. Dyspnea
     h. Cyanosis
     i. Dysphasia
     j. Frequent cough

Rationale

greatest bone marrow activity and blood flow—the vertebrae, pelvis, ribs, skull, and sternum. The most common sites for long bone metastasis are the femur and humerus.

9. Immobilization helps reduce soft tissue damage from dislocations.
10. Devices may be necessary to stabilize bones.

11. Spinal cord compression results from tumor invasion into the epidural space or from bony erosion and altered vertebral alignment secondary to fracture. Symptoms vary depending on the extent and location of compression. Treatments include radiation therapy and corticosteroids for compression resulting from an extradural mass and a decompression laminectomy for compression due to bony erosion.

12. Immobility reduces the risk of injury to the spinal cord.
13. The level of the cord compression influences respiratory (cervical), bowel (lumbar), and bladder (lumbar) functioning.
14. SVCS occurs when the superior vena cava becomes occluded by a tumor or thrombus. Commonly associated with lung cancer, breast cancer, and lymphomas, SVCS causes impaired venous return from the head and upper extremities, resulting in upper body edema and prominent collateral circulation.

▲ **Documentation**

Flow records
    Daily weights
    Vital signs
    Auscultation findings (lung, heart)
    Abdominal girth
    Intake and output
Progress notes
    New complaints

Related Physician-Prescribed Interventions

Medications

Dependent on symptomatology	Chemotherapy
Analgesics	Antiemetics

Intravenous Therapy

Replacement (fluid, electrolytes)	Transfusions
Albumin	

Laboratory Studies

Dependent on history, clinical symptomatology	Serum protein
Complete blood count	Carcinogenic antigens
Blood chemistry	

Diagnostic Studies

Varies according to site, clinical symptomatology	Scans (computed tomography [CT], magnetic resonance imaging [MRI], gallium)
Biopsies	Chest x-ray films

Therapies

Radiation

Nursing Diagnoses

▲ **Outcome Criteria**

The client will:

1. Practice selected noninvasive pain relief measures
2. Report relief after pain relief measures and an increase in activity

Anxiety related to effects of disease process and inadequate relief from pain relief measures

Focus Assessment Criteria	*Clinical Significance*

1. Source of pain:
  a. Obstruction
  b. Effusions (pleural, ascites)
  c. Invasive lines
  d. Immobility
  e. Skeletal source
  f. Muscular source
	1. Pain is caused by destruction of nerves and tissue; other pain may develop from complications or from treatment. Distinguishing the source of pain guides pain relief interventions.

2. Client's perception of pain severity based on a scale of 0 to 10 (0 = no pain, 10 = worst pain), rated as follows:
  a. At its worst
  b. At its best
  c. After each pain relief intervention
	2. This scale provides a good method of evaluating the subjective experience of pain.

3. Physical signs of pain, e.g., increased pulse rate and respirations, elevated blood pressure, restlessness, facial grimacing, guarding	3. In some clients objective signs may be more reliable indicators of pain; for whatever reason, some clients are reluctant to express pain or request pain relief medications.
4. Activity pattern, emotional response	4. This assessment evaluates the effects of pain on functioning.
5. Medications (type, dosage, interval)	5. A medication history can help evaluate effectiveness of pharmacological pain relief.
6. Sedation level, respiratory rate	6. These data establish a baseline for subsequent assessments.
7. Use of noninvasive pain relief techniques	7. Noninvasive measures can promote comfort and relaxation, which reduces pain.

Interventions

1. Assist in identifying the source of pain:
   a. Obstruction
   b. Effusions
   c. Invasive lines
   d. Immobility
   e. Skeletal source
   f. Muscular source
2. Convey that you acknowledge and accept his pain.

3. Provide accurate information:
   a. Explain the cause of the pain, if known.
   b. Explain how long the pain should last, if known.
   c. If indicated, reassure that narcotic addiction is not likely to develop from the pain relief regimen.
4. Provide privacy for the client during acute pain episodes.
5. Provide optimal pain relief with prescribed analgesics.
   a. Determine the preferred route of administration; consult with the physician.

Rationale

1. Do not assume that all pain is related to tissue destruction. Pain of different origins requires different interventions for relief.

2. A client who feels that he must convince skeptical caregivers of the seriousness of his pain experiences increased anxiety, which can increase pain.
3. A client who understands and is prepared for pain by detailed explanations tends to experience less stress—and, consequently, less pain—than a client who receives vague or no explanations.

4. Privacy reduces embarrassment and anxiety and enables more effective coping.
5.

   a. If frequent injections are necessary, the IV route is preferred because it is not painful and absorption is guaranteed.

Interventions

b. Assess vital signs, especially respiratory rate, before and after administration.
c. Consult with a pharmacist for possible adverse interactions with other medications the client is taking, such as muscle relaxants and tranquilizers.
d. Consult with the physician for a regular narcotic administration schedule.

e. If necessary, use the p.r.n. approach to pain medication; administer before treatment procedures or activity, and instruct the client to request pain medications as needed before pain becomes severe.
f. About ½ hour after administration, assess pain relief.

6. Consult with the physician for co-analgesic medications, as necessary:
   a. Bone pain—aspirin or ibuprofen
   b. Increased intracranial pressure—dexamethasone
   c. Postherpetic neuralgia—amitriptyline
   d. Nerve pressure—prednisone
   e. Gastric distention—metoclopramide
   f. Muscle spasm—diazepam
   g. Lymphodermia—diuretics
   h. Infection—antibiotics

7. Explain and assist with noninvasive pain relief measures:
   a. Splinting
   b. Positioning
   c. Distraction
   d. Massage
   e. Relaxation techniques

8. Consult with the physician for other invasive pain relief measures:
   a. Radiation
   b. Nerve block
   c. Surgery

9. Emphasize the need to report unsatisfactory pain relief.

Rationale

b. Narcotics depress the brain's respiratory center.
c. Some medications potentiate the effects of narcotics.

d. The scheduled approach may reduce the total 24-hour drug dose as compared to the p.r.n. approach, and may reduce the client's anxiety associated with having to ask for and wait for p.r.n. medications.
e. The p.r.n. approach is effective for breakthrough pain or to manage additional pain from treatments and procedures.

f. Response to analgesics can vary with stress levels, fatigue, and pain intensity.
6. In addition to narcotics, other medications can help relieve pain and discomfort.

7. Certain measures can relieve pain by preventing painful stimuli from reaching higher brain centers. They also may improve the client's sense of control over pain.

8. Radiation can reduce the tumor size to decrease compression on structures and reduce obstructions. Nerve blocks cause an interruption in nerve function through injection of a local anesthetic (temporary) or a neurodestructive agent (permanent). Surgery can decrease tumor bulk to reduce pressure and obstruction.
9. Prompt reporting enables rapid adjustment to control pain.

▲ **Documentation**

Medication administration record
 Type, dose, time, route of all medications
Progress notes
 Unsatisfactory relief from pain
 Noninvasive relief measures

Grieving related to terminal illness and impending death, functional losses, changes in self-concept, and withdrawal of or from others

Focus Assessment Criteria

1. Response to earlier losses, current losses, and feelings

Clinical Significance

1. End-stage cancer results in many losses; major losses include these:
   a. Loss of functional ability
   b. Change in role
   c. Social isolation
   d. Loss of intimacy
   e. Anticipatory loss of life

▲ Outcome Criteria

The client will:

1. Verbalize losses and changes
2. Verbalize feelings associated with losses and changes
3. Acknowledge that death is imminent

Family members will do the following:

1. Maintain an effective closure relationship, as evidenced in this manner:
   a. Spending time with the client
   b. Maintaining loving, open communication with the client
   c. Participating in care

Focus Assessment Criteria

2. Impact of losses on self

3. Acknowledgment of impending death

4. Grief feelings of family members
5. Distress level of client and family members
6. Client–family relationship and support
7. Family communication

Clinical Significance

2. These losses, like any, are accompanied by grief feelings.
3. A dying person needs to acknowledge impending death so that grief work can begin.
4–7. Family members may need help and support to maintain an effective closure relationship with the client.

Interventions

1. Provide opportunities for the client and family members to ventilate feelings, discuss the loss openly, and explore the personal meaning of the loss. Explain that grief is a common and healthy reaction.

2. Encourage use of positive coping strategies that have proven successful in the past.
3. Encourage the client to express positive self-attributes.
4. Help the client acknowledge and accept impending death; answer all questions honestly.

5. Promote grief work with each response:
   a. Denial:
      • Encourage acceptance of the situation; do not reinforce denial by giving false reassurance.
      • Promote hope through assurances of care, comfort, and support.
      • Explain the use of denial by one family member to other members.
      • Do not push a person to move past denial until he is emotionally ready.
   b. Isolation:
      • Convey acceptance by encouraging expressions of grief.
      • Promote open, honest communication to encourage sharing.
      • Reinforce the client's self-worth by providing for privacy, when desired.
      • Encourage socialization, as feasible (e.g., support groups, church activities).
   c. Depression:
      • Reinforce the client's self-esteem.
      • Employ empathetic sharing and acknowledge grief.
      • Identify the degree of depression and develop appropriate strategies.
   d. Anger:
      • Explain to other family members that anger represents an attempt to control the environment stemming from frustration at the inability to control the disease.
      • Encourage verbalization of anger.
   e. Guilt:
      • Acknowledge the person's expressed self-image.

Rationale

1. The knowledge that no further treatment is warranted and that death is imminent may give rise to feelings of powerlessness, anger, profound sadness, and other grief responses. Open, honest discussions can help the client and family members accept and cope with the situation and their response to it.
2. Positive coping strategies aid acceptance and problem-solving.
3. Focusing on positive attributes increases self-acceptance and acceptance of imminent death.
4. Grief work, the adaptive process of mourning, cannot begin until the impending death is acknowledged.
5. Grieving involves profound emotional responses; interventions depend on the particular response.

Interventions

    • Encourage identification of the relationship's positive aspects.
    • Avoid arguing and participating in the person's system of "I should have . . ." and "I shouldn't have. . . ."
  f. Fear:
    • Focus on the present and maintain a safe and secure environment.
    • Help the person explore reasons for and meanings of the fears.
  g. Rejection:
    • Provide reassurance by explaining what is happening.
    • Explain this response to other family members.
  h. Hysteria:
    • Reduce environmental stressors (e.g., limit personnel).
    • Provide a safe, private area in which to express grief.
6. Encourage the client to engage in a life review, focusing on accomplishments and disappointments. Assist in attempts to resolve unresolved conflicts.
7. Implement measures to support the family and promote cohesiveness:
  a. Help acknowledge losses and impending death.
  b. Explain the grief process.
  c. Encourage verbalization of feelings with the client.
  d. Explain expected behaviors during terminal stages (denial, anger, depression, and withdrawal).
  e. Allow participation in care to promote comfort.
  f. Encourage discussing the significance of the relationship.
  g. Promote adequate rest and nutrition.
  h. Assist with funeral home arrangements, if needed.
  i. Refer to a bereavement support group.
8. Promote hope by assurances of attentive care, relief of discomfort, and support.

Rationale

6. Life review provides an opportunity to prepare for life closure.

7. Family cohesiveness is important to client support.

8. Studies show that terminally ill clients most appreciate the following nursing care measures: assisting with grooming, supporting independent functioning, providing pain medications when needed, and enhancing physical comfort (Skorupka & Bohnet, 1982).

▲ **Documentation**

Progress notes
  Present emotional status
  Interventions
  Response to nursing interventions

▲ **Outcome Criteria**

The client will:
1. Identify factors that can be controlled
2. Participate in decisions regarding care and activities

Powerlessness related to change from curative status to palliative status

Focus Assessment Criteria	*Clinical Significance*
1. Perception of loss of control 2. Feelings of powerlessness and grief 3. Threat of death 4. Inability to make decisions and solve problems 5. Patient strengths and capabilities, available support	1–5. A client's response to loss of control depends on the personal meaning of the loss, individual coping patterns, personal characteristics, and responses of others.

Interventions

1. Determine the client's usual response to problems.

2. Help the client identify personal strengths and assets.
3. Assist in identifying energy patterns and scheduling activities to accommodate these patterns.
4. Help the client prioritize activities and schedule them during usual periods of high energy.

5. Help the client identify components of the situation that can be controlled or maintained:
   a. Comfort
   b. Care schedule
   c. Family interaction and communication
   d. Home care decisions
   e. Death with dignity
   f. Funeral arrangements
6. Promote effective problem-solving by breaking activities down into parts:
   a. Things to be resolved now
   b. Things that require time to resolve
   c. Things that cannot be changed (e.g., impending death)
7. As appropriate, provide opportunities for the client to make decisions about certain aspects of the care plan.
8. Promote communication of feelings and concerns among family members and significant others.
9. If family support is not available, do the following:
   a. Identify possible community resources for home support.
   b. Explain long-term care placement.
   c. Refer to social services or to a clergyman, if appropriate.
   d. Provide social support using volunteer and professional services.

Rationale

1. It is important to determine whether the client usually seeks to change own behaviors to control problems or expects others or external factors to control problems.
2. Discouraging the client from focusing only on limitations can promote self-esteem.
3. A review of the client's daily schedule helps in planning appropriate rest periods.
4. Scheduling can help the client to participate in activities that promote feelings of self-worth and dignity.
5. Loss of power in one area may be counterbalanced by the introduction of other sources of power or control.

6. A sense of control may be established by breaking the situation down into some components that can be controlled.

7. Allowing the client to make decisions reinforces respect for his or her right of self-determination.
8. Open communication can help enlist the support of others.

9. Although end-stage cancer cannot be cured and death will occur, clients and support persons need a sense of hope. The client should believe that he will be comfortable, that his care needs will be met, that he can maintain relationships with others, and he will die with dignity.

▲ **Documentation**

Progress notes
    Participation in self-care, decisions
    Emotional status
    Interactions

▲ **Outcome Criteria**

The client will:
1. Express confidence that he/she will receive the needed care and be comfortable
2. Share his/her suffering openly
3. Die with dignity

Hopelessness related to overwhelming functional losses and impending death

Focus Assessment Criteria	*Clinical Significance*
1. Response to impending death	1,2. Hopelessness is a subjective emotional state that must be validated through assessment.
2. Available support	
3. Spiritual beliefs	3. For some clients, spiritual beliefs can sustain hope for eternal peace when life on earth ends.

Interventions

1. Discuss the medical situation honestly.

2. Redirect the client to identify alternative sources of hope:
   a. Relationships
   b. Faith
   c. Things to accomplish

Rationale

1. Promoting hope for a cure sets the client and support persons up for false hope and despair.
2. Coping with an aspect of one's life that is uncontrollable may be facilitated by recognizing the other positive aspects.

Interventions

3. Help the client to identify realistic hope in his situation:
   a. He will be comfortable.
   b. He will receive needed care.
   c. He will maintain significant relationships.
   d. He will die with dignity.
4. Encourage the client to appreciate the fullness of each moment, each day.
5. Promote a positive psychosocial environment through measures such as the following:
   a. Providing favorite foods
   b. Encouraging personalization of the room
   c. Keeping the room clean and comfortable
6. Help the client to identify purpose in his life, such as in these ways:
   a. Model for others
   b. Love
   c. Advice

Rationale

3. Others can promote hope. Their support can help the client gain confidence and autonomy.

4. Redirecting thoughts can produce growth and strength even in a time of conflict.
5. These techniques show that the client is respected and valued.

6. The dying person can provide others with a gift—an example of how to live with imminent death and how to control one's death.

▲ *Documentation*

Progress notes
  Dialogues
  Emotional, spiritual status

▲ *Outcome Criteria*

The client will:

1. Express feelings regarding beliefs
2. Discuss the meaning and purpose of illness and death

Spiritual Distress related to fear of death, overwhelming grief, belief system conflicts, and unresolved relationship conflicts

Focus Assessment Criteria	*Clinical Significance*
1. Doubting or loss of faith	1–3. The stresses of terminal illness may threaten a client's relationship with a higher being, his beliefs, or others.
2. Religious practices, religious leader (access, visits)	
3. Present response (anger, guilt, self-hate, sadness)	

Interventions

1. Communicate willingness to listen to the client's feelings regarding spiritual distress.

2. Suggest a contact with another spiritual support person—e.g., the hospital chaplain—if the client is reluctant to share feelings with his usual spiritual advisor.
3. Explore if the client desires to engage in a religious practice or ritual, and accommodate his request to the extent possible.
4. Offer to pray with him or read from a religious text.

Rationale

1. The client may view anger at God and a religious leader as a "forbidden" topic, and may be reluctant to initiate discussions of spiritual conflicts.
2. Other contacts may help the client move toward a new spiritual understanding.

3. The client may value prayer and spiritual rituals highly.

4. This can help meet the client's spiritual needs.

▲ *Documentation*

Progress notes
  Dialogues
  Interventions
  Spiritual status
  Referrals

Potential Impaired Home Maintenance Management related to insufficient knowledge of home care, signs and symptoms of complications, pain management, and community resources available

▲ *Outcome Criteria*

The outcome criteria for this diagnosis represent those associated with discharge planning. Refer to the discharge criteria.

Focus Assessment Criteria	*Clinical Significance*
1. Willingness and ability of caregiver(s) to learn treatment measures, manage equipment, and perform needed care	1,2. The wide-ranging aspects and consequences of end-stage cancer require that caregivers be well-versed in all aspects of care.
2. Understanding of home care needs	

Interventions

1. Discuss home care needs:
   a. Treatments
     • Pressure ulcer care

Rationale

1. Each client has specific individual care needs. Understanding can maximize the effectiveness of treatment.

Interventions

- Wound care
- Tube care
- Injections
- Tracheostomy care
- Ostomy care
- Denver shunt management

b. Equipment
- Supplemental oxygen
- Suction equipment
- IV equipment
- Assistive devices (e.g., walker, wheelchair)

c. Care needs
- Positioning
- Feeding and bathing techniques
- Transfer techniques
- Injury prevention strategies

2. Teach home care measures and evaluate ability.
a. Provide written teaching materials for treatments and equipment when feasible.
b. Demonstrate procedures, equipment, and care measures.
c. Have the caregiver return demonstration under supervision until skill is evident.
d. Provide for practice to increase caregiver's skill.
e. Encourage verbalization of questions and concerns.
f. Provide positive reinforcement.

3. Explain the pain management plan to be used at home.

4. Discuss factors besides the disease that can contribute to pain:
a. Positioning
b. Cutaneous stimulation
c. Activity
d. Certain foods
e. Emotional factors

5. Discuss the action, duration, and side effects of prescribed narcotics and co-analgesics.

6. Demonstrate procedures and equipment used to administer pain medication; have the caregiver(s) perform return demonstration to assess competence.

7. Provide caregiver(s) with an opportunity to practice with supervision. Provide positive reinforcement.

8. Explain how and where to obtain needed equipment and supplies.

9. Teach signs and symptoms that must be reported to a health care professional:

a. Change in mental status, visual changes, muscle coordination

Rationale

2. Specific instructions can reduce fear related to lack of knowledge and help the nurse determine what follow-up teaching is needed.

3. The client's particular situation must be considered to develop an effective plan for pain relief.

4. Pain can arise from sources and factors other than the cancer itself. Each source of pain requires specific interventions.

5. Understanding may reduce administration errors and serious side effects.

6. Support persons' ability to perform procedures safely and confidently must be determined before discharge.

7. Practice enables caregivers to refine their skills. Positive reinforcement encourages learning and mastery of skills.

8. Knowledge of access postdischarge can reduce some apprehension and facilitate care.

9. Early reporting may enable prompt interventions to reduce or eliminate certain complications.
a. Neurological changes may indicate cerebral metastasis, which can be sudden or insidious. Cancers of the lung, breast, testicles, thyroid, kidney, prostate, melanoma, and leukemia are associated with cerebral metastasis.

Interventions	*Rationale*
b. Muscle cramps, numbness	**b.** Muscle cramps and numbness may point to calcium imbalance.
c. Increasing dyspnea, edema, abdominal distention	**c.** These symptoms may indicate malignant effusions (pleural, ascites, pericardial).
d. Increasing sedation, decreasing respirations	**d.** Sedation and respiratory depression may indicate narcotic toxicity.
e. Skeletal pain, loss of movement	**e.** Pain and limited movement may indicate pathological fracture.
f. Neck or back pain, motor deficits, sensory deficits (e.g., paresthesias)	**f.** These signs and symptoms may point to cord compression.
g. Change in bowel or bladder function	**g.** Bladder or bowel changes may result from cord compression or ascites.
h. Facial edema, dyspnea, distended neck veins	**h.** These effects may indicate superior vena cava syndrome (SVCS), which is associated with lung cancer, breast cancer, and lymphoma.
10. If skeletal pain, loss of movement, neck or back pain occurs, teach to maintain bed rest and to immobilize the area until a health professional can examine it.	**10.** Immobilization helps prevent further tissue damage.
11. Discuss possible cancer- and death-related stressors with the family, such as financial burdens, role responsibility changes, and dependency. (Refer to Chapter 3, The Ill Adult: Issues and Responses, for information regarding the effects of terminal illness on families.)	**11.** Terminal illness entails a wide range of stressors. Preparing the family for possible problems enables planning to prevent or minimize them.
12. Provide information about or initiate referrals to community resources, e.g., hospice, counselors, home health agencies, American Cancer Society.	**12.** Assistance may be needed with home management and with minimizing the potential destructive effects on the client and family.

▲ Documentation

Discharge summary record
  Client teaching
  Outcome achievement or
    status
  Referrals, if indicated

References/Bibliography

Refer also to references for Cancer (Initial Diagnosis).

Garfield, C. (1978). *Psychosocial care of the dying patient.* New York: McGraw-Hill.
Goldberg, R., & Tull, R.M. (1983). *The psychosocial dimensions of cancer.* New York: Macmillan.
Groenwald, S.L. (1987). *Cancer nursing principles and practice.* New York: Jones and Bartlett.
Hampe, S. (1975). Needs of the grieving spouse in a hospital setting. *Nursing Research, 24*(2), 113–119.
Jones, W.H. (1983). Loss in a hospital setting: Implications for counseling. *The Personnel and Guidance Journal, 22*(4), 359–362.
Kiely, W.F. (1972). Coping with severe illness. *Advances in Psychosomatic Medicine, 8,* 105.
Kirschling, J.M. (1985). Support utilized by caregivers of terminally ill family members: Clinical implications for hospice team members. *American Journal of Hospice Care, 2*(2), 27–31.
Kritek, P.B. (1981). Patient power and powerlessness. *Supervisor Nurse, 12*(6), 26–34.
Lindsey, A.N. (1986). Cancer cachexia effects of disease and its treatment. *Seminars on Oncology Nursing, 6*(4), 19–27.
Miller, J. (1983). *Coping with chronic illness: Overcoming powerlessness.* Philadelphia: F.A. Davis.
Petrosino, B. (Ed.). (1986). Nursing in hospice and terminal care. *The Hospice Journal, 1*(2), 1–9.
Rubin, P. (1983). *Clinical oncology: A multidisciplinary approach* (6th ed.). New York: American Cancer Society.
Skorupka, P., & Bohnet, N. (1982). Primary caregiver's perceptions of nursing behaviors that best meet their needs in a home care hospice setting. *Cancer Nursing, 5*(5), 371–374.

Leukemia

Leukemia is a disease of the bone marrow that causes abnormalities in the blood elements: white blood cells (WBCs), red blood cells (RBCs), and platelets. Immature WBCs, leukemic cells are produced in large numbers in the bone marrow, interfering with RBC and platelet production.

Leukemia is classified according to the cell line involved. Acute myeloblastic leukemia (AML) involves uncontrolled proliferation of myeloblasts. Acute lymphoblastic leukemia (ALL), which occurs primarily in children, involves proliferation of immature lymphocytes. Chronic lymphocytic leukemia (CLL) involves proliferation of long-lived incompetent lymphocytes. Chronic granulocytic leukemia (CGL) involves proliferation of mature granulocytes in the bone marrow.

Diagnostic Cluster

▲ **Time Frame**

Initial diagnosis

Collaborative Problems:

Potential Complications
Myelosuppression
Hepatosplenomegaly
Lymphadenopathy
CNS Involvement
Electrolyte Imbalance

Refer to:

Nursing Diagnoses

Potential for Infection related to increased susceptibility secondary to leukemic process and side effects of chemotherapy

Potential for Injury related to bleeding tendencies secondary to leukemic process and side effects of chemotherapy

Potential Altered Health Maintenance related to insufficient knowledge of disease process, treatment, signs and symptoms of complications, reduction of risk factors, and community resources

Potential Impaired Social Interactions related to fear of rejection or actual rejection of others after diagnosis — Cancer (Initial Diagnosis)

Powerlessness related to inability to control situation — Cancer (Initial Diagnosis)

Potential Altered Sexual Patterns related to fear secondary to potential for infection and injury — Cancer (Initial Diagnosis)

Related Care Plans

Chemotherapy
Cancer (Initial Diagnosis)

▲ **Discharge Criteria**

Before discharge, the client and/or family will:

1. Describe the home care regimen, including restrictions
2. Identify the signs and symptoms of complications that must be reported to a health care professional
3. Describe the necessary follow-up care
4. Verbalize an awareness of available community resources

Collaborative Problems

▲ **Nursing Goal**

The nurse will manage and minimize complication of leukemia.

Potential Complication: Myelosuppression
Potential Complication: Hepatosplenomegaly
Potential Complication: Lymphadenopathy
Potential Complication: CNS Involvement
Potential Complication: Electrolyte Imbalance

Interventions

1. Monitor for signs of myelosuppression:
   a. Decreased WBC count
   b. Decreased hemoglobin and hematocrit

Rationale

1. The client is at high risk for infection, bleeding, and anemia because of WBC immaturity and inadequate RBC and platelet production. Transfu-

Interventions

    c. Decreased platelet count

    d. Decreased granulocyte count

2. Monitor for signs of hepatosplenomegaly:

    a. Weight gain

    b. Elevated liver enzymes

    c. Ascites

3. Monitor for lymphadenopathy (cervical, axillary, and inguinal).

4. Monitor for central nervous system (CNS) involvement:

    a. Altered level of consciousness

    b. Headaches

    c. Blurred vision

    d. Change in coordination, facial symmetry, or muscle strength

5. Monitor for electrolyte imbalance:

    a. Elevated blood urea nitrogen (BUN) and creatinine

    b. Elevated serum potassium

    c. Elevated serum phosphorus

    d. Elevated serum uric acid

    e. Decreased serum calcium

    f. Decreased serum sodium

6. Monitor intake and output.

Rationale

sions generally are required to maintain hemoglobin and platelet counts.

2. Leukemic cells can infiltrate the liver, spleen, lymph nodes, and cerebrospinal fluid, causing abnormalities of these systems and increasing the client's morbidity and mortality. Such infiltrations occur most commonly in ALL and CLL.

3. Leukemic cells can infiltrate the lymph nodes, causing tenderness and obstruction.

4. CNS involvement can result from infiltration of leukemic cells into the cerebrospinal fluid, which increases intracerebral pressure and compresses cerebral tissue.

5. Electrolyte imbalance can occur secondary to tumor lysis, resulting in severe renal, cardiac, and neuromuscular damage. It is most severe in clients with high leukemic cell counts and most common at the initiation of treatment.

6. Careful intake and output monitoring detects fluid imbalance, which can occur secondary to tumor lysis.

▲ **Documentation**

Flow records
    Intake and output
    Vital signs
    Weight
    Physical assessment
Progress notes
    Abnormal assessment findings
    Interventions
    Response to interventions

Related Physician-Prescribed Interventions

Medications

Antineoplastics   Analgesics (nonaspirin)

Antibiotics   Antiemetics

Stool softeners

Intravenous Therapy

Granulocyte transfusion   Platelet transfusion

Blood transfusion

Laboratory Studies

Complete blood count   Urinalysis

Liver enzyme levels   BUN level

Chemistry tests for leukemia   Prothrombin time

Blood cultures   Partial thromboplastin time

Uric acid level

Diagnostic Studies

Bone marrow aspiration   Tomography scan

Chest x-ray film   Liver-spleen scan

Lumbar puncture

Therapies

Nutritional supplements

Nursing Diagnoses

▲ **Outcome Criteria**

The client will:

1. Identify risk factors that can be reduced

2. Relate early signs and symptoms of infection

Potential for Infection related to increased susceptibility secondary to leukemic process and side effects of chemotherapy

Focus Assessment Criteria

1. History of infections

Clinical Significance

1. The client is at high risk for infection owing to WBC immaturity and inadequate numbers of RBCs. Infection is the major cause of death in leukemia.

Focus Assessment Criteria	*Clinical Significance*
2. Vital signs	2. Fever is the hallmark sign of infection in a leukemic client. Changes in vital signs—especially pulse and blood pressure—usually are the first signs of septic shock.
3. Biopsy, puncture, and catheterization sites 4. Respiratory system: cough, sputum, lung fields 5. Gastrointestinal (GI) system: nausea, vomiting, diarrhea, perianal area 6. Genitourinary (GU) system: intake and output, urine characteristics, frequency, burning, perineal area	3–6. Meticulous total body assessment is necessary every shift because usual clues to infection—such as inflammation and pus formation—usually are not present owing to WBC dysfunction.
7. Laboratory values: WBCs, granulocytes, cultures	7. WBCs, particularly granulocytes, are the first line of defense against infection. As levels decrease, susceptibility to infection increases, as follows: a. 2500–2000/mm³: no risk b. 2000–1000/mm³: minimal risk c. 1000–500/mm³: moderate risk d. < 500/mm³: severe risk
8. Medication use, e.g., corticosteroids, antipyretics	8. Corticosteroids and antipyretics mask signs and symptoms of infection, particularly fever.

Interventions	*Rationale*

1. Institute measures to prevent exposure to known or potential sources of infection:
  a. Maintain protective isolation in accordance with institutional policy.
  b. Maintain meticulous handwashing.
  c. Provide scrupulous hygiene.
  d. Restrict visitors with colds, flu, or infections.
  e. Provide good perianal hygiene twice daily and after each bowel movement.
  f. Restrict fresh flowers and plants.
  g. Restrict fresh fruits and vegetables.
  h. Provide good oral hygiene after each meal.
	1. These precautions minimize the client's exposure to bacterial, viral, and fungal pathogens, both exogenous and endogenous.

2. Notify the physician of any changes in vital signs.	2. Subtle changes in vital signs may be only early signs of sepsis.
3. Obtain cultures of sputum, urine, diarrhea, blood, and abnormal body secretions as ordered.	3. Cultures can confirm infection and identify the causative organism.
4. Explain the reasons for precautions and restrictions.	4. The client's understanding may improve compliance and reduce risk factors.
5. Reassure the client and family that the increased susceptibility to infection is only temporary. (Granulocytopenia can persist for 6 to 12 weeks.)	5. Understanding the temporary nature of granulocytopenia may help prevent the client and family from becoming discouraged.
6. Minimize invasive procedures, e.g., rectal and vaginal examinations, indwelling (Foley) catheter insertion.	6. Certain procedures cause tissue trauma, increasing the susceptibility to infection.

▲ **Documentation**

Flow records
  Vital signs
  Intake and output
  Assessments
  WBC/granulocyte count
Progress notes
  Abnormal findings or complaints
Discharge summary record
  Client teaching

▲ **Outcome Criteria**

The client will:
1. Identify risk factors for bleeding that can be reduced
2. Describe early signs and symptoms of bleeding

Potential for Injury related to bleeding tendencies secondary to leukemia process and side effects of chemotherapy

Focus Assessment Criteria	*Clinical Significance*
1. History of bleeding 2. Laboratory values: platelet and WBC counts	1,2. Bleeding is the second leading cause of death in leukemia. As platelet count de-

Focus Assessment Criteria	Clinical Significance
	creases, the risk of bleeding increases, as follows:
	a. > 100,000: no risk
	b. 100,000–50,000: minimal risk
	c. 50,000–20,000: moderate risk
	d. < 20,000: severe risk.
3. Vital signs	3. Hypotension and tachycardia occur with large blood volume loss.
4. Medication history	4. Some medications interfere with platelet functioning, e.g., aspirin, heparin, warfarin (Coumadin), indomethacin (Indocin), ibuprofen.

Interventions

1. Assess for signs of bleeding every day to every shift, as necessary:
   a. Petechiae on skin and mucous membranes
   b. Ecchymoses on skin and mucous membranes
   c. Hematomas on skin and mucous membranes
   d. Bleeding gums
   e. Epistaxis
   f. Conjunctival hemorrhage
   g. Hematemesis or coffee ground emesis
   h. Hemoptysis
   i. Hematuria
   j. Vaginal bleeding
   k. Rectal bleeding or tarry stools
   l. Prolonged bleeding from puncture sites
   m. Changes in neurological status, e.g., headache, blurred vision, loss of vision, disorientation, seizures
   n. Changes in abdominal status, e.g., epigastric pain, absent bowel sounds, abdominal rigidity
2. Transfuse blood components, as ordered.

3. Minimize invasive procedures; avoid the following:
   a. Rectal temperatures
   b. Suppositories
   c. Intramuscular (IM) and subcutaneous (SC) injections
   d. Vaginal douches
   e. Bladder catheterization
4. Apply pressure to puncture sites for 3 to 5 minutes.

5. Provide soft toothbrushes or sponges for oral hygiene.
6. Explain the following to the client and family:
   a. Rationales for precautions
   b. Signs and symptoms that must be reported to a health care professional
   c. The need to avoid medications that interfere with platelet function; provide a list.
7. Take steps to prevent constipation; administer stool softeners as ordered and needed.

Rationale

1. Regular total body assessment is necessary to detect early signs of bleeding.

2. Platelet transfusions are given to maintain platelet count and decrease the risk of bleeding.
3. Invasive procedures can cause tissue trauma.

4. This prevents prolonged bleeding from puncture sites, which can cause damage to underlying structures, such as nerves.
5. This can help prevent damage to oral mucosa, which is susceptible to bleeding.
6. The client's and family's understanding can encourage compliance and reduce anxiety.

7. Constipation can cause stress on the lower GI tract and possibly hemorrhoidal bleeding.

▲ **Documentation**

Flow records
    Vital signs
    Intake and output
    Platelet count
    Assessments
Progress notes
    Abnormal assessment or complaints
Discharge summary record
    Client teaching

▲ Outcome Criteria

The outcome criteria for this diagnosis represent those associated with discharge planning. Refer to the discharge criteria.

Potential Altered Health Maintenance related to insufficient knowledge of disease process, treatment, signs and symptoms of complications, reduction of risk factors, and community resources

Focus Assessment Criteria	*Clinical Significance*
1. Understanding of condition, past experiences with cancer	1. This assessment helps the nurse identify learning needs and plan appropriate teaching strategies.
2. Life style, personal strengths, coping mechanisms, available support systems	2. Health professionals recognize that cancer is a chronic disease that can be cured or controlled with treatment. In the general public, however, the term cancer conjures thoughts of death. Lack of knowledge and negative attitudes about cancer, coupled with the unfamiliarity of medical treatments and the hospital environment, cause most newly diagnosed clients to respond with anxiety and fear, even when the prognosis is good. The physiological and psychological effects of treatments produce changes in body image, life style, and function, which also can contribute to fear and anxiety.

Interventions	*Rationale*

1. Explain leukemia to the client and family, including the following aspects:
  a. Pathophysiology
  b. Function of bone marrow
  c. Potential complications
	1. Providing specific information about leukemia can help the client and family understand the need for treatments and precautions, which may improve compliance.

2. Explain that anemia causes fatigue; stress the need for energy conservation. (Refer to the nursing diagnosis Fatigue in the Inflammatory Joint Disease care plan, page 297, for specific strategies.)	2. Anemia results from inadequate RBC production secondary to increased WBC production. Energy conservation reduces fatigue.
3. Teach the importance of optimal nutrition.	3. Adequate intake of protein, carbohydrates, vitamins, and minerals is required for tissue rebuilding and increased resistance to infection.
4. Provide written information about and applications for registration to the Leukemia Society of America and local leukemia foundations.	4. These resources can provide emotional support and possibly financial assistance.
5. Teach to inspect oral mucous membranes daily and teach the importance of good oral care.	5. Inadequate defense mechanisms (e.g., abnormal WBC count, bone marrow suppression) increase the risk for infection.
6. Teach the importance of good perianal hygiene and of avoiding constipation and rectal trauma (e.g., enemas, thermometers).	6. Rectal abscesses can occur from trauma and constipation, increasing the susceptibility to infection.
7. Teach to avoid all immunizations.	7. An immunosuppressed client must avoid immunization, as he lacks the ability to build antibodies and can contract the disease from the immunization.
8. Teach to avoid over-the-counter (OTC) drugs.	8. Many OTC medications contain guaifenesin, which interferes with platelet function.

9. Teach measures to avoid bacteria in the diet:
  a. Avoid raw fruits and vegetables.
  b. Avoid fried foods in restaurants.
	9. These foods are a potential source of bacterial pathogens.

10. Teach the client to report the following:
  a. Petechiae and ecchymoses
  b. Fever and chills
  c. Increasing malaise
	10. These signs and symptoms may be the only indications of infection.

Interventions

Rationale

▲ *Documentation*

Discharge summary record
  Client teaching
  Outcome achievement or
    status
  Referrals, if indicated

    d. Cough
    e. Rectal pain
    f. Stool changes
11. Explain chemotherapy. (Refer to the Chemo-
    therapy care plan, page 532, for specific inter-
    ventions and rationales.)

References/Bibliography

Campbell, J.B., Preston, R., & Smith, K.Y. (1983). The leukemias. *Nursing Clinics of North America, 18*(3), 523–541.

Cohen, D.G. (1983). Metabolic complications of induction therapy for leukemia and lymphoma. *Cancer Nursing, 6*(4), 307–310.

Harper-Grace Hospitals (1985). *Nursing diagnosis standard care plans.* Detroit: Harper-Grace Hospitals.

Kelly, J.O. (1983). Standards of clinical nursing practice: Neutropenia and thrombocytopenia. *Cancer Nursing, 6*(6), 487–494.

McNally, J.C., Stair, J.C., & Somerville, E.T. (Eds.). (1985). *Guidelines for cancer nursing practice.* Orlando, FL: Grune & Stratton.

Reich, P.R. (1984). *Hematology* (2nd ed.). Boston: Little, Brown.

Simonson, G.M. (1988). Caring for patients with acute myelocytic leukemia. *American Journal of Nursing, 88*(3), 304–309.

Abdominal Aortic Aneurysm Resection

This procedure involves surgical resection of an aneurysm—a localized or diffuse arterial enlargement of an artery—and a replacement graft of the aorta. Aneurysm can result from arteriosclerosis, trauma to the artery, congenital weakness, or previous infections.

Diagnostic Cluster

▲ **Time Frame**

Preoperative and postoperative periods

PREOPERATIVE PERIOD
Collaborative Problems

Potential Complication:
Rupture of aneurysm

POSTOPERATIVE PERIOD
Collaborative Problems

Potential Complications:
Distal Vessel Thrombosis or Emboli
Renal Failure
Mesenteric Ischemia/Thrombosis
Spinal Cord Ischemia

Nursing Diagnoses

Potential Altered Health Maintenance related to insufficient knowledge of home care, activity restrictions, signs and symptoms of complications, and follow-up care
Potential for Infection related to location of surgical incision
Potential Sexual Dysfunction (male) related to possible loss of ejaculate and erections secondary to surgery or atherosclerosis

Related Care Plan

General Surgery Generic Care Plan (Appendix II)

Refer to:

Arterial Bypass Graft
Colostomy

▲ **Discharge Criteria**

Before discharge, the client or family will:

1. State wound care measures to perform at home
2. Verbalize precautions regarding activities
3. State signs and symptoms that must be reported to a health care professional

Preoperative: Collaborative Problems

▲ **Nursing Goal**

The nurse will detect and manage a ruptured aneurysm.

Potential Complication: Ruptured Aneurysm

Interventions

1. Monitor all pulses (carotid, brachial, radial, ulnar, femoral, popliteal, dorsalis pedis, and posterior tibial).

2. Monitor for signs and symptoms of aneurysm rupture:

Rationale

1. A carotid bruit must be evaluated preoperatively to rule out the risk of stroke during the operation. Assessing upper extremity pulses establishes a baseline for follow-up after arterial lines are in place and arterial punctures made for blood gas analysis. Assessing lower extremity pulses establishes a baseline for postoperative assessment. (A potential complication of aneurysm repair is thrombosis or embolus of distal vessels.) Also, clients with abdominal aneurysm have a higher incidence of popliteal aneurysm than the general population.

2. The larger the aneurysm, the greater the risk of rupture. Aneurysms greater than 6 cm in diameter have a high risk of rupture within a year of discovery.

Interventions

   a. Acute abdominal pain with intense back or
      pelvic pain

   b. Shock

   c. Tender, pulsating abdomen

   d. Restlessness
3. Initiate emergency measures as necessary.

Rationale

   a. Pain results from massive tissue hypoxia
      and profuse bleeding into the abdominal cav-
      ity.
   b. Shock may result from massive blood loss
      and tissue hypoxia.
   c. Abdominal pulsations and tenderness result
      from rhythmic pulsations of the artery and
      tissue hypoxia, respectively.
   d. Restlessness is a response to tissue hypoxia.
3. Surgery for ruptured aneurysm carries a mortality rate of 30% to 50%; without immediate
   surgery, however, mortality rate is near 100%.

▲ **Documentation**

Flow records
   Vital signs
Progress notes
   Unusual events
   Interventions

Postoperative: Collaborative Problems

▲ **Nursing Goal**

The nurse will manage and minimize vascular complications.

Potential Complication: Distal Vessel Thrombosis or Emboli
Potential Complication: Renal Failure
Potential Complication: Mesenteric Ischemia/Thrombosis
Potential Complication: Spinal Cord Ischemia

Interventions

1. Monitor for signs of thrombosis in distal vessels:
   a. Diminished distal pulses, decreased capillary
      refill time (< 3 seconds)
   b. Pallor or darkened patches of skin
2. Instruct the client to report numbness or tingling in the distal extremities.

3. If the client complains of pain, evaluate its location and characteristics.

Rationale

1. Comparing pulses, capillary refill, and color
   against preoperative baseline findings aids early
   detection of thrombosis.

2. Thrombosis of an artery supplying the leg results in a cool, pale, numb, or tingling extremity.
3. It is important to differentiate pain of surgical
   manipulation from ischemic pain. Microemboli-
   zation from the aneurysm to the distal skin
   causes skin infarctions, manifested by point discomfort at the infarct and a dark pink-purple
   discoloration.

4. Monitor for signs of renal failure:
   a. Decreased urine output (< 30 mL/hr)
   b. Occult blood in urine
   c. Elevated blood urea nitrogen (BUN), creati-
      nine

5. Monitor for signs and symptoms of mesenteric
   thrombosis:
   a. Decreased bowel sounds

   b. Constipation or diarrhea

   c. Increasing abdominal pain

   d. Elevated WBCs (20,000 to 30,000/mm^3)

6. Monitor for signs and symptoms of spinal cord
   ischemia:
   a. Urinary retention or incontinence

4. During abdominal aorta surgery, the renal arteries are at risk for thrombosis if they are involved in the aneurysm, are clamped for the operation, or are hypoperfused anytime during
   periods of hypotension. Impaired renal function
   can result.
5. The mesenteric artery, like the renal artery, is
   at risk for thrombosis.
   a. Bowel sounds usually are not heard before
      the third postoperative day.
   b. A liquid bowel movement before the third
      postoperative day may point to bowel is-
      chemia.
   c. Normally, postoperative pain decreases each
      day.
   d. Elevated WBC count indicates possible
      bowel necrosis.
6. The spinal arteries are at risk for thrombosis
   for the same reasons as the renal arteries.
   a. Inadequate perfusion above the second lum-
      bar vertebra (L2) can result in bladder dys-
      function.

▲ **Documentation**

Flow records
   Vital signs
   Circulation (distal, pulses,
      color)
   Bowel sounds, presence of
      occult blood
   Lower extremities (sensa-
      tion, motor function)
   Urine (output, occult blood)
Progress notes
   Characteristics of pain
   Unrelieved pain
   Interventions
   Response to interventions

Interventions

b. Changes in sensation and motor function in lower extremities

Rationale

b. Inadequate perfusion also can result in loss of sensation and voluntary motor function below the affected vertebrae.

Related Physician-Prescribed Interventions

Medications
Dependent on underlying etiology

Intravenous Therapy
Fluid and electrolyte replacement

Laboratory Studies
Refer to the General Surgery care plan, Appendix II.

Diagnostic Studies
Fluoroscopy
X-ray film
Abdominal aortography

Ultrasonography
Digital subtraction angiography

Therapies
Refer to the General Surgery care plan, Appendix II.

Postoperative: Nursing Diagnoses

▲ **Outcome Criteria**

The outcome criteria for this diagnosis represent those associated with discharge planning. Refer to the discharge criteria.

Potential Altered Health Maintenance related to insufficient knowledge of home care, activity restrictions, signs and symptoms of complications, and follow-up care

Focus Assessment Criteria	*Clinical Significance*
1. Readiness and ability to learn and retain information	1. A client or family failing to achieve learning goals requires a referral for assistance post-discharge.

Interventions

1. Refer to the General Surgery care plan, Appendix II, for wound care measures and rationales.
2. If an aorto-bifemoral graft was performed, reinforce the need for a slouched position when sitting. (Refer to the Arterial Bypass Grafting care plan, page 364, for more information.)
3. Reinforce activity restrictions, e.g., car riding, stairclimbing, lifting.

4. If the client smokes, reinforce the health benefits of quitting and refer to a smoking cessation program if one is available.
5. Instruct the client to report any changes in color, temperature, or sensation in the legs.

6. Instruct the client to report any GI bleeding immediately.
7. Instruct the client to inform all health care providers about the presence of a prosthetic graft before any invasive procedures.
8. Stress the importance of managing hypertension, if indicated.

Rationale

2. A slouched position helps prevent graft kinking and possible occlusion.

3. About 5 to 6 weeks after the abdominal surgery, if the client is in good nutritional status, the collagen matrix of the wound becomes strong enough to withstand stress from activity. The surgeon may prefer to limit activity for a longer period of time, as certain activities place tension on the surgical site.
4. Tobacco acts as a potent vasoconstrictor, which increases stress on the graft.

5. These signs and symptoms may indicate thrombosis or embolism, requiring immediate evaluation.
6. Duodenal bleeding may point to erosion of the aortic graft into the duodenum.
7. Puncture or exposure of a prosthetic graft risks graft infection, which may compromise the client's life.
8. Hypertension can cause false aneurysms at the anastomosis site.

▲ **Documentation**

Discharge summary record
Client and family teaching
Response to teaching

References/Bibliography

Baum, P.L. (1982). Abdominal aortic aneurysm? *Nursing 82, 12*(12), 34–39.

Berguer, R., & Tintinalli, J.E. (1978). Intestinal infarction. *Journal of the American College of Emergency Practitioners, 7*(11), 412–415.

Doroghazl, R.M. (1986). Aortic dissection. *Primary Cardiology,* 1986, *14*(7), 43–61.

Imparato, A.M. (1983). Abdominal aortic aneurysms. *Hospital Medicine, 20*(2), 211–242.

Jasinkowski, N.L. (1983). Aortic bypass: Trimming the postop risk. *RN, 46*(6), 41–45.

Ricotta, J.J. (1987). Elective resection of abdominal aortic aneurysms. *Cardiology Board Review, 2*(2), 92–95.

Zimmerman, T.A., & Ruplinger, J. (1983). Thoracoabdominal aortic aneurysms: Treatment and nursing interventions. *Critical Care Nurse, 3*(9), 54–63.

Amputation

Surgical severing and removal of a limb, amputation is indicated to prevent severe toxicity from gangrene or to eliminate intractable pain.

Diagnostic Cluster

▲ Time Frame

Preoperative and postoperative periods

▲ Discharge Criteria

Before discharge, the client or family will:

1. Describe daily stump care
2. Explain phantom sensations and interventions to reduce them
3. Describe measures to protect the stump from injury
4. Demonstrate prosthesis application and care, if indicated
5. Demonstrate ability to transfer from bed to chair safely
6. Demonstrate ability to get to the bathroom safely
7. Demonstrate ability to ascend and descend stairs safely
8. Demonstrate exercises taught in physical therapy

PREOPERATIVE PERIOD
Nursing Diagnoses

Anxiety related to insufficient knowledge of postoperative routines, postoperative sensations, and crutch-walking techniques

Related Care Plan

General Surgery Generic Care Plan

POSTOPERATIVE PERIOD
Collaborative Problems

Potential Complications:
Edema of Stump
Hematoma Site
Hemorrhage

Nursing Diagnoses

Potential Body Image Disturbance related to perceived negative effects of amputation and response of others to appearance
Potential for Contractures related to impaired movement secondary to pain
Grieving related to loss of limb and its effects on life style
Altered Comfort: phantom sensations related to nerve stimulation secondary to amputation
Potential for Injury related to altered gait and hazards of assistive devices
Potential Impaired Home Maintenance Management related to architectural barriers
Potential Altered Health Maintenance related to insufficient knowledge of activity of daily living (ADL) adaptations, stump care, prothesis care, gait training, and follow-up care

Refer to:

General Surgery

Preoperative: Nursing Diagnosis

▲ Outcome Criteria

The client will identify his expectations of the postoperative period.

Anxiety related to insufficient knowledge of postoperative routines, postoperative sensations, and crutch-walking techniques

Focus Assessment Criteria	*Clinical Significance*

1. Understanding of the following:
  a. Reason for amputation
  b. Surgical procedure
  c. Postoperative expectations
	1. Amputation poses a threat to body image and life style. The reason for the amputation influences the present response.

Interventions

1. Explore the client's feelings about the impending surgery.

2. Consult with physical therapy to see the client preoperatively.

3. Discuss postoperative expectations, including the following:
   a. Appearance of the stump
   b. Phantom sensations
   c. Immediate physical therapy
   d. Feelings of loss
4. As appropriate, teach crutch-walking preoperatively, if possible.

Rationale

1. Sharing thoughts and feelings provides opportunities to clarify fears and allows the nurse to give realistic feedback and convey that the client's fears and concerns are normal.
2. Preoperative instruction on postoperative activity helps the client focus on rehabilitation instead of on the surgery; this may help reduce anxiety.
3. These explanations can help reduce the fears associated with unknown situations and decrease anxiety.

4. Preoperative practice can increase the client's confidence and reduce fear (and risk) of injury.

▲ *Documentation*

Progress notes
  Assessment of learning
    readiness and ability
  Client teaching
  Response to teaching

Postoperative: Collaborative Problems

▲ *Nursing Goal*

The nurse will manage and minimize vascular complications.

Potential Complication: Edema of Stump
Potential Complication: Hematoma of Site

Interventions

1. Monitor incision for:
   a. Edema along suture line
   b. Areas of compression (if Ace wraps are used)
   c. Areas of pressure (if a splint is used)
   d. Bleeding
2. Monitor for signs of hematoma:
   a. Unapproximated suture line
   b. Ruddy color changes of skin along suture line
   c. Oozing of dark blood from suture line
   d. Point tenderness on palpation
3. Avoid placing a pillow under a leg stump; use a pillow for support only for an arm amputation.

4. Keep the affected leg horizontal and avoid positions of dependency. Use a wheelchair with a leg support and wrap the stump with Ace wraps when ambulating.

Rationale

1. Traumatized tissue responds with lymphedema. Excessive edema must be detected to prevent tension on the suture line, which can cause bleeding. Tissue compression from edema can compromise circulation.
2. Amputation flaps may be pulled over large areas of "space," creating pockets that may contain old blood. Hematoma may compromise flap healing and delay rehabilitation.

3. Placing pillows under the stump puts the proximal joint in a flexed position and promotes flexion contractures at the hip.
4. After leg amputation eliminates the muscle pump action on venous return, gravity's enhancement of venous drainage becomes critical. Dependent positioning causes venous stasis, promoting edema.

▲ *Documentation*

Flow records
  Appearance of suture line
  Appearance of skin around
    suture line
  Drainage
Progress notes
  Abnormal findings

Related Physician-Prescribed Interventions
Medications
  Analgesics
Intravenous Therapy
  Not indicated
Laboratory Studies
  Dependent on underlying condition and symptomatology
Diagnostic Studies
  Dependent on symptomatology
Therapies
  Physical therapy

Postoperative: Nursing Diagnoses

▲ *Outcome Criteria*

The client will communicate feelings about his or her changed appearance.

Potential Body Image Disturbance related to perceived negative effects of amputation and response of others to appearance

Focus Assessment Criteria	*Clinical Significance*
1. Ability to express feelings about appearance	1. Self-concept includes perceptions and feelings about self-worth, attractiveness, lovability, and capacity (Peretz, 1970). The client's ability to express these perceptions and feelings allows the nurse to plan effective interventions to help enhance self-concept.
2. Perception of effects on life style	2. The client's emotional response to the loss is influenced in large part by the extent to which disability interferes with personal goals.
3. Ability to participate in self-care, including dressing changes	3. A client's successful coping with physical loss is manifested by his or her involvement with self-care and care of the surgical site (Hamburg and Adams, 1953).
4. Present response, e.g., denial, mourning, awareness, managing	4. The grieving process in response to a recent disability involves denial or minimal thinking of loss, realization of loss and mourning, and, eventually, managing and incorporating the loss into one's life style (Friedman-Campbell & Hart, 1984).

Interventions	*Rationale*
1. Contact the client frequently, and treat him or her with warm, positive regard.	1. Frequent contact by the caregiver indicates acceptance and may facilitate trust. The client may be hesitant to approach the staff because of negative self-concept; the nurse must reach out.
2. Encourage the client to verbalize feelings about appearance and perceptions of life style impacts.	2,3. Expressing feelings and perceptions increases the client's self-awareness and helps the nurse plan effective interventions to address his needs. Validating the client's perceptions provides reassurance and can decrease anxiety.
3. Validate the client's perceptions and assure the client that they are normal and appropriate.	
4. Assist the client in identifying personal attributes and strengths.	4,5. This can help the client focus on the positive characteristics that contribute to the whole concept of self rather than only on the change in body image. The nurse should reinforce these positive aspects and encourage the client to reincorporate them into his or her new self-concept.
5. Facilitate adjustment through active listening.	
6. Encourage optimal hygiene, grooming, and other self-care activities.	6. Participation in self-care and planning promotes positive coping with the change.
7. Encourage the client to perform as many activities as possible unassisted.	7. Nonparticipation in self-care and overprotection by caregivers tends to promote feelings of helplessness and dependence.
8. When appropriate, do the following: a. Share your perceptions of the injury and the client's response to it. b. Explain the nature of the illness or injury.	8. Open, honest discussions—expressing that changes will occur but that they are manageable—promote feelings of control.

Interventions

    c. Discuss the anticipated changes in life style.

    d. Teach health behaviors that must be learned to facilitate adaptation to life style changes.

9. Encourage visitors.

10. Refer a client at high risk for unsuccessful adjustment to counseling, as appropriate.

Rationale

9. Maintaining social contacts and drawing on support systems is especially important when attempting to cope with a loss.

10. Professional counseling is indicated for a client with poor ego strengths and inadequate coping resources.

▲ *Documentation*

Progress notes
    Present emotional status
    Dialogues

▲ *Outcome Criterion*

The client will demonstrate full range of motion (ROM) of the affected limb.

Potential Impaired Physical Mobility related to limited movement secondary to amputation and pain

Focus Assessment Criteria	*Clinical Significance*
1. ROM of all joints preoperatively	1. This baseline assessment provides data against which to compare postoperative assessment findings.
2. Postoperative ROM after client has received pain medication	2. ROM may be restricted by pain and improved after administration of pain medication.

Interventions

1. Avoid placing pillows under a leg stump to elevate it.

2. Reconsult with physical therapy to begin therapy within 48 hours of surgery.

3. Encourage the abdominal-lying (prone) position for at least 2 hr/day after a leg amputation.

4. Teach the client to perform active ROM exercises on unaffected limbs at least four times a day. (*Note:* perform passive ROM only if the client cannot do it actively.)

5. Teach the client to avoid prolonged sitting.

Rationale

1. Elevating the stump on pillows puts the proximal joint in a flexed position, leading to hip flexion contractures.

2. Joints without ROM develop contractures in 3 to 7 days, because flexor muscles are stronger than extensor muscles.

3. Abdominal lying places the pelvic joints in an extended position, which extends extensor muscles and prevents contractures.

4. Active ROM increases muscle mass, tone, and strength and improves cardiac and respiratory functioning.

5. Prolonged sitting can cause hip flexion contractures.

▲ *Documentation*

Flow records
    Exercises
Progress notes
    Range of motion

▲ *Outcome Criteria*

The client will:

1. Express grief
2. Describe the meaning of the loss
3. Report an intent to discuss feelings with family members or significant others

Grieving related to loss of a limb and its effects on life style

Focus Assessment Criteria	*Clinical Significance*
1. Signs and symptoms of grief reaction, e.g., crying, withdrawal, anxiety, restlessness, decreased appetite, increased dependency	1. Losses related to function and independence usually provoke a profound grief response.

Interventions

1. Provide opportunities for the client and family members to ventilate feelings, discuss the loss openly, and explore the personal meaning of the loss. Explain that grief is a common and healthy reaction.

Rationale

1. Amputation may give rise to feelings of powerlessness, anger, profound sadness, and other grief responses. Open, honest discussions can help the client and family members accept and cope with the situation and their response to it.

Interventions

2. Encourage use of positive coping strategies that have proven successful in the past.
3. Encourage the client to express positive self-attributes.
4. Assess the family's or significant others' response to the situation, focusing on the following:
   a. Their perception of the short- and long-term affects of disability
   b. Past and present family dynamics
5. Help family members and significant others to cope:
   a. Explore their perceptions of how the situation will progress.
   b. Identify behaviors that facilitate adaptation.
   c. Encourage them to maintain usual roles and behaviors.
   d. Encourage including the client in family decision-making.
   e. Discuss the reality of everyday emotions, such as anger, guilt, and jealousy; relate the hazards of denying these feelings.
   f. Explain the dangers of trying to minimize grief and interfering with the normal grieving process.
6. Promote grief work with each response:
   a. Denial:
      • Encourage acceptance of the situation; do not reinforce denial by giving false reassurance.
      • Promote hope through assurances of care, comfort, and support.
      • Explain the use of denial by one family member to other members.
      • Do not push a person to move past denial until he is emotionally ready.
   b. Isolation:
      • Convey acceptance by encouraging expressions of grief.
      • Promote open, honest communication to encourage sharing.
      • Reinforce the client's self-worth by providing for privacy, when desired.
      • Encourage socialization, as feasible (e.g., support groups, church activities).
   c. Depression:
      • Reinforce the client's self-esteem.
      • Employ empathetic sharing and acknowledge grief.
      • Identify the degree of depression and develop appropriate strategies.
   d. Anger:
      • Explain to other family members that anger represents an attempt to control the environment stemming from frustration at the inability to control the disease.
      • Encourage verbalization of anger.

Rationale

2. Positive coping strategies aid acceptance and problem-solving.
3. Focusing on positive attributes increase self-acceptance and acceptance of the loss.
4. Successful adjustment depends on the client's and support persons' realistic perception of the situation.

5. A positive response by the client's family or significant others is one of the most important factors in the client's own acceptance of the loss.

6. Grieving involves profound emotional responses; interventions depend on the particular response.

Interventions

e. Guilt:
- Acknowledge the person's expressed self-image.
- Encourage identification of the relationship's positive aspects.
- Avoid arguing and participating in the person's system of "I should have . . ." and "I shouldn't have. . . ."

f. Fear:
- Focus on the present and maintain a safe and secure environment.
- Help the person explore reasons for and meanings of the fears.

g. Rejection:
- Provide reassurance by explaining what is happening.
- Explain this response to other family members.

h. Hysteria:
- Reduce environmental stressors (e.g., limit personnel).
- Provide a safe, private area in which to express grief.

Rationale

▲ **Documentation**

Progress notes
  Present emotional status
  Interventions
  Response to interventions

▲ **Outcome Criteria**

The client will:

1. State the reasons for phantom sensation
2. Demonstrate techniques for managing phantom sensation

Altered Comfort: Phantom Sensation related to nerve stimulation secondary to amputation

Focus Assessment Criteria	Clinical Significance
1. Presence and character of phantom sensation	1. Often, severed nerves continue to send pain impulses and give the sensation of the limb's presence.

Interventions

1. Explain that the sensations are normal and encourage the client to report them.
2. Explain that phantom sensations may manifest themselves as discomfort, pain, itching, tingling, warmth, or other sensations previously felt on that limb.

3. Avoid administering narcotics or analgesics for phantom pain. Instead, encourage the client to increase activity.

4. Teach measures to reduce phantom sensations:
   a. Application of pressure against the stump, if a cast or bulky dressing is not covering it
   b. Tapping the stump or the remaining limb
   c. Using guided imagery
   d. Using relaxation techniques
5. Refer to physical therapy for transcutaneous electrical nerve stimulation (TENS), if applicable.

Rationale

1. The client may be hesitant to discuss phantom sensations for fear of appearing abnormal.
2. Phantom sensations are caused by stimulation of the nerve proximal to the amputation that previously extended to the limb. The client perceives the stimulation as originating from the absent limb.
3. Narcotics and non-narcotic analgesics are not appropriate for phantom pain, which usually is a fleeting sensation. Activity helps to distract attention from the pain sensation.
4. Stimulation causing a second sensation may override the phantom sensation in the nervous system.

5. In severe cases, electrical stimulation can override phantom sensations.

▲ **Documentation**

Progress notes
  Reports of pain
  Interventions
  Response to interventions

Potential for Injury related to altered gait and hazards of assistive devices

Focus Assessment Criteria	*Clinical Significance*
1. Knowledge of prostheses and assistive devices	1. Assessment guides the nurse in planning appropriate teaching strategies.
2. Fit and comfort of prosthesis	2. Prosthetic devices should not be uncomfortable during use. Over time, weight change or muscle atrophy may necessitate adjustments in a device.
3. Strength (arms, unaffected leg)	3. Upper body strength and the unaffected leg strength influence gait.
4. Ability to perform activities of daily living (ADLs)	4. Use of a leg prosthesis requires an additional 60% to 80% of energy expenditure, which may hinder the client's ability to perform ADLs.

Interventions	*Rationale*
1. Reinforce exercise and activities prescribed in physical therapy.	1. Exercises increase muscle strength needed for transfers and ambulation.
2. Provide an assistive device—e.g., walker, cane—to compensate for altered gait, as necessary.	2. The client may need an assistive device to enable ambulation or reduce the risk of falling.
3. Teach the client to eliminate environmental hazards from the home, such as the following: a. Throw rugs b. Clutter c. Dim lighting d. Uneven or slippery floors	3. Removing hazards can reduce the risk of slipping and falling.
4. Encourage the client to request assistance as needed when in an unfamiliar environment or situation.	4. Assistance may help prevent injury.
5. Encourage the client to report altered gait to the physician or prosthetist.	5. Altered gait may be due to a poorly fitted prosthesis or other reasons; it requires further evaluation.

Impaired Home Maintenance Management related to architectural barriers

Focus Assessment Criteria	*Clinical Significance*
1. Barriers to ADLs in home, e.g., poor access to living quarters (stairs instead of a ramp), insufficient width of doorways if a wheelchair is required	1. Barriers increase dependency and contribute to depression and decreased mobility.

Interventions	*Rationale*
1. Provide the names of commercial and community resources for assistance with home renovations.	1. Assistance may be needed with architectural changes to remove barriers.
2. Refer to social services for information regarding financial assistance, as necessary.	2. Financial assistance may be needed with home renovations.

Potential Altered Health Maintenance related to insufficient knowledge of ADL adaptations, stump care, prosthesis care, gait training, and follow-up care

Focus Assessment Criteria	*Clinical Significance*
1. Self-care limitations imposed by amputation	1–3. Assessment of self-care ability and support system determines whether the client needs assistance at home.
2. Knowledge of self-care activities	
3. Support system	

Interventions	*Rationale*
1. Teach foot care for the remaining foot, including the following:	1. Daily care is necessary to detect or prevent injury, especially if a circulatory disorder was a contributing factor to amputation.
a. Daily foot bath	
b. Thorough drying	
c. Daily inspection for corns, calluses, blisters, and signs of infection	
d. Professional nail cutting	
e. Wearing clean socks daily	
f. Wearing sturdy slippers or shoes	
2. Instruct the client to place a chair or other large object next to the bed at home to prevent him from getting out of bed at night and attempting to stand on the stump when not fully awake.	2. Phantom sensations include a kinesthetic awareness of the absent limb. A client arising during the night, half-asleep, may fall and damage the healing stump.
3. Instruct the client to avoid tobacco; refer to a smoking cessation program, if necessary.	3. Nicotine in tobacco constricts arterial vessels, decreasing the blood flow to the healing stump. If amputation was related to atherosclerosis, tobacco use may threaten the stump's survival.
4. Teach the client to prepare the stump for a prosthesis, as appropriate:	4.
a. Regularly examine the stump for expected changes (e.g., muscle and scar atrophy) and unexpected changes (e.g., skin breakdown, redness, tenderness, increased warmth or coolness, numbness or tingling).	a. Shrinkage occurs as scar tissue retracts. Increasing redness or tenderness may indicate infection.
b. When the incision is closed, perform daily stump care to include the following:	b. Daily cleansing helps prevent infection. Creams and ointments may soften the skin to the point at which it is easily broken down.
(i) Washing with soap and water	
(ii) Drying thoroughly	
(iii) Avoiding creams and ointments	
c. Wrap the stump with Ace bandages.	c. Elastic compression reduces edema in the stump. Edema interferes with wound healing and prolongs the rehabilitation time. Wrapping also helps form the stump into a conical shape for better fit into the prosthesis.
5. Reinforce the need to continue exercises at home. (See the nursing diagnosis Potential Impaired Physical Mobility, page 358, for more information).	5. Active ROM exercises increase muscle mass, tone, and strength and improve cardiac and respiratory function.
6. Evaluate the client's ability to manage the home, shop, prepare food, and do other ADLs. If indicated, initiate referrals to community and social service agencies.	6. Referrals may be indicated to provide additional assistance after discharge.

References/Bibliography

Bourne, B.A., & Kutcher, J.L. (1985). Amputation: Helping the patient face loss of a limb. *RN, 48*(2), 38–44.

Clark, G.S., Blue, B., & Bearer, J.B. (1983). Rehabilitation of the elderly amputee. *Journal of the American Geriatrics Society, 31*(7), 439–448.

Dixon, J.K. (1981). Group self-identification and physical handicap: Implication for patient support groups. *Research in Nursing and Health, 4*(2), 299–308.

Friedman-Campbell, M., & Hart, C.A. (1984). Theoretical strategies and nursing interventions to promote psychological adaptation to spinal cord injuries and disability. *Journal of Neurosurgical Nursing, 16*(6), 335–342.

Hamburg, D.A., & Adams, J.E. (1953). A perspective on coping behaviors. *Archives of General Psychiatry, 17,* 1–20.

Huber, P.M., et al. (1988). Prosthetic problem inventory scale. *Rehabilitation Nursing, 13*(6), 326–329.

Little, J.M. (1975). *Major amputations for vascular disease.* New York: Churchill Livingstone.

Pasnau, R.O., & Pfetterbaum, B. (1986). Post-amputation grief. *Nursing Clinics of North America, 21*(4), 687–690.

Peretz, D. (1970). Reaction to loss. In A.C. Carn & D. Peretz (Eds.). *Loss and grief: Psychological management in medicine.* New York: Columbia University Press.

Ryser, D.K., et al. (1988). Isometric and isokinetic hip abductor strength in persons with above-knee amputations. *Archives of Physical Medical Rehabilitation, 69*(10), 840–845.

Smith, A.G. (1982). Common problems of lower extremity amputees. *Orthopedic Clinics of North America, 13*(3), 569–578.

Stern, P.H. (1988). Occlusive vascular disease of lower limbs: Diagnosis, amputation surgery, and rehabilitation—A review of the Burke experience. *American Journal of Physical Medical Rehabilitation, 67*(4), 145–154.

Walters, J. (1981). Coping with a leg amputation. *American Journal of Nursing, 81*(7), 1349–1352.

Arterial Bypass Grafting in the Lower Extremity

This procedure involves grafting of an autogenous vein or an artificial graft to bypass an arterial occlusion and restore continuous blood flow. Depending on the extent of the occlusion, the bypass graft can reach from the top of the femoral artery to the proximal popliteal artery, the tibioperoneal trunk, or even to the ankle.

Diagnostic Cluster

▲ Time Frame
Preoperative and postoperative periods

▲ Discharge Criteria
Before discharge, the client and/or family will:
1. Demonstrate proper wound care
2. Demonstrate correct pulse palpation technique
4. State the signs and symptoms that must be reported to a health care professional

Collaborative Problems

Potential Complications:
Thrombosis of Graft
Compartment Syndrome
Lymphocele
Disruption of Anastomosis

Nursing Diagnoses

Potential for Infection related to location of surgical incision
Altered Comfort related to increased tissue perfusion to previous ischemic tissue
Potential Impaired Tissue Integrity related to immobility and vulnerability of heels
Potential Altered Health Maintenance related to insufficient knowledge of wound care, signs and symptoms of complications, activity restrictions, and follow-up care

Related Care Plans

General Surgery Generic Care Plan
Abdominal Aortic Aneurysm Resection

Collaborative Problems

▲ Nursing Goal
The nurse will manage and minimize vascular complications.

Potential Complication: Thrombosis of Graft
Potential Complication: Compartment Syndrome
Potential Complication: Lymphocele
Potential Complication: Disruption of Anastomosis

Interventions	Rationale
1. Keep the bed's side rails up.	1. Every practicable measure should be taken to prevent graft trauma from injury.
2. Keep the limb warm, but *do not* use electric heating pads or hot water bottles.	2. Peripheral nerve ischemia causes diminished sensation. High temperatures of heating devices may damage tissue without the client's feeling discomfort.
3. Instruct the client to sit in a "slouched" position. If leg elevation is ordered, elevate the entire leg, including the pelvis.	3. Sharp flexion and pressure on the graft must be avoided to prevent graft damage.
4. Monitor graft patency. Palpate a graft near the skin surface, and assess distal pulses for changes from baseline.	4. Graft patency is essential to arterial circulation.

Interventions

5. Monitor circulatory status, color, temperature, sensation, and motor function in the affected leg.

6. Immediately report changes in color, temperature, sensation, pulses, or pressure to the physician.

7. Monitor for signs and symptoms of compartment syndrome:
   a. Edema of revascularized limb.
   b. Complaints of pain with passive stretching of the muscle
   c. Decreased sensation, motor function, or paresthesias of the distal limb
   d. Increased tension and firmness of muscle

8. Immediately report changes in status to the physician.

9. Monitor for signs and symptoms of lymphocele:
   a. Discomfort accompanied by local swelling
   b. Large amounts of clear or pink-tinged drainage

10. Support the affected leg.
11. Apply compression dressings only if ordered by the physician.

Rationale

5. A sudden change in temperature, drop in pressure, or absence of pulses indicates graft thrombosis. Changes in sensation or motor function can indicate compartment syndrome.

6. Sudden decrease in arterial flow indicating a thrombosed graft is an emergency requiring immediate surgical exploration of the graft.

7. After a period of ischemia comes a period of increased capillary wall permeability. Restoration of arterial flow causes plasma and extracellular fluid to flow into the tissues, producing massive swelling. Pain and muscle tension result as the tissues are prevented from extending outward by the fascia and the inward pressure obliterates the circulation. The nerves become anoxic, causing paresthesias and motor deficits.

8. Postoperative edema is expected in the newly vascularized limb. Careful assessment alerts the nurse to edema severe enough to cause compartment syndrome. Treatment must be initiated within 8 hours to preserve function of the extremity.

9. A major lymphatic channel courses through the inner thigh area. If the lymphatic chain is lacerated during the operation, drainage may occur. The large amount of fluid that accumulates seeks the path of least resistance and usually drains through the incision.

10. Support can reduce muscle spasms.
11. Although compression may possibly halt the flow of lymph long enough for the lymphatic vessel to seal, this usually is not the case, and surgical intervention is required to repair the draining lymphatic chain. Compression should be used only on the physician's order—overly vigorous compression may damage the new graft.

▲ **Documentation**

Flow records
    Vital signs
    Distal pulses
    Circulatory status
Progress notes
    Presence and description of pain
    Unusual events, actions, responses
    Unusual wound drainage or appearance

12. Monitor for disruption of anastomosis:
   a. Decrease in perfusion of distal extremity
   b. Bounding aneurysmal pulsation over the anastomosis site. If bleeding occurs, apply firm constant pressure over the site, and notify the physician.

12. Hemorrhage from anastomotic disruption is an emergency requiring immediate surgical intervention.

Related Physician-Prescribed Interventions

Medications
    Vasodilators   Anticoagulant therapy

Intravenous Therapy
    Fluid/electrolyte replacement

Laboratory Studies
    Prothrombin time   Platelet count

Diagnostic Studies
    Doppler ultrasonography

Therapies
    Refer to the General Surgery care plan (Appendix II).

Nursing Diagnoses

▲ *Outcome Criteria*

The client will exhibit wound healing free of infection.

Potential for Infection related to increased susceptibility to urinary or fecal contamination secondary to location of wound in groin

Focus Assessment Criteria	*Clinical Significance*
1. Groin wound every shift	1. A superficial infection that would be benign in another surgical site can lead to graft failure.

Interventions	*Rationale*
1. If the wound does not have a polyurethane film dressing from the operating room, cover with a dry sterile gauze dressing. Be certain that no skin surfaces come in contact with each other.	1. Minimizing moisture in the groin wound decreases the risk of infection.
2. If the client has a pendulous abdomen, teach him to position himself so that the abdomen does not cover the groin wound.	2. Keeping the wound free of skin overlays decreases moisture, which is a medium for microorganism growth.
3. If tissue becomes macerated, consult with the physician to provide heat lamp therapy (40-watt bulb, 20 inches from wound) for 15 minutes two to three times per day, and increase the frequency of gauze dressing changes.	3. Heat has a drying effect.
4. Teach the client the importance of avoiding wound maceration and graft infection.	4. Graft failure can result from a wound infection

▲ *Documentation*

Flow records
   Interventions
   Response to interventions

▲ *Outcome Criteria*

The client will:
1. Maintain intact skin over heels
2. Describe measures to protect heels

Potential Impaired Tissue Integrity related to immobility and vulnerability of heels

Focus Assessment Criteria	*Clinical Significance*
1. Condition of skin on the feet and heels	1,2. Frequent assessment is needed to detect early signs of tissue ischemia.
2. Condition of underlying tissue	

Interventions	*Rationale*
1. Observe for signs and symptoms of tissue ischemia (e.g., blanching, redness). Palpate for changes in tissue consistency beneath the skin.	1. Pressure ulcer formation may begin deep in the tissue. A client with peripheral vascular disease secondary to atherosclerosis is at high risk for pressure ulcer formation because of the ischemia already present in the tissue.
2. Explain why heels are especially vulnerable to skin breakdown from excessive pressure.	2. A compromised arterial supply may be just enough to maintain viability of a leg but inadequate to heal an ulcer in the leg.
3. Take measures to alleviate pressure on heels, e.g., elevate heels from bed, avoid heel protectors.	3. Skin pressure triggers ulcer formation. Elevation reduces direct pressure; heel protectors are a direct pressure device.

▲ *Documentation*

Flow records
   Skin condition
   Interventions

▲ *Outcome Criteria*

The client will:
1. State the reason for the pain
2. Report pain relief after interventions

Altered Comfort related to increased tissue perfusion to previously ischemic tissue

Focus Assessment Criteria	*Clinical Significance*
1. Comfort level, descriptions of sensations	1–2. The nurse must investigate the underlying cause of pain to rule out an ischemic origin.
2. Operative leg for evidence of ischemia	

Interventions

1. Explain the source of pain and reassure that the sensation is temporary and will decrease each day.
2. Assess carefully to differentiate between the pain of reperfusion and pain of ischemia. (Ischemic tissue is cool; reperfused tissue, warm and edematous.) Notify the physician immediately if you suspect ischemia.
3. Refer to the nursing diagnosis Acute Pain in the General Surgery care plan (Appendix II) for more information.

Rationale

1. Pain occurs as previously ischemic sensory nerve endings are being reperfused and lessens as reperfusion progresses.
2. Ischemic pain may indicate graft failure and warrants immediate evaluation.

▲ *Documentation*

Progress notes
    Unrelieved pain
    Interventions
    Response to interventions

▲ *Outcome Criteria*

The outcome criteria for this diagnosis represent those associated with discharge planning. Refer to the discharge criteria.

Potential Altered Health Maintenance related to insufficient knowledge of wound care, signs and symptoms of complications, activity restrictions, and follow-up care

Focus Assessment Criteria	*Clinical Significance*
1. Readiness and ability to learn and retain information	1. A client or family failing to achieve learning goals requires a referral for assistance post-discharge.

Interventions

1. Teach the client and family wound care techniques. (Refer to the nursing diagnosis Potential Altered Health Maintenance in the General Surgery care plan, Appendix II, for specific measures.)
2. Reinforce teaching regarding activity restrictions and mobility:
   a. Increase activity as prescribed.

   b. Avoid long periods (> 20 minutes) of sitting with legs bent at the groin and knee.

   c. Ambulate as advised; plan a walking program.

   d. Avoid crossing legs.

3. Teach the client and support persons how to assess graft patency:
   a. Assess pulses and capillary refill.
   b. Palpate the graft for pulsations if near the surface.
4. Teach the client and others to recognize signs and symptoms of problems and report them immediately:
   a. Absence of pulses
   b. Change in temperature of leg or foot
   c. Paresthesias and other changes in sensation
   d. Pain
   e. Wound or sore in affected leg
   f. Changes in incision, e.g., redness, drainage
5. Reinforce teaching regarding foot care and prevention of injury to the leg.

Rationale

1. Proper wound care can prevent infection, which delays healing.

2. The client's understanding may encourage compliance with the therapeutic regimen.
   a. Activity should be increased gradually to promote circulation and reduce loss of muscle strength.
   b. Dependent positioning of the legs increases postoperative swelling. Positions of hip and knee flexion impede venous return.
   c. Early ambulation is recommended to restore muscle activity and enhance venous blood return.
   d. Crossing the legs increases the risk of graft kinking and thrombosis.
3. Monitoring of circulatory status must be continued at home.

4. Reporting these signs of compromised circulation, infection, or possible graft failure promptly enables intervention to prevent serious complications. Diminished circulation impedes healing; infection can cause graft failure.

5. Continued care and precautions are necessary at home.

▲ *Documentation*

Discharge summary record
    Client and family teaching
    Response to teaching

References/Bibliography

Andrews-Ekers, M., & Satiani, B. (1982). EAB: A new route for vascular rehabilitation. *Nursing 82, 12*(11), 34–41.

Beasley-Dixon, M., & Nunnelee, J. (1987). Arterial reconstruction for atherosclerotic occlusive disease. *The Journal of Cardiovascular Nursing, 1*(2), 36–49.

Hyde, G.L., Peck, D., & Powell, D.C. (1983). Compartment syndrome: Early diagnosis and a bedside operation. *The American Surgeon, 49*(10), 563–568.

Jones, A.F., & Kempczinski, R.F. (1981). Aortofemoral bypass grafting: A reappraisal. *Archives of Surgery, 116*(3), 301–305.

Patman, D., & Thompson, J.E. (1970). Fasciotomy in peripheral vascular surgery. *Archives of Surgery, 101*(12), 663–672.

Carotid Endarterectomy

The surgical removal of atherosclerotic plaque or thrombus from the carotid artery, carotid endarterectomy is indicated in clients who have experienced a transient ischemic attack, to prevent cerebrovascular accident.

Diagnostic Cluster

▲ **Time Frame**

Preoperative and postoperative periods

PREOPERATIVE PERIOD
Nursing Diagnoses

Anxiety related to anticipated surgery and unfamiliarity with preoperative and postoperative routines and postoperative sensations

POSTOPERATIVE PERIOD
Collaborative Problems

Potential Complications:
Circulatory
  Thrombosis
  Hypotension
  Hypertension
  Hemorrhage
  Cerebral Infarction
Neurological
  Cerebral Infarction
  Cranial Nerve Impairment
    Facial
    Hypoglossal
    Glosspharyngeal
    Vagal
  Local Nerve Impairment
Respiratory Obstruction

Nursing Diagnoses

Potential for Injury related to syncope secondary to vascular insufficiency
Potential Altered Health Maintenance related to insufficient knowledge of home care, signs and symptoms of complications, risk factors, activity restrictions, and follow-up care

Related Care Plan

General Surgery Generic Care Plan

▲ **Discharge Criteria**

Before discharge, the client and/ or family will:

1. Describe wound care techniques
2. State activity restrictions for home care
3. Demonstrate range-of-motion (ROM) exercises
4. State the signs and symptoms that must be reported to a health care professional
5. Identify risk factors and describe their relationship to arterial disease

Preoperative: Nursing Diagnosis

▲ **Outcome Criteria**

The client will relate postoperative expectations.

Anxiety related to anticipated surgery and unfamiliarity with preoperative and postoperative routines and postoperative sensations

Focus Assessment Criteria	Clinical Significance
1. Preoperative facial nerve function	1. This assessment establishes a baseline against which to compare postoperative assessment findings.
2. Anxiety level (mild, moderate, severe, panic)	2. Assessing anxiety level guides the nurse in planning effective interventions.

Interventions	Rationale
1. Discuss with the client the possible effect of surgery on facial nerve function, i.e., numbness and asymmetry. 2. Refer to the nursing diagnosis Anxiety in the General Surgery care plan, Appendix II, for specific interventions and rationales for preoperative anxiety.	1. Alerting the client of what to expect can reduce the anxiety associated with fear of the unknown.

▲ **Documentation**

Progress notes
    Assessment results
    Client teaching

Postoperative: Collaborative Problems

▲ **Nursing Goal**

The nurse will manage and minimize vascular, neurological, and respiratory complications.

Potential Complication: **Circulatory Problems**
        Thrombosis
        Hypotension
        Hypertension
        Hemorrhage
        Cerebral Infarction
Potential Complication: **Neurologic Problems**
        Cerebral Infarction
        Cranial Nerve Impairment
        Local Nerve Impairment
Potential Complication: **Respiratory Obstruction**

Interventions	Rationale

1. Monitor for the following:
  a. Respiratory obstruction (check trachea for deviation from midline, listen for respiratory stridor)
  b. Peri-incisional swelling or bleeding
	1. Edema or hematoma at the surgical site can cause mechanical obstruction.

2. Monitor for changes in neurological function:
  a. Level of consciousness
  b. Pupillary response
  c. Motor/sensory function of all four extremities (check hand grasps, ability to move legs)
	2. Stroke is a possible complication of carotid endarterectomy. Manifestations of cerebral infarction include neuromuscular impairment of the contralateral body side.

3. Monitor for cranial nerve dysfunction:	3. The surgical procedure can temporarily or permanently disrupt cranial nerve functions (Meador and White, 1980).

a. Hypoglossal nerve:
    • Difficulty with speech
    • Dysphagia
    • Upper airway obstruction
	a. The hypoglossal nerve controls intrinsic and extrinsic muscles for tongue movement.

b. Facial nerve: • Upward protrusion of lower lip	b. The facial nerve controls facial motor function and taste.

c. Accessory nerves:
    • Sagging shoulder
    • Difficulty raising arm or shoulder
	c. Accessory nerve controls the trapezius and sternocleidomastoid muscles.

d. Vagus nerve:
    • Loss of gag reflex
    • Hoarseness
    • Asymmetrical movements of vocal cords
	d. The vagus nerve regulates movements of swallowing and sensation to the pharynx and larynx.

Interventions

4. Monitor for hypertension.

5. As necessary, consult with the physician for IV pharmacological management to prevent hypertensive episodes.
6. Monitor for hypotension and bradycardia.

▲ *Documentation*

Flow records
  Vital signs
  Patency of the temporal artery on the operative side
  Level of consciousness
  Pupillary response
  Motor function (hand grasp, leg movement)
  Cranial nerve function
  Wound assessment

7. Consult with the physician for IV lidocaine (Xylocaine) by catheter at the wound.

Related Physician-Prescribed Interventions
Refer to the Atherosclerosis care plan, page 78.

Rationale

4. Hypertension can be anticipated in certain clients exhibiting predisposing factors, such as preoperative hypertension or postoperative hypoxia and excessive fluid replacement.
5. Hypertension can increase the risk of hemorrhage or disruption of arterial reconstruction.

6. The removal of atherosclerotic plaque may cause increased pressure waves on the carotid sinus, leading to hypotension. Bradycardia may result from pressure on the carotid sinus during the operation or from postoperative edema. Postoperative cardiac complications are the leading cause of morbidity following carotid endarterectomy.
7. A catheter placed in the wound with its tip at the carotid sinus may produce hypotension and bradycardia; lidocaine (Xylocaine) reduces catheter tip irritation.

Refer to the General Surgery care plan, Appendix II.

Postoperative: Nursing Diagnosis

Potential for Injury related to syncope secondary to vascular insufficiency

▲ *Outcome Criteria*

The client will:

1. Relate methods of preventing sudden decreases in cerebral blood flow caused by orthostatic hypotension
2. Demonstrate maneuvers to change position to avoid orthostatic hypotension
3. Relate a decrease in episodes of dizziness or vertigo

Focus Assessment Criteria

1. Blood pressure, for postoperative orthostatic hypotension. (To assess, take readings with the client lying down, then immediately on standing.)

Clinical Significance

1. Orthostatic hypotension causes episodes of cerebral hypoxia.

Interventions

1. Remain with the client during initial postoperative activity.
2. Instruct the client to call for assistance when getting out of bed.
3. Teach the client to move slowly from the supine to the upright position to avoid orthostatic hypotension:
   a. Raise the head.
   b. Lower one leg at a time over the side of the bed.
   c. Sit for a few minutes before standing.
   d. Stand for a few minutes before walking.
4. Explain the relationship of dehydration, alcohol intake, and prolonged bed rest to orthostatic hypotension.

▲ *Documentation*

Progress notes
  Complaints of vertigo
Discharge summary record
  Client teaching

Rationale

1,2. Syncope necessitates assistance to prevent injury.

3. Slow movements minimize sudden decrease in cerebral blood flow by reducing the vascular rush to the large muscles.

4. Circulating volume is decreased by dehydration and the vasodilating effects of alcohol. Prolonged bed rest increases venous pooling, contributing to orthostatic hypotension on arising. The client's understanding of these effects may encourage compliance with preventive measures.

Potential Altered Health Maintenance related to insufficient knowledge of home care, signs and symptoms of complications, risk factors, activity restrictions, and follow-up care

▲ **Outcome Criteria**

The outcome criteria for this diagnosis represent those associated with discharge planning. Refer to the discharge criteria.

Focus Assessment Criteria	*Clinical Significance*
1. Knowledge of arteriosclerotic disease, risk factors	1,2. These assessments help identify learning needs and guides the nurse in planning effective teaching strategies.
2. Past experiences with risk factor modification	
3. Readiness and ability to learn and retain information	3. A client or family that fails to achieve learning goals requires a referral for assistance postdischarge.

Interventions

1. Teach the client and family to watch for and report the following:
   a. Swelling or drainage from incision
   b. Numbness or weakness of opposite arm or leg
   c. Changes in speech or swallowing
   d. Changes in vision
2. Discuss the relationship of arterial disease and certain risk factors:
   a. Smoking
   b. High dietary cholesterol intake
   c. Obesity
3. Explore ways in which the client can eliminate or reduce applicable risk factors. (Refer to the Atherosclerosis care plan, page 78, for more information).
4. Explain the need for regular ROM exercises of the head and neck.
5. Refer the client to appropriate resources for assistance with risk factor modification:
   a. Dietician for diet and weight loss counseling
   b. Smoking cessation program
   c. Exercise program (if approved by the physician)

Rationale

1. These signs are indicative of progressive nerve or tissue compression.

2. Smoking causes vasoconstriction with elevated blood pressure. Sustained hypertension injures the vascular lining, increasing plaque adherence. Obesity and high intake of animal fat can contribute to lipid plaques.
3,4. The client's awareness that he can modify risk factors may encourage compliance with the treatment regimen.

5. The client may need assistance for sustained management of risk factors after discharge.

▲ **Documentation**

Discharge summary record
   Client teaching
   Outcome achievement or
     status
   Referrals, if indicated

References/Bibliography

Babu, S.C., Pathanjali Sharma, P.V., Raciti, A., Mayr, C.H., Jr., Elrabie, N.A., Clauss, R.H., Stahl, W.M., & DelQuercio, L.P.M. (1980). Monitor-guided responses. *Archives of Surgery, 115*(9), 1384–1386.

Bove, E.L., Fry, W.J., & Gross, W.S. (1979). Hypotension and hypertension as consequences of dysfunction following carotid endarterectomy. *Surgery, 85*, 633–637.

Cafferata, H.T., Merchant, R.F., & DePalma, R.G. (1982). Avoidance of post-carotid endarterectomy hypertension. *Annals of Surgery, 196*(4), 465–472.

Meador, B., & White, P. (1980). The post-op dangers in carotid endarterectomy. *RN, 30*(4), 54–57.

Pearce, W., Mill, M.R., & Marsch, J.G. (1985). Cerebrovascular insufficiency. *Critical Care Quarterly, 8*(2), 11–24.

Szaflarski, N. (1980). Carotid endarterectomy: After surgery. *AORN, 32*(1), 48–54.

Webb, P.P. (1979). Neurological deficit after carotid endarterectomy. *American Journal of Nursing, 79*(4), 654–658.

Cataract Extraction

Cataract extraction—surgical removal of the lens—can take several forms. The intracapsular procedure leaves an intact capsule; the extracapsular procedure removes the capsule, lens cortex, and nucleus. The phacoemulsification procedure uses ultrasound waves to disintegrate the lens, which is then suctioned out. Regardless of the procedure, extraction allows insertion of an intraocular lens implant.

Diagnostic Cluster

▲ **Time Frame**

Preoperative and postoperative periods

PREOPERATIVE PERIOD
Nursing Diagnoses

Fear related to upcoming surgery and potential failure to regain vision

POSTOPERATIVE PERIOD
Collaborative Problems

Potential Complication:
Hemorrhage

Nursing Diagnoses

Acute Pain related to surgical interruption of body tissues

Potential for Infection related to increased susceptibility: surgical interruption of body surface

Potential for Injury related to visual limitations, presence in unfamiliar environment, limited mobility, and postoperative presence of eye patch

Potential Altered Health Maintenance related to insufficient knowledge of activities permitted and restricted, medications, complications, and follow-up care

Potential Social Isolation related to altered visual acuity, and fear of falling

Potential Impaired Home Maintenance Management related to inability to perform ADL secondary to activity restrictions and visual limitations

Refer to:

Enucleation

Enucleation

▲ **Discharge Criteria**

Before discharge, the client or family will:

1. Discuss management of activities of daily living (ADLs)
2. Verbalize precautions associated with medications and activity
3. State the signs and symptoms that must be reported to a health care professional

Preoperative: Nursing Diagnoses

▲ **Outcome Criteria**

The client will:

1. Express any fears and concerns regarding the upcoming surgery
2. Verbalize an understanding of perioperative routines and care measures

Fear related to upcoming surgery and fear of possible failure to regain vision

Focus Assessment Criteria

1. Verbal and nonverbal indicators of anxiety

Clinical Significance

1. Risks associated with cataract surgery—e.g., potential vision loss or failure to regain useful vision—may trigger anxiety and fear. Other factors also may contribute to anxiety, such as potential changes in work roles or family responsibilities as a result of surgery. Only through discussions with the client can the nurse obtain this information.

2. Understanding of cataract surgery, including the following:
   a. Nature of the procedure
   b. Risks and benefits
   c. Anesthetic agent
   d. Options for visual rehabilitation after surgery, e.g., intraocular lens implant (IOL), contact lenses, cataract glasses (aphakic spectacles)
3. Amount of information the client seeks

2. Assessing the client's knowledge level identifies learning needs and guides the nurse in planning effective teaching strategies.

3. Each client has different learning needs. One client may desire all the information possible about the procedure and its aftermath and may find that it reduces anxiety; another may find too much detailed information overwhelming and anxiety-producing. Assessment allows the nurse to tailor client teaching to fit the client's desires.

Interventions

1. Create a calm, relaxed environment that promotes sharing of feelings and concerns. Encourage verbalization, and listen attentively.
2. Validate the client's feelings and reassure him that anxiety and fear are normal and expected responses to upcoming cataract surgery.
3. Address any misconceptions the client expresses and provide accurate information. Common myths or fears include the following:
   a. Removal of the eye during surgery
   b. Visualization of instruments approaching the eye
   c. Cataract film will be stripped off the eye, causing pain
   d. Suffocation under surgical drapes
   e. Without general anesthesia, surgery will be painful
4. Present information using a variety of instructional methods and media:
   a. Large-print pamphlets
   b. Posters
   c. Audiovisual programs
5. Explain required preadmission activities:
   a. Adherence to dietary instructions provided by anesthesia services
   b. Adjustments in medication regimen as ordered by the surgeon, anesthesiologist, or client's physician
   c. Use of antibiotic eyedrops the day before surgery
6. Discuss expected preoperative care measures:
   a. Preoperative sedation
   b. Dilating drops
   c. Intravenous (IV) infusion
   d. Bladder emptying
7. Provide information about the activities, sights, and sounds associated with the intraoperative period:
   a. Presence and purpose of various personnel

Rationale

1. Verbalizing feelings and concerns increases the client's self-awareness and helps the nurse identify sources of anxiety.
2. Validation and reassurance promote self-esteem and may help reduce anxiety.

3. Misconceptions can contribute to anxiety and fear.

4. Simultaneous stimulation of multiple senses enhances the teaching–learning process. Written materials also provide a source to refer to after discharge.

5. Depending on the client's general health status, presence of concurrent medical problems, time of surgery, and physician's preferences, adjustments may be needed in diet (nothing by mouth for a specified period) and medications (e.g., withholding diuretics, decreasing insulin dose).

6–9. Information about what to expect can help reduce anxiety associated with fear of the unknown. It also enables the client to participate better in care measures.

Interventions

    b. Location, purposes, and noises of equipment

    c. Importance of lying still during the procedure

    d. Importance of communicating the need to move or cough before doing so during surgery

8. For a client receiving general anesthesia, including this information:

    a. Purpose and length of stay in the recovery room

    b. Expected sights and sounds in the recovery room

    c. Postoperative deep breathing and coughing exercises

9. Explain required activities for the immediate postoperative period:

    a. Lying on the nonoperative side

    b. Avoiding bending over at the waist

    c. Requesting assistance with ambulation until instructed otherwise

    d. Avoiding constipation

10. Reinforce the physician's explanations of options for visual rehabilitation after surgery, as appropriate.

    a. Intraocular lenses (IOL): These miniature plastic lenses can be implanted during the surgery or later. They provide the least visual distortion when compared to other methods. Disadvantages include risk of rejection, higher cost, and additional procedures required for accurate fitting.

    b. Contact lenses: These create less image distortion and provide more focused central and peripheral vision than aphakic spectacles. Disadvantages include increased care and maintenance, high replacement costs, and intolerance in some clients.

    c. Aphakic spectacles: This is the least expensive and safest method. Disadvantages include object enlargement (images appear up to 25% larger than actual size), bowing of lines (vertical lines such as doorways and lampposts appear curved), and loss of peripheral vision (only the images viewed through the central part of the lens are in focus).

Rationale

10. Explaining options enables the client to make an informed decision when possible.

▲ **Documentation**

Progress notes
  Client teaching
  Client's understanding of teaching and response

Postoperative: Collaborative Problems

▲ **Nursing Goal**

The nurse will manage and minimize vascular complications.

Potential Complication: Hemorrhage

Interventions

1. Monitor for signs and symptoms of hemorrhage:

    a. Pain in or around eyes

    b. Sudden onset of eye pain

    c. Changes in vision

Rationale

1. Ocular tissue is very vulnerable to bleeding because of its high vascularity and fragile vessels. Blood in vitreous alters vision.

▲ **Documentation**

Flow records
  Vital signs
  Eye assessment (suture
    lines, edema, pupils, vision)

Interventions

2. Remind the client to follow postoperative activity restrictions as explained preoperatively.

Related Physician-Prescribed Interventions

Medications
  Antiemetics
  Cycloplegics
Intravenous Therapy
  Refer to the General Surgery care plan, Appendix II.
Laboratory Studies
  Refer to the General Surgery care plan, Appendix II.
Diagnostic Studies
  Snellen's eye chart
  Gonioscopy
  Visual fields
Therapies
  Eye care

Rationale

2. Postoperative restrictions are aimed at avoiding activities that increase stress on suture lines.

Analgesics
Antibiotics (topical)

Ophthalmoscopic examination
Tonography

Postoperative: Nursing Diagnoses

▲ **Outcome Criteria**

The client will voice progressive pain reduction and pain relief after interventions.

Altered Comfort related to surgical interruption of body tissues

Focus Assessment Criteria

1. Location of pain; severity of pain based on a scale of 0 to 10 (0 = no pain, 10 = greatest pain), rated as follows:
   a. Before pain relief interventions
   b. One half hour after intervention
2. Associated signs and symptoms:
   a. Nausea
   b. Diaphoresis
   c. Vital sign changes
3. Usual response to pain

Clinical Significance

1. This rating scale provides an objective method of evaluating the subjective experience of pain.

2. This assessment helps differentiate normal postoperative pain from pain related to bleeding.

3. Assessing the client's usual response to pain helps the nurse plan effective pain relief interventions.

Interventions

1. Assist the client in identifying effective pain relief measures.

2. Explain that pain may not occur until several hours after surgery.

3. Promote noninvasive and nonpharmacological pain relief measures, such as the following:
   a. Positioning: elevate the head of the bed, alternate between lying on the back and on the nonoperative side
   b. Distraction
   c. Relaxation exercises
4. Support pain relief measures with prescribed analgesics.
5. Notify the physician if pain is unrelieved within ½ hour of drug administration, if pain is accompanied by nausea, or if you note drainage on the eye patch or shield.

Rationale

1. The client has the most intimate knowledge of his pain and the effectiveness of relief measures.
2. Pain may not occur until the local anesthetic wears off; understanding this can help reduce anxiety associated with the unexpected.
3. Noninvasive and nonpharmacological pain relief measures allow the client to gain a sense of control over the pain.

4. For some clients, pharmacological therapy may be needed to provide adequate pain relief.
5. These signs may indicate increased intraocular pressure or other complications.

▲ **Documentation**

Progress notes
  Complaints of pain
  Interventions
  Response to interventions

Potential For Infection related to increased susceptibility secondary to surgical interruption of body surfaces

▲ Outcome Criteria

The client will exhibit healing of incision with no symptoms of infection.

Focus Assessment Criteria

1. Signs of infection:
   a. Redness
   b. Edema
   c. Conjunctival injection (prominent conjunctival blood vessels)
   d. Drainage on eyelids or eyelashes
   e. Purulent matter
   f. Elevated temperature
   g. Laboratory values: increased WBC count, change in WBC differential, abnormal culture and sensitivity results

Clinical Significance

1. Infection following ocular surgery can negatively affect visual acuity and successful surgical outcome. Postoperative care must focus on prevention, early detection, and prompt treatment of infection.

Interventions

1. Promote wound healing:
   a. Encourage a well-balanced diet and adequate fluid intake.
   b. Instruct the client to keep a patch over the eye until the second postoperative day.
2. Use aseptic technique to instill eye drops:
   a. Wash hands before beginning.
   b. Hold the dropper away from the eye slightly.
   c. When instilling, avoid contact between the eye, the drop, and the dropper.
   Teach the technique to the client and family members.
3. Assess for signs and symptoms of infection:
   a. Reddened, edematous eyelids
   b. Conjunctival injection (prominent blood vessels)
   c. Drainage on eyelids and lashes
   d. Purulent material in anterior chamber (between the cornea and iris)
   e. Elevated temperature
   f. Abnormal laboratory values, e.g., elevated WBC count, abnormal culture and sensitivity results
4. Take steps to prevent strain on the suture line, e.g., have the client wear dark glasses and an eyepatch in the daytime and an eye shield at night.
5. Culture and notify the physician of any suspicious-looking drainage.

Rationale

1. Optimal nutrition and hydration improve overall good health, which promotes healing of any surgical wound. Wearing an eye patch promotes healing by decreasing the irritative force of the eyelid against the suture line.
2. Aseptic technique minimizes introduction of microorganisms and reduces the risk of infection.

3. Early detection of infection enables prompt treatment to minimize its seriousness.

4. Strain on the suture line can lead to interruption, creating an entrance point for microorganisms.

5. Abnormal drainage requires medical evaluation and possible initiation of pharmacological treatment.

▲ Documentation

Flow records
    Vital signs
    Condition of eye and suture line
Progress notes
    Abnormal findings

▲ Outcome Criteria

The client will not experience injury or tissue trauma while hospitalized.

Potential for Injury related to visual limitations, unfamiliar environment, limited mobility, and eye patch

Focus Assessment Criteria

1. Visual acuity in each eye
2. Gait, previous history of falls
3. Potential environmental obstacles, such as the following:
   a. Footstools and low furniture
   b. Intravenous (IV) poles
   c. Wastebaskets
   d. Slippers

Clinical Significance

1–3. A client who has undergone ophthalmic surgery may have experienced a sudden loss of vision and is at increased risk of injury. Assessment must include acuity of each eye; acuity of the unaffected eye indicates how the client views the environment, and acuity in the affected eye helps guide the nurse in planning interventions to ensure safety.

Interventions

1. Orient the client to the environment upon arrival.
2. Modify the environment to remove any potential hazards:
   a. Remove obstacles from walking pathways.
   b. Remove straws from trays.
   c. Make sure doors and drawers are kept either completely open or completely closed.
3. Elevate the bed's side rails. Place objects, including the call bell, where the client can see and reach them without stretching too far.
4. Place ambulation aids where the client can see and reach them easily. Instruct the client to request assistance before ambulating. Monitor the use of ambulation aids.
5. Help the client and family evaluate the home environment for potential hazards such as the following:
   a. Throw rugs
   b. Exposed electrical cords
   c. Low furniture
   d. Pets
   e. Stairs

Rationale

1. The client's familiarity with the environment may help reduce accidents.
2. Lost or impaired vision or use of an eye patch also can interfere with depth perception. These measures can help minimize potential hazards and reduce the risk of injury resulting from impaired acuity and depth perception.

3,4. These measures can help reduce the risk of falls.

5. The need to maintain a safe environment continues after discharge.

▲ **Documentation**

Progress notes
   Visual acuity (preoperative and postoperative)
Discharge summary record
   Client teaching

▲ **Outcome Criteria**

The outcome criteria for this diagnosis represent those associated with discharge planning. Refer to the discharge criteria.

Potential Altered Health Maintenance related to insufficient knowledge of activities permitted and restricted, medications, complications, and follow-up care

Focus Assessment Criteria	Clinical Significance
1. Knowledge of the therapeutic regimen	1. Assessing the client's and family's knowledge level guides the nurse in planning teaching strategies.
2. Readiness and ability to learn and retain information	2. A client or family that fails to achieve learning goals requires a referral for assistance postdischarge.
3. Support systems, home environment	3. A client's ability to comply with the therapeutic regimen may be influenced (either positively or negatively) by his home environment and available support systems.

Interventions

1. Discuss permitted activities after surgery:
   a. Reading
   b. Watching TV
   c. Driving
   d. Cooking
   e. Light housekeeping
   f. Sponge or tub bathing
2. Reinforce activity restrictions specified by the physician, which may include avoiding the following activities:
   a. Lying on the operative side
   b. Bending over at the waist
   c. Lifting anything weighing over 20 lb
   d. Showering
   e. Straining during bowel movements

Rationale

1. Beginning your discussions by outlining permitted activities rather than restrictions focuses the client on the positive rather than the negative aspects of recovery.

2. Restrictions are needed to reduce eye movements and prevent increased intraocular pressure. Specific restrictions depend on various factors, including the nature and extent of surgery, the physician's preference, and the client's age and overall health status. The client's understanding of the reasons for these restrictions can encourage compliance with them.

Interventions

3. Reinforce the importance of avoiding rubbing or bumping the eye and of keeping the protective patch and shield in place throughout the first postoperative day.

4. Explain the following information for each prescribed medication:
   a. Name, purpose, and action
   b. Dosage schedule (amount, times)
   c. Administration technique
   d. Special instructions or precautions
5. Instruct the client and family to report the following signs and symptoms:
   a. Vision loss
   b. Eye pain
   c. Vision abnormalities, e.g., light flashes, spots
   d. Redness, increased drainage, elevated temperature
6. Instruct in ocular hygiene measures, i.e., removing crusty drainage by wiping the closed eyelid with a cotton ball moistened with ocular irrigating solution.
7. Stress the importance of adequate follow-up care, with the schedule to be determined by the surgeon. The client should know the date and time of his first scheduled appointment before discharge.
8. Provide written instructions on discharge.

Rationale

3. Rubbing or bumping the eye may interrupt suture line integrity and provide an entry point for microorganisms. Keeping the eye covered reduces the risk of contamination by airborne organisms.

4. Providing accurate information before discharge can promote compliance with the medication regimen and help prevent errors in administration.

5. Early reporting of these signs and symptoms enables prompt intervention to prevent or minimize infection, increased intraocular pressure, hemorrhage, retinal detachment, or other complications.

6. Secretions may adhere to eyelids and eyelashes. Removal promotes comfort and reduces the risk of infection by eliminating a source of microorganisms.
7. Follow-up allows evaluation of healing and enables early detection of complications.

8. Written instructions provide the client and family with a source of information that they can consult as needed.

▲ **Documentation**

Discharge summary record
    Client and family teaching
    Outcome achievement or
      status

References/Bibliography

Bransford, J. (1979). *Human cognition: Learning, understanding, and remembering.* Belmont, CA: Wordsworth Publishing.

Carpenito, L.J. (1989). *Nursing diagnosis: Application to clinical practice* (3rd ed.). Philadelphia: J.B. Lippincott.

Doenges, M., Jeffries, M., & Moorhouse, H. (1984). *Nursing care plans—Nursing diagnosis in planning patient care.* Philadelphia: F.A. Davis.

Keefe, R. (1984). *The cataract book.* Daly City, CA: Krames Communication.

Newell, F. (1983). *Ophthalmology: Principles and concepts.* St. Louis: C.V. Mosby.

McCoy, K. (1981). Intraocular lenses: From cloudy to clear. *Nursing Clinics of North America, 6*(3), 405–414.

Peyman, G., Sanders, D., & Goldberg, M. (1980). *Principles and practice of ophthalmology.* Philadelphia: W.B. Saunders.

Saffle, J., Crandall, A., & Warden, G. (1985). Cataracts: A long-term complication of electrical injury. *The Journal of Trauma, 25*(1), 17–21.

Smith, J., & Nachazel, D. (1980). *Ophthalmic nursing.* Boston: Little, Brown.

Thompson, J., McFarland, G., Hirsch, J., Tucker, S., & Bowers, A. (1986). *Clinical nursing.* St. Louis: C.V. Mosby.

Vaughn, D., & Asbury, J. (1983). *General ophthalmology.* Los Altos, CA: Lange Publishing.

Colostomy

Colostomy entails opening some part of the colon onto the abdominal surface to divert feces, either temporarily or permanently. Indications for colostomy include diverticulitis, carcinoma of the rectosigmoid colon, and congenital anomalies, as well as protection of a more distal suture anastomosis (temporary). *Single-barreled* or end colostomy involves one functioning opening (stoma) on the abdominal surface and is permanent if the portion of the bowel distal to the stoma is removed. *Double-barreled* and loop colostomies involve two openings on the abdominal surface, the ends of the proximal and distal loops. Loop colostomy may be temporary, with closure done later; identification of the proximal and distal loops is needed for proper management (Smith, 1986).

Diagnostic Cluster

▲ Time Frame
Preoperative and postoperative periods

▲ Discharge Criteria
Before discharge, the client and/or family will:

1. State conditions of ostomy care at home: stoma, pouching, irrigation, skin care
2. Discuss strategies for incorporating ostomy management into ADLs.
3. Verbalize precautions for medication use and food intake.
4. State signs and symptoms that must be reported to a health care professional.
5. Verbalize an intent to share feelings and concerns related to ostomy with significant others.
6. Identify available community resources and self-help groups:
   a. Visiting nurse
   b. United Ostomy Association
   c. Recovery of Male Potency: Help for Impotent Male
   d. American Cancer Foundation
   e. Community supplier of ostomy equipment
   f. Financial reimbursement for ostomy equipment

PREOPERATIVE PERIOD
Nursing Diagnoses

Anxiety related to lack of knowledge of colostomy care and perceived negative effects on life style

POSTOPERATIVE PERIOD
Collaborative Problems

Potential Complications:
Peristomal Ulceration/Herniation
Stomal Necrosis, Retraction, Prolapse, Stenosis, Obstruction

Nursing Diagnoses

Potential Self-Concept Disturbance related to effects of ostomy on body image and life style
Potential Altered Sexuality Pattern related to perceived negative impact of ostomy on sexual functioning and attractiveness
Potential Sexual Dysfunction related to physiological impotence secondary to damage to sympathetic nerves (male) or inadequate vaginal lubrication (female)
Potential Social Isolation related to anxiety over possible odor and leakage from appliance
Potential Altered Health Maintenance related to insufficient knowledge of stoma pouching procedure, colostomy irrigation, peristomal skin care, perineal wound care, and incorporation of ostomy care into activities of daily living (ADLs)
Grieving related to implications of cancer diagnosis

Related Care Plan

General Surgery Generic Care Plan

Refer to:

Cancer (Initial Diagnosis)

Preoperative: Nursing Diagnosis

Anxiety related to lack of knowledge of colostomy care and perceived negative effects on lifestyle

Focus Assessment Criteria	Clinical Significance
1. Understanding of underlying disorder necessitating colostomy	1–7. Assessing the client's knowledge of colostomy identifies learning needs and guides

▲ **Outcome Criteria**

The client will:

1. State reason for colostomy
2. Describe anatomical changes following colostomy surgery
3. Identify his or her own type of colostomy
4. Verbalize decreased anxiety related to fear of the unknown

Focus Assessment Criteria

2. Knowledge of structure and function of affected organs
3. Anticipated surgical procedure and stoma location
4. Previous exposure to the client with an ostomy
5. Familiarity with stoma pouching equipment
6. Emotional status, cognitive ability, memory, vision, manual dexterity
7. Life style, strengths, coping mechanisms, available support systems

Clinical Significance

the nurse in planning effective teaching strategies. Assessing emotional status, mental and physical ability, and other factors about the client helps the nurse evaluate the client's ability to accept, adjust to, and manage the ostomy and stoma.

Interventions

1. Identify and dispel any misinformation or misconceptions the client has regarding ostomy.
2. Explain the normal anatomical structure and function of the gastrointestinal (GI) tract.
3. Explain the effects of the client's particular disorder on affected organs.
4. Use an anatomical diagram or model to show the resulting altered route of elimination.

5. Describe the appearance and anticipated location of the stoma. Explain the following about the stoma:
   a. It will be the same color and moistness as oral mucous membrane.
   b. It will not hurt when touched, because it has no sensory endings.
   c. It may bleed slightly when wiped; this is normal and not of concern.
   d. It will become smaller as the surgical area heals; color will remain the same.
   e. It may change in size depending on illness, hormone levels, and weight gain or loss.
6. Discuss the function of the stoma pouch. Explain that it serves as an external receptacle for storage of feces much as the colon acts as an internal storage receptacle.
7. Encourage the client to handle the stoma pouching equipment.

Rationale

1. Replacing misinformation with facts can reduce anxiety.
2. Knowledge increases confidence; confidence produces control and reduces anxiety.
3. Understanding the disorder can help the client accept the need for colostomy.
4. Understanding how body waste elimination occurs after the rectum and anus are removed can help allay anxiety related to altered body function.
5. Explaining expected events and sensations can help reduce anxiety associated with the unknown and unexpected. Accurate descriptions of the stoma appearance help ease shock at the first sight of it after ostomy surgery.

6. Understanding the purpose and need for a pouch encourages the client to accept it and participate in ostomy management.

7. Many clients are relieved to see the actual size and material of a stoma pouch. Often, uninformed clients have visions of large bags and complicated, difficult-to-manage equipment, which can produce anxiety.

▲ **Documentation**

Progress notes
  Present emotional status
  Client teaching

Postoperative: Collaborative Problems

▲ **Nursing Goal**

The nurse will manage and minimize stomal complications.

Potential Complication: Peristomal Ulceration/Herniation
Potential Complication: Stomal Necrosis, Prolapse, Retraction, Stenosis, Obstruction

Interventions

1. Monitor the peristomal area for the following:
   a. Decreased peristomal muscle tone
   b. Bulging beyond the normal skin surface and musculature
   c. Persistent ulceration

Rationale

1. Early detection of ulcerations and herniation can prevent serious tissue damage.

▲ **Documentation**

Flow records
    Intake and output
    Bowel sounds
    Wound status
Progress notes
    Stoma condition
    Changes in physiological
        status

Interventions

2. Monitor the following:
    a. Color, size, and shape of stoma

    b. Color, amount, and consistency of ostomy effluent
    c. Complaints of cramping abdominal pain, nausea and vomiting, abdominal distention
    d. Ostomy appliance and appliance belt fit

Rationale

2.

   a. Changes can indicate inflammation, retraction, prolapse, edema.
   b. Changes can indicate bleeding or infection. Decreased output can indicate obstruction.
   c. These complaints may indicate obstruction.

   d. Improperly fitting appliance or belt can cause mechanical trauma to the stoma.

Related Physician-Prescribed Interventions

Dependent on the underlying problem. Refer also to the General Surgery care plan (Appendix II).

Postoperative: Nursing Diagnoses

▲ **Outcome Criteria**

The client will:

1. Acknowledge change in body structure and function
2. Communicate feelings about the ostomy
3. Participate in stoma care

Potential Self-Concept Disturbance related to effects of ostomy on body image and lifestyle

Focus Assessment Criteria

1. Previous exposure to the client(s) with an ostomy
2. Ability to visualize the stoma
3. Ability to express feelings about the stoma
4. Ability to share feelings about the ostomy with significant others
5. Ability to participate in the stoma pouching procedure
6. Ability to discuss plans to incorporate ostomy management into body image and lifestyle
7. Evidence of negative self-concept

Clinical Significance

1–7. This assessment information helps the nurse evaluate present responses and progress. Participation in self-care and planning indicates positive attempts to cope with the changes.

Interventions

1. Contact the client frequently and treat him or her with warm, positive regard.

2. Incorporate emotional support into technical ostomy self-care sessions.

Rationale

1. Frequent contact by the caregiver indicates acceptance and may facilitate trust. The client may be hesitant to approach the staff because of negative self-concept.
2. This allows resolution of emotional issues during acquisition of technical skills. Shipes (1987) identified four stages of psychological adjustment that ostomy clients experience:
    a. *Narration.* Each client recounts his illness experience and reveals his understanding of how and why he finds himself in this situation.
    b. *Visualization and verbalization.* The client looks at and expresses feelings about his stoma.
    c. *Participation.* The client progresses from observer to assistant and then to independent performer of the mechanical aspects of ostomy care.
    d. *Exploration.* The client begins to explore methods of incorporating the ostomy into his lifestyle.

Use of this adjustment framework helps estab-

Interventions

3. Have the client look at and touch the stoma.

4. Encourage the client to verbalize feelings about the stoma and perceptions of its anticipated effects on his or her lifestyle.
5. Validate the client's perceptions and reassure that such responses are normal and appropriate.
6. Have the client practice using a pouch clamp on an empty pouch.

7. Assist the client with pouch emptying, as necessary.

8. Have the client participate in pouch removal and pouch application. Provide feedback on progress; reinforce positive behavior and proper techniques.
9. Have the client demonstrate the stoma pouching procedure independently in the presence of support persons.
10. Involve support persons in learning ostomy care principles. Assess the client's interactions with support persons.
11. Encourage the client to discuss plans for incorporating ostomy care into his or her lifestyle.
12. Encourage the client to verbalize positive self-attributes.
13. Suggest that the client meet with a person from the United Ostomy Association (UOA) who can share similar experiences.

14. Identify a client at risk for unsuccessful adjustment; look for these characteristics:
    a. Poor ego strength
    b. Ineffective problem-solving ability

    c. Difficulty learning new skills

    d. Lack of motivation
    e. External focus of control

    f. Poor health
    g. Unsatisfactory preoperative sex life
    h. Lack of positive support systems
    i. Unstable economic status
    j. Rejection of counseling (Shipes, 1987).
15. Refer an at-risk client for professional counseling.

Rationale

lish guidelines for planning the client's experiences in an organized manner.
3. The nurse should not make assumptions about a client's reaction to ostomy surgery. He or she may need help in accepting the reality of the altered body appearance and function or in dealing with an overwhelming situation.
4. Sharing gives the nurse an opportunity to identify and dispel misconceptions and allay anxiety and self-doubt.
5. Validating the client's perceptions promotes self-awareness and provides reassurance.

6. Beginning client teaching with a necessary skill that is separate from the body may be less threatening and may ease the fear of failure when performing on his or her own body.
7. During ostomy care procedures, the client will watch health care professionals for signs of revulsion. The nurse's attitude and support are of primary importance (Shipes, 1987).
8. Effective, thorough teaching helps the client learn to master procedures.

9. Return demonstration lets the nurse evaluate the need for any further teaching.

10. Others' response to the ostomy is one of the most important factors influencing the client's acceptance of it.
11. Evidence that the client will pursue his or her goals and lifestyle reflects positive adjustment.

12. Identifying personal strengths promotes self-acceptance and positive self-concept.
13. In addition to the clinical expertise of the professional nurse, the ostomy client may choose to take advantage of a UOA visitor's actual experience with an ostomy (Maklebust, 1985).
14. Successful adjustment to ostomies are influenced by factors such as the following:
    a. Previous coping success
    b. Achievement of developmental tasks pre-surgery
    c. The extent to which the disability interferes with goal-directed activity
    d. Sense of control
    e. Realistic perception of the event by the client and support persons

15. In such a client, follow-up therapy is indicated to assist with effective adjustment.

▲ **Documentation**

Progress notes
　Present emotional status
　Interventions
　Response to interventions

Potential Altered Sexuality Pattern related to perceived negative impact of ostomy on sexual functioning and attractiveness

Focus Assessment Criteria	Clinical Significance
1. Importance of sex to the client 2. Availability of a partner 3. Concerns about resuming intercourse 4. Preferred methods of sexual expression 5. Acceptability of alternative pleasuring activities to the client and partner	1–5. Assessment of current concerns and past sexual patterns provides direction for planning effective nursing interventions.

Interventions	Rationale
1. Reaffirm the need for frank discussion between sexual partners and the need for time for the partner to become accustomed to changes in the client's body.	1. The client may worry about his or her partner's acceptance; the partner may be afraid of hurting the client and needs to know that the stoma is not harmed by sexual activity.
2. Role-play ways for the client and partner to discuss concerns about sex.	2. Role-playing helps a person gain insight by placing him or her in the position of another. It also may promote more spontaneous sharing of fears and concerns.
3. Discuss the possibility that the client may project his or her own feelings onto the partner. Encourage frequent validation of feelings between partners.	3. The client may have erroneous assumptions about the partner, e.g., may erroneously assume that the partner is "turned off" by the ostomy.
4. Reaffirm the need for closeness and expressions of caring; involve the client and partner in touching, stroking, massage, etc.	4. Sexual pleasure and gratification are not limited to intercourse. Other expressions of caring may prove more meaningful.
5. Explore any fears the client may express regarding mutilation, unacceptability, and other concerns that might limit his or her involvement in relationships.	5. These fears might limit involvement in relationships.
6. Discuss the possible availability of a penile prosthesis if the client is physiologically unable to maintain or sustain an erection sufficient for intercourse. Explain that penile implants provide the erection needed for intercourse and do not alter sensations or the ability to ejaculate.	6. Realizing that a prosthesis may be available may reassure the client and reduce anxiety about performance, which actually could help improve function.
7. Refer the client to a certified sex or mental health counselor, if desired.	7. Certain sexual problems require continuing therapy and the advanced knowledge of therapists.

Potential Sexual Dysfunction related to physiological impotence secondary to sympathetic nerve damage (male) or inadequate vaginal lubrication (female)

Focus Assessment Criteria	Clinical Significance
1. Knowledge of the effects of surgery on sexual function. 　a. In men, abdominoperineal resection often damages sympathetic nerves in the presacral area that controls emission. This may result in retrograde ejaculation into the bladder and a "dry" orgasm. During abdominoperineal surgery, the parasympathetic nerves that control blood flow to the penis can be damaged, possibly resulting in erectile dysfunction.	1. Assessing the client's knowledge of possible effects on sexual function guides the nurse in planning effective interventions.

Focus Assessment Criteria

b. In women, there is little objective evidence of sexual dysfunction following abdominoperineal resection. The most common female sexual complaint is dyspareunia, which may result in "female impotence" (Schover, 1985).

Clinical Significance

Interventions

1. In men
   a. Suggest that sexual activity need not always culminate in vaginal intercourse and that orgasm can be reached through noncoital manual or oral stimulation. Remind the client that sexual expression is not limited to intercourse but includes closeness, communication, touching, and giving pleasure to another.
   b. Explain the function of a penile prosthesis. Both semirigid and inflatable penile prostheses have a high rate of success.
   c. Suggest counseling with a certified sex therapist.

2. In women
   a. Suggest using a water-based vaginal lubricant for intercourse.
   b. Teach the client to perform Kegel exercises, and instruct her to do them regularly.

   c. Suggest that she sit astride her partner during intercourse.

Rationale

1a. Alternate methods of sexual expression and gratification promote positive sexual function.

1b. Penile implants provide the erection needed for intercourse and do not alter sensations or the ability to ejaculate.
1c. Certain sexual problems require continuing therapy and the advanced knowledge of therapists.
2a. Water-based lubricant can help prevent dyspareunia related to inadequate vaginal lubrication.
2b. Kegel exercises promote control of the pubococcygeal muscles around the vaginal entrance, which can ease dyspareunia.
2c. A woman on top can control the depth and rate of penetration, which can enhance vaginal lubrication and relaxation.

▲ **Documentation**

Progress notes
   Interventions
   Response to interventions

▲ **Outcome Criteria**

The client will:

1. Discuss methods to control odor and appliance leakage
2. State an intent to reestablish preoperative socialization pattern

Potential Social Isolation related to anxiety about possible odor and leakage from appliance

Focus Assessment Criteria

1. Preoperative socialization pattern
2. Anticipated changes

Clinical Significance

1,2. A client at risk for social isolation must be assessed carefully; the suffering associated with isolation is not always visible. Feelings of rejection and repulsion are common.

Interventions

1. Select an appropriate odor-proof pouching system, and explain to the client how it works.

2. Stress the need for good personal hygiene.
3. Teach the client care of a reusable appliance.
4. Discuss methods for reducing odor:
   a. Avoid odor-producing foods, such as onions, fish, eggs, cheese, asparagus.
   b. Use internal chlorophyll tablets or a liquid appliance deodorant.
   c. Empty or change the ostomy pouch regularly, when one-third to one-half full.

Rationale

1. Fear of accidents and odor can be reduced through effective management. Some pouches have charcoal filters to reduce odor from flatus.
2,3. Proper hygiene and appliance care removes odoriferous retained fecal material.
4. Minimizing odor improves self-confidence and can permit more effective socialization. Bacterial proliferation in retained effluent increases odor over time. A full pouch also puts excessive pressure on seals, increasing the risk of leakage.

Interventions

5. Encourage the client to reestablish his or her preoperative socialization pattern. Help through measures such as progressively increasing the client's socializing time in the hospital and role-playing possible situations that the client feels may cause anxiety, encouraging the client to visualize and anticipate solutions to "worst-case scenarios" for social situations.

6. Suggest that the client meet with a person from the United Ostomy Association (UOA) who can share similar experiences.

Rationale

5. Encouraging and facilitating socialization help prevent isolation. Role-playing can help the client identify and learn to cope with potential anxiety-causing situations in a nonthreatening environment.

6. Others in a similar situation can provide a realistic appraisal of the situation and may provide information to answer the client's unasked questions.

▲ *Documentation*

Progress notes
  Dialogues
Discharge summary record
  Client teaching
  Outcome achievement or
    status

▲ *Outcome Criteria*

The outcome criteria for this diagnosis represent those associated with discharge planning. Refer to the discharge criteria.

Potential Altered Health Maintenance related to insufficient knowledge of stoma pouching procedure, colostomy irrigation, peristomal skin care, perineal wound care, and incorporation of ostomy care into ADLs

Focus Assessment Criteria	*Clinical Significance*
1. Type of colostomy	1. Colostomy care differs according to its type and concurrent therapies. Sigmoid and descending colostomies may be cleansed with irrigation enemas to predict the time of a bowel movement. Colostomies higher in the GI tract produce mushy effluent rather than formed stool; discharge of unformed stool is never predictable. A client receiving radiation or chemotherapy is not able to predict a regular bowel pattern.
2. Desire for control of elimination by irrigation	2. Not every client is a candidate for irrigation. In addition to the type of colostomy, the client's age, physical disabilities, concurrent disease, and personal preference determine the appropriateness of colostomy irrigation. The bowel does empty without irrigation, but not in a predictable pattern.
3. Usual elimination pattern	3. Irrigation should be done within the same 2- or 3-hour period each day so that the bowel becomes regulated. Regular irrigation assists in establishing a normal bowel evacuation pattern. If possible, irrigation should be timed to produce evacuation on a schedule coinciding with the client's preoperative bowel pattern.
4. Home facilities needed for irrigation	4. Adequate and accessible toileting facilities are essential to an effective elimination schedule.
5. Knowledge of colostomy care: diet, activity, hygiene, clothing, sexual expression, community resources, employment, travel, odor, skin care, appliances, and irrigation, if applicable	5. Assessment identifies learning needs and guides the nurse in planning effective teaching strategies.
6. Client's and support persons' readiness and ability to learn and retain information	6. A family or client who fails to achieve learning goals requires a referral for assistance postdischarge.

Interventions

1. Consistently use the same sequence in client teaching.

2. Teach the client basic stoma pouching principles, including the following:
   a. Keeping the peristomal skin clean and dry

   b. Using a well-fitting appliance

   c. Changing the pouch when the least amount of drainage is anticipated (usually on arising)
   d. Emptying the pouch when it is one-third to one-half full and changing routinely before a leak occurs
   e. Changing the pouch if burning or itching occurs under the appliance

   f. Observing the condition of the stoma and peristomal skin during pouch changes
3. Teach the procedure for preparing a stoma pouch:
   a. Select the appropriate stoma pouching system.
   b. Measure the stoma carefully.
   c. Use the appliance manufacturer's stoma measuring card, if possible. If the card does not accommodate stoma size or shape, teach the client to make a customized stoma pattern. Place clear plastic wrap from the skin barrier wafer over the stoma, trace the stoma with a marking pen, and cut a hole in the plastic to accommodate the stoma.
   d. Cut an opening in the center of the skin barrier slightly larger than the stoma (approximately ⅛ inch).
   e. Secure an appropriate odor-proof pouch onto the skin barrier wafer (if using a two-piece appliance system).
4. Teach the procedure for changing a disposable stoma pouch:
   a. Remove the old pouch by gently pushing the skin away from the paper tape and skin barrier wafer.
   b. Fold the old pouch over on itself and discard in a plastic bag.
   c. Cleanse the peristomal skin with a wash cloth and warm tap water.
   d. Blot or pat the skin dry.
   e. Apply the new pouch to the abdomen, carefully centering the hole in the skin barrier wafer over the stoma. Press on the wafer for a few minutes.
   f. Secure the pouch by "picture framing" the wafer with four strips of hypoallergenic paper tape (if the wafer does not already have tape attached).

Rationale

1. Consistency reinforces learning and may enhance the client's sense of control over the situation.
2. Proper pouching techniques can prevent leakage and skin problems.
   a. This ensures that the appliance adheres to the skin.
   b. Proper fit protects the surrounding skin surface from contact with drainage.
   c. This prevents copious drainage from interfering with pouch changes.

   d. A pouch filled more than halfway exerts increased pressure on the seal, increasing the risk of leakage.
   e. Burning or itching may indicate that ostomy effluent has undermined the skin barrier; prompt intervention is necessary to prevent skin breakdown.
   f. Regular observation enables early detection of skin problems.
3. Preparing a new pouch beforehand ensures that it is ready to apply as soon as the used pouch is removed, helping minimize drainage on the skin surface.

4. Correct pouch removal and attachment techniques minimize irritation and injury of peristomal skin and ensure a tight, reliable seal between the pouch and skin.

Interventions

5. Teach the procedure for emptying a stoma pouch:
   a. Put some toilet paper in the toilet bowl and sit on the toilet seat.
   b. Remove the clamp from the tail of the pouch, and carefully empty pouch contents into the toilet.
   c. Clean the inside and outside of the pouch tail with toilet paper and squeeze ostomy appliance deodorant into the end of the pouch.

6. Teach the ostomy irrigation procedure:

   a. Assemble all equipment:
      • Water container and water
      • Irrigating sleeves and stoma
      • Items to clean skin and stoma
      • Way to dispose of old pouch
      • Clean pouch and closure
      • Skin care items
   b. Cleanse the stoma and surrounding skin with water and let dry. Observe their condition and color.
   c. Apply the irrigating sleeve and belt securely. If using karaya washer, dampen and apply this first. You may lubricate the inside of the irrigation sleeve with oil to help the stool slide through the sleeve.
   d. Fill the irrigating container with about 1 quart of tepid water.
   e. Suspend the irrigating container so that the bottom of the container is even with the top of the shoulder.
   f. Remove all air from the tubing.
   g. Gently insert the irrigating cone into the stoma, holding it parallel to the floor. Start the water slowly. If water does not flow easily, try or check the following:
      • Slightly adjust body position or the angle of the cone.
      • Check for kinks in the tubing from the irrigating container.
      • Check the height of the irrigating container.
      • Relax and take some deep breaths.
   h. Instill water into the bowel; the amount of fluid instillation varies. Do not force water into the bowel. If cramping occurs, if the flow of water stops, or if water is forcefully returning around the irrigating cone or catheter, stop the flow.
   i. If bloating or constipation develops, irrigate with about ½ quart more water in the same day, or use a mild laxative.

Rationale

5. Correct techniques can reduce spillage, soiling, and odor. Placing toilet paper in the bowl prevents water from splashing as the pouch contents are emptied.

6. The purpose of colostomy irrigation is to establish a regular bowel evacuation pattern, making a colostomy pouch unnecessary.
   a. Assembling all equipment beforehand prevents delays during the procedure.

   b. Thorough cleansing removes drainage from skin.

   c. Preapplication makes cleaning easier.

   d. Hot water traumatizes the bowel; cold water causes cramping.
   e. At a lower height, the water may not flow easily. Higher height would give too much force to the water, causing cramping or incomplete emptying.
   f. Removing air from the tubing helps prevent gas pains during irrigation.
   g. Gentle and slow movements help reduce tissue trauma. Relaxation decreases muscle tension and resistance.

   h. Forcing water can cause tissue damage.

   i. Increasing the amount of water may promote evacuation.

Interventions	*Rationale*
j. Look for most of the stool to return in about 15 minutes. When most of the stool is expelled, rinse the sleeve with water, dry the bottom edge, roll it up, and close the end.	j. The clamped irrigation sleeve acts as a temporary pouch until all of the stool is expelled.
k. Allow 30 to 45 minutes more for the bowels to finish emptying.	k. Complete emptying helps prevent later leakage.
l. Remove the irrigation sleeve and apply a clean closed-end pouch or a stoma cover.	l. Just a stoma cover is appropriate if the client can achieve total control by irrigation. Manufacturers are currently testing stoma occluding devices that can be inserted and removed intermittently to allow fecal elimination, to serve as an alternative to an external colostomy pouch.
m. Rinse the irrigation sleeve and hang it up to dry.	m. Thorough rinsing and drying decreases odor.
7. Teach strategies for prevention and management of potential peristomal skin problems:	7. A client with a stoma is at increased risk for peristomal skin breakdown. Factors that influence skin integrity include: composition, quantity, and consistency of the ostomy effluent; allergies; mechanical trauma; the underlying disease and its treatment (including medications); surgical construction and location of the stoma; the quality of ostomy and periostomal skin care; availability of proper supplies; nutritional status; overall health status; hygiene; and activity level.
a. Shave the peristomal skin with an electric razor rather than a blade; avoid using shaving cream, soap, and detergents except when showering.	
b. Evaluate all skin products for possible allergic reaction; patch-test all suspect products elsewhere on the abdomen.	
c. Do not change brands of skin barriers and adhesives casually; assess for allergic reaction before using a new brand.	
d. Avoid irritation from contact with ostomy effluent.	
e. Avoid prolonged skin pressure, especially if fair-skinned or having thin, atrophic skin due to long-term corticosteroid therapy.	
f. Use corticosteroid creams sparingly and briefly; they can cause dryness and irritation.	
g. If bacterial or fungal infection is suspected, use a specific antibacterial or antifungal cream or powder.	
h. Use a liquid film barrier; avoid tincture of benzoin compound, which can dry skin.	
i. Avoid aluminum paste and greasy ointments, which can mask skin problems and also interfere with pouch adherence.	
j. Protect the skin with barriers.	
k. Expect the stoma to shrink slightly over time. This necessitates remeasuring the stoma to ensure proper appliance fit.	
8. Teach the procedure for perineal wound care:	8. Removal of the rectum results in a large perineal wound that typically is left open to heal by secondary intention. Some clients with a colostomy do not have the rectum and anus removed but instead have a rectal stump that is sutured across the top. This becomes a nonfunctioning internal pouch (Hartmann's pouch). In this situation, the client continues to expel mucus through the anus that is produced by the remaining rectal mucosa.
a. Take sitz baths or irrigate the area with warm water to cleanse the wound thoroughly.	
b. Wear a peripad to protect the wound and contain drainage until healing occurs.	
c. Watch for and report signs and symptoms of infection or abscess (e.g., pain, purulent drainage).	

Interventions

Rationale

d. Because the rectum is missing, thermometers, suppositories, and other devices cannot be inserted.

9. Address nutrition and diet management:

a. Teach how the ostomy affects absorption and use of nutrients, and discuss dietary implications.

b. Assess food tolerances by adding new foods one at a time and in small amounts.

c. Teach the client to eat regularly and slowly, to chew food well, and to avoid high-fiber foods, which can promote stomal blockage.

d. Discuss dietary modifications that can help decrease odor and flatus.

e. List dietary modifications to prevent or manage diarrhea and constipation, as indicated.

f. Instruct the client to monitor weight and report any loss or gain of more than 10 pounds.

g. Explain the importance of adequate fluid intake (water and juices) to prevent or manage fluid and electrolyte problems related to altered elimination.

10. Explain the effects of certain medications on ostomy function:

a. Antibiotics may induce diarrhea.

b. Narcotics and aluminum- or calcium-containing antacids can promote constipation.

c. Fecal odor may be controlled by internal or external deodorizers. Internal deodorizers may have a mild laxative effect.

d. Suppositories cannot be used after the rectum and anus are removed.

Instruct the client to notify a physician or pharmacist if a drug problem is suspected.

11. Promote measures to help the client incorporate ostomy care into ADLs:

a. Working/traveling: Keep extra supplies at work. When traveling, carry supplies rather than pack them in a suitcase and risk losing them; keep in mind that pectin-based wafers melt in high environmental temperatures. Take a list of ostomy supplies when traveling.

b. Exercise: The only limits involve contact sports during which trauma to the stoma may occur. Normal exercise is beneficial and may help to stimulate bowel evacuation—and, in some cases, can eliminate the need for irrigation. Successful use of exercise to regulate the bowel depends on the presurgical bowel pattern and regularity of elimination. Other contributing factors include the consistency of the fecal contents, motivation, diet, ability to exercise, and practice.

c. Wardrobe: Ostomy appliances are invisible under clothing. Any clothing worn preop-

9. Proper nutritional intake and dietary management are important factors in ostomy management.

10. Counseling the client about the possible harmful effects of home remedies and indiscriminate self-medication may help prevent minor or serious problems.

11. Successful incorporation of ostomy management into ADLs allows the client to resume his precolostomy lifestyle and pursue goals and interests.

Interventions   **Rationale**

eratively may be worn postoperatively.
Dress comfortably.

d. Bathing/showering/swimming: These activities may be done while wearing an ostomy appliance. "Picture-frame" the skin barrier with paper tape to seal the edges and keep the barrier edge from getting wet. Showering may be done without an appliance and, in fact, is recommended on days of appliance changes.

▲ **Documentation**

Discharge summary record
  Client and family teaching
  Response to teaching

References/Bibliography

Alterescu, K.B. (1987). Colostomy. *Nursing Clinics of North America, 22,* 281–289.

Broadwell, D.C. (1987). Peristomal skin integrity. *Nursing Clinics of North America, 22*(2), 321–332.

Broadwell, D.C., & Sorrells, S.L. (1983). *Summary of your colostomy care.* Berkley Heights, NJ: C.R. Bard.

Carpenito, L.J. (1989). *Nursing diagnosis: Application to clinical practice* (3rd ed.). Philadelphia: J.B. Lippincott.

Coe, M., et al. (1988). Concerns of clients and spouses regarding ostomy surgery. *Journal of Enterostomal Therapy, 15*(6), 84–89.

Hedrick, J.K. (1988). Effects of ET nursing intervention on adjustment following ostomy surgery. *Journal of Enterostomal Therapy, 15*(6), 229–239.

Maklebust, J. (1985). United Ostomy Association visits and adjustment following ostomy surgery. *Journal of Enterstomal Therapy, 12*(3), 84–89.

Rideout, B.W. (1987). The patient with an ileostomy. *Nursing Clinics of North America, 22*(1), 253–262.

Schover, L.R. (1985). Sexual rehabilitation of the ostomy patient. In D.B. Smith & D.E. Johnson (Eds.). *Ostomy care and the cancer patient.* Orlando, FL: Grune and Stratton.

Shipes, E. (1987). Psychosocial issues: The person with an ostomy. *Nursing Clinics of North America, 22*(2), 291–302.

Smith, D.B. (1986). *Ostomy care and the cancer patient.* Orlando, FL: Grune and Stratton.

Smith, M.D. (1983). Altered gastrointestinal functioning. In E.A. Mahoney & J.P. Flynn (Eds.). *Handbook of medical-surgical nursing.* New York: John Wiley and Sons.

Thomas, D., et al. (1987). Management of temporary loop ileostomy following colectomy, mucosal protectomy, and ileal pouch-anal anastomosis. *Journal of Enterostomal Therapy, 14*(5), 194–196.

Coronary Artery Bypass Grafting

Indicated for clients with coronary artery disease, coronary artery bypass grafting (CABG) increases blood flow to the heart through anastomosis of a saphenous vein (autograft) to an area proximal and distal to the coronary artery occlusion. Surgery involves cardiopulmonary bypass, or extracorporeal circulation, to circulate and oxygenate the blood while diverting it from the heart and lungs, providing a bloodless operative field for the surgeon.

Diagnostic Cluster

▲ Time Frame
Preoperative and postoperative periods

▲ Discharge Criteria
Before discharge, the client or family will:
1. Demonstrate insertion site care
2. Relate at-home restrictions and follow-up care
3. State signs and symptoms that must be reported to a health care professional
4. Relate a plan to reduce risk factors, as necessary

PREPROCEDURE PERIOD
Nursing Diagnoses

Fear (individual/family) related to the client's health status, need for coronary artery bypass graft surgery, and unpredictable outcome

POSTPROCEDURE PERIOD
Collaborative Problems

Potential Complications:
Cardiovascular Insufficiency
Respiratory Insufficiency
Renal Insufficiency

Nursing Diagnoses

Fear related to transfer from intensive environment of the critical care unit and potential for complications
Altered Family Process related to disruption of family life, fear of outcome (death, disability), and stressful environment (ICU)
Potential Self-Concept Disturbance related to the symbolic meaning of the heart and changes in life style
Potential Altered Health Maintenance related to insufficient knowledge of incisional care, pain management (angina, incisions), signs and symptoms of complications, condition, pharmacological care, risk factors, restrictions, stress management techniques, and follow-up care
Altered Comfort related to surgical incisions, chest tubes, and immobility secondary to lengthy surgery

Related Care Plans

General Surgery Generic Care Plan
Thoracic Surgery

Refer to:

General Surgery

Preoperative: Nursing Diagnosis

Fear (individual, family) related to the client's health status, the need for CABG surgery, and unpredictable outcome

Focus Assessment Criteria	Clinical Significance
1. Understanding of coronary artery disease	1–3. The client's and family's knowledge level guides the nurse in planning appropriate teaching.
2. Understanding of CABG surgery, including:	
a. Reason for surgery	

▲ *Outcome Criteria*

The client or family will:

1. Verbalize, if asked, what to expect before surgery (e.g., routines, tests)
2. Verbalize, if asked, an understanding of the CABG procedure
3. Verbalize, if asked, what to expect post-CABG (e.g., monitoring, care)
4. Demonstrate postoperative exercises, turning, splinting, and respiratory regimen
5. Verbalize concerns regarding surgery

Focus Assessment Criteria

    b. Anticipated outcome
    c. Risks involved
    d. Type of anesthesia to be used
    e. Expected length of recovery period
3. Past experiences with CABG surgery
4. Concerns or fears regarding CABG surgery

5. Readiness and ability to learn and retain information

Clinical Significance

4. Unknown situations produce anxiety and fear. Assessment of the degree of the client's and family's response helps the nurse plan appropriate interventions to decrease it.
5. A client or family failing to meet learning goals requires a referral for assistance post-discharge.

Interventions

1. Reinforce the physician's teaching about coronary artery disease, as necessary.
2. Reinforce the physician's explanation of CABG surgery and why it is needed, as necessary. Notify the physician if additional explanation is indicated.
3. Explain necessary preoperative tests and procedures, such as the following:
   a. 12-Lead electrocardiogram (ECG)
   b. Chest x-ray film
   c. Cardiac catheterization
   d. Urinalysis
   e. Blood work: cardiac enzymes, electrolytes, coagulation studies, complete blood count, type and crossmatch, SMA12, arterial blood gas (ABG) analysis
   f. Nuclear studies
4. Provide instruction about preoperative routines beyond general surgery routines, such as the following:
   a. Chlorhexidine gluconate (Hibiclens) shower the night before and the morning of surgery
   b. Sending belongings home with family members
   c. Measures in the operating room holding area: shave and prep (from chin to ankles), intravenous (IV) and other invasive line insertion, and indwelling (Foley) catheter insertion.
5. Discuss postoperative measures, routines, and expectations, including the following:
   a. Endotracheal intubation and mechanical ventilation
   b. Chest tubes
   c. IV lines
   d. Swan–Ganz catheter
   e. Arterial line
   f. Epidural cardiac pacing
   g. Cardiac monitoring
   h. Indwelling catheter
   i. Autotransfusion
   j. Weight increase
   k. Nasogastric tube
   l. Pain and availability of medications

Rationale

1–6. Preoperative teaching provides information to help reduce the client's and family's fear of the unknown and enhance their sense of control over the situation.

Interventions

    m. Frequent assessment of vital signs, dressing, heart and lung sounds, peripheral pulses, skin, and capillary refill time

  6. Discuss expectations for intensive care:
    a. Environment
    b. Length of stay
    c. Care measures
    d. Visiting policies

  7. Discuss possible emotional and mental reactions post-CABG surgery.

  8. Present information or reinforce learning using written materials (e.g., booklets, posters, instruction sheets) or audiovisual aids (e.g., slides, videotapes, models, diagrams).

Rationale

  7. The heart is a symbol of life; cardiac dysfunction and surgery typically invoke a profound emotional reaction. Anesthesia, fluid loss from surgery, and pain medications can temporarily cloud thinking.

  8. Using various teaching materials and approaches provides multisensory stimulation, which can enhance the effectiveness of teaching and learning and improve retention.

▲ **Documentation**

Progress notes
    Present emotional status
    Interventions
    Response to interventions
Discharge summary record
    Client and family teaching
    Response to teaching
    Outcome achievement or status

Postoperative: Collaborative Problems

▲ **Nursing Goal**

The nurse will manage and minimize cardiac, vascular, and respiratory complications.

Potential Complication: Cardiovascular Insufficiency
Potential Complication: Respiratory Insufficiency
Potential Complication: Renal Insufficiency

Interventions

  1. Monitor for the following:
    a. Dysrhythmias
    b. Abnormal rate
    c. ECG changes: ST segment depression or elevation, PR, QRS, or QT interval changes
    d. Palpitations
    e. Syncope
    f. Cardiac emergencies (e.g., arrest, ventricular fibrillation)

  2. Monitor for signs and symptoms of hypotension and low cardiac output syndrome:
    a. Cardiac index < 2.0
    b. Increased pulmonary capillary wedge pressure (PCWP)
    c. Increased central venous pressure (CVP)
    d. Development of S_3 or S_4
    e. Neck vein distention
    f. Decreased systolic BP (90 mm Hg or 30 mm Hg below baseline)
    g. Irregular pulse
    h. Cool moist skin
    i. Decreased urine output (< 30 mL/hr)
    j. Increased pulse and respirations
    k. Increased restlessness
    l. Lethargy or confusion
    m. Increased rales
    n. Weak peripheral pulses

  3. Monitor for signs and symptoms of cardiac tamponade:
    a. Decreased systolic BP (90 mm Hg or 30 mm Hg below baseline)
    b. Muffled heart sounds
    c. Pericardial friction rub

Rationale

  1. Myocardial ischemia results from reduction of oxygen to myocardial tissue. Ischemic muscle is electrically unstable, leading to dysrhythmias. Dysrhythmias also may result from surgical manipulation, hypothermia, and acidosis.

  2. These effects can result from severe pain or greatly reduced cardiac output secondary to severe tissue hypoxia; inadequate preload and inadequate myocardial contractility; dysrhythmias; and ventricular failure. Decreased circulating volume and cardiac output can lead to kidney hypoperfusion and overall decreased tissue perfusion, triggering a compensatory response of decreased circulation to the extremities and increased heart and respiratory rates. Cerebral hypoperfusion also may result.

  3. Cardiac tamponade results from blood collecting around the heart because of CABG leakage or inadequate chest tube drainage, which compresses the heart and impairs its pumping ability.

Interventions

      d. Pulsus paradoxus

      e. Kussmaul's respirations

      f. Neck vein distention

      g. Narrowing pulse pressure

      h. Anginal pain

      i. Restlessness or stupor

      j. Increasing CVP and pulmonary artery pressure (PAP)

      k. Significant increase in or cessation of chest tube drainage

4. Monitor for signs and symptoms of respiratory failure:

      a. Increased respiratory rate

      b. Dyspnea

      c. Use of accessory muscles of respiration

      d. Cyanosis

      e. Increasing rales, rhonci, or wheezing

      f. Increased pCO_2, decreased O_2 saturation, decreased pH

      g. Restlessness

      h. Decreased capillary refill time

5. Monitor for signs and symptoms of hypertension or hypervolemia:

      a. Systolic blood pressure > 140 mm Hg

      b. Diastolic blood pressure > 90 mm Hg

      c. Increased systemic vascular resistance

6. Monitor for signs and symptoms of hemorrhage or hypovolemia:

      a. Incisional bleeding

      b. Chest tube drainage > 200 mL/hr

      c. Increased heart rate, decreased blood pressure, increased respirations

      d. Weak or absent peripheral pulses

      e. Cool, moist skin

      f. Dizziness

      g. Petechiae

      h. Ecchymoses

      i. Bleeding gums

      j. Decreased hemoglobin and hematocrit

      k. Increased prothrombin time (PT) and partial thromboplastin time (PTT) and decreased platelet count

7. Monitor for signs and symptoms of myocardial infarction:

      a. Chest pain and pressure

      b. Increased heart rate

      c. Hypotension

      d. Tachypnea

      e. Abnormal heart sounds

      f. Restlessness, lethargy, or confusion

      g. Elevated CVP and PCWP

      h. Nausea and vomiting

      i. ECG changes: ST segment elevation, abnormal Q waves

      j. Increased cardiac enzymes

      k. Elevated temperature

      l. Neck vein distention

      m. Weak peripheral pulses

      n. Moist, cool skin

      o. Decreased urine output (< 30 mL/hr)

Rationale

4. In the immediate postoperative period, hypoventilation may result from CNS depression caused by narcotics and anesthesia, impaired respiratory effort due to pain, fatigue, and immobility, or incomplete reinflation of lungs collapsed during surgery.

5. Hypervolemia and hypertension can result from a response to circulating catecholamines and renin secretion following cardiopulmonary bypass, which causes sodium and water retention.

6. Hemorrhage can be caused by inadequate surgical hemostasis, inadequate heparin reversal, or hypertension. It also may result from inadequate cardiac preload. Diuresis usually occurs by the third postoperative day, as fluids shift from interstitial to vascular compartments.

7. Cardiac pain results from cardiac tissue hypoxia secondary to narrowing or blockage of the coronary arteries or collapse of the newly grafted bypass.

▲ **Documentation**

Flow records
    Vital signs
    Cardiac rhythm
    Peripheral pulses
    Skin color, temperature,
      moisture
    Neck vein distention
    Respiratory assessment
    Neurological assessment
    Intake (oral, IVs, blood prod-
      ucts)
    Incisions (color, drainage,
      swelling)
    Output (chest tubes, naso-
      gastric tube)
    Urine specific gravity
    Bowel function (bowel
      sounds, distention)
    Sputum (amount, tenacious-
      ness, color)
Progress notes
    Change in physiological
      status
    Interventions
    Response to interventions

Interventions

8. Monitor for signs and symptoms of renal failure:
   a. Elevated blood urea nitrogen (BUN), creatinine, and potassium
   b. Decreased urine output (< 30 mL/hr)
   c. Elevated urine specific gravity (> 1.030)
   d. Weight gain
   e. Elevated CVP and PAP
9. Monitor for signs and symptoms of cerebrovascular accident (stroke):

   a. Unequal pupil size and reaction
   b. Paralysis or paresthesias in extremities
   c. Decreased level of consciousness
   d. Dizziness
   e. Blurred vision
   f. Seizure activity
10. Monitor for signs and symptoms of postcardiotomy delirium:
   a. Disorientation
   b. Confusion
   c. Hallucinations or delusions

Rationale

8. Cardiopulmonary bypass causes destruction of some RBCs, producing free hemoglobin that may occlude renal arteries. Hypovolemia or poor myocardial contractility may decrease circulation to the kidneys, resulting in hypoperfusion and eventual renal failure.

9. CVA may result from inadequate cerebral perfusion during cardiopulmonary bypass or an embolism.

10. This disorder may result from surgery-related microemboli, sensory overload or deprivation, or altered sleep pattern.

Related Physician-Prescribed Interventions

Medications
Anticoagulants   Analgesics
Diuretics   Beta-blockers
Antidysrhythmics

Intravenous Therapy
Fluid/electrolyte replacement

Laboratory Studies
Complete blood count   ABG analysis
Creatinine   Cardiac enzymes
Electrolytes   BUN
Blood chemistry profile

Diagnostic Studies
Ear/pulse oximetry   Chest x-ray film
ECG

Therapies
Supplemental oxygen   Other dependent on symptomatology

Postoperative: Nursing Diagnoses

▲ **Outcome Criteria**

The client will:

1. Verbalize any concerns regarding the completed surgery, possible complications, and the critical care environment
2. Report a decrease in the level of anxiety or fear

Fear related to transfer from intensive environment of the critical care unit and potential for complications

Focus Assessment Criteria

1. Nature of concerns and fears
2. Perception of progress
3. Understanding of need for transfer from critical care unit
4. Level of anxiety:
   a. Mild
   b. Moderate
   c. Severe
   d. Panic

Clinical Significance

1–4. Assessing the client's fears and anxiety level enables the nurse to plan effective interventions to reduce them. This is especially important to the post-CABG client, as stress, anxiety, and fear can precipitate a sympathetic nervous system response, which increases heart rate, blood pressure, and myocardial oxygen demand.

Interventions

1. Take steps to reduce the client's level of anxiety and fear:
   a. Reassure the client that you or other nurses are always close by and will respond promptly to his call.
   b. Convey a sense of empathy and understanding.
   c. Minimize external stimuli; e.g., close the room door, dim the lights, speak in a quiet voice, decrease the volume level of equipment alarms, position equipment so that alarms are diverted away from the client.
   d. Plan care measures to provide adequate periods of uninterrupted rest and sleep.
   e. Promote relaxation; encourage regular rest periods throughout the day.
   f. Explain each procedure before performing it.
2. Encourage the client to verbalize his concerns and fears. Clarify any misconceptions and provide positive feedback regarding progress.

3. Encourage the client to identify and call on reliable support persons and previously successful coping mechanisms.
4. Consult with the physician for pain medications or other medication, as necessary.

Rationale

1. Reducing anxiety, fear, and stress can decrease the demands made on an already compromised heart.

2. This sharing allows the nurse to correct any erroneous information the client may believe and validate that his concerns and fears are normal, which may help reduce anxiety.
3. Support persons and coping mechanisms are important tools in anxiety reduction.
4. Pharmacological assistance may be necessary if anxiety is at an unmanageable level; severe pain may be interfering with the client's ability to cope.

▲ **Documentation**

Progress notes
   Present emotional status
   Interventions
   Response to interventions

▲ **Outcome Criteria**

The family members or significant others will:

1. Verbalize concerns regarding CABG outcome and client prognosis
2. Verbalize concerns regarding the ICU environment
3. Report continued adequate family functioning during the client's hospitalization

Altered Family Processes related to disruption of family life, fear of outcome (death, disability), and stressful environment (ICU)

Focus Assessment Criteria

1. Specific stressors
2. Nature of concerns
3. Understanding of disease, surgery, and expected outcome
4. Familiarity with the ICU
5. Family coping mechanisms and use of support systems
6. Need for additional resources

Clinical Significance

1–5. A CABG client's family is experiencing a life crisis and is under extreme stress related to separation from the client and the uncertain prognosis. Assessing these factors gives the nurse information on which to base effective interventions.

6. The family may need referrals to assist with coping.

Interventions

1. Spend time with family members or significant others and convey a sense of empathetic understanding.
2. Allow family members or significant others to express their feelings, fears, and concerns.

3. Explain the ICU environment and equipment.
4. Explain the expected postoperative care measures and progress, and provide specific information on the client's progress, as appropriate.
5. Teach family members or significant others ways in which they can be more supportive; e.g., show them how they can touch the client,

Rationale

1. Frequent contact and communicating a sense of caring and concern can help reduce stress and promote learning.
2. Sharing allows the nurse to identify fears and concerns, then plan interventions to address them.
3–4. This information can help reduce anxiety associated with the unknown.

5. This information can ease fears associated with doing or saying the wrong thing and promote normal interaction with the client.

Interventions

encourage them to talk with and touch the client and to maintain a sense of humor.

6. Encourage frequent visitation and participation in care measures, when appropriate.
7. Consult with or provide referrals to community and other resources (e.g., social service agency), as necessary.

Rationale

6. Frequent visitation and participation in care can promote continued family interaction.
7. Families with problems such as financial needs, unsuccessful coping, or unresolved conflicts may need additional resources to help maintain family functioning.

▲ **Documentation**

Progress notes
    Present family functioning
    Interventions
    Response to interventions
Discharge summary record
    Referrals, if indicated

▲ **Outcome Criteria**

The client will begin to accept his new self-concept and the changes in his lifestyle.

Potential Self-Concept Disturbance related to the symbolic meaning of the heart and changes in lifestyle

Focus Assessment Criteria	*Clinical Significance*
1. Expressed self-concept	1. Heart disease and surgery pose a threat to self-concept beyond the obvious threat to life. The heart is a symbol of life and vitality, and any disruption in its function may trigger negative changes in self-concept.
2. Perceptions of and feelings about necessary post-CABG lifestyle changes	2. The client's perception of post-CABG lifestyle changes (e.g., physical, psychological, social, spiritual, financial) influences the extent of his self-concept disturbance.

Interventions

1. Encourage the client to express his feelings and concerns about necessary life style changes and changes in level of functioning.

2. Stress the client's role in preventing recurrence of atherosclerosis. Emphasize the steps he can take and encourage progress.

3. Allow the client to make choices regarding daily activities, when appropriate.

4. Encourage the client to participate actively in the care regimen.

5. Identify a client at risk for poor ego adjustment; look for these characteristics:
    a. Poor ego strength
    b. Ineffective problem-solving ability

    c. Difficulty learning new information or skills

    d. Lack of motivation
    e. External locus of control

    f. Poor health
    g. Unsatisfactory preoperative sex life
    h. Lack of positive support systems
    i. Unstable economic status
    j. Rejection of counseling (Shipes, 1987)
6. Refer an at-risk client for counseling.

Rationale

1. Sharing gives the nurse the opportunity to correct misconceptions, provide realistic feedback, and reassure the client that his concerns are normal.

2. The client's knowledge of his control over the situation can enhance ego strength. Stressing the positive promotes hope and reduces frustration.

3. A decrease in power in one area can be counterbalanced by providing opportunities for choices and control in other areas.

4. Participation in self-care mobilizes the client and promotes decision-making, which enhances self-concept.

5. Successful adjustment to CABG surgery is influenced by factors such as the following:
    a. Previous coping success
    b. Achievement of developmental tasks before surgery
    c. The extent to which resulting lifestyle changes interfere with goal-directed activity
    d. Sense of control over the situation
    e. Realistic perceptions by the client and support persons

6. Follow-up therapy is indicated to assist with effective adjustment.

▲ **Documentation**

Progress notes
    Client's current feelings
        about self and life style
        changes
    Dialogues

▲ *Outcome Criteria*

The outcome criteria for this diagnosis represent those associated with discharge planning. Refer to the discharge criteria.

Potential Altered Health Maintenance related to insufficient knowledge of incisional care, pain management (angina, incisions), signs and symptoms of complications, condition, pharmacological care, risk factors, restrictions, stress management techniques, and follow-up care

Focus Assessment Criteria	*Clinical Significance*
1. Understanding of home care needs	1. This information guides the nurse in planning teaching strategies.
2. Readiness and ability to learn and retain information	2. A client or family failing to meet learning goals requires a referral for assistance post-discharge.

Interventions

1. Explain and demonstrate care of uncomplicated surgical incisions:
   a. Wash with soap and water (bath and shower permitted; use lukewarm water).
   b. Wear loose clothing until incision areas are no longer tender.
2. Provide instruction for pain management:
   a. For incision pain (sore, sharp, stabbing):
      • Take pain medication as prescribed and before activities that cause discomfort.
      • Continue to use the splinting technique as needed.
   b. For angina (tightness, squeezing, pressure, pain, or mild ache in chest; indigestion; choking sensation; pain in jaw, neck, and between shoulder blades; numbness, tingling, and aching in either arm or hand):
      • Stop whatever you are doing and sit down.
      • Take nitroglycerin as prescribed, e.g., one tablet every 5 minutes sublingually until pain subsides or a maximum of three tablets have been taken.
      • If pain is unrelieved by three nitroglycerin tablets, arrange immediate transportation to the emergency room.
3. Provide instruction regarding condition and reduction of risk factors:
   a. Reinforce purpose and outcome of CABG surgery.
   b. Explain the risk factors that need to be eliminated or reduced, e.g., obesity, smoking, high-fat or high-cholesterol diet, sedentary life style, regular heavy alcohol intake, excessive stress, hypertension, uncontrolled diabetes mellitus.
4. Teach the client about safe and effective weight loss methods, if indicated. Consult a dietitian, and refer to appropriate community resources.
5. Provide instruction about smoking cessation, if indicated; refer to a community program.

Rationale

1. Correct technique is needed to reduce the risk of infection.

2.
   a. Adequate instruction in pain management can reduce the fear of pain by providing a sense of control.

   b. Angina is a symptom of cardiac tissue hypoxia. Immediate rest reduces the tissues' oxygen requirements. Nitroglycerin causes coronary vasodilatation, which increases coronary blood flow and relieves symptoms

3. Surgery does not replace the need to reduce risk factors.
   a. Preoperative anxiety may have interfered with retention of preoperative teaching.
   b. Emphasizing those risk factors that can be reduced may decrease the client's sense of powerlessness regarding those factors that cannot be, e.g., heredity.

4. Weight reduction reduces peripheral resistance and cardiac output.

5. Smoking's immediate effects include vasoconstriction and decreased blood oxygenation, elevated blood pressure, increased heart rate and possible dysrhythmias, and increased car-

Interventions

Rationale

diac workload. Long-term effects include an increased risk of coronary artery disease and myocardial infarction. Smoking also contributes to hypertension, peripheral vascular disease (e.g., leg ulcers), and chronically abnormal arterial blood gases (low oxygen, or pO_2, and high carbon dioxide, or pCO_2).

6. Teach about a low-fat, low-cholesterol diet; consult with a dietitian.

6. A low-fat and low-cholesterol diet can reduce or prevent arteriosclerosis in some clients.

7. Provide instruction in a progressive activity program:
   a. Increase activity gradually.

7.

   a. Progressive regular exercise increases cardiac stroke volume, thus increasing the heart's efficiency without greatly altering rate.

   b. Consult with a physical therapist and cardiac rehabilitation specialist.

   b. These professionals can provide specific guidelines.

   c. Schedule frequent rest periods throughout the day for the first 6 to 8 weeks. Balance periods of activity with periods of rest.

   c. Rest periods reduce myocardial oxygen demands.

   d. Consult with the physician before resuming work, driving, strenuous recreational activities (e.g., jogging, golfing, and other sports), and travel (airplane or automobile).

   d. Caution is needed to reduce the risk of myocardial hypoxia from overexertion.

   e. Try to get 8 to 10 hours of sleep each night.

   e. Sleep allows the body restorative time.

   f. Avoid isometric exercises (e.g., lifting anything over 10 lb) for 6 to 8 weeks.

   f. Isometric exercises increase cardiac workload and peripheral resistance.

   g. Avoid pushing anything weighing more than 10 lb (e.g., vacuum cleaner, grocery cart) for 6 to 8 weeks.

   g. Straining increases cardiac workload.

   h. Limit stair climbing to once or twice a day.

   h. Stair climbing increases cardiac workload.

8. Provide instructions for stress management strategies:
   a. Identify stressors.
   b. Avoid stressors if possible.
   c. Use techniques to reduce stress response, e.g., deep breathing, progressive relaxation, guided imagery, exercise within postoperative constraints.

8. Although the relationship of stress and atherosclerotic changes is not clear, stress may increase cardiac workload.

9. Provide instructions for sexual activity:
   a. Consult with the physician about when sexual activity can be resumed.
   b. Rest before and after engaging in sexual activity.
   c. Stop sexual activity if angina occurs.
   d. Try different positions to decrease exertion, e.g., both partners side-lying, client on bottom.
   e. If prescribed, take nitroglycerin before sexual activity.
   f. Avoid sexual activity in very hot or cold temperatures, within 2 hours of eating or drinking, when tired, after alcohol intake, with an unfamiliar partner, and in an unfamiliar environment.

9. Although resumption of sexual activity is encouraged, the client needs specific instructions focusing on reducing cardiac workload and avoiding certain situations that increase anxiety or vasoconstriction.

10. Provide instructions regarding prescribed medications, i.e., purpose, dosage and administration techniques, and possible side effects.

10. Understanding can help improve compliance and reduce the risk of overdose and morbidity.

Interventions

11. Teach the client and family to report these signs and symptoms of complications to the physician:
    a. Redness, drainage, warmth, or increasing pain at incision site
    b. Increasing weakness, fatigue
    c. Elevated temperature
    d. Anginal pain
    e. Difficulty breathing
    f. Weight gain exceeding 3 lb in 1 day or 5 lb in 1 week
    g. Calf swelling, tenderness, warmth, or pain

Rationale

11. Early reporting of complications enables prompt interventions to minimize their severity.
    a,b,c. These signs and symptoms may indicate infection.

    d. Anginal pain indicates myocardial hypoxia.
    e,f. Difficulty breathing and abnormal weight gain may point to fluid retention.

    g. These signs and symptoms may indicate thrombophlebitis.

▲ **Documentation**

Discharge summary record
  Client and family teaching
  Response to teaching
  Referrals, if indicated

References/Bibliography

Gilliss, C., Sparacino, P., Gatner, S., & Kenneth, H. (1985). Events leading to the treatment of coronary artery disease: Implications for nursing care. *Heart & Lung, 14*(3), 350–356.

Gregersen, R.A. (1988). Fatigue in the cardiac surgical patient. *Progressive Cardiovascular Nursing, 3*(3), 106–111.

Gurevich, I. (1984). Infectious complications after open heart surgery. *Heart & Lung, 13*(4), 472–481.

Guzzetta, C., & Dossey, B. (1984). *Cardiovascular nursing: Body-mind tapestry.* St Louis: C.V. Mosby.

Jansen, K., & McFadden, P. (1982). Postoperative nursing management in patients undergoing myocardial revascularization with the internal mammary artery bypass. *Heart & Lung, 15*(1), 48–54.

Raymond, M., Conklin, C., Schaeffer, J., Newstadt, G., Mattoff, J., & Gray, R. (1984). Coping with transient intellectual dysfunction after coronary bypass surgery. *Heart & Lung, 13*(4), 531–539.

Shipes, E. (1987). Psychosocial issues: The person with an ostomy. *Nursing Clinics of North America, 22*(2), 291–302.

Stanton, B., Jenkins, D., Savageau, J., Harken, D., & Auioin, R. (1984). Perceived adequacy of patient education and fears and adjustment after cardiac surgery. *Heart & Lung, 13*(4), 525–531.

Underhill, S., Woods, S., Sivarajan, E., & Halpenny, C. (1982). *Cardiac nursing.* Philadelphia: J.B. Lippincott.

Weiland, A., & Walker, W. (1986). Physiologic principles and clinical sequelae of cardiopulmonary bypass. *Heart & Lung, 15*(1), 34–39.

Cranial Surgery

Involving surgical access through the skull to the intracranial structures, cranial surgery is indicated to remove a tumor, control hemorrhage, remove hematomas, or reduce increased intracranial pressure.

Diagnostic Cluster

▲ **Time Frame**

Preoperative and postoperative periods
Post-intensive care unit

PREOPERATIVE PERIOD
Nursing Diagnoses

Anxiety related to impending surgery and perceived negative effects on life style

POSTOPERATIVE PERIOD
Collaborative Problems

Potential Complications:
Increased Intracranial Pressure
Brain Hemorrhage, Hematomas, Hygroma
Cranial Nerve Dysfunctions
Fluid/Electrolyte Imbalances
Meningitis/Encephalitis
Sensory/Motor Losses
Cerebral/Cerebellar Dysfunction
Hypo- or Hyperthermia
Antidruretic Hormone (ADH) Secretion Disorders
Cerebrospinal Fluid (CSF) Leaks
Seizures

Nursing Diagnoses

▲ **Discharge Criteria**

Before discharge, the client or family will:

1. Explain surgical site care
2. Discuss management of activities of daily living (ADLs)
3. Verbalize precautions to take for medication use
4. State the signs and symptoms that must be reported to a health care professional

Altered Comfort related to compression/displacement of brain tissue and increased intracranial pressure
Potential Impaired Corneal Tissue Integrity related to inadequate lubrication secondary to tissue edema
Potential Altered Health Maintenance related to insufficient knowledge of wound care, signs and symptoms of complications, restrictions, and follow-up care

Related Care Plan

General Surgery Generic Care Plan

Preoperative: Nursing Diagnosis

▲ **Outcome Criteria**

The client will:

1. State the reason for surgery
2. Describe postoperative restrictions
3. Verbalize decreased anxiety related to impending surgery

Anxiety related to impending surgery and perceived negative affects on life style

Focus Assessment Criteria

1. Understanding of condition
2. Knowledge of structure and function of affected area
3. Understanding of anticipated surgical procedure
4. Previous exposure to person(s) experiencing cranial surgery

Clinical Significance

1–3. Assessing the client's knowledge level guides the nurse in planning effective teaching strategies.

4. Often, a client is positively or negatively influenced by information from others who have undergone cranial surgery.

Interventions

1. Explain the effects of disease on the affected brain area and the need for surgery.

2. Explain the specific postoperative experience, which may include the following:
   a. A large head dressing
   b. Swollen eyes
   c. Tracheostomy or endotracheal intubation

3. Inform the client if an alternate form of communication to speech (e.g., note pad and pencil, hand signals) will be necessary postoperatively.

▲ **Documentation**

Progress notes
    Present emotional status
    Interventions
    Response to interventions

4. Refer to the General Surgery care plan, Appendix II, for more interventions and rationales.

Rationale

1. This information can help the client accept the need for surgery and ready himself psychologically, which may reduce anxiety.

2. Information about what to expect can reduce anxiety associated with the unknown.

3. The client may require another means of communication if large head dressings inhibit hearing, periorbital edema impairs sight, or speech is prevented by tracheostomy or endotracheal intubation. Preoperative teaching prepares the client for this possibility and may decrease anxiety.

Postoperative: Collaborative Problems

▲ **Nursing Goal**

The nurse will manage and minimize complications of abnormal cranial pressure.

Potential Complication: Increased Intracranial Pressure
Potential Complication: Brain Hemorrhage, Hematoma, Hygroma
Potential Complication: Cranial Nerve Dysfunction
Potential Complication: Fluid and Electrolyte Imbalances
Potential Complication: Meningitis or Encephalitis
Potential Complication: Sensory and Motor Losses
Potential Complication: Cerebral or Cerebellar Dysfunction
Potential Complication: Hypothermia or Hyperthermia
Potential Complication: Antidiuretic Hormone Secretion Disorders
Potential Complication: Cerebrospinal Fluid Leakage
Potential Complication: Seizure Activity

Interventions

1. Monitor for signs and symptoms of increased intracranial pressure (ICP).

   a. Assess the following:
   - Best eye opening response: spontaneously, to auditory stimuli, to painful stimuli, or no response
   - Best motor response: obeys verbal commands, localizes pain, flexion-withdrawal, flexion-decorticate, extension-decerebrate, or no response
   - Best verbal response: oriented to person, place, and time; confused conversation, inappropriate speech, incomprehensible sounds, or no response

   b. Assess for changes in vital signs:

   - Pulse changes: slowing rate to 60 or below or increasing rate to 100 or above

   - Respiratory irregularities: slowing of rate with lengthening periods of apnea

Rationale

1. Cerebral tissue is compromised by deficiencies of cerebral blood supply caused by hemorrhage, hematoma, cerebral edema, thrombus, or emboli. Monitoring intracranial pressure (ICP) serves as an indicator of cerebral perfusion.

   a. These responses evaluate the client's ability to integrate commands with conscious and involuntary movement. Cortical function can be assessed by evaluating eye opening and motor response. No response may indicate damage to the midbrain.

   b. These vital sign changes may reflect increasing ICP.
   - Changes in pulse may indicate brainstem pressure, slowed at first, then increasing to compensate for hypoxia.
   - Respiratory patterns vary with impairments at various sites. Cheyne-Stokes breathing (a gradual increase followed by

Interventions

Rationale

- Rising blood pressure or widening pulse pressure

c. Assess pupillary response:

- Inspect the pupils with a flashlight to evaluate size, configuration, and reaction to light. Compare both eyes for similarities and differences.
- Evaluate gaze to determine whether it is conjugate (paired, working together) or if eye movements are abnormal.
- Evaluate ability of the eyes to adduct and abduct.

d. Note the presence of the following:
- Vomiting

- Headache (constant, increasing in intensity, or aggravated by movement or straining)
- Subtle changes, e.g., lethargy, restlessness, forced breathing, purposeless movements, and changes in mentation
2. Elevate the head of the bed 15 to 30 degrees unless contraindicated. Avoid changing position rapidly.
3. Avoid the following:

a. Carotid massage

b. Neck flexion or extreme rotation

c. Digital anal stimulation
d. Breath holding
e. Straining

f. Extreme flexion of hips and knees
4. Consult with the physician for stool softeners, if needed.
5. Maintain a quiet, calm, softly lit environment. Plan activities to minimize interruptions.
6. Assess cranial nerve function by evaluating the following:
   a. Pupillary responses
   b. Corneal reflex
   c. Gag reflex
   d. Cough
   e. Swallow
   f. Facial movements
   g. Tongue movements

a gradual decrease, then a period of apnea) points to damage in both cerebral hemispheres, midbrain, and upper pons. Ataxic breathing (irregular with random sequence of deep and shallow breaths) indicates medullar dysfunction.
- Blood pressure and pulse pressure changes are late signs indicating severe hypoxia.

c. Pupillary changes indicate pressure on oculomotor or optic nerves.
- Pupil reactions are regulated by the oculomotor nerve (cranial nerve III) in the brain stem.

- Conjugate eye movements are regulated from parts of the cortex and brain stem.

- Cranial nerve VI, or the abducens nerve, regulates abduction and adduction of the eyes. Cranial nerve IV, or the trochlear nerve, also regulates eye movement.

d.
- Vomiting results from pressure on the medulla, which stimulates the brain's vomiting center.
- Compression of neural tissue movement increases ICP and increases pain.

- These changes may be early indicators of ICP changes.

2. Slight head elevation can aid venous drainage to reduce cerebrovascular congestion.

3. These situations or maneuvers can increase ICP.
   a. Carotid massage slows heart rate and reduces systemic circulation, which is followed by a sudden increase in circulation.
   b. Neck flexion or extreme rotation disrupts circulation to the brain.
   c,d,e. These activities initiate Valsalva's maneuver, which impairs venous return by constricting the jugular veins and increases ICP.

4. Stool softeners prevent constipation and straining, which initiates Valsalva's maneuver.
5. These measures promote rest and decrease stimulation, helping decrease ICP.
6. Cranial nerve pathways may be damaged directly by ischemia, trauma, or increased pressure.

Interventions

7. Assess cerebellar function by observing for the following:
   a. Ataxic movements
   b. Loss of equilibrium
8. Monitor intake and administer necessary IV fluids via infusion pump.
9. Monitor for signs and symptoms of diabetes insipidus:
   a. Excessive urinary output
   b. Dilute urine
10. Monitor urinary output and urine specific gravity.

11. Monitor the wound site for the following:
    a. Bleeding
    b. Bulging
    c. CSF leakage
    d. Infection
12. Consult with the physician if the client experiences seizure activity.

13. Teach the client to avoid the following:
    a. Coughing
    b. Neck hyperextension
    c. Neck hyperflexion
    d. Neck turning

Rationale

7. Cerebellar function may be affected by ischemia, trauma, or increased pressure.

8. Strict control of infusion is imperative to prevent fluid overload or dehydration.
9. Surgery around the pituitary gland and hypothalamus can cause a deficiency of ADH, resulting in diabetes insipidus.

10. Trauma to the brain results in increased aldosterone production and sodium retention, which intensifies hypertonicity and decreases urine output.
11. A visible bulge under the wound may indicate localized bleeding or hygroma (collection of CSF). CSF leakage through the incision must be dealt with using strict asepsis to avoid ascending infection.
12. Seizures must be controlled to avoid hypoxia and resultant increased pCO_2 and increased ICP.
13. Head and neck alignment must be maintained to prevent jugular vein compression, which can inhibit venous return and result in increased ICP. Coughing increases intrathoracic pressure, which also has these effects.

▲ **Documentation**

Flow records
  Vital signs
  Intake and output
  Body systems assessment findings
  Neurological assessment findings
Progress notes
  Assessment findings deviating from normal
  Seizures
  Complaints of vomiting, headache

Related Physician-Prescribed Interventions

Medications
  Antihypertensives
  Peripheral vasodilators
  Anticoagulants

  Stool softeners
  Corticosteroids

Intravenous Therapy
  Fluid and electrolyte replacement

Laboratory Studies
  Complete blood count
  Blood chemistry profile

  Prothrombin time
  Urinalysis

Diagnostic Studies
  Computed tomography (CT) scan of head
  Cerebral angiography
  Positron emission tomography (PET)
  Brain scan
  Electroencephalography

  Lumbar puncture
  Magnetic resonance imaging (MRI)
  Tomography scan
  Doppler ultrasonography
  Skull x-ray film

Therapies
  Antiembolism stockings
  Physical therapy

  Speech therapy

Postoperative: Nursing Diagnoses

▲ **Outcome Criteria**

The client will report progressive pain reduction after pain-relief measures.

Altered Comfort related to compression/displacement of brain tissue and increased intracranial pressure

Focus Assessment Criteria

1. Complaints of pain: location, description, intensity, duration
2. Effects of pain relief interventions

Clinical Significance

1,2. The client is the best source of information about his pain and the degree of relief obtained from interventions.

Interventions

1. Ascertain the location, nature, and intensity of the pain.

2. If the pain is a headache, slightly raise the head of the bed, reduce bright lights and room noise, and loosen head dressings if constrictive.
3. Provide nonpharmacological relief measures, as appropriate:
   a. For eye edema: eye patches
   b. For immobility: frequent position changes and back rubs
4. Observe for a decrease in level of consciousness (LOC) and respiratory rate after narcotic administration. (*Note:* you must be able to arouse the client fully to ascertain actual LOC.)

Rationale

1. Pressure exerted on the baroreceptors in blood vessel walls causes generalized headache. Other sources of discomfort may include dressings, IV lines, edema, and poor positioning.
2. These measures may help reduce increased ICP and relieve headache.

3. The nurse should make every attempt to minimize the use of narcotic analgesics.

4. Narcotics constrict pupils, they may mask eye sign changes, and they depress respiration.

▲ **Documentation**

Medication administration record
   Type, dosage, and route of
    all medications
Progress notes
   Unsatisfactory pain relief

▲ **Outcome Criteria**

The client will demonstrate continued corneal integrity.

Potential Impaired Corneal Tissue Integrity related to inadequate lubrication secondary to tissue edema

Focus Assessment Criteria	*Clinical Significance*
1. Eyes: moisture, lid closure, drainage, abrasions	1. Assessment is indicated to establish a baseline and detect early changes.

Interventions

1. Loosen any tight dressings over the eyes.
2. Instill hydroxyethylcellulose (Artificial Tears), as necessary.
3. Assess for irritation and drainage.

4. Apply cool compresses to the eye area, if necessary.

Rationale

1. Direct pressure on eyes should be reduced.
2. Artificial Tears provide lubrication and prevent dryness.
3. Early recognition of inflammation enables prompt intervention to prevent serious damage.
4. This can help reduce periocular edema by decreasing lymphatic response to injured tissue.

▲ **Documentation**

Flow records
   Eye assessment findings
    (vision, edema)

▲ **Outcome Criteria**

The outcome criteria for this diagnosis represent those associated with discharge planning. Refer to the discharge criteria.

Potential Altered Health Maintenance related to insufficient knowledge of wound care, signs and symptoms of complications, restrictions, and follow-up care

Focus Assessment Criteria	*Clinical Significance*
1. Readiness and ability to learn and retain information	1. A client or family failing to meet learning goals requires a referral for assistance post-discharge.

Interventions

1. Explain that mild headaches will persist but will gradually decrease.
2. Explain surgical site care;

   a. Wear a cap after bandages are removed.
   b. Hair can be shampooed after suture removal, but avoid scrubbing near the incision.
   c. Pat the incision area dry.

3. Explain the need to avoid hair dryers or hot curlers until hair has regrown.

Rationale

1. Explaining what to expect can reduce the anxiety associated with headaches.
2. This knowledge enables the client and family to participate in care.
   a. This helps protect the incision site.
   b. Hair regrowth indicates adequate wound closure.

   c. Vigorous rubbing can separate the wound edges.
3. Direct heat can burn the unprotected surgical site.

Interventions

4. Teach the client not to do the following:
   a. Hold his breath
   b. Strain during defecation
   c. Lift heavy objects
   d. Blow his nose
5. Teach the client and family to watch for and report the following:
   a. Drainage from surgical site, nose, or ear

   b. Increasing headaches

   c. Elevated temperature, stiff neck, photophobia, hyperirritability
6. If motor–sensory deficits remain, refer to the index for specific nursing diagnoses, e.g., Impaired Communication.

Rationale

4. These activities activate Valsalva's maneuver, which impairs venous return by compressing the jugular veins and can increase ICP.

5. Early detection enables prompt intervention to prevent serious complications.
   a. Leakage may be CSF, which represents an entry route for microorganisms.
   b. Increasing headaches may point to increasing ICP.
   c. These signs may indicate infection or meningitis.

▲ **Documentation**

Discharge summary record
    Client and family teaching
    Outcome achievement or status

References/Bibliography

Hannegan, L. (1989). Transient cognitive changes after craniotomy. *Journal of Neuroscience Nursing, 21*(3), 165–170.

Henning, R.J., & Jackson, D.L. (1986). *Handbook of critical care neurology and neurosurgery.* New York: Praeger Scientific.

Hickey, J.V. (1986). *The clinical practice of neurological and neurosurgical nursing* (2nd ed.). Philadelphia: J.B. Lippincott.

Houston, C.S. (1985). Intracranial aneurysms: Diagnosis, treatment, and nursing implications. *Perioperative Nursing Quarterly, 1*(2), 39–48.

Walleck, C. (1987). Intracranial hypertension: Interventions and outcomes. *Critical Care Nursing Quarterly, 10*(1), 45–57.

Enucleation

Surgical removal of the eyeball, enucleation is indicated for post-trauma, severe infections, malignant tumors, or cosmetic improvement (blind eye). After the eyeball is excised, the ocular muscles are sutured over a plastic sphere inserted in the ocular cavity, and a temporary conformer is inserted to maintain the natural shape of the eye socket. Between 2 and 6 weeks after surgery, an ocular prosthesis can be fixed to the sphere, restoring natural appearance and movement.

Diagnostic Cluster

▲ Time Frame

Preoperative and postoperative periods

▲ Discharge Criteria

Before discharge, the client or family will:

1. Demonstrate eye care
2. Verbalize precautions to take regarding activities
3. State the signs and symptoms that must be reported to a health care professional
4. Verbalize an intent to share feelings and concerns related to surgery with significant others
5. Identify available community resources and self-help groups

---

PREOPERATIVE PERIOD
Nursing Diagnoses

Fear related to upcoming surgery, uncertain outcome of surgery, and others expressed by individual

POSTOPERATIVE PERIOD
Collaborative Problems

Potential Complications:
Abscess
Hemorrhage

Nursing Diagnoses

Potential for Infection related to increased susceptibility secondary to surgical interruption of body surface and use of prosthesis (ocular)

Potential for Injury related to visual limitations and presence in unfamiliar environment

Altered Comfort related to surgical interruption of body surfaces

Grieving related to loss of eye and its effects on life style

Potential Self-Concept Disturbance related to effects of change in appearance on life style

Potential Social Isolation related to changes in body image and altered vision

Potential Impaired Home Maintenance Management related to inability to perform activities of daily living (ADLs) secondary to change in visual abilities

Potential Altered Health Maintenance related to insufficient knowledge of activities permitted, self-care activities, medications, complications, and plans for follow-up care

Refer to:

General Surgery

Preoperative: Nursing Diagnosis

▲ Outcome Criteria

The client will express concerns regarding upcoming surgery during dialogues.

Fear related to upcoming surgery, uncertain outcome of surgery, and other concerns expressed by the client

Focus Assessment Criteria	*Clinical Significance*
1. Verbal and nonverbal indicators of anxiety	1. Most surgical clients express anxiety and fear. A client awaiting enucleation also may have additional fears related to the impact of surgery on his appearance and life style

Focus Assessment Criteria	Clinical Significance
	(e.g., occupation, financial status), the underlying reason for the procedure (e.g., cancer), and other concerns. The nurse needs to delve into the source of the fears to plan effective interventions to reduce them.
2. Knowledge of the surgical procedure and its risks and benefits	2. This assessment guides the nurse in planning teaching strategies.
3. Amount of information the client seeks	3. Providing just the amount of information sought by the client affords him a measure of control over the situation. Some clients may find detailed information overwhelming and confusing; others may experience reduced anxiety from detailed information.

Interventions

1. Promote an environment in which the client will express his feelings and concerns. Listen actively, validate the client's fears, and reassure him that anxiety and fear is a normal and expected response to the upcoming surgery.
2. Present information using a variety of instructional methods and media, such as the following:
   a. Large-print pamphlets
   b. Posters
   c. Audiovisual programs
   d. Anatomical models
   e. Sample prosthesis
3. Explain required preadmission activities:
   a. Adherence to dietary instructions provided by anesthesia services
   b. Adjustments in medication regimen as ordered by the surgeon, anesthesiologist, or client's physician
4. Discuss expected preoperative care measures, including the following:
   a. Preoperative sedation
   b. IV fluid infusion
   c. Bladder emptying
5. Explain postoperative activities to be avoided:
   a. Lying on the operative side
   b. Bending over at the waist
   c. Ambulating without assistance
   d. Removing the pressure dressing
6. Explain general postoperative care measures, such as these:
   a. Deep breathing exercises
   b. Early ambulation

Rationale

1. Verbalizing feelings and concerns increases the client's self-awareness and helps the nurse identify sources of anxiety. Validation and reassurance promote self-esteem and may help reduce anxiety.
2. Simultaneous stimulation of multiple senses enhances the teaching–learning process. Written materials also provide a source to refer to after discharge.

3. Depending on the client's general health status, presence of concurrent medical problems, time of surgery, and physician's preferences, adjustments may be needed in diet (nothing by mouth for a specified period) and medications (e.g., withholding diuretics, decreasing insulin dose).
4. Information about what to expect can help reduce anxiety associated with fear of the unknown. It also enables the client to participate better in care measures and enhances his sense of control.
5,6. Information about what to expect can reduce fear of the unknown. Explaining postoperative care before surgery allows the client to absorb the information while not under the effects of sedation. It also can help improve compliance and facilitates the discharge planning process. Postoperative restrictions aim to prevent increased intraocular pressure and avoid injury resulting from decreased vision secondary to loss of a visual field.

▲ **Documentation**

Progress notes
  Client teaching
  Client's understanding of
    teaching and response
Progress notes
  Dialogues

Postoperative: Collaborative Problem

▲ **Nursing Goal**

The nurse will detect and manage abscesses.

▲ **Documentation**

Flow records
  Vital signs
Progress notes
  Unusual complaints

Potential Complication: Abscess

Interventions

1. Monitor for signs and symptoms of abscess formation:
   a. Increasing pain, headache on affected side
   b. Temperature elevation

Rationale

1. Because of the nature of the surgery and the creation of a cavity, infection can lead to abscess and possible meningitis.

Related Physician-Prescribed Interventions

Medications
Antibiotics

Intravenous Therapy
Not indicated

Laboratory Studies
Refer to the General Surgery care plan (Appendix II).

Diagnostic Studies
Dependent on underlying etiology

Therapies
Eye care

Postoperative: Nursing Diagnoses

▲ **Outcome Criteria**

The client will demonstrate evidence of wound healing without infection.

Potential for Infection related to increased susceptibility secondary to surgical interruption of body surface and use of ocular prosthesis

Focus Assessment Criteria	*Clinical Significance*

1. Signs of infection:
    a. Periorbital redness
    b. Drainage on eyelids or eyelashes
    c. Drainage from eye socket
    d. Elevated temperature
    e. Laboratory values: increased WBC count, change in WBC differential, abnormal culture and sensitivity results
	1. A client receiving a prosthetic device, such as a ball implant inserted immediately after enucleation and a conformer placed between the eyelids and conjunctiva, is at high risk for infection. Severe infection can negatively affect the ocular support structures and cause difficulty with prosthesis fitting. Postoperative care must focus on prevention, early detection, and prompt treatment of infection.

Interventions

1. Promote wound healing:
   a. Encourage a well-balanced diet and adequate fluid intake.
   b. Instruct the client to keep a continuous dressing over the eye for 24 to 48 hours postoperatively.
2. Take steps to prevent strain on the suture line, e.g., have the client wear dark glasses and an eyepatch in the daytime and an eye shield at night.
3. Instruct the client to use aseptic technique to care for the socket and prosthesis:
   a. Wash hands first.
   b. Rinse the cavity, as instructed, then insert the prosthesis.
   c. Once the prosthesis is in place, remove it weekly and clean as ordered.
   d. With the prosthesis removed, inspect the cavity for signs of infection or other problems.
4. Culture and notify the physician of any suspicious-looking drainage.

Rationale

1. Optimal nutrition and hydration improve overall good health, which promotes healing of any surgical wound. Wearing an eye patch promotes healing by decreasing the irritative force of the eyelid against the suture line.

2. Strain on the suture line can lead to interruption, creating an entrance point for microorganisms.

3. Aseptic technique minimizes introduction of microorganisms and reduces the risk of infection.

4. Drainage may signify an infection; a culture identifies organisms and guides treatment. Early detection of infection enables prompt treatment to minimize its seriousness.

▲ **Documentation**

Progress notes
   Client teaching
   Signs of infection

▲ Outcome Criteria

The client will not experience injury or tissue trauma while hospitalized.

Potential for Injury related to visual limitations and presence in unfamiliar environment

Focus Assessment Criteria

1. Visual acuity in the remaining eye
2. Gait, previous history of falls
3. Potential environmental obstacles, such as the following:
   a. Footstools and low furniture
   b. IV poles
   c. Wastebaskets
   d. Slippers

Clinical Significance

1–3. A client who has undergone enucleation has experienced a sudden loss of vision and is at increased risk of injury as he adjusts to seeing with only one eye.

Interventions

1. Orient the client to the environment upon arrival.
2. Modify the environment to remove any potential hazards:
   a. Remove obstacles from walking pathways.
   b. Remove straws from trays.
   c. Make sure doors and drawers are kept either completely open or completely closed.
3. Explain the vision loss resulting from surgery. Point out that he has lost about 50 degrees of his normal 180-degree peripheral visual field, and that depth perception also may be affected.
4. Place objects, including the call bell, where the client can see and reach them without stretching too far.
5. Place ambulation aids where the client can see and reach them easily. Instruct the client to request assistance before ambulating. Monitor the use of ambulation aids.
6. Help the client and family evaluate the home environment for potential hazards such as the following:
   a. Throw rugs
   b. Exposed electrical cords
   c. Low furniture
   d. Pets
   e. Stairs
   Instruct them to eliminate all identified hazards.

Rationale

1. The client's familiarity with the environment may help reduce accidents.
2. Loss of an eye narrows peripheral vision and can interfere with depth perception. These measures can help minimize potential hazards and reduce the risk of injury resulting from these impairments.

3. The client's understanding of vision deficits encourages compliance with precautions to prevent injury.

4,5. These measures can help reduce the risk of falls.

6. The need to maintain a safe environment continues at home after discharge.

▲ Documentation

Progress notes
    Visual acuity (preoperative and postoperative)
Discharge summary record
    Client teaching

▲ Outcome Criteria

The client will voice progressive pain reduction and pain relief after interventions.

Altered Comfort related to surgical interruption of body surfaces

Focus Assessment Criteria

1. Location of pain

2. Severity of pain based on a scale of 0 to 10 (0 = no pain, 10 = greatest pain), rated as follows:
   a. Before pain relief interventions
   b. One-half hour after intervention

Clinical Significance

1. Incising ocular tissues during enucleation injures surrounding tissues as well. Generally, the greater the tissue manipulation, the greater the postoperative pain.
2. This rating scale provides an objective method of evaluating the subjective experience of pain.

Focus Assessment Criteria

3. Previous experiences with and usual response to pain
4. Verbal and nonverbal indicators of pain, such as the following:
   a. Grimacing
   b. Rubbing the eye
   c. Withdrawal
   d. Vital sign changes
   e. Altered disposition

Clinical Significance

3,4. Each client responds to pain in a personal manner. Assessing the client's usual response to pain helps the nurse plan effective pain relief interventions.

Interventions

1. Assist the client in identifying effective pain relief measures.

2. Provide information to allay anxiety and fear, such as the following:
   a. Give reassurance that pain is not always directly related to the development of complications.
   b. Explain how and when pain reduction interventions will begin working.
3. Promote noninvasive and nonpharmacological pain relief measures:
   a. Positioning: elevate the head of the bed, alternate between lying on the back and on the nonoperative side.
   b. Dressing: leave in place for 24 to 48 hours.
   c. Distraction
   d. Relaxation exercises
4. Support pain relief measures with prescribed analgesics as necessary.
5. Notify the physician if pain is unrelieved within ½ hour of drug administration, if pain is accompanied by nausea, or if you note drainage on the eye patch or shield.

Rationale

1. The client has the most intimate knowledge of his pain and the effectiveness of relief measures.
2. This information can help reduce anxiety associated with the unexpected; anxiety and fear actually can increase pain.

3. Noninvasive and nonpharmacological pain relief measures allow the client to gain a sense of control over the pain.

4. For some clients, pharmacological therapy may be needed to provide adequate pain relief.
5. These signs may indicate increased intraocular pressure or other complications.

▲ **Documentation**

Progress notes
   Complaints of pain
   Interventions
   Response to interventions

▲ **Outcome Criteria**

The client will:

1. Express grief
2. Report an intent to discuss feelings with significant others

Grieving related to loss of eye and its effects on life style

Focus Assessment Criteria

1. Response to loss of eye

2. Independence in activities

Clinical Significance

1. Grieving over the loss of vision secondary to removal of an eye is a difficult situation through which to assist a client
2. Increased dependency can indicate depression.

Interventions

1. Provide opportunities for the client and family members to ventilate feelings, discuss the loss openly, and explore the personal meaning of the loss. Explain that grief is a common and healthy reaction.

2. Encourage use of positive coping strategies that have proven successful in the past.

Rationale

1. Loss of an eye and vision may give rise to feelings of powerlessness, anger, profound sadness, and other grief responses. Open, honest discussions can help the client and family members accept and cope with the situation and their response to it.
2. Positive coping strategies can help decrease feelings of hopelessness and aid problem-solving.

Interventions

3. Encourage the client to express positive self-attributes.
4. Implement measures to support the family and promote cohesiveness:
   a. Support the family at its level of functioning.
   b. Encourage members to reevaluate their feelings and to support one another.
5. Promote grief work with each response:
   a. Denial:
      - Encourage acceptance of the situation; do not reinforce denial by giving false reassurance.
      - Promote hope through assurances of care, comfort, and support.
      - Explain the use of denial by one family member to other members.
      - Do not push a person to move past denial until he is emotionally ready.
   b. Isolation:
      - Convey acceptance by encouraging expressions of grief.
      - Promote open, honest communication to encourage sharing.
      - Reinforce the client's self-worth by providing for privacy when desired.
      - Encourage socialization as feasible (e.g., support groups, church activities).
   c. Depression:
      - Reinforce the client's self-esteem.
      - Employ empathetic sharing and acknowledge grief.
      - Identify the degree of depression and develop appropriate strategies.
   d. Anger:
      - Explain to other family members that anger represents an attempt to control the environment stemming from frustration at the inability to control the disease.
      - Encourage verbalization of anger.
   e. Guilt:
      - Acknowledge the person's expressed self-image.
      - Encourage identification of the relationship's positive aspects.
      - Avoid arguing and participating in the person's system of "I should have . . ." and "I shouldn't have. . . ."
   f. Fear:
      - Focus on the present and maintain a safe and secure environment.
      - Help the person explore reasons for and meanings of the fears.
   g. Rejection:
      - Provide reassurance by explaining what is happening.
      - Explain this response to other family members.

Rationale

3. Focusing on positive attributes increases self-acceptance.
4. Family cohesiveness is important to client support.

5. Grieving involves profound emotional responses; interventions depend on the particular response.

▲ **Documentation**

Progress notes
  Present emotional status
  Interventions
  Response to interventions

▲ **Outcome Criteria**

The client will:

1. Acknowledge the change in appearance
2. Communicate feelings regarding the effects on his life style of loss of an eye and changes in appearance

Interventions

h. Hysteria:
  • Reduce environmental stressors (e.g., limit personnel).
  • Provide a safe, private area in which to express grief.

Rationale

Potential Self-Concept Disturbance related to effects of change in appearance on life style

Focus Assessment Criteria	*Clinical Significance*
1. Client's expressed self-concept before and after enucleation	1–3. Appearance is a critical component of self-concept; any change in appearance affects self-concept to some degree. Enucleation can have a dramatic negative impact on self-concept. Assessing the client's self-concept before surgery allows the nurse to evaluate adaptation to the change. Others' perceptions of the client's self-concept and any change after surgery may provide even more useful information than that obtained from the client himself. Others may provide insight into factors that may have affected the client's self-concept development and, from their more objective viewpoint, be sensitive to subtle changes.
2. Support persons' perceptions of client's self-concept	
3. Reaction to changes in self-concept	

Interventions

1. Encourage the client to verbalize feelings about the underlying illness, surgery, and altered appearance and self-concept.

2. Help the client identify personal attributes and strengths.

3. Facilitate adjustment through active listening.

4. Encourage regular hygiene, grooming, and other self-care activities; assist as necessary. Allow the client to make decisions about care and participate in planning as appropriate.

5. Encourage visitors and telephone conversations.

6. Reinforce that an ocular prosthesis (usually fitted 2 to 6 weeks after surgery) restores natural appearance.

7. Discuss strategies for socialization, as necessary, e.g., continued involvement in presurgical activities, exploring new activities and interests.

8. Assess for signs of negative adjustment to change in appearance:
  a. Refusal to look at face in the mirror
  b. Refusal to discuss the loss

Rationale

1. Interactions seeking to improve a client's self-concept must begin with assessing how the client feels about the illness, surgery, and self at this stress-producing time.

2. This may help the client shift focus from the change in appearance to all the positive aspects that contribute to self-concept.

3. By doing so, the nurse can reinforce positive attributes and help the client reincorporate them into his or her new self-concept.

4. Participation in self-care and planning helps facilitate positive coping with the change.

5. Maintaining social contacts can promote positive coping.

6. This information can minimize anxiety related to fear of a radical change in appearance.

7. Minimizing life style changes promotes adjustment and coping. Isolation can contribute to negative self-concept.

8. These signs may indicate that the client is at high risk for unsuccessful adjustment.

Interventions

   c. Denial of change in body
   d. Decrease in self-care ability
   e. Withdrawal and isolation
   f. Refusal to discuss future care, including prosthesis fitting
9. Refer an at-risk client for professional counseling.

Rationale

9. The client may need follow-up counseling to assist with successful adjustment.

▲ Documentation

Progress notes
   Present emotional status
   Interventions
   Response to interventions

▲ Outcome Criteria

During the recovery process, the client will identify ways to increase socialization considering altered appearance and vision.

Potential Social Isolation related to changes in body image and altered vision

Focus Assessment Criteria

1. Presurgical socialization patterns:
   a. Hobbies and other interests
   b. Friends and family
   c. Community
   d. Church
   e. Work
   f. School
2. Concerns regarding socialization

Clinical Significance

1,2. This assessment provides information to evaluate the client's life style and the effects of enucleation on socialization patterns.

Interventions

1. Help the client understand the need for socialization.

2. Provide emotional support, and validate that fears and concerns are normal.

3. Discuss alternative opportunities for socialization, such as these:
   a. Having telephone conversations
   b. Receiving visitors at home
   c. Visiting familiar environments
4. Allow the client's support persons opportunities to share their feelings and concerns also.

5. Help reduce barriers to social contact:
   a. Encourage good hygiene and grooming.
   b. Suggest wearing sunglasses.
   c. Reinforce that the ocular prosthesis (usually fitted within 2 to 6 weeks) restores normal appearance.
   d. Encourage support persons to help the client resume activities.
6. Encourage the client to participate in a support group or seek other community resources, as necessary.

Rationale

1. A client with an altered body image and limited vision may lack self-confidence in his ability to fulfill previous roles and may withdraw from family, friends, and society. Withdrawal can lead to isolation.

2. Emotional support can help the client cope with the often difficult adjustment to altered self-concept and resocialization.

3. These alternatives can promote limited socialization as the client gradually adjusts to the change and is awaiting an ocular prosthesis.

4. Socialization patterns of family and other support persons also may be disrupted by the client's surgery, e.g., withdrawal from social circle, especially sports- or other activity-related groups. Giving them the chance to express their concerns and doubts can help them adjust to the change as well.

5. Maintaining appearance and grooming helps promote a positive self-concept and reduces anxiety about appearance that can interfere with socialization.

6. Interacting with persons with similar problems can promote a realistic appraisal of the situation and provide answers for unasked questions. It also provides another opportunity for socialization.

▲ Documentation

Progress notes
   Client's concerns
   Interventions
   Response to interventions

▲ *Outcome Criteria*

Before discharge, the client and family will verbalize ways to adjust the home environment to accommodate the client's current abilities.

Potential Impaired Home Maintenance Management related to inability to perform ADLs secondary to change in visual ability

Focus Assessment Criteria	*Clinical Significance*

1. Home environment:
  a. Layout
  b. Stairs
  c. Obstacles or hazards to ambulation, e.g., throw rugs, low furniture, pets, clutter
2. Available support systems, e.g., family, friends, visiting nurse, Meals-on-Wheels, Lions Club, Center for the Visually Impaired
3. Services currently used
	1–3. This assessment identifies whether home adaptations or referral to community resources is indicated.

Interventions	*Rationale*
1. Help the client identify problem areas, such as transportation, food shopping and preparation, and safety.	1. A client experiencing a vision loss needs to adapt the home environment to his or her current ability. As the client adjusts to altered depth perception and other changes, home maintenance abilities will improve.

2. Assist with adaptations to address problems:
  a. Transportation needs: Call on family, friends, or public transportation.
  b. Shopping: Arrange for delivery from the market, call on community resources.
  c. Food preparation: Obtain assistance from friends and family; arrange for Meals-on-Wheels.
	2. The nurse should make every feasible attempt to promote self-care and independence.

3. Refer the client to community agencies as necessary.	3. Specialized assistance may be required.

▲ *Documentation*

Progress notes
    Needs identified
    Interventions
    Response to interventions

▲ *Outcome Criteria*

The outcome criteria for this diagnosis represent those associated with discharge planning. Refer to the discharge criteria.

Potential Altered Health Maintenance related to insufficient knowledge of activities permitted, self-care activities, medications, complications, and plans for follow-up care

Focus Assessment Criteria	*Clinical Significance*
1. Knowledge of and ability to comply with the therapeutic regimen	1. The client's understanding of the regimen and physical ability to perform necessary activities is essential to optimal compliance.
2. Readiness and ability to learn and retain information	2. A client or family failing to achieve learning goals requires a referral for assistance postdischarge.

Interventions	*Rationale*

1. Reinforce postoperative activity restrictions, such as avoiding the following:
  a. Lying on the operative side
  b. Bending over at the waist
  c. Driving
  d. Lifting anything weighing more than 5 lb
	1. Activity restrictions are aimed at reducing strain on the suture line and, in the case of driving, at eliminating situations that could be hazardous owing to impaired depth perception and visual field loss.

2. Reinforce required self-care activities:
  a. Wear eye protection at all times during waking hours. Suggest wearing glasses even when no vision correction is required.
  b. Cleanse the eyelids and eyelashes of drainage as necessary.
	2.
	  a. Because only one operative eye remains, that eye must be protected to preserve vision.
	  b. Weekly cleaning reduces the risk of infection.

Interventions

    c. Remove and clean the prosthesis and clean the ocular cavity at least once a week.

    d. After removal, store the prosthesis in water or contact lens solution.

3. Instruct to notify the physician of the following:
    a. Periorbital redness and edema
    b. Purulent drainage
    c. Pain

4. Provide information about scheduled follow-up care. Stress the importance of keeping appointments with the surgeon and ocular prosthetist. Make sure the client has the date and time of the first scheduled appointment before discharge.

Rationale

    c. Regular cleansing and inspection for rough surfaces can help prevent irritation and possible infection.

    d. Storage in liquid protects the prosthesis from damage and maintains the condition of the plastic.

3. These signs and symptoms can indicate infection; early detection enables prompt intervention to prevent serious infection.

4. Follow-up care enables early detection of problems.

▲ **Documentation**

Discharge summary record
    Client teaching
    Outcome achievement or
       status

References/Bibliography

Beyers, H., & Duda, S. (1977). *The clinical practice of medical–surgical nursing.* Boston: Little, Brown.

Carpenito, L.J. (1989). *Nursing diagnosis: Application to clinical practice* (3rd ed.). Philadelphia: J.B. Lippincott.

Doenges, M., Jeffries, M., & Moorhouse, H. (1985). *Nursing care plans–nursing diagnosis in planning patient care.* Philadelphia: F.A. Davis.

Nador, C., Harrison, J., & Schaeffer, S. (1985). Ocular trauma and the sudden impact of vision loss. *Ophthalmic Nursing Forum, 1*(1), 1–7.

Newell, F. (1983). *Ophthalmology: Principles and concepts.* St. Louis: C.V. Mosby.

McCoy, K. (1981). Intraocular lenses: From cloudy to clear. *Nursing Clinics of North America, 6*(3), 405–414.

Peyman, G., Sanders, D., & Goldberg, M. (1980). *Principles and practice of ophthalmology.* Philadelphia: W.B. Saunders.

Smith, J., & Nachazel, D. (1980). *Ophthalmic nursing.* Boston: Little, Brown.

Thompson, J., McFarland, G., Hirsch, J., Tucker, S., & Bowers, A. (1986). *Clinical nursing.* St. Louis: C.V. Mosby.

Vaughn, D., & Asbury, J. (1983). *General ophthalmology.* Los Altos, CA: Lange Publishing.

Fractured Hip and Femur

A fractured hip may be intracapsular, involving the neck of the femur, or extracapsular, involving the trochanteric region. Intracapsular fractures tend to heal poorly because the fracture damages circulation to the area. Elderly persons are more vulnerable to hip fractures because of osteoporosis and mobility problems.

Diagnostic Cluster

▲ **Time Frame**

Preoperative and postoperative periods

▲ **Discharge Criteria**

Before discharge, the client or family will:

1. Demonstrate care of the surgical site and use of assistive devices
2. Relate at-home restrictions and follow-up care
3. State the signs and symptoms that must be reported to a health care professional

PREOPERATIVE PERIOD

Nursing Diagnoses

Anxiety related to recent trauma, upcoming surgery and insufficient knowledge of preoperative routines, postoperative routines, and postoperative sensations

POSTOPERATIVE PERIOD

Collaborative Problems

Potential Complications:
Fat Emboli
Compartment Syndrome
Peroneal Nerve Palsy
Displacement of Hip Joint
Venous Stasis/Thrombosis
Avascular Necrosis of Femoral Head
Sepsis
Hemorrhage/Shock
Pulmonary Embolism

Nursing Diagnoses

Pain related to trauma and muscle spasms
(Specify) Self-Care Deficit related to prescribed activity restrictions
Fear related to anticipated dependence postoperatively
Potential Sensory–Perceptual Alteration related to increased age, pain, and immobility
Potential Altered Health Maintenance related to insufficient knowledge of activity restrictions, assistive devices, home care, follow-up care, and supportive services
Potential Altered Bowel Elimination:
Constipation related to immobility
Potential Impaired Skin Integrity related to immobility and urinary incontinence secondary to inability to reach toilet quickly enough between urge to void and need to void

Related Care Plan

General Surgery Generic Care Plan

Refer to:

General Surgery
General Surgery

Immobility or
Unconsciousness
Immobility or
Unconsciousness

Postoperative: Collaborative Problems

▲ *Nursing Goal*

The nurse will manage and minimize vascular and orthopedic complications.

Potential Complication: Fat Emboli
Potential Complication: Compartment Syndrome
Potential Complication: Peroneal Nerve Palsy
Potential Complication: Hip Joint Displacement
Potential Complication: Venous Stasis/Thrombosis
Potential Complication: Avascular Necrosis of the Femoral Head
Potential Complication: Sepsis

Interventions

1. Monitor for signs and symptoms of fat emboli:
   a. Fever
   b. Tachycardia
   c. Dyspnea
   d. Cough
   e. Petechiae on upper trunk and axillae
2. Monitor for signs and symptoms of compartment syndrome:
   a. Deep, throbbing pain at the fracture site
   b. Increasing pain with passive movement
   c. Decreased sensation to light touch
   d. Inability to distinguish between sharp and dull sensation in first web space of toes, sole, and dorsum and lateral aspect of foot
   e. Diminished or absent pedal pulses
   f. Increased edema and induration in extremity
3. Monitor for signs and symptoms of peroneal nerve palsy:
   a. Decreased sensation to light touch
   b. Inability to distinguish between sharp and dull sensations
   c. Tingling in extremity
   d. Paralysis
4. Monitor for signs and symptoms of hip joint displacement:
   a. External rotation of affected extremity
   b. Affected extremity shorter than unaffected extremity
   c. Increased pain
5. Monitor for signs and symptoms of avascular necrosis of the femoral head:
   a. Redness
   b. Warmth
6. Monitor for signs and symptoms of sepsis:
   a. Temperature > 101° F or < 98.6° F
   b. Abnormal laboratory values: increased creatinine, decreased pH, increased WBC count
   c. Decreased urine output

Rationale

1. Fat emboli most commonly occur after long bone fractures, especially in older clients. Signs and symptoms indicate an inflammatory response or obstruction.

2. Edema at the fracture site can compromise muscular vascular perfusion. Stretching of the damaged muscle causes pain. Sensory deficit is an early sign of nerve ischemia; the specific area of change indicates the affected compartment.

3. Pressure of the strap from skeletal traction (Buck's traction) over the fibular head can compress the peroneal nerve, resulting in paresthesias and, ultimately, paralysis due to nerve ischemia. (Buck's traction is not commonly used in acute care settings.)

4. Damaged tissue and muscles may not provide adequate support of the hip joint, resulting in displacement.

5. Hematoma formation results from tearing and rupture of blood vessels within the bone. Extensive blood loss with disruption of blood supply can result in bone death.
6. Sepsis results in massive vasodilatation and hypovolemia, leading to tissue hypoxia with decreased renal function and cardiac output. This triggers a compensatory response of increased heart and respiratory rates in an attempt to correct hypoxia and acidosis.

▲ *Documentation*

Flow records
    Vital signs
    Distal limb sensation, paresthesias, circulation
    Intake (oral, parenteral)
    Output (urine, urine specific gravity)
    Wound (color, drainage, swelling, rate of healing)

Related Physician-Prescribed Interventions

Medications
    Refer to the General Surgery care plan (Appendix II).

Intravenous Therapy
    Refer to the General Surgery care plan (Appendix II).

Related Physician-Prescribed Interventions (Continued)
Laboratory Studies
    Refer to the General Surgery care plan (Appendix II).
Diagnostic Studies
    Femur x-ray film
Therapies
    Wound care   Physical therapy

Postoperative: Nursing Diagnoses

▲ **Outcome Criteria**

The client will report pain relief after pain relief measures.

Pain related to trauma and muscle spasms

Focus Assessment Criteria	Clinical Significance

1. Source of pain:
  a. Fracture site with hematoma
  b. Groin
  c. Medial aspect of knee
	1. External rotation resulting from a shortened leg after fracture may cause muscle spasms. These spasms are more pronounced in intracapsular fracture because of the greater extent of external rotation involved.

Interventions

1. Position the client in proper alignment.

2. Use a trochanter roll to support the involved extremity in the neutral position.
3. Take steps to maintain the effectiveness of Buck's traction:
    a. Evaluate for appropriate use of weights.
    b. Ensure that weights hang freely.
    c. Ensure proper pulley functioning.
    d. Ensure that the heel does not rest on the mattress.
    e. Assess for paresthesias in the involved extremity.
4. Provide an orthopedic (fracture) bedpan rather than a standard bedpan.
5. Refer to the General Surgery care plan (Appendix II) for general pain relief interventions.

Rationale

1. Optimal alignment reduces pressure on nerves and tissue, reducing pain.
2. The trochanter roll prevents or minimizes external rotation.
3. Proper use of Buck's traction immobilizes the involved extremity, reducing muscle spasms and minimizing further tissue destruction from bone fragments.

4. Use of an orthopedic bedpan helps maintain proper body alignment during elimination.

▲ **Documentation**

Medication administration record
    Type, dosage, route of all
        medications
Progress notes
    Unsatisfactory response
    Positioning

▲ **Outcome Criteria**

The client will participate in self-care to the greatest extent possible considering his condition and status.

(Specify) Self-Care Deficit related to prescribed activity restrictions

Focus Assessment Criteria	Clinical Significance
1. Preoperative self-care ability 2. Preoperative endurance level 3. Preoperative mobility 4. Home environment: barriers to access	1–4. Pain and limited mobility affect a client's self-care ability. An elderly client may have had mobility problems before surgery (e.g., arthritis), further compromising self-care ability.

Interventions

1. Collaborate with the client to prioritize self-care tasks.

2. Encourage the client to participate in doable high-priority self-care tasks to the fullest extent possible.

Rationale

1. The client is more likely to participate in the self-care activities that he or she values. Prioritizing activities also gives the client a sense of control over the situation.
2. Achieving success at some tasks encourages the client to attempt other activities, which can promote progression in self-care ability.

Interventions

3. Provide physical therapy (e.g., range-of-motion [ROM] exercises, instruction in proper transfer techniques, and use of assistive devices). *Note:* the client, particularly if he is elderly, may have other problems that require modifications to standard assistive devices.
4. Pace activities to ensure adequate rest periods.

5. Evaluate progression of ability, and refer to a rehabilitation center if necessary.
6. As necessary, consult with occupational therapy for assistance in adapting self-care activities such as dressing and cooking.
7. Instruct the client or family in ways to modify the home environment to ease access to the bathroom, kitchen, and other areas.

Rationale

3. This can help increase muscle strength, endurance, and mobility.

4. Pacing activities helps avoid fatigue and ensure sufficient energy to perform tasks.
5. The client needs referral if he or she is unable to return to his or her former setting safely.
6,7. Assistance with tasks can help the client perform them, which promotes independence. In turn, independence increases motivation and decreases feelings of helplessness.

▲ **Documentation**

Flow records
    Participation in self-care

▲ **Outcome Criteria**

The client will express a progressive reduction in fear.

Fear related to anticipated postoperative dependence

Focus Assessment Criteria	*Clinical Significance*
1. Emotional status	1. Assessment is needed to establish a baseline and to determine interventions needed.

Interventions

1. Encourage the client to express his or her feelings regarding the impact of the fracture and surgery on self-care ability and life style.

2. Stress the importance of complying with the treatment regimen.

3. Encourage the highest possible level of independent functioning.
4. Involve family members or significant others in the care regimen to the fullest extent possible.

5. Plan diversional activities for stress management.

Rationale

1. Fear of adverse health impacts and loss of independence has a significant impact on a client's psychosocial functioning. Encouraging the client to share these fears gives the nurse the opportunity to validate them and possibly to correct any misconceptions.
2. Compliance can decrease the length of rehabilitation and promote a return to preoperative functioning.
3. Self-care promotes self-esteem and reduces feeling of dependency.
4. Others' involvement in care can provide the client with both physical and emotional support.
5. Diversional activities can help the client refocus on matters other than his or her condition and associated fears.

▲ **Documentation**

Progress notes
    Interventions
    Response to interventions

▲ **Outcome Criteria**

The client will resume presurgical orientation postoperatively.

Potential Sensory–Perceptual Alteration related to increased age, pain, and immobility

Focus Assessment Criteria	*Clinical Significance*
1. Preoperative level of orientation 2. Age 3. Preoperative level of activity	1–3. Elderly clients, who tend to have a lowered preinjury activity pattern and have some errors in mental tests on admission, are at high risk for confusion postsurgery (Williams and coworkers, 1985).

Interventions

1. Orient the client to all three spheres (person, place, time). Introduce yourself frequently.

2. Specifically request the client's perception of the situation.
3. Explain all activities.
4. Promote movement to the fullest extent possible. Encourage the client to eat meals sitting in a chair rather than in bed.
5. If the client becomes confused, direct him back to reality.
6. Encourage the client to use glasses and hearing aids, if necessary.
7. Provide meaningful sensory input, e.g., clock, calendar, window, familiar objects from home.

8. Encourage the client to wear his own clothes rather than a hospital gown.

Rationale

1. The trauma, surgery, and medications can decrease the efficiency of the sensory organs for reception and perception.
2. The nurse can correct misperceptions.

3. Explanations can reduce misinterpretations.
4. The quality and quantity of sensory input are reduced by immobility.

5. Ignoring confusion reinforces it as reality.

6. Aids reduce visual or auditory misinterpretation.
7. Familiar objects and orientation to daylight, time, and date reduce disorientation and can spark appropriate discussions.
8. Wearing one's own clothes can provide familiarity and security.

▲ **Documentation**

Progress notes
    Level of orientation

▲ **Outcome Criteria**

The outcome criteria for this diagnosis represent those associated with discharge planning. Refer to the discharge criteria.

Potential Altered Health Maintenance related to insufficient knowledge of activity restrictions, assistive devices, home care, follow-up care, and supportive services

Focus Assessment Criteria	*Clinical Significance*
1. Readiness and ability to learn and retain information	1. A client or family failing to meet learning goals requires a referral for assistance post-discharge.

Interventions

1. Evaluate the client's ability to ambulate and perform activities of daily living (ADLs).

2. Initiate appropriate referrals—e.g., home care agency, social services—if necessary.

3. Provide instruction on postoperative exercises per physician's order; these may include the following:
   a. Quadriceps setting
   b. Gluteal strengthening
   c. Dorsiplantar flexion
   d. Range-of-motion for upper and nonaffected lower extremities.
4. Teach the client how to ambulate without weightbearing using crutches or a walker; request a return demonstration to evaluate ability. Consult with the physician regarding the amount of weightbearing allowed.

5. Teach the client and family to do the following:

   a. Use proper transfer techniques to a chair: Place the chair on the affected side, abduct and support the affected leg, and pivot on the unaffected leg.
   b. Use pillows to maintain abduction while seated

Rationale

1. The nurse must evaluate the client's self-care abilities before discharge, to determine the need for referrals.
2. Community resources and other agencies can provide needed additional therapy or other assistance.
3. Exercises facilitate use of assistive devices by maintaining or enhancing present level of muscle function in unaffected limbs.

4. The client—particularly if elderly—may have impaired balance or decreased upper body strength, necessitating the use of a walker to maintain mobility. This need may persist for 3 to 7 days after surgery, depending on the internal fixation device used.

5. These measures may help reduce the risk of injury.
   a. Proper transfer technique prevents weightbearing on the affected side.

   b. Leg abduction relieves stress on the internal fixation device and fracture site.

Interventions

c. Sit without flexing the hip more than 60 degrees for 5 to 10 days after surgery.
d. Avoid adducting the affected extremity beyond the midline for at least 2 months after surgery
e. Use proper body mechanics within limitations
f. Use an elevated toilet seat

6. Present information or reinforce learning using written materials (e.g., booklets, instruction sheets) or audiovisual aids (e.g., slides, videotapes, models, diagrams).
7. Explain the importance of progressive care, i.e., early nonweightbearing ambulation, self-care within abilities.
8. Teach the client and family to watch for and report subtle signs of infection:
   a. Increased temperature, chills
   b. Malaise

Rationale

c. Hip flexion puts stress on the internal fixation device and fracture site.
d. Leg adduction puts stress on the internal fixation device and fracture site.

e. Proper body mechanics prevent injury to muscles and ligaments.
f. Using an elevated toilet seat decreases flexion and minimizes stress on fracture site. It also facilitates independent toileting.

6. Using a variety of teaching materials stimulates learning and enhances retention, particularly for an elderly client, who may have visual or hearing impairment.
7. The risk for complications increases with each day of immobility, particularly in an elderly client.
8. Hip fracture typically affects elderly clients, who have a decreased ability to compensate for physiological changes and immunological system changes that may mask pronounced signs and symptoms of infection.

▲ **Documentation**

Discharge summary record
    Client and family teaching
    Outcome achievement or
      status
    Referrals, if indicated

References/Bibliography

Callahan, J. (1985). Compartment syndrome. *Orthopedic Nursing, 4*(4), 11–15.

Ceccio, C.M. (1984). Postoperative pain relief through relaxation in elderly patients with fractured hips. *Orthopedic Nursing, 3*(3), 11–19.

Cummings, S.R., et al. (1988). Recovery of function after hip fracture: The role of social supports. *Journal of the American Geriatric Society, 36*(9), 801–806.

Dubrovski, V., et al. (1988). Hip fracture in the elderly: Program planning puts these patients on their feet again. *Canadian Nurse, 84*(5), 20–22.

Duerksen, J.R. (1982). Hip fractures: Special considerations in the elderly. *Orthopedic Nursing, 1*(1), 11–19.

Hansell, M.J. (1988). Fractures and the healing process. *Orthopedic Nursing, 7*(1), 43–50.

Mossey, J.M., et al. (1989). Determinants of recovery 12 months after hip fracture: The importance of psychosocial factors. *American Journal of Public Health, 79*(3), 279–286.

Reinhard, S.C. (1988). Case managing community services for hip fractured elders. *Orthopedic Nursing, 7*(5), 42–49.

Sanford, M., & Fowler, C. (1989). Positioning the patient with an abductor pillow. *Orthopedic Nursing, 8*(5), 21–23.

White, L., et al. (1984). Who's at risk? Hip fracture epidemiology report. *Journal of Gerontologic Nursing, 10*(10), 26–28.

Williams, M., et al. (1985). Predicators of acute confusional states in hospitalized elderly patients. *Research in Nursing and Health, 8*(1), 31–40.

Hysterectomy

The surgical removal of the internal female reproductive organs, hysterectomy is classified according to the organs removed. *Subtotal hysterectomy* involves removal of the uterus only; *total hysterectomy*, removal of the uterus and cervical stump; *salpingectomy*, removal of these structures plus the fallopian tubes; and *oophorectomy*, removal of the uterus, cervix, fallopian tubes, and ovaries. Surgery is performed either through a lower abdominal incision or through the vagina.

Diagnostic Cluster

▲ Time Frame

Preoperative and postoperative periods

▲ Discharge Criteria

Before discharge, the client and/or family will:

1. State wound care procedures to follow at home
2. Verbalize precautions to take regarding activities
3. State the signs and symptoms that must be reported to a health care professional
4. Verbalize an intent to share feelings and concerns with significant others

---

PREOPERATIVE PERIOD
Refer to General Surgery Generic Care Plan

POSTOPERATIVE PERIOD
Collaborative Problems

Potential Complications:
Ureter, Bladder, Rectal Trauma
Vaginal Bleeding
Deep Vein Thrombosis
Fistula Formation

Nursing Diagnoses

Potential Self-Concept Disturbance related to significance of loss
Potential Altered Health Maintenance related to insufficient knowledge of perineal/incisional care, signs of complications, activity restrictions, loss of menses, hormone therapy, and follow-up care

---

Postoperative: Collaborative Problems

▲ Nursing Goal

The nurse will manage and minimize complications post-hysterectomy.

Potential Complication: Ureter, Bladder, Rectal Trauma
Potential Complication: Vaginal Bleeding
Potential Complication: Deep Venous Thrombosis
Potential Complication: Fistula Formation

Interventions

1. Monitor for signs and symptoms of ureter, bladder, or rectal trauma:
   a. Urinary retention
   b. Prolonged diminished bowel sounds
   c. Bloody, cloudy urine
   d. Absence of flatus
2. Monitor for signs and symptoms of deep venous thrombosis:
   a. Leg pain
   b. Leg swelling
   c. Referred pain in abdomen or buttocks
3. Provide frequent position changes; avoid high Fowler's position and putting pressure under the knees.

Rationale

1. Proximity of these structures to the surgical site may predispose them to atony due to edema or nerve trauma.

2. Positioning during surgery and postoperative edema contribute to vascular stasis and thrombosis formation.

3. Movement reduces stasis and vascular pooling in legs. High Fowler's position leads to decreased circulation in the pelvis; pressure under knees can interfere with peripheral circulation.

▲ Documentation

Flow records
  Vital signs
  Perineal drainage
  Intake and output
  Turning, ambulation

Interventions

4. Monitor for signs and symptoms of fistula formation:
   a. Fecal-colored urine
   b. Abdominal distention

Related Physician-Prescribed Interventions

Medications
  Estrogen therapy (selected cases)

Intravenous Therapy
  Refer to the General Surgery care plan (Appendix II).

Laboratory Studies
  Refer to the General Surgery care plan (Appendix II).

Diagnostic Studies
  Ultrasound or computed tomography (CT) scan   Hysterosalpingography

Therapies
  Refer to the General Surgery care plan (Appendix II).

Rationale

4. A tract may develop from the surgical site to the bladder and bowel.

Postoperative: Nursing Diagnoses

▲ Outcome Criteria

The client will:

1. Acknowledge change in body structure and function
2. Communicate feelings about the hysterectomy
3. Participate in self-care

Potential Self-Concept Disturbance related to perceived effects on sexuality and feminine role

Focus Assessment Criteria	Clinical Significance
1. Exposure to others who have undergone hysterectomy	1,2. This information can be used to measure present response and progress. Discussions can detect misinformation and fears.
2. Ability to express feelings about the hysterectomy	
3. Evidence of negative self-concept	3. A client with a previous negative self-concept is at higher risk for impaired adjustment.
4. Participation in self-care	4. Participation in self-care indicates an attempt to cope positively with the changes.

Interventions

1. Contact the client frequently and treat her with warm, positive regard.

2. Incorporate emotional support into technical care teaching sessions, e.g., wound care, bathing.

3. Encourage the client to verbalize her feelings about surgery and perceptions of life style impact. Validate her perceptions and reassure her that the responses are normal and appropriate.

4. Replace myths with facts, e.g., hysterectomy usually does not affect physiological sexual response.

5. Discuss the surgery and its effects on functioning with family members or significant others; correct any misconceptions. Encourage the client to share her feelings and perceptions with them also.

6. Refer a client at high risk for unsuccessful adjustment for professional counseling.

Rationale

1. Frequent contact by the caregiver indicates acceptance and may facilitate trust. The client may be hesitant to approach staff because of a negative self-concept.

2. This encourages resolution of emotional issues while teaching technical skills.

3. Sharing concerns and ventilating feelings provides an opportunity for the nurse to correct any misinformation. Validating the client's perceptions increases self-awareness.

4. Misinformation may contribute to unfounded anxiety and fear. Providing accurate information can help reduce these emotional stressors.

5. The support of family members or significant others often is critical to the client's acceptance of changes and positive self-concept.

6. Follow-up therapy to assist with effective adjustment may be indicated.

▲ Documentation

Progress notes
  Present emotional status
  Interventions
  Response to interventions

▲ **Outcome Criteria**

The outcome criteria for this diagnosis represent those associated with discharge planning. Refer to the discharge criteria.

Potential Altered Health Maintenance related to insufficient knowledge of perineal/incisional care, signs of complications, activity restrictions, loss of menses, hormone therapy, and follow-up care

Focus Assessment Criteria	*Clinical Significance*
1. Readiness and ability to learn and retain information	1. A client or family failing to meet learning goals requires a referral for assistance postdischarge.

Interventions

1. Discuss expectations for recovery based on the type and extent of surgery. Explain that vaginal hysterectomy generally affords more rapid recovery and causes less postoperative discomfort, but that it has several disadvantages, including:
   a. Greater risk of postoperative infection
   b. Reduced ability (as compared to abdominal hysterectomy) to deal with unexpected difficulties of surgery or complications.
   Explain that abdominal hysterectomy allows better visualization during surgery and has fewer contraindications, but it involves longer recovery periods, increased use of anesthesia, and increased postoperative pain.
2. Explain care of an uncomplicated wound (abdominal hysterectomy); teach the client to do the following:
   a. Wash with soap and water (bath or shower when able)
   b. Towel-dry thoroughly, separating skin folds to ensure complete drying.
   Consult with a physician for care of a complicated wound.
3. Explain perineal care (vaginal hysterectomy); teach the client to do the following:
   a. Maintain good hygiene
   b. Wash thoroughly with soap and water
   c. Change the peripad frequently
   d. After elimination, wipe from the front to back, using a clean tissue for each front-to-back pass
4. Explain the need to increase activity as tolerated.

5. Teach the client and family to watch for and report the following:
   a. Changes in perineal drainage (e.g., unusual drainage, bright red bleeding, foul odor)
   b. Urinary retention, burning, frequency
   c. Cloudy, foul-smelling urine
   d. Blood in urine
   e. Change in bowel function (constipation, diarrhea)

Rationale

1. Understanding expectations for recovery can help the client and family plan strategies for complying with the postoperative care regimen.

2. Proper wound care helps reduce microorganisms at the incision site and prevent infection.

3. Proper perineal care reduces microorganisms around the perineum, minimizing their entry into the vagina.

4. Physical activity, especially early and frequent ambulation, can help prevent or minimize abdominal cramps, a common complaint during recovery from abdominal hysterectomy.
5. Because of the abundance of blood vessels in the female pelvis, hysterectomy carries a higher risk of postoperative bleeding than most other surgeries. Bleeding most often occurs within 24 hours after surgery, but high risk also occurs on the fourth, ninth, and 21st postoperative days, when sutures dissolve. A small amount of pink, yellow, or brown serous drainage, or even minor frank vaginal bleeding (no heavier than normal menstrual flow), is normal and expected.

Interventions

6. Explain the effects of surgery on menstruation and ovulation. Instruct the client to report symptoms of the climacteric (cessation of menses):
   a. Hot flashes
   b. Headache
   c. Nervousness
   d. Palpitations
   e. Fatigue
   f. Depression, feelings of uselessness, and other emotional reactions

7. Explain activity restrictions; teach the client to do the following:
   a. Expect fatigue and weakness during the recovery period
   b. Delegate tasks to others (e.g., vacuuming, lifting) for at least 1 month
   c. Walk in moderation; gradually increase distance and pace
   d. Resume driving 2 weeks after surgery, if the car is equipped with an automatic transmission
   e. Avoid sitting for prolonged periods

8. Explore the client's concerns regarding the impact of surgery on sexual feelings and function. Explain that she should be able to resume intercourse anywhere from 3 weeks (with a vaginal hysterectomy) to 16 weeks after surgery; confirm a specific time frame with the physician.

9. If a subtotal hysterectomy was performed, explain that menses will continue because a portion of the uterus and its endometrial lining remain.

10. Explain that total removal of the uterus prevents pregnancy and results in loss of menses, but that as long as even a portion of an ovary remains, she may experience monthly premenstrual symptoms, such as bloating and abdominal cramps.

11. If estrogen replacement therapy is indicated, provide client teaching:
    a. Explain that estrogen typically is administered in low doses on a cyclical basis—5 days on, 2 days off—until she reaches the average age of menopause.
    b. Discuss the rationale for therapy: to provide a feeling of well-being, to decrease the risk of cardiovascular disease, to decrease the risk of osteoporosis.
    c. Explain the risks associated with therapy: thrombophlebitis, cancer. A study on the long-term effects of estrogen use found a decreased death rate from myocardial infarction and cancer, but an increased incidence of breast cancer (although a decrease

Rationale

6. Removal of the uterus (leaving the ovaries) theoretically should not produce menopausal symptoms; however, the client may experience them temporarily, apparently because of increased estrogen levels resulting from surgical manipulation of the ovaries. Removal of both ovaries artificially induces menopause, causing more severe symptoms than typically experienced in a normal climacteric. To help reduce these symptoms, a portion of the ovary often is left in place, unless contraindicated. Estrogen therapy relieves symptoms and may be indicated except in cases of malignancy.

7. Adequate rest allows the body to repair surgical tissue trauma. Walking improves muscle strength and endurance, speeding recovery. Prolonged sitting may cause pelvic congestion and thrombosis formation.

8. In most cases, hysterectomy should not affect sexual response or functioning. For 3 to 4 months after surgery, intercourse may be painful owing to abdominal soreness and temporary shrinking of the vagina. Intercourse helps stretch the vaginal walls and eventually relieve the discomfort.

9,10. Explanations of what to expect from surgery can help reduce anxiety associated with the unknown and allow effective coping.

11. The client's understanding of estrogen therapy may encourage compliance with the prescribed regimen.

Interventions   *Rationale*

in breast cancer–related death rate) and osteoporosis. Nulliparous women were found
to be at high risk for breast cancer during
the first 10 years of therapy. Women over
age 55 and women experiencing late menopause also were found to be at increased
risk for breast cancer. The study recommended that physicians give these clients
special consideration before prescribing estrogen therapy.

   d. Teach the client to report the following:
- Mood changes, especially depression
- Signs and symptoms of thrombo-
  phlebitis (warmth and pain in the
  calf, abdominal pain, and pain,
  numbness, or stiffness in the legs
  and buttocks)
- Excessive fluid retention
- Jaundice
- Excessive nausea and vomiting
- Dizziness, frequent headaches
- Hair loss
- Visual disturbances
- Breast lumps

   e. Explain the need for regular follow-up visits (at least yearly) and monthly breast self-
examination.

▲ **Documentation**

Discharge summary record
   Client and family teaching
   Outcome achievement or
     status

12. Discuss follow-up care; explain that discharge
usually occurs in 5 to 7 days, and that a postoperative check is scheduled for 4 to 6 weeks
after discharge. Reinforce the importance of
keeping scheduled appointments.

12. Regular follow-up care is necessary to evaluate the results of surgery and estrogen therapy, if indicated, and to detect any complications.

References/Bibliography

Moore, J. (1988). Vaginal hysterectomy: Its success as an outpatient procedure. *AORN Journal, 48*(6), 1114–
   1120.
Webb, C., & Wilson-Barnet, J. (1983). Self-concept, social support, and hysterectomy. *International Journal
   of Nursing Studies, 20*(2), 97–107.
Wells, M.P., & Vilano, K. (1985). Total abdominal hysterectomy. *AORN Journal, 42*(3), 368–373.

Ileostomy

A traditional ileostomy is the surgical diversion of the ileum through an opening onto the abdominal surface. If indicated, the colon, rectum and anus may also be removed. A collection device must be worn continuously with a traditional ileostomy. Ileostomy is typically indicated for clients with inflammatory bowel conditions.

Another type of ileostomy is the Kock continent ileostomy. A *Kock continent ileostomy* pouch is an internal fecal reservoir constructed of ileum and containing a nipple valve that maintains continence of stool and flatus. An *ileoanal reservoir* is an ileal pouch located in the pelvis. Various pouch configurations are possible, the most common being an S- or J-shaped pouch. The pouch is drained periodically with a catheter.

Continent ileostomy surgery is done in two stages. The first operation involves an abdominal colectomy, construction of an ileal pouch, mucosectomy of the rectum, ileoanal anastomosis, and creation of a diverting ileostomy. The second operation is performed to take down the temporary ileostomy in order to restore the continuity of the fecal stream.

Diagnostic Cluster

▲ Time Frame
Preoperative and postoperative periods

▲ Discharge Criteria
Before discharge, the client or family will:

1. State conditions of ostomy care at home: stoma, pouching, irrigation, skin care
2. Discuss strategies for incorporating ostomy management into ADLs
3. Verbalize precautions for medication use and food intake
4. State signs and symptoms that must be reported to a health care professional
5. Verbalize an intent to share feelings and concerns related to ostomy with significant others
6. Identify available community resources and self-help groups:
   a. Visiting nurse
   b. United Ostomy Association
   c. Recovery of Male Potency; Help for Impotent Male
   d. American Cancer Foundation
   e. Community supplier of ostomy equipment
   f. Financial reimbursement for ostomy equipment
7. If the client has a Kock continent ileostomy, he or she should demonstrate ability to perform intermittent self-intubation.

PREOPERATIVE PERIOD
Nursing Diagnoses

Anxiety related to lack of knowledge of ileostomy care and perceived negative effects on life style

POSTOPERATIVE PERIOD
Collaborative Problems

Potential Complications:
Peristomal Ulceration/Herniation
Stomal Necrosis, Retraction Prolapse, Stenosis, Obstruction
Fluid and Electrolyte Imbalances
Ileal Reservoir Pouchitis (Kock Pouch)
Failed Nipple Valve (Kock Pouch)
Ileoanal Pouchitis

Nursing Diagnoses

Potential Self-Concept Disturbance related to effects of ostomy on body image
Potential Altered Sexuality Pattern related to perceived negative impact of ostomy on sexual functioning and attractiveness
Potential Sexual Dysfunction related to physiological impotence secondary to damaged sympathetic nerves (male) or inadequate vaginal lubrication (female)
Potential Social Isolation related to anxiety over possible odor and leakage from appliance
Potential Altered Health Maintenance related to insufficient knowledge of stoma pouching procedure, peristomal skin care, perineal wound care, and incorporation of ostomy care into activities of daily living (ADLs)
Potential Altered Health Maintenance related to insufficient knowledge of care of ileoanal reservoir

---

Nursing Diagnoses, cont'd.

Potential Altered Health Maintenance related to insufficient knowledge of intermittent intubation of Kock continent ileostomy

Related Care Plan

General Surgery Generic Care Plan

Preoperative: Nursing Diagnosis

▲ Outcome Criteria

The client will:

1. State reason for ileostomy
2. Describe anatomical changes following ileostomy surgery
3. Identify his or her own type of ileostomy
4. Verbalize decreased anxiety related to fear of the unknown

Anxiety related to lack of knowledge of ostomy care and perceived negative effects on life style

Focus Assessment Criteria

1. Understanding of underlying disorder necessitating ileostomy
2. Knowledge of structure and function of affected organs
3. Anticipated surgical procedure and stoma location
4. Previous exposure to a client with an ostomy
5. Familiarity with stoma pouching equipment
6. Emotional status, cognitive ability, memory, vision, manual dexterity
7. Life style, strengths, coping mechanisms, available support systems

Clinical Significance

1–7. Assessing the client's knowledge of ileostomy identifies learning needs and guides the nurse in planning effective teaching strategies. Assessing emotional status, mental and physical ability, and other factors about the client helps the nurse evaluate the client's ability to accept, adjust to, and manage the ostomy and stoma.

Interventions

1. Identify and dispel any misinformation or misconceptions the client has regarding ostomy.
2. Explain the normal anatomical structure and function of the gastrointestinal (GI) tract.
3. Explain the effects of the client's particular disorder on affected organs.
4. Use an anatomical diagram or model to show the resultant altered route of elimination.

5. Describe the appearance and anticipated location of the stoma. Explain the following about the stoma:
   a. It will be the same color and moistness as oral mucous membrane.
   b. It will not hurt when touched, because it has no sensory endings.
   c. It may bleed slightly when wiped; this is normal and not of concern.
   d. It will become smaller as the surgical area heals; color will remain the same.
   e. It may change in size depending on illness, hormone levels, and weight gain or loss.
6. Discuss the function of the stoma pouch. Explain that it serves as an external receptacle for storage of feces much as the colon acts as an internal storage receptacle.

Rationale

1. Replacing misinformation with facts can reduce anxiety.
2. Knowledge increases confidence; confidence produces control and reduces anxiety.
3. Understanding the disorder can help the client accept the need for ileostomy.
4. Understanding how body waste elimination occurs after the rectum and anus are removed can help allay anxiety related to altered body function.
5. Explaining expected events and sensations can help reduce anxiety associated with the unknown and unexpected. Accurate descriptions of the stoma appearance help ease shock at the first sight of it after ostomy surgery.

6. Understanding the purpose and need for a pouch encourages the client to accept it and participate in ostomy management.

Interventions

Rationale

▲ **Documentation**

Progress notes
    Present emotional status
Teaching records
    Client teaching

7. Encourage the client to handle the stoma pouching equipment.

7. Many clients are relieved to see the actual size and material of a stoma pouch. Often, uninformed clients have visions of large bags and complicated, difficult-to-manage equipment, which can produce anxiety.

Postoperative: Collaborative Problems

▲ **Nursing Goal**

The nurse will manage and minimize complications post-ileostomy.

Potential Complication: Peristomal Ulceration/Herniation
Potential Complication: Stomal Necrosis, Retraction, Prolapse, Stenosis, Obstruction
Potential Complication: Fluid and Electrolyte Imbalances
Potential Complication: Ileal Reservoir Pouchitis (Kock Pouch)
Potential Complication: Failed Nipple Valve (Kock Pouch)
Potential Complication: Ileoanal Pouchitis

Interventions

1. Monitor for signs of peristomal ulceration or herniation:
    a. Decreased peristomal muscle tone
    b. Bulging beyond the normal skin surface and musculature
    c. Persistent ulceration
2. Monitor for stomal necrosis, prolapse, retraction, stenosis, and obstruction. Assess the following:
    a. Color, size, and shape of stoma

    b. Color, amount, and consistency of ostomy effluent
    c. Complaints of cramping, abdominal pain, nausea and vomiting, abdominal distention
    d. Ostomy appliance and appliance belt fit

3. Monitor for signs of fluid and electrolyte imbalance:
    a. High volume of watery ostomy output (more than five one-third to one-half filled pouches or > 1000 mL daily)
    b. Decreased serum sodium, potassium, and magnesium levels
    c. Weight loss
    d. Nausea and vomiting, anorexia, abdominal distention
4. Administer fluid and electrolyte replacement therapy, as ordered.
5. Monitor for signs and symptoms of ileal reservoir or ileoanal pouchitis:
    a. Acute increase in effluent flow
    b. Evidence of dehydration
    c. Abdominal pain and bloating, nausea and vomiting
    d. Fever
6. Connect an indwelling catheter to continuous straight drainage.
7. Monitor for stool leakage from a stoma with a nipple valve.

8. Irrigate the ileoanal reservoir daily to flush out mucus.

Rationale

1. Early detection of ulcerations and herniation can prevent serious tissue damage.

2. Daily assessment is necessary to detect early changes in stoma condition.

    a. Changes can indicate inflammation, retraction, prolapse, edema.
    b. Changes can indicate bleeding or infection. Decreased output can indicate obstruction.
    c. These complaints may indicate obstruction.

    d. Improperly fitting appliance or belt can cause mechanical trauma to the stoma.
3. Fluid and electrolyte imbalance most commonly results from diarrhea. Major causes of acute diarrhea include infection, diuretic therapy, obstruction, and hot weather. Chronic diarrhea can result from ileal resection or "short gut syndrome," radiation therapy, or chemotherapy.

4. Replacement therapy may be needed to prevent serious electrolyte imbalance or fluid deficiency.
5. Pouchitis or ileitis involves inflammation of the ileal pouch. The cause is unknown, but bacterial growth in the pouch is a suspected causative factor. Insufficiently frequent pouch emptying increases the risk; it occurs in about 10% of clients with a Kock ileostomy.

6. This measure promotes continuous urine drainage of the Kock Pouch

7. Nipple valve failure—pulling apart of the bowel segment forming the valve—most commonly occurs within the first 3 months after surgery.
8. Daily irrigation helps prevent stomal obstruction.

▲ **Documentation**

Flow records
    Intake and output
    Bowel sounds
    Wound status
Progress notes
    Stoma condition
    Changes in physiological
        status

Related Physician-Prescribed Interventions
Dependent on the underlying problem. Refer also to the General Surgery care plan in Appendix II.

Postoperative: Nursing Diagnoses

▲ Outcome Criteria

The client will:

1. Acknowledge change in body structure and function
2. Communicate feelings about the ostomy
3. Participate in stoma care

Potential Self-Concept Disturbance related to effects of ostomy on body image and life style

Focus Assessment Criteria	Clinical Significance
1. Previous exposure to person(s) with an ostomy	1–7. This assessment information helps the nurse evaluate present responses and progress. Participation in self-care and planning indicates positive attempts to cope with the changes.
2. Ability to visualize the stoma	
3. Ability to express feelings about the stoma	
4. Ability to share feelings about the ostomy with significant others	
5. Ability to participate in the stoma pouching procedure	
6. Ability to discuss plans to incorporate ostomy management into body image and life style	
7. Evidence of negative self-concept	

Interventions	Rationale
1. Contact the client frequently and treat him or her with warm, positive regard.	1. Frequent contact by the caregiver indicates acceptance and may facilitate trust. The client may be hesitant to approach the staff because of negative self-concept.
2. Incorporate emotional support into technical ostomy self-care sessions.	2. This allows resolution of emotional issues during acquisition of technical skills. Shipes (1987) identified four stages of psychological adjustment that ostomy clients experience:
	a. *Narration.* Each client recounts his illness experience and reveals his understanding of how and why he finds himself in this situation.
	b. *Visualization and verbalization.* The client looks at and expresses feelings about his stoma.
	c. *Participation.* The client progresses from observer to assistant and then to independent performer of the mechanical aspects of ostomy care.
	d. *Exploration.* The client begins to explore methods of incorporating the ostomy into his life style.
	Use of this adjustment framework helps establish guidelines for planning the client's experiences in an organized manner.
3. Have the client look at and touch the stoma.	3. The nurse should not make assumptions about a client's reaction to ostomy surgery. He or she may need help in accepting the reality of the altered body appearance and function, or in dealing with an overwhelming situation.
4. Encourage the client to verbalize feelings about the stoma and perceptions of its anticipated effects on his or her life style.	4. Sharing gives the nurse an opportunity to identify and dispel misconceptions and allay anxiety and self-doubt.

Interventions

5. Validate the client's perceptions and reassure that such responses are normal and appropriate.
6. Have the client practice using a pouch clamp on an empty pouch.

7. Assist the client with pouch emptying, as necessary.

8. Have the client participate in pouch removal and pouch application. Provide feedback on progress; reinforce positive behavior and proper techniques.
9. Have the client demonstrate the stoma pouching procedure independently in the presence of support persons.
10. Involve support persons in learning ostomy care principles. Assess the client's interactions with support persons.
11. Encourage the client to discuss plans for incorporating ostomy care into his or her life style.
12. Encourage the client to verbalize positive self-attributes.
13. Suggest that the client meet with a person from the United Ostomy Association (UOA) who can share similar experiences.

14. Identify a client at risk for unsuccessful adjustment; look for these characteristics:
   a. Poor ego strength
   b. Ineffective problem-solving ability

   c. Difficulty learning new skills

   d. Lack of motivation
   e. External focus of control

   f. Poor health
   g. Unsatisfactory preoperative sex life
   h. Lack of positive support systems
   i. Unstable economic status
   j. Rejection of counseling (Shipes, 1987)
15. Refer an at-risk client for professional counseling.

Rationale

5. Validating the client's perceptions promotes self-awareness and provides reassurance.

6. Beginning client teaching with a necessary skill that is separate from the body may be less threatening and may ease the fear of failure when performing on his or her own body.
7. During ostomy care procedures, the client watches health care professionals for signs of revulsion. The nurse's attitude and support are of primary importance (Shipes, 1987).
8. Effective, thorough teaching helps the client learn to master procedures.

9. Return demonstration lets the nurse evaluate the need for any further teaching.

10. Others' response to the ostomy is one of the most important factors influencing the client's acceptance of it.
11. Evidence that the client will pursue his or her goals and life style reflects positive adjustment.
12. Identifying personal strengths promotes self-acceptance and positive self-concept.
13. In addition to the clinical expertise of the professional nurse, the ostomy client may choose to take advantage of a UOA visitor's actual experience with an ostomy (Maklebust, 1985).
14. Successful adjustment to ostomies is influenced by factors such as the following:
   a. Previous coping success
   b. Achievement of developmental tasks pre-surgery
   c. The extent to which the disability interferes with goal-directed activity
   d. Sense of control
   e. Realistic perception of the event by the client and support persons

15. In such a client, follow-up therapy is indicated to assist with effective adjustment.

▲ **Documentation**

Progress notes
   Present emotional status
   Interventions
   Response to interventions

▲ **Outcome Criteria**

The client will:

1. Discuss own feelings and partner's concerns regarding the effect of ostomy surgery on sexual functioning
2. Verbalize an intent to discuss concerns with partner before discharge

Potential Altered Sexuality Pattern related to perceived negative impact of ostomy on sexual functioning and attractiveness

Focus Assessment Criteria	*Clinical Significance*
1. Importance of sex to the client	1–5. Assessing current concerns and past sexual patterns provides direction for planning effective nursing interventions.
2. Availability of a partner	
3. Concerns about resuming intercourse	
4. Preferred methods of sexual expression	
5. Acceptability of alternative pleasuring activities to the client and partner	

Interventions

1. Reaffirm the need for frank discussion between sexual partners and the need for time for the partner to become accustomed to changes in the client's body.
2. Role-play ways for the client and partner to discuss concerns about sex.

3. Discuss the possibility that the client may project his or her own feelings onto the partner. Encourage frequent validation of feelings between partners.
4. Reaffirm the need for closeness and expressions of caring; involve the client and partner in touching, stroking, massage, etc.
5. Explore any fears the client may express regarding mutilation, unacceptability, and other concerns that might limit his or her involvement in relationships.
6. Discuss the possible availability of a penile prosthesis if the client is physiologically unable to maintain or sustain an erection sufficient for intercourse. Explain that penile implants provide the erection needed for intercourse and do not alter sensations or the ability to ejaculate.
7. Refer the client to a certified sex or mental health counselor, if desired.

Rationale

1. The client may worry about his or her partner's acceptance; the partner may be afraid of hurting the client and needs to know that the stoma is not harmed by sexual activity.
2. Role-playing helps a person gain insight by placing him or her in the position of another. It also may promote more spontaneous sharing of fears and concerns.
3. The client may have erroneous assumptions about the partner; e.g., he or she may erroneously assume that the partner is "turned off" by the ostomy.
4. Sexual pleasure and gratification are not limited to intercourse. Other expressions of caring may prove more meaningful.
5. These fears might limit involvement in relationships.

6. Realizing that a prosthesis may be available may reassure the client and reduce anxiety about performance, which actually could help improve function.

7. Certain sexual problems require continuing therapy and the advanced knowledge of therapists.

▲ **Documentation**

Progress notes
    Assessment data
    Interventions
    Response to interventions
    Referrals, if indicated

▲ **Outcome Criteria**

The client will state alternatives to deal with physiological impotence.

Potential Sexual Dysfunction related to physiological impotence secondary to sympathetic nerve damage (male) or inadequate vaginal lubrication (female)

Focus Assessment Criteria

1. Knowledge of the effects of surgery on sexual function:
   a. In men, a wide resection for Crohn's disease occasionally damages sympathetic nerves in the presacral area that control emission. This may result in retrograde ejaculation into the bladder and a "dry" orgasm. During abdominoperineal surgery, the parasympathetic nerves that control blood flow to the penis can be damaged, possibly resulting in erectile dysfunction.
   b. In women, there is little objective evidence of sexual dysfunction following ileostomy surgery. The most common female sexual complaint is dyspareunia, which may result in "female impotence" (Schover, 1986).

Clinical Significance

1. Assessment of the client's knowledge of possible effects on sexual function guides the nurse in planning effective interventions.

Interventions

1. In men
   a. Suggest that sexual activity need not always culminate in vaginal intercourse and that orgasm can be reached through noncoital manual or oral stimulation. Remind the

Rationale

1.
   a. Alternate methods of sexual expression and gratification promote positive sexual function.

Interventions

      client that sexual expression is not limited to intercourse but includes closeness, communication, touching, and giving pleasure to another.

    b. Suggest counseling with a certified sex therapist.

2. In women
    a. Suggest using a water-based vaginal lubricant for intercourse.

    b. Teach the client to perform Kegel exercises, and instruct her to do them regularly.

    c. Suggest that she sit astride her partner during intercourse.

Rationale

    b. Certain sexual problems require continuing therapy and the advanced knowledge of therapists.

2.
    a. Water-based lubricant can help prevent dyspareunia related to inadequate vaginal lubrication.

    b. Kegel exercises promote control of the pubococcygeal muscles around the vaginal entrance, which can ease dyspareunia.

    c. A woman on top can control the depth and rate of penetration, which can enhance vaginal lubrication and relaxation.

▲ **Documentation**

Progress notes
   Interventions
   Response to interventions

▲ **Outcome Criteria**

The client will:

1. Discuss methods to control odor and appliance leakage
2. State an intent to reestablish preoperative socialization pattern

Potential Social Isolation related to anxiety about possible odor and leakage from appliance

Focus Assessment Criteria	*Clinical Significance*
1. Preoperative socialization pattern 2. Anticipated changes	1,2. A client at risk for social isolation must be assessed carefully; the suffering associated with isolation is not always visible. Feelings of rejection and repulsion are common.

Interventions

1. Select an appropriate odorproof pouching system, and explain to client how it works.

2. Stress the need for good personal hygiene.
3. Teach the client care of a reusable appliance.
4. Discuss methods for reducing odor:
    a. Avoid odor-producing foods, such as onions, fish, eggs, cheese, asparagus.
    b. Use internal chlorophyll tablets or a liquid appliance deodorant.
    c. Empty or change the ostomy pouch regularly; when one third to one half full.
5. Encourage the client to reestablish his or her preoperative socialization pattern. Help through measures such as progressively increasing the client's socializing time in the hospital and role-playing possible situations that the client feels may cause anxiety, encouraging the client to visualize and anticipate solutions to "worst-case scenarios" for social situations.
6. Suggest that the client meet with a person from the United Ostomy Association (UOA) who can share similar experiences.

Rationale

1. Fear of accidents and odor can be reduced through effective management. Some pouches have charcoal filters to reduce odor from flatus.
2,3. Proper hygiene and appliance care remove odoriferous retained fecal material.
4. Minimizing odor improves self-confidence and can permit more effective socialization. Bacterial proliferation in retained effluent increases odor over time. A full pouch also puts excessive pressure on seals, increasing the risk of leakage.

5. Encouraging and facilitating socialization help prevent isolation. Role-playing can help the client identify and learn to cope with potential anxiety-causing situations in a nonthreatening environment.

6. Others in a similar situation can provide a realistic appraisal of the situation and may provide information to answer the client's unasked questions.

▲ **Documentation**

Progress notes
   Dialogues
Discharge summary record
   Client teaching
   Outcome achievement or
     status

▲ **Outcome Criteria**

The outcome criteria for this diagnosis represent those associated with discharge planning. Refer to the discharge criteria.

Potential Altered Health Maintenance related to insufficient knowledge of stoma pouching procedure, ileostomy irrigation, peristomal skin care, perineal wound care, and incorporation of ostomy care into ADLs

Focus Assessment Criteria	Clinical Significance
1. Knowledge of ileostomy care: diet, activity, hygiene, clothing, sexual expression, community resources, employment, travel, odor, skin care, appliances, and irrigation, if applicable	1. Assessment identifies learning needs and guides the nurse in planning effective teaching strategies.
2. Client's and support persons' readiness and ability to learn and retain information	2. A family or client failing to achieve learning goals requires a referral for assistance postdischarge.

Interventions

1. Teach the client basic stoma pouching principles:
   a. Keeping the peristomal skin clean and dry

   b. Using a well-fitting appliance

   c. Changing the pouch when the least amount of drainage is anticipated (usually on arising)
   d. Emptying the pouch when it is one-third to one-half full and changing routinely before a leak occurs
   e. Changing the pouch if burning or itching occurs under the appliance

   f. Observing the condition of the stoma and peristomal skin during pouch changes
2. Teach the procedure for preparing a stoma pouch:
   a. Select the appropriate stoma pouching system.
   b. Measure the stoma carefully.
   c. Use the appliance manufacturer's stoma measuring card, if possible. If the card does not accommodate stoma size or shape, teach the client to make a customized stoma pattern. Place clear plastic wrap from the skin barrier wafer over the stoma, trace the stoma with a marking pen, and cut a hole in the plastic to accommodate the stoma.
   d. Cut an opening in the center of the skin barrier slightly larger than the stoma (approximately ⅛ inch).
   e. Secure an appropriate odorproof pouch onto the skin barrier wafer (if using a two-piece appliance system).
3. Teach the procedure for changing a disposable stoma pouch:

   a. Remove the old pouch by gently pushing the skin away from the paper tape and skin barrier wafer.

Rationale

1. Proper pouching techniques can prevent leakage and skin problems.
   a. This ensures that the appliance adheres to the skin.
   b. Proper fit protects the surrounding skin surface from contact with drainage.
   c. This prevents copious drainage from interfering with pouch changes.

   d. A pouch filled more than halfway exerts increased pressure on the seal, increasing the risk of leakage.
   e. Burning or itching may indicate that ostomy effluent has undermined the skin barrier; prompt intervention is necessary to prevent skin breakdown.
   f. Regular observation enables early detection of skin problems.
2. Preparing a new pouch beforehand ensures that it is ready to apply as soon as the used pouch is removed, helping minimize drainage on the skin surface.

3. Correct pouch removal and attachment techniques minimize irritation and injury of peristomal skin and ensure a tight, reliable seal between the pouch and skin.

Interventions

    b. Fold the old pouch over on itself and discard in a plastic bag.

    c. Cleanse the peristomal skin with a wash cloth and warm tap water.

    d. Blot or pat skin dry.

    e. Apply the new pouch to the abdomen, carefully centering the hole in the skin barrier wafer over the stoma. Press on the wafer for a few minutes.

    f. Secure the pouch by "picture framing" the wafer with four strips of hypoallergenic paper tape (if the wafer does not already have tape attached).

4. Teach the procedure for emptying a stoma pouch:

    a. Put some toilet paper in the toilet bowl and sit on the toilet seat.

    b. Remove the clamp from the tail of the pouch, and carefully empty pouch contents into the toilet.

    c. Clean the inside and outside of the pouch tail with toilet paper and squeeze ostomy appliance deodorant into the end of the pouch.

5. Teach strategies for prevention and management of potential peristomal skin problems:

    a. Shave the peristomal skin with an electric razor rather than a blade; avoid using shaving cream, soap, and detergents except when showering.

    b. Evaluate all skin products for possible allergic reaction; patch-test all suspect products elsewhere on the abdomen.

    c. Do not change brands of skin barriers and adhesives casually; assess for allergic reaction before using a new brand.

    d. Avoid irritation from contact with ostomy effluent.

    e. Avoid prolonged skin pressure, especially if fair-skinned or having thin, atrophic skin due to long-term corticosteroid therapy.

    f. Use corticosteroid creams sparingly and briefly; they can cause dryness and irritation.

    g. If bacterial or fungal infection is suspected, use a specific antibacterial or antifungal cream or powder.

    h. Use a liquid film barrier; avoid tincture of benzoin compound, which can dry skin.

    i. Avoid aluminum paste and greasy ointments, which can mask skin problems and also interfere with pouch adherence.

    j. Protect the skin with barriers.

    k. Expect the stoma to shrink slightly over time. This will necessitate remeasuring the stoma to ensure proper appliance fit.

6. Teach the procedure for perineal wound care:

    a. Take sitz baths or irrigate the area with warm water to cleanse the wound thoroughly.

Rationale

4. Correct techniques can reduce spillage, soiling, and odor. Placing toilet paper in the bowl prevents water from splashing as the pouch contents are emptied.

5. A client with a stoma is at increased risk for peristomal skin breakdown. Factors that influence skin integrity include the following: composition, quantity, and consistency of the ostomy effluent; allergies; mechanical trauma; the underlying disease and its treatment (including medications); surgical construction and location of the stoma; the quality of ostomy and periostomal skin care; availability of proper supplies; nutritional status; overall health status; hygiene; and activity level.

6. Some clients with an ileostomy have the rectum and anus removed. Removal of the rectum results in a large perineal wound that typically is left open to heal by secondary intention.

Interventions

    b. Wear a peripad to protect the wound and contain drainage until healing occurs.

    c. Watch for and report signs and symptoms of infection or abscess (e.g., pain, purulent drainage).

    d. Because the rectum is missing, thermometers, suppositories, and other devices cannot be inserted.

7. Address nutrition and diet management:

    a. Teach how the ostomy affects absorption and use of nutrients, and discuss dietary implications.

    b. Assess food tolerances by adding new foods one at a time and in small amounts.

    c. Teach the client to eat regularly and slowly, to chew food well, and to avoid high-fiber foods, which can promote stomal blockage.

    d. Discuss dietary modifications that can help decrease odor and flatus.

    e. List dietary modifications to prevent or manage diarrhea and constipation, as indicated.

    f. Instruct the client to monitor weight and report any loss or gain of more than 10 pounds.

    g. Explain the importance of adequate fluid intake (water and juices) to prevent or manage fluid and electrolyte problems related to altered elimination.

8. Explain the effects of certain medications on ostomy function:

    a. Antibiotics may induce diarrhea.

    b. Narcotics and aluminum- or calcium-containing antacids can promote constipation.

    c. Fecal odor may be controlled by internal or external deodorizers. Internal deodorizers may have a mild laxative effect.

    d. Suppositories cannot be used after the rectum and anus are removed.
Instruct the client to notify a physician or pharmacist if a drug problem is suspected.

9. Promote measures to help the client incorporate ostomy care into ADLs:

    a. Working/traveling: Keep extra supplies at work. When traveling, carry supplies rather than pack them in a suitcase and risk losing them; keep in mind that pectin-based wafers melt in high environmental temperatures. Take a list of ostomy supplies when traveling.

    b. Exercise: The only limits involve contact sports during which trauma to the stoma may occur. Normal exercise is beneficial and may help to stimulate bowel evacuation— and, in some cases, can eliminate the need for irrigation. Successful use of exercise to regulate the bowel depends on the presurgical bowel pattern and regularity of elimination. Other contributing factors include the consistency of the fecal contents, motivation, diet, ability to exercise, and practice.

Rationale

7. Proper nutritional intake and dietary management are important factors in ostomy management.

8. Counseling the client about the possible harmful effects of home remedies and indiscriminate self-medication may help prevent minor or serious problems.

9. Successful incorporation of ostomy management into ADLs allows the client to resume his pre-ileostomy life style and pursue goals and interests.

Interventions

    c. Wardrobe: Ostomy appliances are invisible under clothing. Any clothing worn preoperatively may be worn postoperatively. Dress comfortably.

    d. Bathing/showering/swimming: These activities may be done while wearing an ostomy appliance. "Picture-frame" the skin barrier with paper tape to seal the edges and keep the barrier edge from getting wet. Showering may be done without an appliance and, in fact, is recommended on days of appliance changes.

Rationale

▲ **Documentation**

Discharge summary record
    Client and family teaching
    Outcome achievement or
        status

▲ **Outcome Criteria**

The outcome criteria for this diagnosis represent those associated with discharge planning. Refer to the discharge criteria.

Potential Altered Health Maintenance related to insufficient knowledge of care of ileoanal reservoir

Focus Assessment Criteria	*Clinical Significance*
1. Perianal skin condition 2. Anal sphincter competence 3. Frequency and consistency of stools	1–3. Because stools are loose and frequent (initially 10 to 20/day, progressively decreasing to 3 to 4/day after the first postoperative year), good sphincter control is essential to bowel management.
4. Readiness and ability to learn and retain information	4. A client or family failing to achieve learning goals requires a referral for assistance post-discharge.

▲ **Documentation**

Discharge summary record
    Client teaching
    Outcome achievement or
        status

Interventions

1. Instruct the client to practice Kegel exercises regularly.
2. Teach the client how to intubate the anus and irrigate the ileoanal pouch.
3. Teach to protect perianal skin by using liquid skin sealant prophylactically and wearing mini-pads at night to absorb anal drainage.

Rationale

1. Regular performance of Kegel exercises can strengthen sphincter muscle tone.
2. Irrigation is needed to remove mucus and prevent clogging.
3. These measures can help protect against perianal skin denudation resulting from frequent stools.

▲ **Outcome Criteria**

The outcome criteria for this diagnosis represent those associated with discharge planning. Refer to the discharge criteria.

Potential Altered Health Maintenance related to insufficient knowledge of intermittent intubation of Kock continent ileostomy

Focus Assessment Criteria	*Clinical Significance*
1. Readiness and ability to learn and retain information	1. A client or family failing to achieve learning goals requires a referral for assistance post-discharge.

Interventions

1. Explain the reason for continuous drainage postoperatively.
2. If indicated, teach the client intermittent self-intubation to drain the pouch, covering such measures as the following:
    a. Gradually decreasing the number of intubations to 3 to 4 times/day
    b. Irrigating if stool is thick
    c. Using lubricant on a large-bore catheter
3. Encourage through chewing of food before swallowing, and caution against eating high-fiber foods.
4. Notify the physician immediately if unable to intubate the client.

Rationale

1. Continuous drainage is needed to decrease pressure on the suture line.
2. Proper intubation technique helps maximize pouch capacity, provides complete drainage, and prevents tissue trauma.

3. Bulk in diet increases irritation to the bowel and the risk of obstruction.

4. Inability to intubate puts the client at high risk for bowel obstruction.

▲ **Documentation**

Discharge summary record
    Client teaching
    Response to teaching
    Outcome achievement or
        status

References/Bibliography

Alterescu, K.B. (1987). Colostomy. *Nursing Clinics of North America, 22*(2), 281–289.

Broadwell, D.C. (1987). Peristomal skin integrity. *Nursing Clinics of North America, 22*(2), 321–332.

Broadwell, D.C., & Sorrells, S.L. (1983). *Summary of your ileostomy care.* Berkley Heights, NJ: C.R. Bard.

Carpenito, L.J. (1989). *Nursing diagnosis: Application to clinical practice* (3rd ed.). Philadelphia: J.B. Lippincott.

Church, J.M. (1986). The current status of the Kock continent ileostomy. *Ostomy/Wound Management, 10,* 32–35.

Coe, M., et al. (1988). Concerns of clients and spouses regarding ostomy surgery. *Journal of Enterostomal Therapy, 15*(6), 84–89.

Kenny, R.M. (1986). Conventional versus continent ileostomy. *World Council of Enterostomal Therapists Journal, 6*(4), 13.

Maklebust, J. (1985). United Ostomy Association visits and adjustment following ostomy surgery. *Journal of Enterostomal Therapy, 12*(3), 84–89.

McLead, R.D., & Fazio, V.W. (1984). The continent ileostomy: An acceptable alternative. *Journal of Enterostomal Therapy, 11*(4), 140–146.

Rideout, B.W. (1987). The patient with an ileostomy. *Nursing Clinics of North America, 22*(1), 253–262.

Rolstad, B.S. (1987). Innovative surgical procedures and stoma care in the future. *Nursing Clinics of North America, 22*(2), 341–356.

Schover, L.R. (1986). Sexual rehabilitation of the ostomy patient. In D.B. Smith & D.E. Johnson (Eds.). *Ostomy care and the cancer patient.* Orlando, FL: Grune and Stratton.

Shipes, E. (1987). Psychosocial issues: The person with an ostomy. *Nursing Clinics of North America, 22*(2), 291–302.

Thomas, D., et al. (1987). Management of temporary loop ileostomy following colectomy, mucosal protectomy, and ileal pouch–anal anastomosis. *Journal of Enterostomal Therapy, 14*(5), 194–196.

Laminectomy

In laminectomy, the surgeon excises the lamina to expose the neural components of the spinal canal, then resects diseased or damaged tissue. This procedure is commonly performed to treat herniation or rupture of a intervertebral disc by reducing compression of nerve roots.

Diagnostic Cluster

▲ Time Frame
Preoperative and postoperative periods

▲ Discharge Criteria
Before discharge, the client or family will:
1. Describe proper wound care at home
2. Verbalize necessary activity precautions
3. State signs and symptoms that must be reported to a health care professional

---

PREOPERATIVE PERIOD
Nursing Diagnoses

Potential for Injury related to lack of knowledge of postoperative position restrictions and log-rolling technique

POSTOPERATIVE PERIOD
Collaborative Problems

Potential Complications:
Neurosensory Impairments
Urinary Retention
Paralytic Ileus
Cerebrospinal Fistula

Nursing Diagnoses

Pain related to muscle spasms (back, thigh) secondary to nerve irritation during surgery, skeletal malalignment, and bladder distention
Potential Altered Health Maintenance related to insufficient knowledge of home care, activity restrictions, and exercise program

Related Care Plan

General Surgery Generic Care Plan

Preoperative: Nursing Diagnosis

▲ Outcome Criteria
The client will demonstrate correct positioning and log-rolling technique.

Potential for Injury related to lack of knowledge of postoperative position restrictions and log-rolling technique

Focus Assessment Criteria	*Clinical Significance*
1. Readiness and ability to learn and retain information	1. A client failing to achieve learning goals requires a referral for assistance postdischarge.

Interventions

1. Teach the client correct body alignment to maintain while lying in bed, sitting, and standing. Teach the correct log-rolling technique to use to get in and out of bed; show the client how to do the following:
   a. Roll to the edge of the bed, keeping the lower back flat and the spine straight

Rationale

1. Maintaining proper positioning and good posture and using the proper procedure for getting in and out of bed will minimize back strain, muscle spasms, and discomfort.

Interventions

▲ **Documentation**

Discharge summary record
  Client teaching
  Outcome achievement or
    status

   b. Raise the head and simultaneously swing
      both legs (bent at the knees) over the side of
      the bed
   c. Use the upper hand to support the stomach
      muscles, and the lower arm to push himself
      away from the mattress.

Rationale

Postoperative: Collaborative Problems

▲ **Nursing Goal**

The nurse will manage and minimize complications post-
laminectomy.

Potential Complication: Neurosensory Impairment
Potential Complication: Urinary Retention
Potential Complication: Paralytic Ileus
Potential Complication: Cerebrospinal Fistula

Interventions

1. Monitor symmetry of sensory and motor function in extremities:
   a. To touch, pin scratch
   b. Strength (Have the client push your hand
      away from the soles and then pull up
      against resistance.)
   Compare findings from side to side.
2. Monitor bladder function:
   a. Ability to void sufficient quantities and
      empty bladder completely
   b. Ability to sense sensation of bladder fullness
3. If possible, stand a male client 8 to 12 hours after surgery to void.

4. Monitor bowel function:
   a. Bowel sounds in all quadrants returning
      within 24 hours of surgery
   b. Flatus and defecation resuming by the sec-
      ond or third postoperative day
5. Monitor for signs and symptoms of cerebrospinal fistula:
   a. Clear or pink ring around bloody drainage
   b. Positive glucose test of drainage
   c. Headache

Rationale

1. Cord or nerve root edema, pressure on a nerve
   root from herniated disc fragments, or hematoma at the operative site can cause or exacerbate deficits in motor and sensory function
   postoperatively. Surgical manipulation can result in nerve damage causing paresthesias, paralysis, and possibly respiratory insufficiency.
2. Cord edema can interfere with autonomic innervation of the bladder, causing a temporary loss
   of bladder tone.

3. Edema at the operative site and general anesthesia enhance voiding problems, especially
   when the client lies flat. Standing takes advantage of gravity to promote urination.
4. Surgery on the lumbosacral spine decreases innervation of the bowels, reducing peristalsis
   and possibly leading to transient paralytic ileus

5. Incomplete closure of the dura causes cerebrospinal fluid (CSF) drainage. Glucose is present
   in CSF, but not in normal wound drainage.
   Changes in CSF volume cause headache.

▲ **Documentation**

Flow records
  Vital signs
  Intake and output
  Circulation (color, peripheral
    pulses)
  Neurosensory status (re-
    flexes, sensory and motor
    function)
  Bowel function (bowel
    sounds, defecation)
  Wound condition (color,
    drainage, swelling)
Progress notes
  Changes in status

Related Physician-Prescribed Interventions
Medications
  Corticosteroids
Intravenous Therapy
  Refer to the General Surgery care plan (Appendix II).
Laboratory Studies
  Refer to the General Surgery care plan (Appendix II).
Diagnostic Studies
  Computed tomography (CT) scan
  Spinal x-ray film
  Myelography
Therapies
  Refer to the General Surgery care plan (Appendix II).

Electromyelography
Magnetic resonance imaging (MRI)

Postoperative: Nursing Diagnoses

▲ Outcome Criteria

The client will report progressive pain reduction and relief after pain relief interventions.

Pain related to muscle spasms (back, thigh) secondary to nerve irritation during surgery, skeletal misalignment, and bladder distention

Focus Assessment Criteria	Clinical Significance
1. Pain at operative site 2. Muscle spasms radiating to thigh, lower leg, foot, or arm; or to hand, in cervical spinal laminectomy 3. Voiding patterns (times, amounts)	1–3. Nerve root irritation from surgery is the primary cause of postoperative pain. Pain management should focus on proper positioning and activity in conjunction with narcotic or antispasmodic agents. The nurse must differentiate pain due to bladder distention from operative site pain and muscle spasms.

Interventions

1. Explain to the client that muscle spasms and paresthesias commonly occur after laminectomy.

2. Teach the client to use his arms and legs to transfer weight properly when getting out of bed.

3. Encourage walking, standing, and sitting for short periods from the first postoperative day, or as soon as possible after surgery. Assess the client carefully the first few days after surgery to ensure proper use of body mechanics and to detect any gait or posture problems.

4. Teach the client the following precautions to maintain proper body alignment:
   a. Use the log-rolling technique with the help of two persons for the first 48 hours after surgery. (Refer to the nursing diagnosis Potential for Injury in this care plan for details.)
   b. Avoid stress or strain on the operative site.
   c. Use the side-lying position in bed, with the legs bent up evenly and the abdomen and back supported by pillows.
   d. Avoid the prone position; after the bulky dressing is removed, he may lie on his back with the legs evenly elevated and knees slightly higher than the sacrum, using a small pillow to elevate the head no higher than 30 degrees.
   e. Sit with the knees higher than the hips.
   f. When standing, regularly shift weightbearing from one foot to the other.

5. Refer to the General Surgery care plan in Appendix II, for general pain-relief techniques.

Rationale

1. Surgical trauma and edema cause pain and muscle spasms. Spasms may begin on the third or fourth postoperative day. Postoperative paresthesias in the affected leg and back may result from impaired neural function due to edema. As edema subsides, normal sensation returns.

2. Using the stronger muscles of the arms and legs can reduce strain on the back.

3. Activity goals depend on the client's pain level and functional ability. Gait or posture problems can contribute to pain on walking, standing, or sitting.

4. Proper body alignment avoids tension on the operative site and reduces spasms. Techniques are taught to keep the lower spine as flat as possible and prevent twisting, flexing, or hyperextending.

▲ Documentation

Medication administration record
  Type, dose, route, frequency
    of all medications
Progress notes
  Activity level
  Unsatisfactory pain relief

▲ **Outcome Criteria**

The outcome criteria for this diagnosis represent those associated with discharge planning. Refer to the discharge criteria.

Potential Altered Health Maintenance related to insufficient knowledge of home care, activity restrictions, and exercise program

Focus Assessment Criteria	Clinical Significance
1. Readiness and ability to learn and retain information	1. A client or family failing to achieve learning goals requires a referral for assistance post-discharge.

Interventions

1. Explain the rationale for activity restrictions and for gradual activity progression as tolerance increases.

2. Teach the client to avoid the following:
   a. Prolonged sitting
   b. Twisting the spine
   c. Bending at the waist
   d. Climbing stairs
   e. Automobile trips

3. Teach the proper use of a back brace, if indicated.

4. Explain the importance of following a regular exercise program after recovery.

5. Encourage the use of heat on the operative area, as indicated.

6. Teach the client precautions for after recovery, such as the following:
   a. Sleeping on a firm mattress
   b. Maintaining proper body mechanics
   c. Wearing only moderately high-heeled shoes
   d. Avoiding lifting heavy objects

7. As appropriate, explain the connection between obesity and lower back problems; encourage weight loss.

8. Teach the client and family to report the following:
   a. Change in mobility, sensation, color, or pain in extremities
   b. Increased pain at the operative site
   c. Persistent headaches
   d. Elevated temperature
   e. Change in bowel or bladder function

Rationale

1. Activity restrictions allow the spinal supporting structures time to heal. Complete healing of ligaments and muscles takes approximately 6 weeks.

2. These activities increase spinal flexion and create tension at the surgical site.

3. A brace may be indicated to stabilize the spine and reduce pain; instruction in proper use is necessary.

4. Regular, safe exercise increases spinal muscle strength and flexibility, helping protect against future injury.

5. Heat increases circulation to the operative site, promoting healing and removal of wound exudate.

6. Techniques that reduce stress and strain on the lumbosacral spine can decrease spasms and help prevent other disc herniations.

7. Excess weight, particularly in the abdomen, strains and stretches the muscles that support the spine, predisposing the client to spinal injury. Explaining these effects may encourage the client to lose weight.

8. Early detection and reporting enable prompt intervention to prevent or minimize serious complications, such as infection (marked by headache, fever, and increased pain) and cord compression (indicated by changes in bowel and bladder function, movement, and sensation).

▲ **Documentation**

Discharge summary record
  Client and family teaching
  Outcome achievement or
    status

References/Bibliography

See also Cranial Surgery, page 402.

Hickey, J. V. (1986). *The clinical practice of neurological and neurosurgical nursing* (2nd Ed.). Philadelphia: J. B. Lippincott.

Neatherlin, J.S., et al. (1988). Factors determining length of hospitalization for patients having laminectomy surgery. *Journal of Neuroscience Nursing, 20*(1), 39–41.

Laryngectomy

The surgical excision of the larynx and the removal of affected structures, laryngectomy is classified according to the degree of tissue removal as partial, hemi-vertical, supraglottic, or total. (The table below provides more information on these different types.) Laryngectomy is indicated for tumors of the vocal cords and surrounding area.

Diagnostic Cluster

▲ Time Frame
Preoperative and postoperative periods

▲ Discharge Criteria
Before discharge, the client or family will:

1. Describe and demonstrate proper wound care techniques
2. Discuss strategies for performing activities of daily living (ADLs)
3. State the signs and symptoms that must be reported to a health care professional
4. Verbalize an intent to share feelings and concerns with significant others
5. Identify appropriate community resources and self-help groups

---

PREOPERATIVE PERIOD
Nursing Diagnoses

Anxiety related to lack of knowledge of impending surgical experience and implications of condition on life style

POSTOPERATIVE PERIOD
Refer to Tracheostomy care plan.
Refer to Radical Neck Dissection care plan.

Related Care Plan

Surgery Generic care plan

Procedure	Structures Removed	Structures Remaining	Effects on Function
Total laryngectomy	Hyoid bone Entire larynx Epiglottis, false, true cords Cricoid cartilage Two/three tracheal rings	Tongue Pharyngeal walls Lower trachea	Loss of voice Normal swallowing
Supraglottic/horizontal laryngectomy	Hyoid bone Epiglottis False cords	True cords Cricoid cartilage Trachea	Normal voice Normal airway Increased risk of aspiration
Hemi-vertical laryngectomy	One true/false cord Arytenoid One-half thyroid Cartilage	Epiglottis One true/false cord Cricoid	Hoarse but serviceable voice Normal airway Swallowing within normal limits
Partial laryngectomy	One vocal cord	All other structures	Hoarse but serviceable voice Normal airway Normal swallowing

Preoperative: Nursing Diagnosis

▲ **Outcome Criteria**

The client will:

1. State the reason for surgery and its expected outcome
2. Describe expected limitations on speech and swallowing
3. Describe immediate postoperative care and self-care measures

Anxiety related to lack of knowledge of impending surgical experience and implications of condition on life style

Focus Assessment Criteria	*Clinical Significance*
1. Understanding of condition, surgery, expected outcome, expected postoperative limitations, and care measures	1,2. Disfigurement from a permanent stoma with a tracheostomy or laryngectomy tube can pose a significant threat to a client's body image and self-esteem. Assessing the client's level of understanding allows the nurse to identify learning needs and plan effective teaching strategies. A client who does not achieve learning goals requires a referral for assistance postdischarge.
2. Readiness and ability to learn and retain information	

Interventions

1. Explain commonly used terms and procedures. Provide written information to reinforce teaching, and introduce actual equipment. Cover these topics:
   a. Laryngectomy tube
   b. Stoma
   c. Suctioning and suction catheter
   d. Mucus
   e. Humidity collar
   f. Pharynx
   g. Laryngectomy ties
   h. Trachea

2. Explain the postoperative changes in appearance and body function that the client can expect—e.g., loss of ability to blow nose, suck, gargle, and whistle, and decreased smell and taste sensation. If possible, arrange for a visit by a person who has already undergone laryngectomy.

3. Instruct the client in alternative communication techniques, e.g., flip chart, picture board, electrolarynx, and esophageal speech. Request return demonstration to ensure the client's mastery of the chosen technique(s).

Rationale

1. Effective client teaching enhances positive coping mechanisms, provides an opportunity for the client to express concerns and ask questions, and enables the nurse to correct misconceptions—all of which can help decrease preoperative anxiety.

2. This information and contact with a person who has successfully adapted to the postoperative changes in appearance and functioning may help reduce anxiety associated with fear of the unknown.

3. Learning alternative communication techniques to speech lets the client maintain the ability to communicate. This can help decrease a sense of alienation and isolation, enhance the client's sense of control over the situation, and decrease anxiety. Evaluating the client's performance of these techniques can also alert the nurse to possible cognitive or motor deficits (e.g., vision or hearing problems, facial nerve impairment, altered mentation) that may require further evaluation by a specialist.

▲ **Documentation**

Progress notes
   Current knowledge level
   Ability to use alternative communication technique
   Response to laryngectomee visit
Discharge summary record
   Client teaching

References/Bibliography

See also Radical Neck Dissection, page 472.

Hancher, K. (1988). Social adjustment of laryngectomy patients. *Journal of the Society of Otorhinolaryngol-Head-Neck Nurses, 6*(2), 4–8.

Mastectomy

Surgical removal of the breast, portions of the breast, or adjacent structures, mastectomy is indicated for treatment of breast cancer. It is classified according to the extent of tissue removal as *radical* (removal of the breast, lymph nodes, and major and minor pectoral muscles), *total* (breast and axillary nodes), *simple* (breast only), *lumpectomy* (cancerous tissue and a small amount of adjacent healthy tissue), and *subcutaneous* (subcutaneous breast tissue with skin and areola left intact). Following mastectomy, adjunctive chemotherapy, radiation therapy, or hormonal therapy is recommended for some clients.

Diagnostic Cluster

▲ Time Frame
Preoperative and postoperative periods

▲ Discharge Criteria
Before discharge, the client or family will:

1. Demonstrate hand and arm exercises
2. Describe hand and arm precautions
3. Demonstrate breast self-examination
4. State care measures to perform at home
5. Discuss strategies for performing activities of daily living (ADLs)
6. State necessary precautions
7. State the signs and symptoms that must be reported to a health care professional
8. Verbalize an intent to share feelings and concerns with significant others
9. Identify available community resources and self-help groups

PREOPERATIVE PERIOD
Nursing Diagnoses

Anxiety/Fear related to perceived effects of mastectomy (immediate: pain, edema; postdischarge: relationships, work) and prognosis

POSTOPERATIVE PERIOD
Collaborative Problems

Potential Complication:
Neurovascular Compromise

Nursing Diagnoses

Potential Impaired Physical Mobility (shoulder, arm) related to lymphedema, nerve/muscle damage, and pain
Potential for Injury related to compromised lymph, motor, and sensory function in affected arm
Potential Altered Health Maintenance related to insufficient knowledge of wound care, exercises, breast prosthesis, signs and symptoms of complications, hand/arm precautions, community resources, and follow-up care
Potential Self-Concept Disturbance related to perceived negative effects of loss on functioning
Grieving related to loss of breast and change in appearance

Related Care Plan

General Surgery Generic Care Plan

Refer to:

Radical Vulvectomy

Cancer (Initial Diagnosis)

Preoperative: Nursing Diagnosis

▲ Outcome Criteria
The client will:

1. Share concerns regarding the surgery and its outcome
2. Describe actions that can help reduce postoperative edema and immobility

Anxiety/Fear related to perceived immediate and long-term effects of mastectomy and prognosis

Focus Assessment Criteria	*Clinical Significance*
1. Nature of concerns and fears	1. Mastectomy poses a threat to body image; breast cancer may pose a threat to life. The client's emotional reaction to surgery depends in large part on her perception of its effects (e.g., physical, psychological, social, spiritual, financial) on her life.

Focus Assessment Criteria	Clinical Significance
2. Understanding of mastectomy, including past experience and information from others who have undergone the surgery	2. Assessment of the client's knowledge level identifies learning needs and guides the nurse in planning effective teaching strategies.
3. Support systems, coping patterns	3. Assessment of available support and coping skills identifies needs in these areas.
4. Anxiety level (mild, moderate, severe, panic)	4. High anxiety impairs learning.

Interventions

1. Encourage the client to verbalize her concerns and fears. Stay with the client and family as much as possible, and convey empathy and concern.

2. Initiate dialogue regarding concerns about the cancer diagnosis.

3. If agreeable, arrange for a visitor from Reach for Recovery.

4. Explain expected events, such as the following:
   a. Preoperative and postoperative routines
   b. Development of lymphedema and sensory changes after surgery
   c. Postoperative positioning and exercises
   d. Presence of drainage tubes
5. Explain that a temporary soft prosthesis can be worn immediately.

6. Allow the client's partner to share his concerns alone.
7. Validate to the client and partner that their concerns and fears are normal and expected.

Rationale

1. Encouraging the client to share concerns allows the nurse to identify and correct any misconceptions, which can reduce fear. Many women have heard "horror stories" about mastectomy. Many of these stories involve older types of surgery that often did involve widespread tissue destruction. By comparison, today's procedures are much less destructive.
2. Open, honest dialogue can help instill realistic hope. Avoiding the topic only promotes feelings of despair and isolation.
3. A person who has undergone successful mastectomy can give the client insights into the emotional aspects of the procedure and offer hope for a successful outcome.
4. Explaining what to expect can help reduce fear of the unknown and anxiety over unexpected events.

5. A temporary prosthesis enhances appearance and reduces the sense of imbalance that can result from breast removal. Understanding that a prosthesis can be worn immediately after recovery can help allay anxiety associated with altered body image.
6. Male significant others may need special encouragement to share their fears.
7. Validation can help reduce fear associated with such feelings as rejection, repulsion, abandonment, and loss of attractiveness.

▲ **Documentation**

Progress notes
　Dialogues
　Interventions
　Response to interventions

Postoperative: Collaborative Problems

▲ **Nursing Goal**

The nurse will manage and minimize neurovascular complications.

Potential Complication: Neurovascular compromise

Interventions

1. Monitor for signs and symptoms of neurovascular compromise, comparing findings between limbs:
   a. Diminished or absent radial pulse
   b. Numbness or tingling in hand
   c. Capillary refill time > 3 seconds
   d. Pallor, blanching, or cyanosis, and coolness of extremity
   e. Inability to flex or extend fingers

Rationale

1. Removal of lymph nodes causes edema, leading to entrapment of peripheral nerves at the cervical outlet or wrist, marked by decreased sensation, movement, and circulation.

▲ **Documentation**

Flow records
　Radial pulse assessment
　Affected arm: color, sensation, capillary refill time, movement

Related Physician-Prescribed Interventions

Medications

Refer to the Cancer (Initial Diagnosis) care plan, page 322.

Refer to the General Surgery care plan, Appendix II.

Intravenous Therapy

None indicated

Laboratory Studies

None indicated

Diagnostic Studies

Mammography
Ultrasonography
Xeroradiography

Thermography
Computed tomography (CT) scan
Breast biopsy

Therapies

Back brace
Temporary soft prosthesis

Physical therapy

Postoperative: Nursing Diagnoses

▲ **Outcome Criteria**

The client will demonstrate progressive mobility to the extent possible within limitations imposed by the surgery.

Potential Impaired Physical Mobility (arm, shoulder) related to lymphedema, nerve or muscle damage, and pain

Focus Assessment Criteria	Clinical Significance
1. Motion in the affected arm and shoulder	1. Assessment is needed to determine the baseline and to gauge progress.
2. Level of pain and fatigue	2. Pain and fatigue can interfere with ability and motivation to participate in self-care.
3. Balance	3. Postoperative factors (e.g., large dressing, limited use of one arm) can impair balance and predispose to injury.

Interventions

1. Explain the need to increase mobility to the maximum extent tolerated, and specify the hazards of immobility.
2. Provide appropriate pain relief. (Refer to the General Surgery care plan in Appendix II, for specific interventions.)
3. Explain the reasons for poor balance; accompany the client while she walks.

4. Instruct the client to elevate the affected arm on a pillow when sitting or reclining.
5. Teach hand exercises.
6. Initiate passive range-of-motion (ROM) exercises on the affected arm, as prescribed.
7. Teach selected exercises, such as the following:
   a. Clasping hands behind the head and attempting to touch elbows in front
   b. Turning a rope tied to a doorknob
   c. Wall hand climbing (keeping palms flat with elbows slightly bent)

▲ **Documentation**

Progress notes
   Level of function
   Exercises (type, frequency)

8. As activities are increased, encourage the client to use the affected arm as much as possible.

Rationale

1. Explanations can help to elicit cooperation despite discomfort or fear of falling.

2. Pain reduces the ability and motivation to perform ROM and other exercises and to walk.

3. A large compression bandage and impaired arm movement can interfere with balance and increase the risk of falling.
4. Elevation facilitates lymphatic drainage and prevents pooling.
5–7. These exercises increase circulation and help maintain function.

8. Frequent arm movement prevents lymphedema and contractures.

Potential for Injury related to compromised lymph drainage, motor and sensory function in affected arm

Focus Assessment Criteria	Clinical Significance
1. Edema 2. Sensory and motor function in the affected arm 3. Pain	1–3. Extensive mastectomy involving surgery to soft tissue, muscles, and nerves can create slight to profound changes in the lymphatic system. The resultant edema causes tissue compression, decreasing circulation, and impairing sensorimotor function.

Interventions	Rationale

1. Monitor for signs and symptoms of sensorimotor impairment:
  a. Impaired joint movement
  b. Muscle weakness
  c. Numbness or tingling
	1. These signs can indicate entrapment of nerves at the cervical outlet or wrist from lymphedema or damage to thoracodorsal nerve.

2. Monitor regular measurements of arm circumference for changes.	2. Regular measurements can detect increasing lymphedema.
3. Consult with the physician for additional interventions, as needed, e.g., diuretics, elastic wraps, intermittent pneumatic compression.	3. If lymphedema increases, more aggressive therapy may be indicated.

4. Teach the client to avoid the following:
  a. Blood pressure measurements in the affected arm
  b. Constrictive jewelry and clothing
  c. Carrying a shoulder bag or heavy object with the affected arm
  d. Brassieres with thin shoulder straps. (Wear ones with wide straps or no straps instead.)
	4.
	
	  a,b. Constriction to the arm can exacerbate lymphedema.
	
	  c. Shoulder bags and heavy objects increase pressure at the shoulder joint.
	  d. Thin straps also produce constriction on the shoulder.

5. Teach precautions to prevent trauma to the affected arm and hand:
  a. Using long glove potholders
  b. Avoiding cuts and scratches
  c. Avoiding injections and venipunctures of any kind
  d. Using a thimble when sewing
  e. Avoiding strong detergents or other chemical agents
  f. Gardening in thorny plants
	5. Trauma to tissue with compromised lymphatic drainage exacerbates lymphedema.

6. Teach to cleanse wounds to the arm or hand promptly and to observe carefully for early signs of infection (e.g., redness, increased warmth). Stress the need to report any signs promptly.	6. Compromised lymph drainage compromises the body's defense against infection, necessitating increased emphasis on infection prevention.

Potential Altered Health Maintenance related to insufficient knowledge of wound care, exercises, breast prosthesis, signs and symptoms of complications, hand/arm precautions, community resources, and follow-up care

Focus Assessment Criteria	Clinical Significance
1. Readiness and ability to learn and retain information	1. A client or family failing to achieve learning goals requires a referral for assistance post-discharge.

Interventions

1. Teach breast self-examination techniques; instruct the client to examine both breasts periodically.
2. Teach wound care measures. (Refer to the General Surgery care plan in Appendix II for details.)
3. Teach to massage the healed incision gently with an emollient.
4. Provide information about breast prostheses. Emphasize the importance of a properly fitted prosthesis.

5. Provide written instructions for exercises to perform at home, and reemphasize their importance.
6. Instruct the client to report promptly any signs and symptoms of complications, including these:
   a. Increasing edema
   b. Numbness or tingling
   c. Impaired hand or arm movement
7. Discuss available community resources (e.g., Reach for Recovery, ENCORE). Encourage contact and initiate referrals if appropriate.

8. As appropriate, explore the client's feelings concerning radiation therapy or chemotherapy.

Rationale

1. Periodic, careful breast self-examination can detect problems early, improving the likelihood of successful treatment.
2. Proper wound care is essential to reduce the risk of infection.

3. Massage stimulates circulation and promotes skin elasticity.
4. A prosthesis of optimal contour, size, and weight provides normal appearance, promotes good posture, and helps prevent back and shoulder strain.
5. Written materials provide a reference that the client can consult after discharge, which can help increase compliance.
6. These signs and symptoms point to increasing lymphedema, which can lead to impaired sensorimotor function.

7. Community resources can provide unique, specific assistance with adjustment and adaptation after mastectomy (e.g., prostheses, clothing, exercise programs).
8. Both radiation therapy and chemotherapy carry side effects that necessitate client teaching to enhance self-care and coping.

▲ **Documentation**

Discharge summary record
Client and family teaching
Outcome achievement or status
Referrals, if indicated

References/Bibliography

Feather, B.L., & Wainstock, J.M. (1989). Perceptions of postmastectomy patients, Part 1: The relationships between social support and network providers. *Cancer Nursing, 12*(5), 293–300.

Feather, B.L., & Wainstock, J.M. (1989). Perceptions of postmastectomy patients, Part II: Self-esteem: Social support and attitudes towards mastectomy. *Cancer Nursing, 12*(5), 301–309.

Hailey, B.J. (1988). The mastectomy experience: Patients' perspectives. *Women's Health, 14*(1), 75–88.

Lierman, L.M. (1988). Discovery of breast changes: Women's responses and nursing implications. *Cancer Nursing, 11*(6), 352–361.

Northouse, L.L. (1989). The impact of breast cancer on patients and husbands. *Cancer Nursing, 12*(5), 276–284.

Williams, P.D., et al. (1988). Effects of preparation for mastectomy/hysterectomy on women's post-operative self-care behaviors. *International Journal of Nursing Studies, 25*(3), 191–206.

Ophthalmic Surgery

Ophthalmic surgery encompasses a variety of surgical procedures on the eye (e.g., vitrectomy, photocoagulation, cryosurgery, electrodiathermy, and scleral-buckle surgery). This care plan presents predictive nursing diagnoses and collaborative problems for clients undergoing ophthalmic surgery.

Diagnostic Cluster

▲ **Time Frame**

Preoperative and postoperative periods

PREOPERATIVE PERIOD
Nursing Diagnoses

Anxiety/Fear related to loss of vision, potential failure to regain vision, lack of time to adjust to need for surgery, and insufficient knowledge of preoperative and postoperative routines

POSTOPERATIVE PERIOD
Collaborative Problems

Potential Complications:
Wound Dehiscence/Evisceration
Increased Intraocular Pressure
Retinal Detachment
Dislocation of Lens Implant
Choroidal Hemorrhage
Endophthalmitis
Hyphema
Hypopyon
Blindness

Nursing Diagnoses

Potential for Infection related to increased susceptibility secondary to interruption of body surfaces
Altered Comfort related to surgical interruption of eye structure
Potential for Injury related to visual limitations, presence in unfamiliar environment and presence of eye patches postoperatively
Potential Feeding, Hygiene Self-Care Deficit related to activity restrictions, visual impairment, or presence of eye patches
Potential Sensory/Perceptual Alteration related to insufficient input secondary to impaired vision or presence of unilateral/bilateral eye patches
Potential Altered Health Maintenance related to insufficient knowledge of activities permitted and restricted, medications, complications, and follow-up care

▲ **Discharge Criteria**

Before discharge, the client and/or family will:

1. Demonstrate eye care
2. Describe activity restrictions
3. Relate signs and symptoms that must be reported to a health care professional

Preoperative: Nursing Diagnosis

▲ **Outcome Criteria**

The client will:

1. Express concerns regarding surgery and recovery
2. Before surgery, verbalize understanding of perioperative routines and care measures

Anxiety/Fear related to loss of vision, potential failure to regain vision, lack of time to adjust to need for surgery, and insufficient knowledge of preoperative and postoperative routines

Focus Assessment Criteria

1. Verbal and nonverbal indicators of anxiety and fear
2. Expressed fears and concerns regarding upcoming surgery
3. Understanding of the surgery and of any preoperative tests and procedures
4. Previous coping mechanisms
5. Available support systems

Clinical Significance

1–5. The retina converts visual images to electrical impulses for transmission to the brain. Any alteration in the medium through which light passes (vitreous) or in the retina itself may affect vision. Restoration of visual function depends on the successful outcome of surgery. Faced with this threat to vision, the client understandably may be extremely anxious about the surgery—particularly if vision in the nonoperative eye is impaired or if the surgery is to be performed on the "better" eye. Often contributing to anxiety and fear is the short amount of time the client may have to prepare for the surgery. Retinal repairs, excluding scleral buckling procedures, commonly are performed on an emergency basis, which does not give the client much time to mobilize support systems and coping mechanisms. Although additional time is available for a client scheduled to undergo vitrectomy, the condition necessitating the procedure may be bilateral in nature, contributing to increased anxiety and fear.

Interventions

1. Help the client express concerns and fears through active listening.
2. Promote an environment conducive to sharing concerns.
3. Validate the client's expressed concerns as a source of anxiety and fear. Explore other factors that may be contributing to fear, such as these:
   a. Perceived role changes
   b. Concern about meeting family, business, and other responsibilities
   c. Financial concerns
4. Assist the client to view his fears and concerns as a normal response.
5. Provide information about the scheduled surgery and about preoperative tests and procedures such as the following:
   a. Health history and physical examination
   b. Chest x-ray film
   c. Electrocardiogram (ECG)
   d. Dietary restriction
   e. Preoperative sedation
   f. Intravenous (IV) fluid infusion
   g. Instillation of dilating eyedrops
   If presurgical time is limited, prioritize the information presented.
6. Present information using various instructional methods, such as large-print pamphlets and audiovisual programs.

Rationale

1–4. The nurse must be sensitive to the client's level of anxiety as the therapeutic relationship is initiated. Encouraging the client to ventilate fears provides an opportunity to examine their source and correct any misconceptions that may be contributing to them. Validating that fear is a normal and expected response helps bolster the client's self-esteem and may enhance coping abilities.

5. Accurate information can help reduce fear of the unknown and enhance the client's sense of control over the situation. Prioritizing enables the nurse to present the most important information in a short amount of time.

6. Simultaneous stimulation of multiple senses augments the learning process. Written information also provides a resource for the client and support persons to consult at home after discharge.

Interventions

7. Describe postoperative activity restrictions, which may include avoiding the following:
   a. Bending at the waist
   b. Making sudden head movements
   c. Rubbing eyes
   d. Straining during bowel movements
8. Explain the importance of preventing vomiting, coughing, and sneezing after surgery; explain precautions such as the following:
   a. Avoiding use of narcotics
   b. Avoiding pepper and spices on food, and talcum powder on skin
   c. Requesting antiemetic agents if nauseated
   d. Avoiding persons with upper respiratory infections
   e. Avoiding known allergy-producing substances

Rationale

7,8. The client's understanding of postoperative restrictions and precautions can help him plan strategies for compliance, which enhances his sense of control and may reduce anxiety and fear.

▲ **Documentation**

Discharge summary record
  Client teaching
  Outcome achievement or status

Postoperative: Collaborative Problems

▲ **Nursing Goal**

The nurse will manage and minimize ophthalmic complications.

Potential Complication: Wound Dehiscence/Evisceration
Potential Complication: Increased Intraocular Pressure
Potential Complication: Retinal Detachment
Potential Complication: Dislocation of Lens Implant
Potential Complication: Choroidal Hemorrhage
Potential Complication: Endophthalmitis
Potential Complication: Hyphema
Potential Complication: Hypopyon
Potential Complication: Blindness

Interventions

1. Monitor the surgical site for bleeding, dehiscence, and evisceration.

2. Monitor for severe, unrelieved eye pain.

3. Reinforce compliance with precautions and restrictions as explained preoperatively.
4. Provide an entiemetic if nausea develops.

5. Monitor visual acuity.

Rationale

1. Ocular tissue is very vulnerable to these problems because of its high vascularity and fragility of vessels.
2. Severe pain may indicate increased intraocular pressure.
3. Compliance is necessary to prevent stress and pressure on the suture site.
4. Vomiting increases intraocular pressure and must be avoided.
5. Factors that can alter vision include blood in the vitreous or from the incision, infection, dislocation of the lens implant redetachment of the retina, and increased intraocular pressure.

▲ **Documentation**

Flow Records
  Vital signs
  Eye assessment (edema, drainage, suture line, pupils)

Related Physician-Prescribed Interventions

Medications
  Antiemetics
  Cycloplegics
  Analgesics
  Antibiotics (topical)

Intravenous Therapy
  Refer to the General Surgery care plan, Appendix II.

Laboratory Studies
  Refer to the General Surgery care plan, Appendix II.

Diagnostic Studies
  Snellen's eye chart
  Visual field testing
  Ophthalmoscopic examination
  Gonioscopy
  Tonography

Therapies
  Eye care

Postoperative: Nursing Diagnoses

▲ Outcome Criteria

The client will exhibit healing with no evidence of infection.

Potential for Infection related to increased susceptibility secondary to interruption of body surfaces

Focus Assessment Criteria	Clinical Significance
1. Eye (edema, drainage) 2. Suture line	1,2. Frequent assessment enables early detection of problems and prompt treatment to prevent serious complications.

Interventions

1. Promote wound healing:
   a. Encourage a well-balanced diet and adequate fluid intake.
   b. Instruct the client to keep a patch over the eye until the second postoperative day.
2. Use aseptic technique to instill eye drops:
   a. Wash hands before beginning.
   b. Hold the dropper away from the eye slightly.
   c. When instilling, avoid contact between the eye, the drop, and the dropper.
   Teach the technique to the client and family members.
3. Assess for signs and symptoms of infection:
   a. Reddened, edematous eyelids
   b. Conjunctival injection (prominent blood vessels)
   c. Drainage on eyelids and lashes
   d. Purulent material in anterior chamber (between the cornea and iris)
   e. Elevated temperature
   f. Abnormal laboratory values, e.g., elevated WBC count, abnormal culture and sensitivity results
4. Take steps to prevent strain on the suture line; e.g., have the client wear dark glasses and an eye patch in the daytime, and an eye shield at night.
5. Notify the physician of any suspicious-looking drainage.

Rationale

1. Optimal nutrition and hydration improve overall good health, which promotes healing of any surgical wound. Wearing an eye patch promotes healing by decreasing the irritative force of the eyelid against the suture line.
2. Aseptic technique minimizes introduction of microorganisms and reduces the risk of infection.

3. Early detection of infection enables prompt treatment to minimize its seriousness.

4. Strain on the suture line can lead to interruption, creating an entrance point for microorganisms.

5. Abnormal drainage requires medical evaluation and possible initiation of pharmacological treatment.

▲ Documentation

Flow records
  Vital signs
  Condition of eye
  Condition of suture line

▲ Outcome Criteria

The client will report progressive decline in pain and relief following specific interventions.

Altered Comfort related to surgical interruption of eye structure

Focus Assessment Criteria	Clinical Significance
1. Location of pain 2. Severity of pain 3. Nonverbal indicators of pain, e.g., grimacing, covering eye with hand, restlessness 4. Associated symptoms, e.g., vital sign changes, nausea, changes in visual acuity	1–4. The degree of pain depends in part on the extent of tissue manipulation during surgery. During retinal surgery, ocular tissues are mobilized, incised, and retracted to various degrees, depending on the location and extent of surgery. Scleral buckling requires greater manipulation than a vitrectomy and thus typically causes more pain. However, each client has his or her own individual pain perception and reacts differently to surgery. The nurse must evaluate all factors contributing to the client's pain experience to plan effective interventions.

Interventions

1. Explain the nature of the pain and when it should resolve, if known.
2. Have the client evaluate his pain on a scale of 1 to 10 (1 = no pain; 10 = the most severe pain), and rate it both before and after initiation of pain relief measures.
3. Consult with the client to determine the most effective methods of alleviating pain.
4. Encourage nonpharmacological pain relief measures such as the following:
   a. Maintaining proper positioning, per physician's order
   b. Using relaxation techniques
   c. Using distraction, e.g., music (TV may not be permitted.)
   d. Maintaining a calm, quiet environment
   e. Providing optimum comfort
5. Administer prescribed pain relief medications as needed. Notify the physician if pain is not relieved within 30 minutes of administration.

Rationale

1. This information may help reduce the client's anxiety level, which can reduce pain.
2. A rating scale provides an objective means of evaluating the subjective experience of pain.

3. The client has the best insight into his pain and the effectiveness of pain relief measures.
4. Effective nonpharmacological pain relief measures can help reduce the need for narcotics and increase the client's sense of control over the situation.

5. Increasing pain may indicate increasing intraocular pressure.

▲ *Documentation*

Medication administration record
  Type, dose, route of all medications
Progress notes
  Description of pain
  Unsatisfactory relief

▲ *Outcome Criteria*

The client will not experience injury or tissue trauma while hospitalized.

Potential for Injury related to visual limitations, presence in unfamiliar environment, and presence of eye patch(es) postoperatively

Focus Assessment Criteria

1. Visual acuity in each eye; have the client describe ability (e.g., "I can see the chair and the table with my right eye, but only the chair with my left eye").
2. Potential environmental obstacles such as footstools and low furniture, IV poles, wastebaskets, and slippers.

Clinical Significance

1,2. A client who has undergone ophthalmic surgery may have experienced a sudden loss of vision and is at increased risk of injury. This client requires careful evaluation because of several factors:
   a. Lack of time to develop strategies for adapting self-care abilities to vision loss
   b. Potential for further vision loss from complications or injury. Assessment must include acuity of each eye; acuity of the unaffected eye indicates how the client views the environment, and acuity in the affected eye helps guide the nurse in planning interventions to ensure safety.

Interventions

1. Orient the client to the environment upon arrival.
2. Modify the environment to remove any potential hazards:
   a. Remove obstacles from walking pathways.
   b. Remove straws from trays.
   c. Make sure doors and drawers are kept either completely open or completely closed.
3. Elevate the bed's siderails. Place objects where the client can see and reach them without stretching too far.
4. Place ambulation aids where the client can see and reach them easily. Monitor the use of ambulation aids.

Rationale

1. The client's familiarity with the environment may help reduce accidents.
2. Lost or impaired vision or use of an eye patch also can interfere with depth perception. These measures can help minimize potential hazards and reduce the risk of injury resulting from impaired acuity and depth perception.
3,4. These measures can help reduce the risk of falls.

Interventions

5. Check the client every hour.

Rationale

5. Frequent contact allows the nurse to meet the client's needs, limiting his need for unsupervised ambulation and reducing the risk of injury.

▲ *Documentation*

Progress notes
    Visual acuity (preoperative and postoperative)
Discharge summary record
    Client teaching

6. Help the client and family evaluate the home environment for potential hazards:
   a. Throw rugs
   b. Exposed electrical cords
   c. Low furniture
   d. Pets
   e. Stairs

6. The need to maintain a safe environment continues after discharge.

▲ *Outcome Criteria*

The client will demonstrate self-care abilities appropriate for activity restrictions.

Potential Feeding, Hygiene Self-Care Deficit related to activity restrictions, visual impairment, or presence of eye patch(es)

Focus Assessment Criteria	*Clinical Significance*

1. Preadmission self-care ability
2. Factors limiting self-care ability:
   a. Immobility
   b. Unilateral or bilateral eye patch(es)
	1,2. Adequate vision is important to self-care ability. A client commonly experiences reduced self-care ability after ocular surgery.

Interventions

1. Investigate the client's emotional response to reduced self-care ability; provide emotional support.
2. Encourage participation in self-care to the limits imposed by vision deficit or the recovery process. Schedule activities to allow time for self-care, and identify strategies to maximize current abilities, such as maintaining a consistent environment and storing needed objects and utensils within easy reach.
3. Allow the client to control the environment as much as possible; assist only as requested.

4. Explain how long the reduced self-care abilities are expected to persist, if known.

Rationale

1. The change in self-care ability may provoke feelings of anxiety and frustration, which can further impair ability.
2. The client's participation in self-care promotes self-esteem and decreases feelings of dependency.

3. Providing opportunities for control can enhance the client's self-esteem and promote improved self-care.
4. This can help reduce fear of long-term or permanent dependence.

▲ *Documentation*

Flow records
    Level of participation

▲ *Outcome Criteria*

The client will have sensory stimulation needs met while hospitalized.

Potential Sensory/Perceptual Alteration related to insufficient input secondary to impaired vision or presence of unilateral or bilateral eye patch(es)

Focus Assessment Criteria	*Clinical Significance*
1. Presurgical activities and interests 2. Emotional response to sensory/perceptual loss	1,2. Most sensory input is through vision. Impaired vision can easily lead to insufficient sensory stimulation. Clients all have different sensory input needs; assessing an individual client's particular needs and desires allows the nurse to plan to ensure the maximum amount and appropriate types of sensory input.

Interventions

1. Institute measures to increase sensory stimulation:
   a. Scheduling regular discussion periods

Rationale

1. Promoting regular and varied sensory stimulation can help prevent alterations from prolonged sensory deprivation.

Interventions

    b. Encouraging frequent visits from others, optimally at regular intervals to avoid long periods between visitors

    c. Encouraging telephone conversations

    d. Reading to the client

    e. Playing a radio or television

2. Monitor for symptoms of sensory deprivation:
     a. Anxiety
     b. Withdrawal and isolation
     c. Disorientation
     d. Restlessness
     e. Flat affect

3. Consult with occupational or physical therapy, as necessary.

4. Explain available community resources that may be able to provide help postdischarge, e.g., Lion's Club, church groups.

Rationale

2. Detection of subtle behavioral changes can enable prompt intervention to prevent serious problems.

3. Additional sensory stimulation activities beyond the scope of nursing practice may be indicated.

4. Participation in activities outside the home should be encouraged to reduce isolation. Community service organizations may have established visiting programs or contribute monies toward sensory stimulation devices for persons in need.

▲ **Documentation**

Progress notes
    Activities performed
    Unusual symptoms

▲ **Outcome Criteria**

The outcome criteria for this diagnosis represent those associated with discharge planning. Refer to the discharge criteria.

Potential Altered Health Maintenance related to insufficient knowledge of activities permitted and restricted medications, complications, and follow-up care

Focus Assessment Criteria	*Clinical Significance*
1. Knowledge of the therapeutic regimen	1. Assessing the client's and family's knowledge level guides the nurse in planning teaching strategies.
2. Readiness and ability to learn and retain information	2. A client or family failing to achieve learning goals requires a referral for assistance postdischarge.
3. Support systems, home environment	3. A client's ability to comply with the therapeutic regimen may be influenced (either positively or negatively) by his home environment and available support systems.

Interventions

1. Reinforce activity restrictions specified by the physician, which may include avoiding the following:
     a. Lying on the operative side
     b. Bending over at the waist
     c. Shaving
     d. Activities associated with rapid eye movement, e.g., watching TV or sports, reading
     e. Showers
     f. Heavy lifting

2. Instruct in proper positioning:
     a. Postvitrectomy: Keep the head of the bed elevated at all times.
     b. Post–retinal reattachment: Requirements depend on the location of detachment and technique used for reattachment.

Rationale

1. Restrictions are needed to reduce eye movements and prevent increased intraocular pressure. Specific restrictions depend on various factors, including the nature and extent of surgery, the physician's preference, and the client's age and overall health status. The client's understanding of the reasons for these restrictions can encourage compliance with them.

2. Postvitrectomy, elevating the head of the bed helps prevent rebleeding into the vitreous and settling of blood out of the visual field. After retinal reattachment, positioning focuses on promoting retinal reattachment. For example, if air or gas was injected during surgery, the client is positioned to allow pressure from the air or gas bubble to tamponade the reattachment site.

Interventions	*Rationale*
3. Reinforce the importance of not rubbing or bumping the eye and of keeping the protective patch and shield in place throughout the first postoperative day.	3. Rubbing or bumping the eye may interrupt suture line integrity and provide an entry point for microorganisms. Keeping the eye covered reduces the risk of contamination by airborne organisms.

4. Explain the following information for each prescribed medication:
  a. Name, purpose, and action
  b. Dosage schedule (amount, times)
  c. Administration technique
  d. Special instructions or precautions
	4. Providing accurate information before discharge can promote compliance with the medication regimen and help prevent errors in administration.

5. Instruct the client and family to report the following signs and symptoms:
  a. Vision loss
  b. Eye pain
  c. Vision abnormalities, e.g., light flashes, spots
  d. Redness, increased drainage, elevated temperature
	5. Early reporting of these signs and symptoms enables prompt intervention to prevent or minimize infection, retinal detachment, or other complications.

6. Stress the importance of adequate follow-up care.	6. Follow-up allows evaluation of healing and enables early detection of complications.

7. Help the client and family identify potential problem areas after discharge.
  a. Home environment:
    • Floor plan
    • Stairs
    • Obstacles in walking paths, e.g., throw rugs, low furniture, pets, cords, and wires
  b. Cooking:
    • Kitchen layout
    • Food and equipment storage
    • Waste removal
    • Safety
  c. Shopping:
    • Ability to obtain food
    • Access to grocery store
    • Transportation
  d. Medications:
    • Ability to obtain prescribed medications
    • Administration
  e. Bathing and grooming:
    • Ability to perform self-care activities
    • Available assistance
  f. Safety:
    • Presence of telephone
    • Emergency plan in place
	7. This evaluation can promote problem-solving before discharge, to maximize the client's self-care ability, independence, and ability to comply with the therapeutic regimen.

8. Help the client and family adapt the home environment to the client's altered abilities. Strategies may include the following:
  a. Removing all obstacles to safe ambulation
  b. Keeping all necessary cooking and eating utensils within easy reach
  c. Making use of Meals-on-Wheels and other appropriate community services
  d. Buying groceries in small amounts
  e. Using public transportation when necessary
  f. Requesting assistance from support persons when necessary
	8. Enhancing the client's self-care ability promotes independence and self-esteem, and also improves his ability to comply with the therapeutic regimen.

▲ **Documentation**

Discharge summary record
  Client and family teaching
  Outcome achievement or
    status

References/Bibliography

Bovino, J., & Marcus, D. (1984). Physical activity after retinal detachment surgery. *American Journal of Ophthalmology, 98*(8), 171–179.

Boyd, M.H. (1981). Retinal detachment and vitrectomy: Nursing care. *Nursing Clinics of North America, 16,* 433–452.

Carpenito, L. (1989). *Nursing diagnosis: Application to clinical practice* (3rd ed.). Philadelphia: J.B. Lippincott.

Cavender, J. (1984). *The retina book.* Daly City, CA: Krames Communication.

Newell, F. (1982). *Ophthalmology: Principles and concepts.* St. Louis: C.V. Mosby.

Smith, J., & Nachazel, D. (1980). *Ophthalmic nursing.* Boston: Little, Brown.

Thompson, J., McFarland, G., Hirsch, J., Tucker, S., & Bauers, A. (1986). *Clinical nursing.* St Louis: C.V. Mosby.

Vaughn, D., & Asbury, T. (1983). *General ophthalmology.* Los Altos, CA: Lange Publishing.

Whitton, S., & Liebman, G. (1986). Managing complex retinal detachment using retinal tacks. *Ophthalmic Nursing Forum, 2*(3), 1–7.

Penetrating Keratoplasty (Corneal Transplant)

Involving the surgical transplant of corneal tissue from a cadaver donor, penetrating keratoplasty is indicated for clients with aphakic bullous keratopathy, keratoconus, corneal scars, Fuch's dystrophy, keratitis, or severe chemical burns.

Diagnostic Cluster

▲ **Time Frame**

Preoperative and postoperative periods

▲ **Discharge Criteria**

Before discharge, the client and/ or family will:

1. Demonstrate eye care
2. Describe activity restrictions
3. Relate signs and symptoms that must be reported to a health care professional

---

PREOPERATIVE PERIOD
Nursing Diagnoses

Fear related to surgical experience, loss of control, and the unpredictable outcome

POSTOPERATIVE PERIOD
Collaborative Problems

Potential Complications:
Endophthalmitis
Increased Intraocular Pressure
Epithelial Defects
Graft Failure

Nursing Diagnoses

Potential for Infection related to nonintact ocular defense mechanisms secondary to surgery or previous eye disorder
Altered Comfort related to surgical procedure
Potential Altered Health Maintenance related to insufficient knowledge of eye care, resumption of activities, medications or medication administration, signs and symptoms of complications, and long-term follow-up care

Related Care Plan

General Surgery Generic Care Plan (Appendix II)

Preoperative: Nursing Diagnoses

▲ **Outcome Criteria**

The client will communicate feelings regarding the upcoming surgery.

Fear related to the surgical experience, loss of control, and unpredictable outcome

Focus Assessment Criteria	*Clinical Significance*

1. Specific stressors, such as the following:
  a. Visual impairment of unoperated eye
  b. Past unsuccessful penetrating kerato-plasty or other ophthalmic surgeries or procedures
	1. Any potential change in vision provokes anxiety and fear. Past unsuccessful experiences heighten these feelings.

2. Nature of fears and concerns, such as these:
  a. Quality and source of donor tissue
  b. Potential for infectious organisms in do-nor tissue, e.g., hepatitis, human immu-nodeficiency virus (HIV)
  c. Long-term follow-up care
  d. Infection
	2. Current public awareness of acquired immu-nodeficiency syndrome (AIDS) has led to in-creased concern over the potential risk of transmission via donor corneal tissue. The client should be made aware of the fact that eye-banking organizations are continually improving quality control of donor selection

Focus Assessment Criteria

   e. Graft failure

   f. Poor vision even after successful surgery

3. Anxiety level: mild, moderate, severe, or panic

4. Understanding of the surgery, the reason for it, and its anticipated outcome. (Before hospitalization, the client's physician should have explained the procedure.)

Clinical Significance

and tissue storage. In addition, the client may have misconceptions about the rapid return of vision; unrealistic expectations can lead to disappointment and frustration at gradual progress.

3. High anxiety impairs learning ability and can increase the risks of surgery and anesthesia.

4. The physician is legally responsible for providing the patient with information concerning surgery; the nurse determines level of understanding and reinforces information as necessary.

Interventions

1. Reinforce the physician's explanations. Notify the physician if additional information is needed.

2. As necessary, review the anatomy and physiology of the eye and cornea and the nature of the existing eye disease.

3. Present information using various media, including written information, anatomical models, and audiovisual programs.

4. Explain procedures, their rationales, and their importance.

   a. Preoperative
- Laboratory studies: blood work, electrocardiogram (ECG)
- Nothing-by-mouth (NPO) status
- Ophthalmic medications
- Intravenous (IV) line

   b. Intraoperative
- Anesthesia
- Operating room (OR) environment, personnel, and equipment
- Surgical procedure
- Positioning

   c. Postoperative
- Sensations during recovery from sedation
- Length of stay on recovery room
- Recovery room environment
- Eye patch and shield
- Deep breathing exercises, avoidance of coughing and strenuous activity
- Frequent vital sign assessments
- IV fluid infusion until NPO status is lifted
- Availability of analgesia and antiemetics as needed
- Availability of call bell
- Changes in proprioception due to eye patch
- Importance of resuming self-care as soon as condition permits

Rationale

1–4. Understanding the underlying disease, reason for surgery, and expected preoperative, intraoperative, and postoperative events and sensations can help reduce fear of the unknown and enhance the sense of control. The client may need repeated explanations to ensure complete understanding. Teaching strategies that stimulate multiple senses facilitates learning.

▲ **Documentation**

Teaching record
   Client teaching
   Outcome achievement or
      status

Related Physician-Prescribed Interventions
Medications

Miotics (preoperatively)	Topical antivirals
Topical antibiotics	Corticosteroids

Related Physician-Prescribed Interventions (Continued)

Intravenous Therapy
Not indicated

Laboratory Studies
Not indicated

Diagnostic Studies
Snellen's eye chart   Visual fields
Tonography   Gonioscopy

Therapies
Eye patch or shield

Postoperative: Collaborative Problems

▲ **Nursing Goal**

The nurse will manage and minimize ophthalmic complications.

Potential Complication: **Increased Intraocular Pressure**
Potential Complication: **Epithelial Defects**
Potential Complication: **Graft Failure**
Potential Complication: **Endophthalmitis**

Interventions

1. Monitor for signs and symptoms of complications:
   a. Increased intraocular pressure
   b. Graft failure
   c. Endophthalmitis
   d. Changes in visual acuity

▲ **Documentation**

Flow records
    Vital signs
Progress notes
    Change in external appearance of operative eye
    Visual acuity
    Wound status
    Persistent eye pain or headache

2. Reinforce the need to wear eye protection (patch and shield) to protect the surgical site.

Rationale

1. Early detection of complications enables prompt intervention to prevent serious damage. Increased intraocular pressure may result from poor wound closure technique, inflammatory sequelae, or long-term corticosteroid therapy. Corneal allograft rejection is a complex immune response involving host sensitization followed by generation of a specific efferent immune response to antigens, localization of foreign cells, and subsequent destruction of the graft. Epithelial defects or cell loss may result from improper storage of the donor cornea before transplant or from intraoperative or postoperative trauma to the eye. Changes in visual acuity can indicate increased intraocular pressure or graft defect or rejection.
2. Reinforcement may help encourage compliance, which helps protect the eye from postoperative trauma.

Postoperative: Nursing Diagnoses

Potential for Infection related to nonintact ocular defense mechanisms secondary to surgery or previous eye disorder

Focus Assessment Criteria

1. Signs and symptoms of infection:
   a. Purulent discharge
   b. Increased conjunctival hyperemia
   c. Suppurative infiltrate in the host or donor corneal tissue
   d. Abrupt onset of pain in the operative eye
   e. Decreased visual acuity

▲ **Outcome Criteria**

The client will demonstrate optimal wound healing without incidence of postoperative infection.

Clinical Significance

1. The cornea acts as the eye's protective membrane; the corneal epithelium provides a barrier against microorganism entrance into the cornea. Trauma to the avascular epithelium not only promotes entry of microorganisms but also provides a favorable culture medium for a variety of microorganisms. Nonintact ocular defense mechanisms caused by eye disease increase the risk of infection.

Interventions

1. Use aseptic technique when cleansing eyelids and performing dressing changes. Teach the client this technique, and stress the importance of cleansing the eyelids only when necessary.
2. Teach the client and family members to watch continually for and promptly report signs and symptoms of infection:
   a. Eye pain
   b. Eye and periorbital redness and swelling
   c. Altered vision
   d. Increased tearing or drainage
3. Teach the client to avoid touching, rubbing, or scratching the operative eye.

Rationale

1. Aseptic technique and minimizing contact with the eye can reduce the risk of infection.

2. Until the epithelium is completely healed, the incision site provides a possible entry point for microorganisms. Corticosteroid therapy can prolong the healing process, increasing the length of time requiring careful surveillance. Early detection enables prompt intervention to prevent serious infection.
3. Eye tissue injury increases the risk of infection.

▲ **Documentation**

Progress notes
  Condition of wound
  Appearance of eye
  Complaints of pain

▲ **Outcome Criteria**

The client will:

1. Report relief from pain relief measures
2. Acknowledge the importance of reporting severe pain immediately

Altered Comfort related to surgical procedure

Focus Assessment Criteria

1. Source of pain:
   a. Localized to operative eye, foreign body sensation
   b. Radiating throughout the cranium accompanied by nausea and vomiting
2. Onset and duration of pain
3. Severity of pain, based on a scale of 0 to 10 (0 = no pain; 10 = most severe pain), rated as follows:
   a. At its best
   b. At its worst
   c. After pain relief interventions
4. Client's expectations of postoperative discomfort

Clinical Significance

1–4. Assessing the location and nature of pain helps identify its source and guides interventions. After penetrating keratoplasty, only mild pain is expected because of the minimal nerve disruption associated with the surgery. Foreign-body sensation could indicate complications such as suture disruption, microbial keratitis, infection, and wound dehiscence.

Interventions

1. Inform the client that mild discomfort is expected as the effects of local anesthetic wear off. Explain that analgesics are available for pain relief as needed, and instruct him to report pain or discomfort as soon as it occurs.

2. Notify the physician of client complaints of severe pain, pain accompanied by nausea and vomiting, or pain not relieved by analgesic administration.
3. Convey to the client your acceptance of his pain, acknowledge and listen attentively to his descriptions of the pain, and explain that you are assessing his pain because you want to understand it better (not to determine whether it really exists).
4. Explain the cause of the pain and how long it should last, if known. Provide accurate information about pain relief medications.

5. Provide nonpharmacological pain relief measures in conjunction with medications:
   a. Proper positioning

Rationale

1. Use of a long-acting retrobulbar anesthetic before surgery reduces the discomfort experienced during the first postoperative day. Explanations of what to expect and the availability of pain relief can help reduce anxiety related to fear of the unknown.
2. Prompt treatment is needed to prevent serious infections, increased intraocular pressure, or graft rejection.

3. A client who feels that he must convince caregivers of his pain experiences increased anxiety and frustration, which can contribute to pain.

4. A client who is prepared for pain through detailed explanations tends to experience less stress than a client receiving vague or no explanations.
5. Nonpharmacological pain relief measures can prevent painful stimuli from reaching higher brain centers by introducing another stimulus.

▲ **Documentation**

Medication administration record
  Type, route, and dosage of all medications
Progress notes
  Status of pain
  Effectiveness of pain relief measures

Interventions	Rationale
b. Relaxation exercises c. Distraction d. Quiet, calm, dimly lit environment	Relaxation reduces muscle tension and enhances the client's sense of control over the pain.

▲ **Outcome Criteria**

The outcome criteria for this diagnosis represent those associated with discharge planning. Refer to the discharge criteria.

Potential Altered Health Maintenance related to insufficient knowledge of eye care, resumption of activities, medications or medication administration, signs and symptoms of complications, and long-term follow-up care

Focus Assessment Criteria	Clinical Significance
1. Readiness and ability to learn and retain information 2. Understanding of home and long-term follow-up care 3. Available resources for assistance with home care and transportation to follow-up appointments	1. A client or family failing to achieve learning goals requires a referral for assistance postdischarge. 2,3. Assessing understanding of and ability to comply with the postdischarge regimen identifies needs and guides interventions.

Interventions	Rationale

1. Explain and demonstrate proper cleansing of the eyelids; emphasize the need for handwashing and aseptic technique.
2. Consult with the physician for care instructions for complicated wounds.
3. Reinforce postoperative activity instructions as indicated:
  a. Avoid strenuous activities such as contact sports, diving, racket sports, and skiing.
  b. Avoid dusty environments and swimming and other situations that increase the risk of eye contamination until the epithelium is completely healed.
  c. Activities such as hair washing, reading, and driving may be resumed as soon as comfort and vision permit.
  d. Avoid bending over at the waist for several months after surgery.
  e. Avoid touching, rubbing, or scratching the operative eye.
4. Review the purpose, action, dosage schedule, and possible side effects of prescribed medications, which may include corticosteroids or antibiotics.
5. Review proper administration of eye drops. For a client with poor vision, review ways of distinguishing eye drop containers, e.g., by size, shape, or color.
6. Explain the purpose and use of an eye patch and shield. Reinforce that he should wear them until the first postoperative follow-up visit, and that he should wear eye protection—e.g., glasses—for at least 2 weeks after surgery.
7. Teach to watch for and promptly report signs and symptoms of complications:
  a. Redness and swelling
  b. Pain
	1. Proper technique is needed to reduce the risk of infection.
	
	2. Complicated wounds may require irrigation and pharmacological intervention.
	3. Compliance with specific instructions is necessary to help prevent eye injury and contamination, prevent increased intraocular pressure, and ensure safety in the presence of impaired vision.
	
	4. Explanations can promote compliance with the medication regimen and help reduce the incidence of serious side effects.
	
	5. This teaching can help prevent injury by ensuring safe instillation of the correct medication at the scheduled dose and correct time.
	
	6. The operative eye must be protected from injury and environmental contaminants until healing is complete.
	
	7. Early detection enables prompt intervention to prevent serious complications.

Interventions

c. Altered vision

d. Purulent discharge

e. Severe or persistent headache

8. Validate understanding of the physician's explanations of long-term follow-up care. (Corrective refraction for astigmatism begins about 2 months after surgery. Prescription for glasses or contact lenses is provided as soon as the refraction seems to be stabilizing, which may take as long as 6 months.)

Rationale

8. Understanding may reduce anxiety and frustration and promote compliance.

▲ **Documentation**

Discharge summary record
  Client and family teaching
  Status at discharge (eye pain, wound integrity)
  Outcome achievement or status

References/Bibliography

American Academy of Ophthalmology. (1984). *Ophthalmology basic and clinical science course, Section 7: External disease and cornea.* San Francisco: American Academy of Ophthalmology.

Barraquer, J., & Rustlan, J. (1984). *Microsurgery of the cornea: An atlas and textbook.* Barcelona, Spain: Ediciones Scriba.

Brightbill, F.S. (Ed.) (1986). *Corneal surgery: Theory, technique, and tissue.* St. Louis: C.V. Mosby.

Buxton, J.N. (1982). Corneal surgery. In J.F. Collins (Ed.). *Handbook of clinical ophthalmology.* New York: Marson Publishing USA.

Engelstein, J.M. (1984). *Cataract surgery: Current options and problems.* Orlando, FL: Grune & Stratton.

Shapiro, M., Mandel, M., & Krachmer, J. (1986). Rejection. In F.S. Brightbill (Ed.). *Corneal surgery.* St Louis: C.V. Mosby.

Stark, W., Terry, A., & Maumenee, A.E. (1987). *Anterior segment surgery, IOLs, lasers, and refractive keratoplasty.* Baltimore: Williams and Wilkins.

Vaughan, D., & Asbury, T. (1980). *General ophthalmology* (9th ed.). Los Altos, CA: Lange Medical Publications.

Prostatectomy

Indicated for prostatic hyperplasia and cancer, prostatectomy involves surgical removal of all or part of the prostate gland. The surgical approach can be transurethral (through the urethra), or through a suprapubic (lower abdomen and bladder neck), perineal (anterior to rectum), or retropubic (lower abdomen, no bladder neck resection) incision.

Diagnostic Cluster

▲ **Time Frame**

Preoperative and postoperative periods

▲ **Discharge Criteria**

Before discharge, the client and/or family will:

1. Identify the need for increased oral fluid intake
2. Demonstrate care of the indwelling (Foley) catheter
3. Explain wound care at home
4. Verbalize necessary precautions for activity and urination
5. State the signs and symptoms that must be reported to a health care professional
6. Verbalize an intent to share feelings and concerns related to sexual function with significant others

PREOPERATIVE PERIOD
Nursing Diagnoses

Anxiety related to upcoming surgery and insufficient knowledge of routine and postoperative activities

POSTOPERATIVE PERIOD
Collaborative Problems

Potential Complications:
Hemorrhage
Clot Formation
Hyponatremia

Nursing Diagnoses

Altered Comfort related to bladder spasms, clot retention, or back and leg pain
Potential Altered Sexuality Patterns related to fear of impotence resulting from surgical intervention
Potential Altered Health Maintenance related to insufficient knowledge of fluid restrictions, catheter care, activity restrictions, urinary control, and signs and symptoms of complications

Related Care Plan

General Surgery Generic Care Plan

Preoperative: Nursing Diagnosis

▲ **Outcome Criteria**

The client will state the reasons for activity restrictions, indwelling catheterization, and increased fluid intake

Anxiety related to upcoming surgery and insufficient knowledge of routine preoperative and postoperative activities

Focus Assessment Criteria	*Clinical Significance*
1. Understanding of the surgical procedure and related preoperative and postoperative routines	1. Assessing the client's knowledge level guides the nurse in planning appropriate teaching strategies.
2. Readiness and ability to learn and retain information	2. Anxiety can interfere with learning.

Interventions

1. Reinforce the physician's explanation of the scheduled surgery, and answer any questions.
2. Explain expected postoperative procedures, such as the following:
   a. Indwelling (Foley) catheterization

Rationale

1–3. The client's understanding can help reduce anxiety related to fear of the unknown. Preoperative education has been shown to reduce anxiety and also help improve compliance.

Interventions

    b. Continuous and manual irrigation
    c. Intravenous (IV) infusions
  3. Explain expected activity restrictions:
    a. Bed rest for the first postoperative day
    b. Progressive ambulation beginning on the first postoperative day
    c. Avoiding activities that put strain on the bladder area
  4. Explain that transient hematuria is normal in the immediate postoperative period.

  5. Explain the need for increased fluid intake.
  6. Provide teaching aids (e.g., pamphlets, video tapes) as available.

Rationale

  4. Preparing the client for postoperative hematuria prevents him from being shocked at its appearance.
  5. Dilute urine deters clot formation.
  6. A multisensory approach to teaching enhances learning and retention.

▲ **Documentation**

Discharge summary record
  Client teaching
  Outcome achievement or status

Postoperative: Collaborative Problems

▲ **Nursing Goal**

The nurse will manage and minimize vascular and electrolyte complications.

Potential Complication: Hemorrhage
Potential Complication: Clot formation
Potential Complication: Hyponatremia

Interventions

  1. Monitor for signs and symptoms of hemorrhage:
    a. Abnormal urine characteristics, e.g., highly viscous, clots, bright red or burgundy color
    b. Increased pulse rate
    c. Urine output < 30 mL/hr
    d. Restlessness, agitation
    e. Cool, pale, or cyanotic skin

  2. Monitor dressings, catheters, and drains, which vary depending on the type of surgery performed:
    a. Transurethral approach (TURP)
      • Urethral catheter
    b. Suprapubic approach
      • Urethral catheter
      • Suprapubic tube
      • Abdominal drain
    c. Retropubic approach
      • Urethral catheter
      • Abdominal drain
    d. Perineal approach
      • Urethral catheter
      • Perineal drain
  3. Encourage the client to avoid straining for bowel elimination.

  4. Provide bladder irrigation, as ordered:
    a. Continuous (closed)
    b. Manual: Using a bulb syringe, irrigate the catheter with 30 to 60 mL normal saline solution every 3 to 4 hours, as needed.

Rationale

  1. The prostate gland is highly vascular, receiving its blood supply from the internal iliac artery. Elderly clients and those who have had prolonged urinary retention are vulnerable to rapid changes in bladder contents and fluid volume. During the first 24 hours after surgery, the urine should be pink or clear red, gradually becoming amber to pink-tinged by the fourth day. Bright red urine with clots indicates arterial bleeding. Burgundy-colored urine indicates venous bleeding, which usually resolves spontaneously. Clots are expected; their absence may point to blood dyscrasias.

  2. Heavy venous bleeding is expected the first 24 hours for all approaches except the perineal approach. Blood loss can occur from the catheter or incision. The TURP approach results in the heaviest bleeding.

  3. Straining to defecate may stress the suture line and cause bleeding, especially with retropubic or perineal incisions.
  4. Continuous bladder irrigation with normal saline dilutes the blood in the urine to prevent clot formation. Manual irrigation provides the negative pressure needed to remove obstructive clots or tissue particles.

Interventions

5. Ensure adequate fluid intake (oral, parenteral).

6. Monitor catheter traction: Note the time that traction was initiated and the time it is to be released.

7. Monitor for signs and symptoms of hyponatremia:
   a. Agitation
   b. Decreased pulse rate, increased blood pressure
   c. Nausea
   d. Confusion
   e. Decreased serum sodium level

Rationale

5. Optimal hydration dilutes urine to prevent clot formation.

6. Catheter traction causes the inflated balloon to wedge against the prostatic fossa, decreasing bleeding. Constant traction may cause ischemia and necrosis, however; generally, it should be released within 3 to 6 hours after surgery.

7. Hyponatremia can result from the use of glycine irrigant solution; this solution is hypotonic, allowing absorption through open veins in the prostate and leading to an increase in circulating volume and a decrease in sodium concentration. Failure to intervene promptly after detecting early signs of hyponatremia can result in rapid blood pressure drop after the initial rise, possibly leading to pulmonary edema, renal failure, seizures, coma, and eventual death.

▲ *Documentation*

Flow records
  Vital signs
  Intake and output
  Urine (color, viscosity, presence of clots)
  Continuous irrigations
  Manual irrigations (times, amounts)

Related Physician-Prescribed Interventions

Medications
  Antispasmodics

Intravenous Therapy
  Refer to the general surgery care plan, Appendix II.

Laboratory Studies
  Acid phosphates
  Alkaline phosphatase

Diagnostic Studies
  Cystoscopy
  Prostatic biopsy

Therapies
  Indwelling catheterization
  Catheter traction

  Bladder irrigation (manual, continuous)
  Sitz baths

Postoperative: Nursing Diagnoses

▲ *Outcome Criteria*

The client will report decreased pain after pain relief interventions.

Altered Comfort related to bladder spasms, clot retention, or back and leg pain

Focus Assessment Criteria

1. Location, characteristics, and duration of pain

Clinical Significance

1. Postoperative pain may result from surgical manipulation, obstruction, or bladder spasms.

Interventions

1. Monitor for intermittent suprapubic pain: bladder spasms, burning sensation at the tip of the penis.
2. Monitor for persistent suprapubic pain: bladder distention with sensations of fullness and tightness, inability to void.
3. Monitor for lower back and leg pain. Provide gentle massage to the back and heat to the legs, if necessary.
4. Anchor the catheter to the leg with tape or a catheter leg strap.

Rationale

1. Irritation from the indwelling catheter can cause bladder spasms and pain in the penis.

2. Catheter obstruction can cause urinary retention, leading to increased bladder spasms and increased risk of infection.

3. During surgery, the client lies in the lithotomy position, which can stretch and aggravate muscles that normally may be underused.

4. Pressure from a dangling catheter can damage the urinary sphincter, resulting in urinary incontinence after catheter removal. Catheter movement also increases the likelihood of bladder spasms.

▲ *Documentation*

Medication administration record
  Type, dose, route of all medications
Progress notes
  Complaints of pain (type, site, duration)
  Unsatisfactory pain relief

Interventions	Rationale
5. Encourage adequate oral fluid intake (at least 2000 mL/day, unless contraindicated).	5. Adequate hydration promotes dilute urine, which helps to flush out clots.
6. Manually irrigate the indwelling catheter only when indicated.	6. Each time the closed system is opened for manual irrigation, the risk of bacterial contamination increases.

Potential Altered Sexuality Patterns related to fear of impotence resulting from surgical intervention

▲ **Outcome Criteria**

The client will:

1. Discuss his and his partner's feelings and concerns regarding the effect of surgery on sexuality and sexual functioning
2. Verbalize an intention to discuss concerns with partner after discharge from hospital

Focus Assessment Criteria	Clinical Significance
1. Usual pattern of sexual functioning 2. Perceived effects of surgery on sexual functioning	1,2. Misconceptions related to inaccurate information can lead to undue anxiety and stress, which may result in decreased libido and psychological impotence.

Interventions	Rationale
1. Provide a private, confidential setting for discussion, and encourage the client to express his concerns. Introduce the subject in a nonthreatening manner, e.g., "Many men undergoing this procedure are concerned about how it may affect them sexually."	1. The nurse should not assume that the client understands the ramifications of surgery just because he asks no questions. Many clients are reluctant to discuss sexual concerns. Privacy may encourage sharing.

2. Provide information regarding sexual functioning postoperatively. Explain the following:
  a. The remaining prostate tissue can provide sufficient prostatic fluid for sperm passage and nourishment.
  b. The ability to maintain an erection is unchanged.
  c. Because the bladder neck is opened during surgery, semen will flow through the larger opening into the bladder, rather than through the urethra. As a result, retrograde ejaculation or "dry ejaculation" may occur, resulting in a milky appearance of the urine after intercourse.
  d. The ability to have children decreases as long as retrograde ejaculation is present; otherwise, the ability to reproduce remains unaltered.
	2. Specific, accurate information can help reduce the anxiety stemming from misinformation and lack of knowledge.

▲ **Documentation**

Progress notes
  Usual sexual patterns
  Expressed concerns
Discharge summary record
  Client teaching
  Response to teaching

Interventions	Rationale
3. Use familiar terms when possible, and explain unfamiliar terms.	3. Unfamiliar medical terminology may cause confusion and misunderstanding.
4. Encourage the client to ask the physician questions during hospitalization and follow-up visits.	4. An open dialogue with the physician is encouraged to clarify concerns and to provide access to specific explanations.

Potential Altered Health Maintenance related to insufficient knowledge of fluid restrictions, catheter care, activity restrictions, urinary control, and signs and symptoms of complications

Focus Assessment Criteria	Clinical Significance
1. Readiness and ability to learn and retain information	1. A client or family failing to achieve learning goals requires a referral for assistance postdischarge.

▲ **Outcome Criteria**

The outcome criteria for this diagnosis represent those associated with discharge planning. Refer to the discharge criteria.

Interventions

1. Reinforce the need for adequate oral fluid intake (at least 2000 mL/day, unless contraindicated).

2. Teach indwelling catheter care:
   a. Wash the urinary meatus with soap and water twice a day.
   b. Increase the frequency of cleansing if drainage is evident around the catheter insertion site.
3. Reinforce activity restrictions, which may include the following:
   a. Avoid straining with bowel movements; increase intake of dietary fiber or take stool softeners, if indicated.
   b. Avoid sitting for extended periods.
   c. Avoid heavy lifting and strenuous activity.
   d. Avoid sexual intercourse until the physician advises otherwise (usually within 6 to 8 weeks after surgery).
4. Explain expectations for urinary control once catheter is removed.
   a. Dribbling, frequency, and urgency may occur initially but gradually subside.
   b. Perineal exercises (tense buttocks, hold, and release) can help speed return of urinary control.
   c. Voiding as soon as the urge occurs can help prevent urinary retention.
   d. Avoiding caffeine and alcohol can help prevent problems.
   e. Transient hematuria is normal and should decrease with increased fluid intake.
5. Review signs and symptoms of complications:

   a. Inability to void for more than 6 hours

   b. Fever, chill, flank pain

   c. Increased hematuria

Rationale

1. Optimal hydration helps to reestablish bladder tone after catheter removal by stimulating voiding, diluting the urine, and decreasing susceptibility to urinary tract infections and clot formation.
2. The indwelling catheter provides a route for bacteria normally found on the urinary meatus to enter the urinary tract. These measures help reduce the risk of urinary tract infection.

3. These restrictions are necessary to reduce the risk of internal bleeding.

4. Difficulty in resuming normal voiding patterns may be related to bladder neck trauma, urinary tract infection, or catheter irritation. While the indwelling catheter is in place, constant urine drainage decreases muscle control and increases flaccidity. Caffeine acts as a mild diuretic, making it more difficult to control the urine. Alcohol may increase burning on urination.

5. Early detection enables prompt intervention to minimize the severity of complications.
   a. Inability to void may indicate clot or tissue blockage.
   b. These symptoms may indicate urinary tract infection.
   c. Increased hematuria points to bleeding or hemorrhage.

▲ **Documentation**

Discharge summary record
 Client teaching
 Outcome achievement or
  status
 Referrals, if indicated

References/Bibliography

Carpenito, L.J. (1989). *Nursing diagnosis: Application to clinical practice* (3rd ed.). Philadelphia: J.B. Lippincott.
Clark, N., & O'Connell, S. (1984). Prostatectomy: A guide to answering your patient's unspoken questions. *Nursing 84, 14*(4), 48–51.
Lawler, P. (1984). Benign prostatic hyperplasia. *AORN Journal, 40*(5), 745–748.
McConnell, E., & Zimmerman, M. (1983). *Care of patients with urologic problems.* Philadelphia: J.B. Lippincott.
Payton, T.R. (1988). Impotence: a nonprosthetic approach. *Nursing, 9*(1), 10–12.

Radical Neck Dissection

Surgical removal of tissue for treatment of head and neck cancer, radical neck dissection may be classical or modified. *Classical* radical neck dissection includes removal of the sternocleidomastoid muscle, the carotid artery or branch(es), lymphatics, and portions of the spinal accessory nerve supplying the trapezius muscle on the back. *Modified* neck dissection involves removal of the sternocleidomastoid muscle, omohyoid, lymphatics, and carotid artery and other vasculature if involved with the tumor. Because the spinal accessory nerve is left intact, scapular instability typically does not occur.

Diagnostic Cluster

▲ Time Frame
Preoperative and postoperative periods
Postintensive care

▲ Discharge Criteria
Before discharge, the client and/or family will:

1. Demonstrate wound care
2. Verbalize the need to continue exercises and follow-up care
3. Discuss management of activities of daily living (ADLs)
4. State signs and symptoms that must be reported to a health care professional
5. Verbalize an intent to share feelings and concerns related to appearance with significant others
6. Identify available community resources and self-help groups

---

POSTOPERATIVE PERIOD
Collaborative Problems

Potential Complications:
Flap Rejection
Carotid Artery Rupture
Hemorrhage

Nursing Diagnoses

Potential Impaired Physical Mobility: Shoulder, Head related to removal of muscles, nerves, flap graft reconstruction, trauma secondary to surgery
Potential Self-Concept Disturbance related to change in appearance
Potential Altered Health Maintenance related to insufficient knowledge of wound care, signs and symptoms of complications, exercises, and follow-up care

Related Care Plan

General Surgery Generic Care Plan (Appendix II)
Tracheostomy

Postoperative: Collaborative Problems

▲ Nursing Goal
The nurse will manage and minimize vascular and graft complications.

Potential Complication: Flap Rejection
Potential Complication: Carotid Artery Rupture
Potential Complication: Hemorrhage

Interventions

1. Monitor the pectoralis myocutaneous flap and surrounding tissue every 2 hours for the first 72 hours postsurgery and then every 4 hours thereafter for the following:
   a. Color: redness, pallor, blackness, cyanosis
   b. Vascularity; presence or absence of blanching
   c. Temperature changes, edema, turgor, drainage (type, amount, color)
2. Monitor vital signs.

Rationale

1. Abnormal findings may indicate impending flap rejection and call for immediate medical evaluation. Maximum redness should occur within the first 8 to 12 hours postsurgery and slowly decrease over the next 2 to 3 days. A healthy flap is pink and warm to the touch, has minimal edema, and recovers color slowly after exposure to blanching.

2. Vital signs are monitored to determine circulatory and respiratory status.

Interventions	*Rationale*
3. Monitor surgical drainage tubes for presence of air, milky or bloody drainage, or excessive or absent drainage.	3. Drains prevent development of dead space (air or fluid accumulation between the flap and underlying tissue) and help prevent approximation. Air in the drains indicates dead space. Milky drainage may point to a fistula within the thoracic duct, which can lead to severe fluid and electrolyte imbalance. Continuous bloody drainage may indicate small vessel rupture requiring surgical ligation. Over the first 24 hours postsurgery, drainage should be between 200 and 300 mL and should decline daily thereafter.

4. Maintain proper body positioning:
  a. Elevate the head of bed 30 to 45 degrees.
  b. Use pillows or sandbags to maintain proper alignment.
  c. Instruct the client not to lay on the operative side.
	4. With the client positioned so that the base of the flap is dependent to the tip of the flap, gravity promotes venous drainage through the flap.

5. Monitor for external pressure on the reconstruction/flap from any of these:
  a. Intravenous (IV) lines
  b. Feeding tubes
  c. Drainage tubes
  d. Tracheostomy or laryngectomy ties
	5. External pressure on the flap compromises circulation, promotes venous congestion, and can lead to increased permeability and occlusion of the lymphatics.

6. Monitor for signs of carotid artery rupture:
  a. Evidence of arterial erosion
  b. Change in color: redness, pallor, blackness
  c. Evidence of bleeding or bruising, pulsations, arterial exposure
  d. Temperature changes
	6. Exposure of the adventitial layer of the artery to the atmosphere causes drying and interrupts the blood supply to the flap. Once the artery is exposed to air, arterial destruction occurs in approximately 6 to 10 days. Factors contributing to arterial erosion include poor wound healing, exposure of the artery during surgery, tumor growth or invasion, radiation therapy, fistula formation, and infection.

7. Observe strict aseptic dressing technique using nonocclusive, fine-mesh, nonadherent gauze dressings with nonporous tape.	7. Dressings protect the wound from trauma and contamination, absorb drainage, and provide an aesthetic covering. Fine-mesh gauze inhibits interweaving of granulation tissue into dressing material, thus preventing mechanical débridement. Nonadherent dressings prevent growth of fungus and yeast infections, which require a dark, moist environment.
8. Change a saturated external dressing over draining wounds every 24 hours.	8. Dressings over wounds with extensive tissue loss should be changed frequently, because the lack of a skin barrier increases the risk of infection.

9. Promote efforts to clear secretions without coughing:
  a. Position to maximize respiratory excursion.
  b. Encourage deep breathing.
  c. Provide gentle nasotracheal, tracheal, or oropharyngeal suctioning only when absolutely needed.
	9. Coughing increases intrathoracic pressure, which stresses the wound. Because suctioning also increases intrathoracic pressure, suction only when the presence of secretions is identified on chest auscultation.

10. Monitor for nausea and vomiting.	10. Contraction of the diaphragm and abdominal muscles during vomiting raises intra-abdominal and intrathoracic pressure, which stresses the wound.
11. Monitor for constipation/abdominal distention, and take steps to prevent or treat constipation:	11.

Interventions	*Rationale*
a. Administer stool softener with wetting agent or glycerine suppository or gentle laxative.	**a.** Valsalva's maneuver, which accompanies straining on defecation related to constipation or fecal impaction, increases intrathoracic pressure, which stresses the wound.
b. Encourage adequate dietary fiber and fluid intake.	**b.** Adequate fiber and fluid intake helps decrease the potential for constipation.
12. Monitor for bleeding at the wound site.	12. A small amount of blood or pink-tinged drainage at the wound site or on the dressing may herald major rupture. Typically, a small prodromal bleed occurs 24 to 48 hours before a major rupture.
13. Monitor for complaints of sternal or high epigastric distress.	13. These complaints may indicate carotid rupture.
14. During episodes of bleeding, maintain a patent airway and prevent aspiration.	14. These measures aim to facilitate drainage and prevent aspiration.
a. For external hemorrhage:	
• Position the client in high Fowler's position with the head turned to the affected side. If unable to turn the head to the side, turn the entire body.	
• Provide continuous suctioning.	
b. For internal hemorrhage:	
• Pack the site with absorptive pressure dressing.	
• Position the client to facilitate drainage from the airway.	
• Provide continuous suctioning.	
• If a tracheostomy is in place, inflate the cuff.	

▲ **Documentation**

Flow records
    Vital signs
    Intake and output
    Wound site and drainage
      tube assessment

Related Physician-Prescribed Interventions

Medications
  Refer to the General Surgery care
  plan, Appendix II.

Intravenous Therapy
  Refer to the General Surgery care
  plan, Appendix II.

Laboratory Studies
  Arterial blood gas analysis

Diagnostic Studies
  Pulmonary function studies   Computed tomography (CT) scan
  Chest X-ray film

Therapies
  Oxygen with humidification   Irrigations
  Speech therapy   Nasogastric intubation
  Donor site care

Postoperative: Nursing Diagnoses

Potential Impaired Physical Mobility: Shoulder, Head, related to removal of muscles, nerves, flap graft reconstruction, trauma secondary to surgery

Focus Assessment Criteria (Preoperative and Postoperative)	*Clinical Significance*
1. Ability to perform activities of daily living (ADLs): feeding, bathing, etc; also, fine motor hand skill and vision	1–3. Assessing function identifies limitations and guides realistic goal-setting. Documentation of baseline functional levels

▲ Outcome Criteria

The client will:

1. State limitations on shoulder and head mobility and surgical factors that influence mobility postoperatively
2. Demonstrate optimal head and shoulder mobility postoperatively
3. Demonstrate measures to prevent complications of decreased mobility

Focus Assessment Criteria (Preoperative and Postoperative)

2. Head and neck movements (passive and active):
   a. Flexion
   b. Extension
   c. Rotation
   d. Lateral turning
3. Shoulder movements:
   a. Flexion
   b. Extension
   c. Internal rotation
   d. External rotation
   e. Scapular elevation
4. Factors that impair mobility:
   a. Arthritis
   b. Previous injuries
   c. Previous surgeries
   d. Vertebral deformities
   e. Peripheral vascular disease
   f. Pain

Clinical Significance

preoperatively enables comparison with postoperative findings to track developments.

4. Passive and active muscle movement is necessary to maintain skin integrity, range of motion, and adequate circulation, and to prevent contractures.

Interventions

1. Consult with the physician regarding an exercise program.

2. Teach the client to do the following:
   a. Maintain good posture at all times; pull the shoulders back frequently

   b. Avoid sitting for prolonged periods

   c. Avoid putting pressure on the arm of the operative side; use the other arm to lift, pull, and press
   d. When reclining, lie in the supine position (avoid lying on the operative side); place the involved arm to the side of the body with the elbow bent, and support it with pillows
   e. Avoid lifting or carrying objects weighing more than 3 lb with the involved arm
   f. Avoid injury to the involved side

3. Provide pain medication, as ordered, before the client begins prescribed exercises.

4. Consult with physical therapy as appropriate.

Rationale

1. The physician determines when the exercise program should be initiated and recommends a program based on the extent of tissue excision and reconstruction and progression of healing. Generally, exercise is initiated once drains are removed, the suture line is intact, and postoperative edema resolves.

2.
   a. Good posture is essential to prevent the chest muscles from tightening and pulling against the weaker muscles on the back of the shoulder, e.g., the rhomboids and levator.
   b. Prolonged sitting tires the muscles that provide good posture.
   c. These measures decrease stress on the remaining neuromuscular structures.

   d. Maintaining neutral alignment helps prevent contractures.

   e. This restriction can prevent strain and pain in the involved arm
   f. Minor injuries to the involved arm can compromise circulation and lymph drainage.
3. Pain can make the client reluctant to perform prescribed exercises. Adequate pain relief can increase compliance with the therapeutic regimen.
4. A physical therapist can suggest specific exercises to strengthen the remaining musculature and increase support and stability of the shoulder joint.

▲ Documentation

Progress notes
  Client teaching
  Therapeutic exercises performed

Potential Self-Concept Disturbance related to change in appearance

▲ *Outcome Criteria*

The client will:
1. Acknowledge changes in body structure and function
2. Communicate feelings about the surgery and its outcome
3. Participate in self-care

Focus Assessment Criteria

1. Exposure to others who have undergone radical neck dissection
2. Ability to visualize the operative area
3. Ability to express feelings about the surgery
4. Ability to share feelings and concerns with family and others
5. Participation in self-care

Clinical Significance

1–5. This assessment information helps the nurse evaluate current response and measure progress. Discussions can identify misinformation and fears. Participation in self-care indicates an attempt to cope positively with the changes.

Interventions

1. Contact the client frequently and treat him or her with warm, positive regard.

2. Incorporate emotional support into technical care teaching sessions, e.g., wound care, bathing.

3. Encourage the client to look at the operative site.

4. Encourage the client to verbalize feelings about surgery and perceptions of life style impacts. Validate his or her perceptions and reassure that the responses are normal and appropriate.

5. Encourage the client to participate in self-care. Give feedback and reinforce positive techniques and progress.

6. Have the client demonstrate proper wound care and teach the procedure to a support person.

7. Encourage support persons to become involved with wound care and to provide emotional support.

8. Encourage the client to identify and verbalize personal strengths and positive self-attributes, and to verbalize an intent to resume normal activities as soon as possible.

9. Provide information about measures to help improve appearance:
   a. Wearing clothes with high collars, e.g., turtleneck sweaters
   b. Wearing ascots or scarves
   c. Wearing clothing with shoulder padding
   d. Wearing accessories that draw attention away from the neck, e.g., hats

10. Identify clients at high risk for unsuccessful adjustment; look for these characteristics:
    a. Poor ego strength
    b. Ineffective problem-solving ability
    c. Difficulty learning new skills
    d. Lack of motivation
    e. External focus of control
    f. Poor health
    g. Unsatisfactory preoperative sex life

Rationale

1. Frequent contact by the caregiver indicates acceptance and may facilitate trust. The client may be hesitant to approach staff because of a negative self-concept.

2. This encourages resolution of emotional issues while teaching technical skills.

3. Accepting the reality of the body change is the first step in successful adjustment to it.

4. Sharing concerns and ventilating feelings provide an opportunity for the nurse to correct any misinformation. Validating the client's perceptions increases self-awareness.

5. Participation in self-care is a sign of successful adjustment.

6. Successful return demonstration and ability to teach the skill to others indicate mastery.

7. Support persons' acceptance is a critical factor in the client's own acceptance and adjustment.

8. Evidence of positive self-concept and desire to pursue goals and life style reflect successful adjustment.

9. Improving appearance can boost self-confidence and aid successful adjustment.

10. Successful adjustment to appearance changes is influenced by factors such as these:
    a. Previous coping success
    b. Achievement of developmental tasks before surgery
    c. The extent to which the change interferes with goal-directed activity
    d. Sense of control
    e. Realistic perception of the change by the client and others

▲ Documentation

Progress notes
  Present emotional status
  Interventions
  Response to interventions

▲ Outcome Criteria

The outcome criteria for this diagnosis represent those associated with discharge planning. Refer to the discharge criteria.

Interventions

h. Lack of effective support systems
i. Unstable economic status
j. Rejection of counseling (Shipes, 1987)
11. Refer a client at high risk for unsuccessful adjustment for professional counseling.

Rationale

11. Follow-up therapy may be indicated to assist with effective adjustment.

Potential Altered Health Maintenance related to insufficient knowledge of wound care, signs and symptoms of complications, exercises, and follow-up care

Focus Assessment Criteria

1. Readiness and ability to learn and retain information

Clinical Significance

1. A client or family failing to achieve learning goals requires a referral for assistance post-discharge.

Interventions

1. Teach wound care measures. (Refer to the General Surgery care plan, Appendix II, for specific interventions.)
2. Explain the normal function of neuromuscular structures and how they have been disrupted by surgery.
3. Discuss the importance of complying with the prescribed exercise regimen. Reinforce teaching, and provide written instructions.

4. Instruct the client to report the following promptly:
   a. Increased temperature
   b. New or increasing pain
   c. Change in amount or color of drainage
   d. Leakage around the prosthetic insertion site

Rationale

1. *Note,* no rationale needed here.

2. The client's understanding of the impairment can encourage compliance with postoperative instructions.
3. The postoperative exercise program aims to strengthen the levator scapulae and rhomboid muscles to compensate for the loss of the trapezius. If these muscles are not strengthened, the pectoralis muscle will pull the shoulder forward and down and cause pain. Explanations and written instructions can encourage compliance.
4. Early detection of complications enables prompt intervention to reduce their severity. Increased temperature, pain, and a change in drainage typically point to infection. Leakage around the prosthetic insertion may indicate a tracheo-esophageal fistula.

▲ Documentation

Discharge summary record
  Client and family teaching
  Outcome achievement or status

References/Bibliography

Burke, J. (1989). Maintaining adequate nutrition in the head and neck patient undergoing radiation therapy. *Journal of the Society of Otorhinolaryngology Head–Neck Nurses, 7*(1), 8–12.

Kane, K.K. (1983). Carotid artery rupture in advanced head and neck cancer patients. *Oncology Nursing Forum, 10*(1), 14–18.

Shipes, E. (1986). Psychosocial issues: The person with an ostomy. *Nursing Clinics of North America, 22*(2), 291–302.

Shumrick, D.A. (1973). Carotid artery rupture. *Laryngoscope, 83*(7), 1051–1061.

Swartz, S.L., & Barr, N.J. (1979). Carotid catastrophe. *American Journal of Nursing, 79*, 1566–1567.

Radical Vulvectomy

Extensive surgery, radical vulvectomy involves removing the vulva and also some or all of the urethra, vagina, rectum, and lymph glands. This surgery is indicated for invasive cancer of the vulva.

Diagnostic Cluster

▲ **Time Frame**

Preoperative and postoperative periods

PREOPERATIVE PERIOD
Nursing Diagnoses

Anxiety related to insufficient knowledge of preoperative and postoperative routines and perceived negative effects on life style

POSTOPERATIVE PERIOD
Collaborative Problems

Potential Complications:
Hemorrhage/Shock
Urinary Retention
Sepsis
Pulmonary Embolism
Thrombophlebitis

Nursing Diagnoses

Altered Comfort related to effects of surgery and immobility
Grieving related to loss of body function and its effects on life style
Potential Altered Sexuality Pattern related to perceived negative impact of surgery on sexual functioning and attractiveness
Potential Altered Health Maintenance related to insufficient knowledge of home care, wound care, self-catheterization, and follow-up care

Related Care Plans

General Surgery Generic Care Plan (Appendix II)
Anticoagulant Therapy

▲ **Discharge Criteria**

Before discharge, the client and/ or family will:

1. Describe wound care measures
2. Demonstrate correct self-catheterization
3. Describe a plan for resumption of self-care
4. State signs and symptoms that must be reported to a health care professional
5. Verbalize an intent to share feelings and concerns related to surgery with significant others

Preoperative: Nursing Diagnoses

▲ **Outcome Criteria**

The client will:

1. State the reason for surgery
2. Describe anatomical changes following surgery
3. Verbalize decreased anxiety related to fear of the unknown

Anxiety related to insufficient knowledge of preoperative and postoperative routines and perceived negative effects on life style

Focus Assessment Criteria	*Clinical Significance*
1. Understanding of underlying disease and need for surgery	1–3. Assessing knowledge level guides the nurse in planning effective teaching strategies.
2. Knowledge of structure and function of affected organs	
3. Understanding of anticipated surgical procedure	
4. Life style, strengths, coping mechanisms, and available support systems	4. Discussions can help determine the client's and support persons' past ability to manage stress.

Interventions

1. Provide opportunities for the client to share feelings. Promote a calm, relaxed atmosphere, convey a nonjudgmental attitude, and listen attentively. Encourage verbalization of fears to nurses, physicians, and family members.

2. Explore with the client her feelings about the upcoming surgery. Identify her support systems, resources, and coping strategies.

3. Explain preoperative and postoperative routines, covering the following information as applicable:
   a. Equipment: intravenous (IV)-line, indwelling (Foley) catheter, Jackson-Pratt drains, nasogastric tube, air flotation bed, Ace wraps, antiembolic hose
   b. Medication regimen: analgesics, antibiotic therapy
   c. Dietary changes: clear liquid diet initially, advanced as tolerated
   d. Dressings: bulky abdominal dressing for 10 days, daily wrapping for pressure
   e. Activity modification: bed rest for 10 days, then progressive activity as tolerated; leg elevation; possible change in activity because of restrictive dressing
   f. Exercises: incentive spirometry, coughing and deep breathing exercises, respiratory treatments, ankle rotation, relaxation techniques

4. Identify a client at risk for unsuccessful adjustment; look for these traits:
   a. Poor ego strength
   b. Ineffective problem-solving ability
   c. Lack of motivation
   d. External focus of control
   e. Poor health
   f. Unsatisfactory preoperative sex life
   g. Lack of positive support systems
   h. Unstable economic status
   i. Rejection of counseling (Shipes, 1987)

Rationale

1. Frequent contact by the caregiver indicates acceptance and may facilitate trust. The client may be hesitant to approach the staff because of negative self-concept. Assumptions cannot be made about a client's reaction to a situation. The reality of the altered body function may be overwhelming.

2. The client may need assistance to identify available resources and support persons.

3. Accurate descriptions of postoperative sensations and procedures help ease anxiety related to fear of the unknown.

4. Successful adjustment is influenced by factors such as these:
   a. Previous coping success
   b. Achievement of developmental tasks before surgery
   c. The extent to which the disability interferes with goal-directed activity
   d. Sense of control
   e. Realistic perception of the event by the client and support persons.

A client at risk for unsuccessful adjustment requires referral for counseling.

Postoperative: Collaborative Problems

▲ **Nursing Goal**

The nurse will manage and minimize vascular and urinary complications.

Potential Complication: Hemorrhage/Shock
Potential Complication: Urinary Retention
Potential Complication: Sepsis
Potential Complication: Pulmonary Embolism
Potential Complication: Thrombophlebitis

Interventions

1. Monitor for urinary retention.

Rationale

1. The proximity of the surgical site may cause obstruction from edema or nerve trauma.

Interventions	*Rationale*

2. Monitor for signs of sepsis:
  a. Temperature >101° F or < 98.6° F
  b. Abnormal laboratory values: serum creatinine, pH, WBC count, arterial blood gas (ABG) analysis
  c. Decreased urine output
	2. An abdominal pressure dressing is kept in place for approximately 10 days, providing a reservoir for microorganism growth. Sepsis involves massive vasodilatation and hypovolemia, resulting in tissue hypoxia, impaired renal function, and decreased cardiac output. The compensatory response increases heart rate and respirations in an attempt to correct hypoxia and acidosis.

3. Monitor for signs and symptoms of pulmonary embolism:
  a. Chest pain
  b. Dyspnea, tachypnea
  c. Hemoptysis
  d. Hypotension, tachycardia
  e. Cyanosis
  f. Altered level of consciousness
	3. Pulmonary embolism interferes with perfusion, increasing the work of breathing and leading to hypoxia.

4. Monitor for signs and symptoms of thrombophlebitis:
  a. Ischemia
  b. Decreased capillary refill time and warmth
  c. Edema
  d. Redness, pallor, or cyanosis
  e. Pain
  f. Paresthesias
	4. Prolonged prescribed immobility (approximately 10 days) and the edema resulting from the extensive surgery increase risk.

5. Maintain adequate hydration status.	5. Optional hydration reduces hyperviscosity of blood and decreases the risk of thrombus formation.
6. Apply and reapply support hose to legs every shift.	6. Support hose provide constant pressure, which promotes venous return and reduces venous pooling.

▲ **Documentation**

Flow records
  Intake and output
  Vital signs
  Wound status
  Circulatory status

Related Physician-Prescribed Interventions

Medications
  Refer to the General Surgery care plan, Appendix II.
Intravenous Therapy
  Refer to the General Surgery care plan, Appendix II.
Laboratory Studies
  Refer to the General Surgery care plan, Appendix II.
Diagnostic Studies
  Refer to the General Surgery care plan, Appendix II.
Therapies
  Antiembolic hose
  Wound irrigations

Postoperative: Nursing Diagnoses

▲ **Outcome Criteria**

The client will verbalize effectiveness of pain-reducing measures.

Altered Comfort related to effects of surgery and immobility

Focus Assessment Criteria	*Clinical Significance*

1. Source of pain:
  a. Surgical site
  b. Constriction of bulky dressing, tubes, or Ace wrap
  c. Other sources
	1. Pain could have many sources, including urinary retention, abdominal distention, thrombophlebitis, pulmonary embolism, and stiffness due to immobility from restrictive position during surgery or from an abdominal pressure dressing. Determining the source guides the nurse in planning effective interventions.

Interventions

1. Assist the client to change position and perform range-of-motion (ROM) exercises.
2. When the client is side-lying, place a pillow between her legs and at the lumbar region.
3. Explain the need to take pain medications regularly and before dressing changes, incision scrub, or other activities that could cause pain.

4. Provide an over-bed trapeze.

5. Refer to the General Surgery care plan, Appendix II, for general pain relief interventions.

Rationale

1. Frequent position changes and ROM exercises reduce muscle tension and spasms.
2. This support reduces tension on the wound.

3. The preventive approach to pain relief involves regularly administering medication before pain becomes severe, rather than following the p.r.n. approach.
4. The trapeze allows more movement with less pain.

▲ **Documentation**

Medication administration record
 Type, route, and dosage of
 all medications
Progress notes
 Unsatisfactory response

▲ **Outcome Criteria**

The client will:

1. Express her grief
2. Describe the personal meaning of her loss
3. Report an intent to discuss her feelings with significant others

Grieving related to loss of body function and its effects on life style

Focus Assessment Criteria

1. Signs and symptoms of grief reaction, e.g., crying, withdrawal, anxiety, restlessness, decreased appetite, increased dependency

Clinical Significance

1. Losses related to sexual identity, sexual function, and possibly even life usually provoke a profound grief response.

Interventions

1. Provide opportunities for the client and family members to ventilate feelings, discuss the loss openly, and explore the personal meaning of the loss. Explain that grief is a common and healthy reaction.

2. Encourage use of positive coping strategies that have proven successful in the past.
3. Encourage the client to express positive self-attributes.
4. Implement measures to support the family and promote cohesiveness:
   a. Explain the grieving process.
   b. Encourage verbalization of feelings with the client.
   c. Allow participation in care to promote comfort.
   d. Support the family at its level of functioning.
5. Promote grief work with each response:
   a. Denial:
      • Encourage acceptance of the situation; do not reinforce denial by giving false reassurance.
      • Promote hope through assurances of care, comfort, and support.
      • Explain the use of denial by one family member to other members.
      • Do not push a person to move past denial until she is emotionally ready.
   b. Isolation:
      • Convey acceptance by encouraging expressions of grief.
      • Promote open, honest communication to encourage sharing.
      • Reinforce the client's self-worth by providing for privacy, when desired.
      • Encourage socialization, as feasible (e.g., support groups, church activities).

Rationale

1. Cancer and this extensive surgery may give rise to feelings of powerlessness, anger, profound sadness, and other grief responses. Open, honest discussions can help the client and family members accept and cope with the situation and their response to it.
2. Positive coping strategies aid acceptance and problem-solving.
3. Focusing on positive attributes increases self-acceptance and acceptance of imminent death.
4. Family cohesiveness is important to client support.

5. Grieving involves profound emotional responses; interventions depend on the particular response.

Interventions

  c. Depression:
  - Reinforce the client's self-esteem.
  - Employ empathetic sharing and acknowledge grief.
  - Identify the degree of depression and develop appropriate strategies.
  d. Anger:
  - Explain to other family members that anger represents an attempt to control the environment stemming from frustration at the inability to control the disease.
  - Encourage verbalization of anger.
  e. Guilt:
  - Acknowledge the person's expressed self-image.
  - Encourage identification of the relationship's positive aspects.
  - Avoid arguing and participating in the person's system of "I should have . . ." and "I shouldn't have. . . ."
  f. Fear:
  - Focus on the present and maintain a safe and secure environment.
  - Help the person explore reasons for and meanings of the fears.
  g. Rejection:
  - Provide reassurance by explaining what is happening.
  - Explain this response to other family members.
  h. Hysteria:
  - Reduce environmental stressors (e.g., limit personnel).
  - Provide a safe, private area in which to express grief.

Rationale

▲ **Documentation**

Progress notes
  Present emotional status
  Interventions
  Response to interventions

▲ **Outcome Criteria**

The client will:
1. Express her feelings and discuss her partner's concerns regarding the effect of surgery on sexual functioning
2. Verbalize an intention to discuss concerns with her partner before discharge

Potential Altered Sexuality pattern related to perceived negative impact of surgery on sexual functioning and attractiveness

Focus Assessment Criteria	*Clinical Significance*
1. Sexual patterns 2. Concerns about resuming intercourse	1,2. Identifying sexual patterns and concerns guides the nurse in planning effective interventions.

Interventions

1. Reaffirm the need for frank discussion between sexual partners and the need for time for the partner to become accustomed to changes in the client's body.
2. Explain how the client and partner can use role-playing to discuss concerns about sex.

3. Discuss the possibility that the client may be projecting her own feelings onto the partner; encourage validation of feelings with partner.

Rationale

1. Both partners will have some doubts and concerns about resuming sexual activity. Repressing these feelings would negatively affect the relationship.
2. Role-playing can help partners gain insight by placing each in the other's position. It also may encourage more spontaneous sharing of doubts and concerns.
3. Worried about acceptance, the client may have erroneous perceptions of her partner's response and may assume that the partner is "turned off" by her altered appearance when in fact that may not be the case.

Interventions

4. Reaffirm the need for closeness and expressions of caring; encourage touching, massage, and other nongenital contact.
5. Explore the client's fear of mutilation and unacceptability and other concerns that might limit involvement in relationships.
6. Consult with the physician regarding the intactness of the client's sexual organs.
7. Explain the need to use a water-soluble vaginal lubricant when resuming intercourse after surgery.
8. Refer to a certified sex or mental health counselor, if desired.

Rationale

4. Sexual pleasure and gratification are not limited to intercourse. Other expressions of caring may prove even more meaningful.
5. These fears might limit the client's involvement in relationships.
6. If vulvectomy was extensive, the client may need vaginal reconstructive surgery.
7. After recovery, the vagina is shorter, narrower, and drier. Removal of the clitoris diminishes sexual response.
8. Certain sexual problems necessitate continuing therapy and the advanced knowledge of specialists.

▲ *Documentation*

Progress notes
  Assessment data
  Interventions
  Response to interventions
  Referrals, if indicated

▲ *Outcome Criteria*

The outcome criteria for this diagnosis represent those associated with discharge planning. Refer to the discharge criteria.

Potential Altered Health Maintenance related to insufficient knowledge of home care, wound care, self-catheterization, and follow-up care

Focus Assessment Criteria	*Clinical Significance*
1. Readiness and ability to learn and retain information	1. A client or family failing to achieve learning goals requires referral for assistance postdischarge.

Interventions

1. Explain that healing is a slow, gradual process.

2. Teach wound care and irrigation techniques.

3. Teach the home use of support hose and the need for leg elevation.

4. Teach self-catheterization, if indicated.

5. Teach to monitor for and report signs and symptoms of complications:
   a. Temperature changes, increased wound drainage
   b. Increased edema in the legs or feet

   c. Weight gain > 5 lb in 2 days
   d. Calf pain
6. Refer the client to a home health or visiting nurse agency.

Rationale

1. Explaining the gradual nature of the healing process decreases the client's anxiety over perceived slow healing.
2. Daily wound cleansing with warm saline irrigations promotes débridement and helps protect against contamination.
3. These measures reduce venous pooling and increase venous return—especially critical when deep node dissection compromises lower extremity circulation and aggravates edema.
4. Postoperative edema or surgical removal of the urethra necessitates self-catheterization to empty the bladder. Proper technique helps ensure success and prevent injury.
5. The slow-healing wound is very vulnerable to infection and other complications.
   a. These signs may indicate infection.

   b. Edema indicates compromised venous return.
   c. Weight gain points to fluid retention.
   d. Calf pain may be a sign of thrombosis.
6. The client requires a follow-up visit in the home to evaluate self-care ability.

▲ *Documentation*

Discharge summary record
  Client teaching
  Outcome achievement or status
  Referrals

References/Bibliography

Barber, H. (1980). *Manual of gynecologic oncology.* Philadelphia: J.B. Lippincott.
Carpenito, L.J. (1989). *Nursing diagnosis: Application to clinical practice* (3rd ed.). Philadelphia: J.B. Lippincott.
McConnell, E., et al. (1983). *Care of patients with urologic problems.* Philadelphia: J.B. Lippincott.
Nordmark, M., et al. (1975). *Scientific foundations of nursing.* Philadelphia: J.B. Lippincott.
Servatius, D., et al. (1975). Easing the shock of a radical vulvectomy. *Nursing 75, 5*(8), 26–31.
Shipes, E. (1987). Psychosocial issues: The person with an ostomy. *Nursing Clinics of North America, 22*(2), 291–302.

Renal Surgery (Nephrostomy, Nephrectomy, Extracorporeal, Ureteral Stents)

The term renal surgery encompasses various procedures. *Nephrostomy* involves an opening into the kidney with placement of a permanent or temporary drainage tube. *Nephrectomy* is the surgical removal of a kidney owing to disease or malfunction or for donation. Insertion of *ureteral stents* is done to maintain urinary flow in cases of ureteral obstruction. *Extracorporeal renal surgery* involves removing the kidney, preserving it by continuous flushing with a cold solution, surgically repairing it, and then reimplanting it. This surgery is indicated to remove obstructions (tumors, calculi) and to repair vascular lesions.

Diagnostic Cluster

▲ **Time Frame**

Preoperative and postoperative periods

▲ **Discharge Criteria**

Before discharge, the client and/or family will:

1. Demonstrate nephrostomy tube care
2. State measures for at-home wound care
3. Share feelings regarding loss of kidney
4. State signs and symptoms that must be reported to a health care professional

POSTOPERATIVE PERIOD
Collaborative Problems

	Refer to:
Potential Complications:	
Hemorrhage/Shock	
Paralytic Ileus	
Renal Insufficiency	
Pyelonephritis	
Ureteral Stent Dislodgement	
Pneumothorax Secondary to Thoracic Approach	Thoracic Surgery

Nursing Diagnoses

Potential Altered Health Maintenance related to insufficient knowledge of hydration requirements, nephrostomy care, and signs and symptoms of complications	
Impaired Physical Mobility related to distention of renal capsule and incision	General Surgery
Potential Altered Respiratory Function related to pain on breathing and coughing secondary to location of incision	General Surgery

Related Care Plan

General Surgery Generic Care Plan (Appendix II)

Postoperative: Collaborative Problems

▲ **Nursing Goal**

The nurse will manage and minimize complications of renal surgery.

Potential Complication: Hemorrhage/Shock
Potential Complication: Paralytic Ileus
Potential Complication: Renal Insufficiency
Potential Complication: Pyelonephritis
Potential Complication: Ureteral Stent Dislodgement

Interventions

1. Monitor for signs and symptoms of hemorrhage/shock:
   a. Increasing pulse rate with normal or slightly decreased blood pressure
   b. Urine output < 30 mL/hr
   c. Restlessness, agitation, change in mentation

Rationale

1. Since the renal capsule is very vascular, massive blood loss can occur. The compensatory response to decreased circulatory volume is to increase blood oxygen by increasing heart and respiratory rates and decreasing circulation to extremities (manifested by decreased

Interventions	*Rationale*

Interventions

    d. Increasing respiratory rate

    e. Diminished peripheral pulses

    f. Cool, pale, or cyanotic skin

    g. Thirst

2. Monitor fluid status:

    a. Intake (parenteral, oral)

    b. Output and loss (urinary, drainage, vomiting)

3. Monitor the surgical site for bleeding, dehiscence, and evisceration.

4. Teach the client to splint the incision site with a pillow when coughing.

5. Monitor for signs and symptoms of paralytic ileus:

    a. Decreased or absent bowel sounds

    b. Abdominal distention

    c. Abdominal discomfort

6. Do not initiate fluids until bowel sounds are present. Begin with small amounts. Note the client's response and the type and amount of emesis, if any.

7. Monitor for early signs and symptoms of renal insufficiency:

    a. Sustained elevated urine specific gravity

    b. Elevated urine sodium level

    c. Sustained insufficient urine output ($<$ 30 mL/h)

    d. Elevated blood pressure

    e. Elevated blood urea nitrogen (BUN) and serum creatinine, potassium, phosphorus, and ammonia, and decreased creatinine clearance

8. Monitor for signs and symptoms of pyelonephritis:

    a. Chills, fever

    b. Costovertebral angle (CVA) pain (a dull, constant backache below the 12th rib)

    c. Leukocytosis

    d. Bacteria and pus in urine

    e. Dysuria, frequency

Rationale

pulses and cool skin). Diminished cerebral oxygenation can cause changes in mentation.

2. Fluid loss due to surgery and nothing-by-mouth (NPO) status can disrupt fluid balance in some clients. Stress can produce sodium and water retention.

3. Frequent monitoring enables early detection of complications.

4. Splinting reduces stress on suture lines by equalizing the pressure across the incision site.

5,6. Reflex paralysis of intestinal peristalsis and manipulation of the colon to gain access make this client at high risk for ileus. The depressive effects of narcotics and anesthetics on peristalsis can also cause paralytic ileus. Ileus can occur between the third and fifth postoperative day. Pain can be localized, sharp, and intermittent.

7. Renal insufficiency can result from edema caused by surgical manipulation, urethral edema after stent insertion, or a nonpatent nephrostomy tube.

    a,b. Decreased ability of the renal tubules to rebsorb electrolytes results in increased urine sodium levels and urine specific gravity.

    c,d. Decreased glomerular filtration rate eventually leads to insufficient urine output and increased renin production, resulting in elevated blood pressure in an attempt to increase renal blood flow.

    e. These changes result from decreased excretion of urea and creatinine in urine.

8. Microorganisms can be introduced into the body during surgery or through incision. Urinary tract infections can be caused by urinary stasis (e.g., from a nonpatent nephrostomy tube) or irritation of tissue by calculi.

    a. Bacteria can act as pyrogen by raising the hypothalamic thermostat through the production of endogenous pyrogen, which may mediate through prostaglandins. Chills can occur when the temperature set-point of the hypothalamus changes rapidly.

    b. CVA pain results from distention of the renal capsule.

    c. Leukocytosis reflects an increase in WBCs to fight infection through phagocytosis.

    d. Bacteria and pus in the urine indicate a urinary tract infection.

    e. Bacteria irritates bladder tissue, causing spasms and frequency.

▲ ***Documentation***

Flow records
    Vital signs
    Circulatory status
    Intake (oral, parenteral)
    Output (urinary, drainage tubes)
    Bowel function (bowel sounds, defecation pattern, abdominal distention)
    Wound status (color, drainage)

Interventions	Rationale
9. Monitor for signs and symptoms of ureteral stent dislodgement: a. Sudden, sharp, pain radiating anteriorly and downward to bladder b. Nausea and vomiting c. Decreased urine output d. Fever, chills	9. Dislodgment of the ureteral stent causes an afferent stimuli in the renal capsule, producing pylorospasm of the smooth muscle of the enteric tract and adjacent structures. Disruption of ureter patency decreases urine output.

Related Physician-Prescribed Interventions

Refer to the care plan for the underlying disorder, e.g., urolithiasis, chronic renal failure.

Postoperative: Nursing Diagnosis

▲ **Outcome Criteria**

The outcome criteria for this diagnosis represent those associated with discharge planning. Refer to the discharge criteria.

Potential Altered Health Maintenance related to insufficient knowledge of hydration requirements, nephrostomy care, and signs and symptoms of complications

Focus Assessment Criteria	Clinical Significance
1. Readiness and ability to learn and retain information	1. A client or family failing to achieve learning goals requires a referral for assistance post-discharge.

Interventions	Rationale
1. Explain the need to maintain optimal hydration.	1. Optimal hydration reduces urinary stasis, decreasing the risk of infection and calculi formation.
2. Teach and have the client perform a return demonstration of nephrostomy care measures, including these: a. Aseptic technique b. Skin care c. Stabilization of tube	2. Proper techniques can reduce the risk of infection. Movement of the tube can cause dislodgement or tissue trauma.
3. Teach the client to report the following: a. Decreased urine output b. Fever, malaise c. Purulent, cloudy drainage from or around the tube	3. Early detection enables prompt intervention to prevent serious complications, such as renal insufficiency and infection.
4. Refer the client and family to a home health agency for follow-up care.	4. The home care nurse evaluates the client's ability for home care and provides periodic assessment of renal function and development of infection.

▲ **Documentation**

Discharge summary record
 Client and family teaching
 Outcome achievement or
  status
 Referrals

References/Bibliography

Blandy, J. (1986). *Operative urology.* Boston: Blackwell Scientific.

MacFarlane, D.E. (1985). Prevention and treatment of catheter-associated urinary tract infection. *Journal of Infection, 10*(2), 96–106.

McConnell, E.A., & Zimmerman, M.F. (1983). *Care of patients with urologic problems.* Philadelphia: J.B. Lippincott.

Schoengrund, L., & Balzer, P. (1985). *Renal problems in critical care.* New York: John Wiley & Sons.

Thoracic Surgery

A term encompassing various procedures involving a surgical opening into the chest cavity, thoracic surgery may be a pneumonectomy (removal of entire lung), lobectomy (removal of a lobe), segmentectomy (removal of a segment), wedge resection (removal of a lesion), or exploratory thoracotomy (diagnostic).

Diagnostic Cluster

▲ **Time Frame**

Preoperative and postoperative periods

PREOPERATIVE PERIOD
Nursing Diagnoses

Refer to:

Anxiety related to impending surgery and insufficient knowledge of preoperative routines, intraoperative activities, and postoperative self-care activities

POSTOPERATIVE PERIOD
Collaborative Problems

Potential Complications:
Mediastinal Shift
Subcutaneous Emphysema
Acute Pulmonary Edema
Respiratory Insufficiency

Coronary Artery Bypass Grafting

Pneumothorax, Hemothorax

Abdominal Aortic Aneurysm Resection

Pulmonary Embolism

Abdominal Aortic Aneurysm Resection

Thrombophlebitis

Abdominal Aortic Aneurysm Resection

Nursing Diagnoses

Ineffective Airway Clearance related to increased secretions and diminished cough secondary to pain and fatigue
Impaired Physical Mobility related to restricted arm and shoulder movement secondary to pain and muscle dissection and imposed position restrictions
Altered Comfort related to surgical incision, chest tube sites, and immobility secondary to lengthy surgery

General Surgery

Grieving related to loss of body part and its perceived effects on life style

Enucleation

Related Care Plan

General Surgery Generic Care Plan (Appendix II)

▲ **Discharge Criteria**

Before discharge, the client or family will:

1. Describe wound care at home
2. Relate the need to continue exercises at home
3. Verbalize precautions for activities
4. State signs and symptoms that must be reported to a health care professional
5. Identify appropriate community resources and self-help groups

Preoperative: Nursing Diagnosis

▲ **Outcome Criteria**

The client will:

1. Verbalize knowledge of perioperative routines and care before surgery
2. Share concerns and fears

Anxiety related to impending surgery and insufficient knowledge of preoperative routines, intraoperative activities, and postoperative self-care activities

Focus Assessment Criteria

1. Anxiety level (mild, moderate, severe, panic)
2. Readiness and ability to learn and retain information

Clinical Significance

1,2. Anxiety can interfere with learning. Assessing anxiety level guides the nurse in planning appropriate teaching strategies.

Interventions

1. Explain the expected postoperative events, such as the following:

   a. Presence of chest tubes and drainage tubes

   b. Oxygen therapy

   c. Pain and available relief measures

2. Teach postoperative respiratory exercises and reinforce their importance. Refer to the General Surgery care plan, Appendix II, for instructions on coughing and deep breathing exercises. Also teach "huffing" breathing:
   a. Take a deep diaphragmatic breath and exhale forcefully against the hand with a "huff."
   b. Start with small huffs and progress to one strong huff.

3. Instruct the client to refrain from smoking postoperatively.

Rationale

1. Preoperative education improves the client's ability to participate postoperatively and decreases anxiety associated with the unknown.
   a. Drainage tubes remove liquids and gas from the surgical site (thoracic cavity, pleural space, mediastinal cavity). Chest tubes re-expand the lungs by reestablishing negative intrapleural pressures. Chest tubes are not indicated after a pneumonectomy, for it is desired that the space accumulate with fluid.
   b. Supplemental oxygen is indicated to compensate for impaired ventilation.
   c. Moderate to severe pain is expected; the client should be aware of this possibility.

2. Surgery on the lung reduces the surface area for oxygen exchange, and trauma to the tracheobronchial tree produces excessive secretions and a diminished cough reflex. Respiratory exercises stimulate pulmonary expansion and assist in alveolar inflation.

3. Irritants from smoking increase pulmonary secretions.

▲ **Documentation**

Teaching record
 Instructional method used
 Outcome achievement or
  status

Postoperative: Collaborative Problems

▲ **Nursing Goal**

The nurse will manage and minimize complications of thoracic surgery.

Potential Complication: Acute Pulmonary Edema
Potential Complication: Mediastinal Shift
Potential Complication: Subcutaneous Emphysema

Interventions

1. Monitor for signs of acute pulmonary edema:
   a. Severe dyspnea
   b. Tachycardia
   c. Adventitious breath sounds
   d. Persistent cough
   e. Productive cough of frothy sputum
   f. Cyanosis
2. Cautiously administer intravenous (IV) fluids. Consult with the physician if the ordered rate exceeds 125 mL/hr.
3. Be sure to include all additional IV fluids (e.g., antibiotic agents) in the hourly allocation.
4. Encourage and assist the client to get adequate rest and conserve strength.
5. Monitor for signs of mediastinal shift:
   a. Increased, irregular pulse rate
   b. Severe dyspnea
   c. Increased restlessness
   d. Deviation of larynx or trachea from midline
   e. Shift in the point of apical impulse

Rationale

1. Circulatory overload can result from the reduced size of the pulmonary vascular bed caused by the removal of pulmonary tissue and the yet-unexpanded lung postoperatively. Hypoxia produces increased capillary permeability, causing fluid to enter pulmonary tissue and triggering signs and symptoms.
2. Caution is needed to prevent circulatory overload.

3. Administration of even an extra 50 mL of fluid for dilution of antibiotics can create overload.
4. Rest reduces oxygen consumption and decreases hypoxia.
5. Increased intrapleural pressure on the operative side from fluid and air accumulation or excessive negative pressure on the operative side from inadequate fluid accumulation provides a space for the contents of the mediastinum (heart, trachea, esophagus, pulmonary vessels) to shift. Constriction of vessels (aorta, vena cava) creates hypoxia and its resultant signs and symptoms.

Interventions

6. If signs and symptoms of a mediastinal shift occur, do the following:
   a. Position the client in a semi-Fowler's position.
   b. Maintain oxygen therapy.
7. Monitor the status of subcutaneous emphysema:

   a. Mark the periphery of the emphysematous tissue with a skin-marking pencil; reevaluate frequently.
   b. Monitor for neck involvement.

Rationale

6.

   a. Sitting upright reduces mediastinal shifting.

   b. Oxygen therapy reduces hypoxia.
7. Subcutaneous emphysema occurs commonly after thoracic surgery as air leaks out of incised pulmonary tissue.
   a. Serial markings help the nurse evaluate the rate of progression.

   b. Severe subcutaneous emphysema can indicate air leakage through the bronchial stump and can compress the trachea.

▲ **Documentation**

Flow records
   Vital signs
   Intake and output records

Related Physician-Prescribed Interventions
Medications
   Bronchodilators
   Expectorants
Intravenous Therapy
   Refer to the General Surgery care plan, Appendix II.
Laboratory Studies
   Arterial blood gas analysis
Diagnostic Studies
   Chest x-ray film   Pulmonary function studies
   Fiberoptic bronchoscopy   Computed tomography (CT) scan
Therapies
   Intermittent positive-pressure   Chest drainage system
      breathing (IPPB) treatments
   Chest physiotherapy

Postoperative: Nursing Diagnoses

▲ **Outcome Criteria**

The client will demonstrate effective coughing and increased air exchange.

Ineffective Airway Clearance related to increased secretions and diminished cough secondary to pain and fatigue

Focus Assessment Criteria

1. Breath sounds (before and after coughing exercises)

2. Pain level

Clinical Significance

1. Assessing breath sounds before and then after coughing helps the nurse evaluate the effectiveness of the client's coughing effort.
2. Pain can interfere with effective coughing.

Interventions

1. Teach the client to sit as erect as possible, using pillows for support if needed.
2. Teach the proper method of controlled coughing:
   a. Breathe deeply and slowly while sitting up as high as possible.
   b. Use diaphragmatic breathing.
   c. Hold the breath for 3 to 5 seconds and then slowly exhale as much as possible through the mouth. (The lower rib cage and abdomen should sink down.)

Rationale

1. Slouching and cramping positions of the thorax and abdomen interfere with air exchange.
2. Deep breathing dilates the airways, stimulates surfactant production, and expands the lung tissue surface; thus improving respiratory gas exchange. Coughing loosens secretions and forces them into the bronchus to be expectorated or suctioned. In some clients, "huffing" breathing may be effective and is less painful.

Interventions

    d. Take a second breath, hold, and cough forcefully from the chest (not from the back of the mouth or throat), using two short, forceful coughs.

    e. If indicated, use the "huffing" breathing technique as taught preoperatively.

3. Assess the lung fields before and after coughing exercises.

4. If breath sounds are moist-sounding, instruct the client to rest briefly, then repeat the exercises.

5. Assess the current analgesic regimen:

    a. Administer pain medication as needed.

    b. Assess its effectiveness: Is the client still in pain? If not, is he too lethargic?

    c. Note times when the client seems to obtain the best pain relief with an optimal level of alertness and physical ability. This is the time to initiate breathing and coughing exercises.

6. Provide emotional support:

    a. Stay with the client for the entire coughing session.

    b. Explain the importance of coughing after pain relief is obtained.

    c. Reassure the client that the suture lines are secure and that splinting by hand or pillow will minimize pain on movement.

    d. Offer sips of warm water prior to coughing exercises.

7. Maintain adequate hydration and adequate humidity of inspired air.

8. Provide motivation and plan strategies to avoid overexertion:

    a. Plan and bargain for adequate rest periods (e.g., "Work hard now, then I'll let you rest.").

    b. Vigorously coach and encourage coughing, using positive reinforcement.

    c. Plan coughing sessions for periods when the client is obtaining optimal pain relief and is alert.

    d. Allow for rest after coughing sessions and before meals.

9. Evaluate the need for tracheobronchial suctioning.

Rationale

3. Comparison assessments help evaluate the effectiveness of coughing.

4. Rales indicate trapped secretions.

5. Pain or fear of pain can inhibit participation in coughing and breathing exercises. Adequate pain relief is essential.

6. Coughing exercises are fatiguing and painful. Emotional support provides encouragement; warm water can aid relaxation.

7. These measures help decrease the viscosity of secretions. Tenacious secretions are difficult to mobilize and expectorate.

8. The client's cooperation enhances the effectiveness of the exercises.

9. Suctioning will be needed if the client is unable to cough effectively.

▲ **Documentation**

Flow records
    Auscultation findings (before and after coughing exercises)
Progress notes
    Effectiveness of coughing

▲ **Outcome Criteria**

The client will:

1. Return or progress to preoperative arm and shoulder function
2. Relate the need to maintain certain positions

Impaired Physical Mobility related to restricted arm and shoulder movement secondary to pain and muscle dissection and imposed position restrictions

Focus Assessment Criteria	*Clinical Significance*
1. Range of motion (ROM) of arm and shoulder	1. Surgical resection reduces the ability to move the arm and shoulder actively.
2. Tolerance to repositioning	2. Certain positions may compromise diaphragmatic movements.

Interventions

1. Position the client as indicated or prescribed:
   a. Supine position until consciousness is regained
   b. Semi-Fowler's position (30 to 45°) thereafter

2. Explain the need for frequent turning. Gently turn from side to side every 1 to 2 hours, unless contraindicated.

3. Avoid extreme lateral turning following a pneumonectomy.

4. Avoid traction on chest tubes during movement; check for kinks after repositioning.

5. Explain the need for frequent exercises of the arms, shoulders, and trunk even in the presence of some pain and discomfort.

6. Initiate passive ROM exercises on the operative arm and shoulder within 4 hours after recovery from anesthesia. Begin with two times every 4 hours for the first 24 hours, and progress to 10 to 20 times every 2 hours.

7. Consult with a physical therapist for active ROM exercises for the client to perform starting 1 to 2 days after surgery:
   a. Hyperextending the arms, to strengthen the latissimus dorsi
   b. Adducting and forward flexing the arms and shoulders, to maintain shoulder girdle motion
   c. Adducting the scapula, to strengthen the trapezius

8. Encourage use of the affected arm in activities of daily living (ADLs), and stress the need to continue exercises at home.

Rationale

1.
   a. The supine position prevents aspiration.

   b. This position allows the diaphragm to resume its normal position, which reduces the effort of respiration.

2. Turning mobilizes drainage of secretions, promotes circulation, inhibits thrombus formation and aerates all parts of the remaining lung tissue. Lying on the operative side can be contraindicated following a wedge resection and pneumonectomy.

3. This can cause a mediastinal shift (refer to Potential Complication: Mediastinal Shift in this entry for more information.)

4. Traction can cause dislodgment; kinks can inhibit drainage or negative pressure.

5. The muscle groups transcended by a thoracotomy form the shoulder girdle and maintain the trunk's posture. Failure to perform exercises can result in muscle adhesions, contractures, and postural deformities.

6. Passive ROM exercises help prevent ankylosis of shoulder and contractures of arm.

7. Active ROM exercises help prevent adhesions of two incised muscle layers.

8. Regular use increases ROM and decreases contractures.

▲ **Documentation**

Progress notes
    Limitations on performing activities
    Therapeutic exercises performed
Flow records
    Turning, positioning
Discharge summary record
    Client teaching
    Response to teaching

References/Bibliography

Burkhart, C. (1983). Pneumonectomy. *American Journal of Nursing, 83*(11), 1562–1565.

Burton, G.G., & Hodgkin, J.E. (Eds.). (1984). *Respiratory care: A guide to clinical practice* (2nd ed.). Philadelphia: J.B. Lippincott.

Carpenito, L.J. (1989). *Nursing diagnosis: Application to clinical practice* (3rd ed.). Philadelphia: J.B. Lippincott.

Connolly, J.E. (1980). Thoracotomy and pulmonary resection. *Surgical Clinics of North America, 60*(6), 1481–1496.

Hughes, J.M. (1983). Postoperative pulmonary care: Past, present, future. *Critical Care Quarterly, 6*(2), 67–71.

Total Joint Replacement (Hip, Knee)

Prosthetic replacement may be indicated for joint degeneration caused by rheumatoid arthritis, osteoarthritis, trauma, or congenital deformities. Joint prostheses of metal or high-density polyethylene are implanted into the prepared bone using cement, or a porous, coated prosthesis is implanted that allows bone growth into the implant.

Diagnostic Cluster

▲ **Time Frame**

Preoperative and postoperative periods

PREOPERATIVE PERIOD
Nursing Diagnoses

Anxiety related to scheduled surgery and lack of knowledge of preoperative and postoperative routines, postoperative sensations, and use of assistive devices

Refer to:
Fractured Hip and Femur

POSTOPERATIVE PERIOD
Collaborative Problems

Potential Complications:
Dislocation of Joint
Neurovascular Compromise
Fat Emboli
Hemorrhage/Hematoma Formation
Sepsis
Thromboemboli

Fractured Hip and Femur
Fractured Hip and Femur
Fractured Hip and Femur
Fractured Hip and Femur

Nursing Diagnoses

Impaired Physical Mobility related to pain, stiffness, fatigue, restrictive equipment and prescribed activity restrictions
Potential Impaired Skin Integrity related to pressure and immobility secondary to pain and restrictions
Potential Altered Health Maintenance related to insufficient knowledge of activity restrictions, use of assistive devices, signs of complications, and follow-up care
Potential for Injury related to altered gait and use of assistive devices

Amputation

Related Care Plans

General Surgery Generic Care Plan
Anticoagulant Therapy

▲ **Discharge Criteria**

Before discharge, the client and/or family will:

1. Describe activity restrictions
2. Describe a plan for resuming activities of daily living (ADLs)
3. Regain mobility while adhering to weightbearing restrictions
4. State signs and symptoms that must be reported to a health care professional

Postoperative: Collaborative Problems

▲ **Nursing Goal**

The nurse will manage and minimize vascular and joint complications.

Potential Complication: Dislocation of Joint
Potential Complication: Neurovascular Compromise

Interventions

1. Maintain correct positioning:

   a. Hip: Keep in abduction, at 45° or less. Do not cross legs.
   b. Knee: Slightly elevate from hip; do not flex or hyperextend.

Rationale

1. Specific positions are used to prevent prosthesis dislocation.

Interventions

2. Monitor for signs of joint dislocation:
   a. Shortening of leg
   b. Inability to move
   c. Misalignment
   d. Abnormal rotation
   e. Bulge at the surgical site
3. Maintain bed rest as ordered. Keep the affected joint in a neutral position with rolls, pillows, or specified devices.
4. Turn the client to the unaffected side only; limit the use of Fowler's position.

5. Monitor for signs and symptoms of neurovascular compromise, comparing findings to the unaffected limb:
   a. Diminished or absent pedal pulses

   b. Capillary refill time > 3 seconds

   c. Pallor, blanching, cyanosis, coolness of extremity
   d. Complaints of abnormal sensations (e.g., tingling, numbness)
   e. Increasing pain not controlled by medication

6. Instruct the client to report numbness, tingling, coolness, or change in skin color.

Rationale

2. Until the surrounding muscles and joint capsule heals, joint dislocation may occur if positioning exceeds the limits of the prosthesis, as in flexing or hyperextending the knee or abducting the hip more than 45 degrees.

3. Bed rest typically is ordered for 1 to 3 days after surgery to allow stabilization of the prosthesis.
4. Pressure on the affected side can disrupt the prosthesis in the acetabular component. Prolonged Fowler's position can dislocate the prosthesis.

5.
   a. Surgical trauma causes swelling and edema, which can compromise circulation and compress nerves.
   b. Prolonged capillary refill time points to diminished capillary perfusion.
   c. These signs may indicate compromised circulation.
   d. These symptoms may result from nerve compression.
   e. Tissue and nerve ischemia produces a deep, throbbing, unrelenting pain.
6. Early detection of neurovascular compromise enables prompt intervention to prevent serious complications.

▲ **Documentation**

Flow records
  Positioning
  Peripheral circulation status

Related Physician-Prescribed Interventions
Medications
  Anticoagulants
Intravenous Therapy
  Refer to the General Surgery care plan, Appendix II.
Laboratory Studies
  Refer to the General Surgery care plan, Appendix II.
Diagnostic Studies
  X-ray films
  Bone scans
Therapies
  Antiembolic hose

Postoperative: Nursing Diagnoses

▲ **Outcome Criteria**

The client will increase activity to a level consistent with abilities.

Impaired Physical Mobility related to pain, stiffness, fatigue, restrictive equipment, and prescribed activity restrictions

Focus Assessment Criteria	*Clinical Significance*
1. Endurance level 2. Mobility	1,2. Pain and limited range of motion affect mobility. The client, particularly if elderly, may have a chronic disease that affects endurance.

Interventions

1. Establish an exercise program tailored to the client's ability; consult with a physical therapist.
   a. For hip: quadriceps and gluteal settings, plantar flexion of foot, leg lifts
   b. For knee: quadriceps setting, isometrics, leg lifts
2. Develop a plan for range-of-motion (ROM) exercise at regular intervals, increasing the use of involved extremity as ordered.
3. Teach body mechanics and transfer techniques; ensure proper body alignment.
4. Encourage the client's independence and reward progress. Include him in care planning and contracting.
5. Schedule progressive and paced activities, as appropriate. Consult with the physical therapist for weightbearing regimen.
6. Teach the correct use and supervise the use of ambulatory aids, as necessary.

Rationale

1. Exercises are needed to improve circulation and strengthen muscle groups needed for ambulation.

2. Active ROM increases muscle mass, tone, and strength and improves cardiac and respiratory functioning.
3. Proper mechanics and alignment help prevent dislocation of the prosthesis.
4. The client's participation in decision-making about care increases self-esteem and can encourage compliance.
5. The amount of weightbearing depends on the type of prosthesis used and on the client's condition and abilities.
6. Such devices must be used correctly and safely to ensure effectiveness and prevent injury.

▲ *Documentation*

Progress notes
    Activity level
    Response to activity

▲ *Outcome Criteria*

The client will exhibit intact skin.

Potential Impaired Skin Integrity related to pressure and immobility secondary to pain and restrictions

Focus Assessment Criteria	*Clinical Significance*
1. Skin and circulation 2. Hydration and nutrition status 3. Ability to change positions	1,2,3. This assessment determines skin condition and identifies risk factors that contribute to pressure ulcer development.

Interventions

1. Use a pressure-relieving device, e.g., alternating mattress, specialized bed pad.
2. Turn and reposition the client every 2 hours. Teach the client ways to shift position in bed, e.g., lifting buttocks and legs.
3. Assess pressure points—shoulder blades, heals, elbow, sacrum, and hips—each shift.

4. Lightly massage bony prominences with lotion. Protect vulnerable areas with film dressings.

5. Stress the importance of optimal nutritional intake and hydration.
6. Encourage ambulation, as indicated.

Rationale

1. These and other devices can help distribute pressure uniformly over the skin surface.
2. Frequent repositioning allows circulation to return to tissues where pressure has inhibited it.

3. Bony prominences are covered with minimal skin and subcutaneous fat, and thus are more prone to skin breakdown from pressure.
4. Light massage stimulates circulation. Film dressings provide more structure to prevent injury from shearing force.
5. Inadequate nutrition and hydration reduce circulation and increase tissue wasting.
6. Ambulation improves circulation and reduces pressure on vessels.

▲ *Documentation*

Flow records
    Turning and repositioning
    Skin assessment

▲ *Outcome Criteria*

The outcome criteria for this diagnosis represent those associated with discharge planning. Refer to the discharge criteria.

Potential Altered Health Maintenance related to insufficient knowledge of activity restrictions, use of assistive devices, signs of complications, and follow-up care

Focus Assessment Criteria	*Clinical Significance*
1. Readiness and ability to learn and retain information.	1. A client or family failing to achieve learning goals requires a referral for assistance post-discharge.

Interventions

1. Explain restrictions, which typically include avoiding the following:
   a. Sitting for long periods
   b. Excessive bending and lifting
   c. Crossing the legs
   d. Jogging and jumping
2. Explain the need to continue prescribed exercises at home.
3. Teach wound care and assessment techniques.

4. Teach and encourage the safe use of assistive devices and therapeutic aids. Request return demonstration of correct use.
5. Explain the need to continue leg exercises (5 to 10 times an hour) and use of antiembolic hose at home.
6. Teach to report signs and symptoms of complications:
   a. Increased temperature
   b. Red, swollen, draining incision
   c. Coolness of skin on affected limb or numbness
   d. Pain in calf or upper thigh
7. If anticoagulants are prescribed, refer to the Anticoagulant Therapy care plan, page 507, for specific interventions.

Rationale

1. These activities can put great stress on the implant.

2. Exercises increase muscle strength and joint mobility.
3. Instructions are needed to prevent infection and to detect early signs.
4. Assistive devices may be needed. Return demonstration allows the nurse to evaluate proper, safe use.
5. The risk of thrombophlebitis continues after discharge.

6. Early detection enables prompt interventions to prevent serious complications.
   a. Fever may indicate an infection or phlebitis.
   b. Incision changes may indicate infection.
   c. These signs indicate compromised circulation.
   d. Leg pain may point to thrombophlebitis.

▲ **Documentation**

Discharge summary record
   Client teaching
   Outcome achievement or
     status

References/Bibliography

Cox, J. (1987). A plan for preoperative preparation of patients having total joint replacement surgery. *Washington Nurse, 17*(10), 14–15.

Nolde, T., et al. (1989). Teaching patients how to use a new hip: What elders said they needed to know and how nurses made sure they understood the information. *Geriatric Nursing, 10*(2), 69–70.

National Association of Orthopedic Nurses. (1988). Total hip arthroplasty. *Orthopedic Nursing, 7*(4), 8–9.

National Association of Orthopedic Nurses. (1988). Total knee arthroplasty. *Orthopedic Nursing, 7*(4), 56–57.

Urostomy

There are several methods of urostomy or urinary diversion e.g. ileal conduit, ureterostomy, continent ileal urinary reservoir (Kock pouch). In ureterostomy, the surgeon diverts the ureters external to the abdomen. For an ileal or colon conduit, the ureters are diverted to a resected segment of the bowel, then one end of the bowel segment is brought to the abdominal surface as a urinary stoma. Both a ureterostomy and an ileal or colon conduit require urinary collection appliance. The Kock continent urostomy pouch, an internal low-pressure urinary reservoir constructed of ileum, contains two nipple valves, one on the loop of ileum entering the pouch and one directly behind the abdominal stoma. The ureters are anastomosed to this loop; the valves prevent reflux of urine into the renal collecting system. The client, if able, can learn to perform periodic ileal bladder emptying via intermittent self-catheterization.

Diagnostic Cluster

▲ *Time Frame*

Preoperative and postoperative periods

▲ *Discharge Criteria*

Before discharge, the client and/ or family will:

1. Describe routine ostomy care
2. Demonstrate the proper stoma pouching procedure
3. Identify measures to help maintain peristomal skin integrity
4. Demonstrate self-catheterization of Kock pouch
5. State conditions of ostomy care at home: stoma, pouching, skin care
6. Discuss strategies for incorporating ostomy management into activities of daily living (ADLs)
7. Verbalize measures for maintaining fluid intake and acidic urine
8. State signs and symptoms that must be reported to a health care professional
9. Verbalize an intent to share feelings and concerns related to ostomy with significant others
10. Identify available community resources and self-help groups:
    a. Visiting nurse
    b. United Ostomy Association
    c. Recovery of Male Potency; Help for Impotent Male
    d. American Cancer Foundation
    e. Community supplier of ostomy equipment
    f. Financial reimbursement for ostomy equipment

PREOPERATIVE PERIOD
Nursing Diagnoses

Refer to:

Anxiety related to lack of knowledge of urostomy care and perceived negative effects on life style

POSTOPERATIVE PERIOD
Collaborative Problems

Potential Complications:
Internal Urine Leakage
Urinary Tract Infection
Peristomal Skin Ulceration
Paralytic Ileus

Renal Surgery

Nursing Diagnoses

Potential Altered Sexuality Patterns related to erectile dysfunction (male) or inadequate vaginal lubrication (female)
Potential Social Isolation related to anxiety over possible odor and leakage from appliance
Potential Altered Health Maintenance related to insufficient knowledge of stoma pouching procedure, colostomy irrigation, peristomal skin care, perineal wound care, and incorporation of ostomy care into activity of daily living (ADL)
Potential Altered Health Maintenance related to insufficient knowledge of intermittent self-catheterization of Kock continent urostomy
Potential Self-Concept Disturbance related to effects of ostomy on body image
Potential Altered Sexuality Pattern related to perceived negative impact of ostomy on sexual functioning and attractiveness

Ileostomy

Ileostomy

Related Care Plan

General Surgery Generic Care Plan

Outcome Criteria

The client will:

1. State reason for urostomy
2. Describe anatomical changes following urostomy surgery
3. Identify his or her own type of urostomy
4. Verbalize decreased anxiety related to fear of the unknown

1. Understanding of underlying disorder necessitating urostomy
2. Knowledge of structure and function of affected organs
3. Anticipated surgical procedure and stoma location
4. Previous exposure to a client with an ostomy
5. Familiarity with stoma pouching equipment
6. Emotional status, cognitive ability, memory, vision, manual dexterity
7. Life style, strengths, coping mechanisms, available support systems

1–7. Assessing the client's knowledge of urostomy identifies learning needs and guides the nurse in planning effective teaching strategies. Assessing emotional status, mental and physical ability, and other factors about the client helps the nurse evaluate the client's ability to accept, adjust to, and manage the ostomy and stoma.

1. Identify and dispel any misinformation or misconceptions the client has regarding ostomy.
2. Explain the normal anatomical structure and function of the genitourinary (GU) tract.
3. Explain the effects of the client's particular disorder on affected organs.
4. Use an anatomical diagram or model to show the resultant altered route of elimination.

5. Describe the appearance and anticipated location of the stoma. Explain the following facts about the stoma:
   a. It will be the same color and moistness as oral mucous membrane.
   b. It will not hurt when touched because it has no sensory endings.
   c. It may bleed slightly when wiped; this is normal and not of concern.
   d. It will become smaller as the surgical area heals; color will remain the same.
   e. It may change in size depending on illness, hormone levels, and weight gain or loss.
6. Discuss the function of the stoma pouch. Explain that it serves as an external receptacle for storage of urine much as the bladder acts as an internal storage receptacle.
7. Encourage the client to handle the stoma pouching equipment.

1. Replacing misinformation with facts can reduce anxiety.
2. Knowledge increases confidence; confidence produces control and reduces anxiety.
3. Understanding the disorder can help the client accept the need for urostomy.
4. Understanding how urine elimination occurs after the bladder removal can help allay anxiety related to altered body function.
5. Explaining expected events and sensations can help reduce anxiety associated with the unknown and unexpected. Accurate descriptions of the stoma appearance help ease shock at the first sight of it after ostomy surgery.

6. Understanding the purpose and need for a pouch encourages the client to accept it and participate in ostomy management.

7. Many clients are relieved to see the actual size and material of a stoma pouch. Often, uninformed clients have visions of large bags and complicated, difficult-to-manage equipment, which can produce anxiety.

Documentation

Progress notes
    Presence of dysfunctional anxiety
Teaching records
    Client teaching

Nursing Goal

The nurse will manage and minimize urinary and stomal complications.

Interventions

1. Monitor for signs of internal urine leakage:
   a. Abdominal distention with adynamic ileus
   b. Fever
   c. Elevated serum creatinine level
   d. Decreased urine output despite adequate hydration

2. Monitor for signs and symptoms of urinary tract infection:
   a. Fever
   b. Flank pain
   c. Malodorous, cloudy urine
   d. Alkaline urine *p*H
3. Consult with the physician for a urine culture from a double-lumen catheter specimen.
4. Consult with a clinical specialist or ostomy therapist regarding skin irrigation
5. Monitor

   a. Color, size, and shape of stoma

   b. Color and amount of urine from the urostomy or from each stent
   c. Ostomy appliance and appliance belt fit

Rationale

1. Urine leakage either from the ureter-ileal anastomosis or from the base of the conduit occurs in as many as 8% of clients with a urostomy. Leakage is confirmed through fluoroscopy. Small leaks may seal themselves with continuous drainage of the conduit via a stomal catheter.
2. Between 10% and 20% of clients with a urinary diversion develop pyelonephritis. The major cause is poor urine flow through the conduit, leading to urinary stasis and bacterial contamination through the stoma.

3. Cultures enable identification of the causative organism and guide pharmacological therapy.
4. Expert assistance may be needed for persistent skin problems.
5. Daily assessment is necessary to detect early changes in stoma condition.
   a. Changes can indicate bleeding or infection Decreased output can indicate obstruction
   b. Decreased urine output can indicate an anastamosis leak.
   c. Improperly fitting appliance or belt can cause mechanical trauma to the stoma.

▲ **Documentation**

Flow records
    Vital signs
    Intake and output
    Abdomen (girth, bowel sounds)
    Condition of peristomal area

Related Physician-Prescribed Interventions

Medications
Refer to the General Surgery care plan, Appendix II.
Intravenous Therapy
Refer to the General Surgery care plan, Appendix II.
Laboratory Studies
Refer to the General Surgery care plan, Appendix II.
Diagnostic Studies
Intravenous pyleography
Cystoscopy
Computed tomography (CT) scan
Conduitography
Therapies
Sitz baths

Postoperative: Nursing Diagnoses

Potential Altered Sexuality Patterns related to erectile dysfunction (male) or inadequate vaginal lubrication (female)

▲ **Outcome Criteria**

The client will:
1. Describe the possible effects of urostomy surgery on sexual function
2. Identify available community resources, if necessary

Focus Assessment Criteria

1. Knowledge of the effects of surgery on sexual function
   a. In men, after radical cystectomy, penile

Clinical Significance

1. Assessing the client's knowledge of possible effects on sexual function guides the nurse in planning effective interventions.

Focus Assessment Criteria

Clinical Significance

sensation and the ability to reach orgasm remain intact. However, semen production ceases because the prostate, seminal vesicles, and proximal vas deferens are removed with the bladder. The incidence of erectile dysfunction associated with urostomy is 85%; few clients can achieve an erection of sufficient rigidity for intercourse.

b. In women, satisfactory intercourse after radical cystectomy depends on vaginal preservation. Surgery typically involves removing the bladder, ovaries, fallopian tubes, uterus, cervix, and the anterior one-third to one-half of the vagina. The surgeon may rebuild the vagina; a common problem in a client with a rebuilt vagina is dyspareunia related to vaginal tightness and lack of lubrication.

Interventions

1. In men
   a. Suggest that sexual activity need not always culminate in vaginal intercourse, and that orgasm can be reached through noncoital manual or oral stimulation. Remind the client that sexual expression is not limited to intercourse, but includes closeness, communication, touching, and giving pleasure to another.
   b. Explain the function of a penile prothesis. Both semirigid and inflatable penile protheses have a high rate of success.
   c. Suggest counseling with a certified sex therapist.

2. In women
   a. Suggest using a water-based vaginal lubricant for intercourse.

   b. Teach the client to perform Kegel exercises, and instruct her to do them regularly.

   c. Suggest that she sit astride her partner during intercourse.

Rationale

1.
   a. Alternative methods of sexual expression and gratification promote positive sexual function.

   b. Penile implants provide the erection needed for intercourse and do not alter sensations or the ability to ejaculate.
   c. Certain sexual problems require continuing therapy and the advanced knowledge of therapists.

2.
   a. Water-based lubricant can help prevent dyspareunia related to inadequate vaginal lubrication.
   b. Kegel exercises promote control of the pubococcygeal muscles around the vaginal entrance, which can ease dyspareunia.
   c. A woman on top can control the depth and rate of penetration, which can enhance vaginal lubrication and relaxation.

▲ *Documentation*

Progress notes
Interventions
Response to interventions

▲ *Outcome Criteria*

The client will:

1. Discuss methods to control odor and appliance leakage
2. State an intent to reestablish preoperative socialization pattern

Potential Social Isolation related to anxiety about possible odor and leakage from appliance

Focus Assessment Criteria

1. Preoperative socialization pattern
2. Anticipated changes

Clinical Significance

1,2. A client at risk for social isolation must be assessed carefully; the suffering associated with isolation is not always visible. Feelings of rejection and repulsion are common.

1. Select an appropriate odorproof pouching system, and explain to the client how it works.

2. Stress the need for good personal hygiene.
3. Teach the client care of a reusable appliance.
4. Discuss methods for reducing odor:
   a. Avoid odor-producing foods such as asparagus, cabbage
   b. Drink cranberry juice or use a liquid appliance deodorant.
   c. Empty or change the ostomy pouch regularly when one-third to one-half full.
5. Encourage the client to reestablish his or her preoperative socialization pattern. Help through measures such as progressively increasing the client's socializing time in the hospital, and role-playing possible situations that the client feels may cause anxiety, encouraging the client to visualize and anticipate solutions to "worst-case scenarios" for social situations.
6. Suggest that the client meet with a person from the United Ostomy Association (UOA) who can share similar experiences.

1. Fear of accidents and odor can be reduced through effective management. Some pouches have charcoal filters to reduce urine odor.
2,3. Proper hygiene and appliance care remove odoriferous retained urine.
4. Minimizing odor improves self-confidence and can permit more effective socialization. Bacterial proliferation in retained urine increases odor over time. A full pouch also puts excessive pressure on seals, increasing the risk of leakage.

5. Encouraging and facilitating socialization helps prevent isolation. Role-playing can help the client identify and learn to cope with potential anxiety-causing situations in a nonthreatening environment.

6. Others in a similar situation can provide a realistic appraisal of the situation and may provide information to answer the client's unasked questions.

Documentation

Progress notes
   Dialogues and interactions
Teaching record
   Client teaching

Outcome Criteria

The outcome criteria for this diagnosis represent those associated with discharge planning. Refer to the discharge criteria.

1. Type of urostomy

2. Knowledge of urostomy care: fluid intake, activity, hygiene, clothing, sexual expression, community resources, employment, travel, odor, skin care, appliances
3. Client's and support persons' readiness and ability to learn and retain information

1. Urostomy care differs according to its type and concurrent therapies.
2. Assessment identifies learning needs and guides the nurse in planning effective teaching strategies.
3. A family or client failing to achieve learning goals requires a referral for assistance postdischarge.

1. Teach the client basic stoma pouching principles:
   a. Keeping the peristomal skin clean and dry

   b. Using a well-fitting appliance

   c. Changing the pouch when the least amount of drainage is anticipated (usually on arising)

1. Proper pouching techniques can prevent leakage and skin problems.
   a. This ensures that the appliance adheres to the skin.
   b. Proper fit protects the surrounding skin surface from contact with drainage.
   c. This prevents copious drainage from interfering with pouch changes.

Interventions

    d. Emptying the pouch when it is one-third to one-half full and changing routinely before a leak occurs

    e. Changing the pouch if burning or itching occurs under the appliance

    f. Observing the condition of the stoma and peristomal skin during pouch changes

2. Teach the procedure for preparing a stoma pouch:

    a. Select the appropriate stoma pouching system; avoid Karaya gum and pectin-based skin barriers.

    b. Measure the stoma carefully.

    c. Use the appliance manufacturer's stoma measuring card, if possible. If the card does not accommodate stoma size or shape, teach the client to make a customized stoma pattern: Place clear plastic wrap from the skin barrier wafer over the stoma, trace the stoma with a marking pen, and cut a hole in the plastic to accommodate the stoma.

    d. Use this pattern to trace the opening onto the reverse side of a skin barrier wafer.

    e. Cut an opening in the center of the skin barrier slightly larger than the stoma (approximately ⅛ inch).

    f. Secure an appropriate odorproof pouch onto the skin barrier wafer (if using a two-piece appliance system). The pouch should have an antireflux valve to prevent urine from bathing the stoma.

3. Teach the procedure for changing a disposable stoma pouch:

    a. Remove the old pouch by gently pushing the skin away from the paper tape and skin barrier wafer.

    b. Fold the old pouch over on itself and discard in a plastic bag.

    c. Hold gauze or toilet paper over the stoma.

    d. Cleanse the peristomal skin with a wash cloth and warm tap water.

    e. Blot or pat skin dry.

    f. Apply the new pouch to the abdomen, carefully centering the hole in the skin barrier wafer over the stoma. Press on the wafer for a few minutes.

    g. Secure the pouch by "picture framing" the wafer with four strips of hypoallergenic paper tape (if the wafer does not already have tape attached).

4. Teach the procedure for emptying a stoma pouch:

    a. Put some toilet paper in the toilet bowl and sit on the toilet seat.

    b. Remove the plug or turn valve to open pouch and carefully empty pouch contents into the toilet.

Rationale

    d. A pouch filled more than halfway exerts increased pressure on the seal, increasing the risk of leakage.

    e. Burning or itching may indicate that urine has undermined the skin barrier; prompt intervention is necessary to prevent skin breakdown.

    f. Regular observation enables early detection of skin problems.

2. Preparing a new pouch beforehand ensures that the new pouch is ready to apply as soon as the used pouch is removed, helping minimize drainage on the skin surface.

3. Correct pouch removal and attachment techniques minimize irritation and injury of peristomal skin and ensure a tight, reliable seal between the pouch and skin.

4. Correct techniques can reduce spillage, soiling, and odor. Placing toilet paper in the bowl prevents water from splashing as the pouch contents are emptied.

Interventions	Rationale
5. Connect the appliance to straight drainage when the client is sleeping in bed.	5. Bacteria multiply rapidly as urine collects in the pouch. Bacterial contamination of the urinary tract can result from backflow of urine from a full pouch. Nighttime drainage systems hold large amounts of urine and drain the urine away from the stoma.

6. Teach strategies for preventing and managing peristomal skin problems:
  a. Shave the peristomal skin with an electric razor rather than a blade; avoid using shaving cream, soap, and detergents except when showering.
  b. Evaluate all skin products for possible allergic reaction; patch-test all suspect products elsewhere on the abdomen.
  c. Do not change brands of skin barriers and adhesives casually; assess for allergic reaction before using a new brand.
  d. Avoid irritation from contact with urine; clean the skin regularly. Cleanse urine encrustation on the stoma or peristomal skin with a 1:1 solution of vinegar and water.
  e. Avoid prolonged skin pressure, expecially if fair-skinned or having thin, atrophic skin due to long-term corticosteroid therapy.
  f. Use corticosteroid creams sparingly and briefly; they can cause dryness and irritation.
  g. If bacterial or fungal infection is suspected, use a specific antibacterial or antifungal cream or powder.
  h. Use a liquid film barrier; avoid tincture of benzoin compound, which can dry skin.
  i. Avoid aluminum paste and greasy ointments, which can mask skin problems and also interfere with pouch adherence.
  j. Protect the skin with barriers.
  k. Expect the stoma to shrink slightly over time. This necessitates remeasuring the stoma to ensure proper appliance fit.
	6. A client with a stoma is at increased risk for peristomal skin breakdown. Factors that influence skin integrity include allergies; mechanical trauma; the underlying disease and its treatment (including medications); the quality of ostomy and periostomal skin care; availability of proper supplies; nutritional status; overall health status; hygiene; and activity level.

7. Promote measures to help the client incorporate ostomy care into ADLs:
  a. Fluid management: Drink 2 to 3 liters of fluids per day to dilute urine and flush the urinary tract. Drink cranberry juice to help acidify urine; avoid or limit coffee, tea, colas, and other caffeine-containing beverages.
  b. Working/traveling: Keep extra supplies at work. When traveling, carry supplies rather than pack them in a suitcase and risk losing them; keep in mind that pectin-based wafers melt in high environmental temperatures. Take a list of ostomy supplies when traveling.
  c. Exercise: The only limits involve contact sports during which trauma to the stoma may occur. Normal exercise is beneficial and may help to stimulate urine excretion.
	7. Successful incorporation of ostomy management into ADLs allows the client to resume his preurostomy life style and pursue goals and interests.

Interventions

    d. Wardrobe: Ostomy appliances are invisible under clothing. Any clothing worn preoperatively may be worn postoperatively. Dress comfortably.

    e. Bathing/showering/swimming: These activities may be done while wearing an ostomy appliance. "Picture-frame" the skin barrier with paper tape to seal the edges and keep the barrier edge from getting wet. Showering may be done without an appliance and, in fact, is recommended on days of appliance changes.

8. Teach measures to help prevent urinary calculi:

    a. Ensure optimal hydration.

    b. Avoid sulfa drugs and vitamin C supplements.

    c. Engage in regular physical activity.

Rationale

8. Inadequate hydration promotes urinary stasis and calculi formation. Certain drugs and inactivity can predispose to calculi formation.

▲ **Documentation**

Discharge summary record
    Client and family teaching
    Outcome achievement or
      status

▲ **Outcome Criteria**

The outcome criteria for this diagnosis represent those associated with discharge planning. Refer to the discharge criteria.

Potential Altered Health Maintenance related to insufficient knowledge of intermittent self-catheterization of Kock continent urostomy

Focus Assessment Criteria	*Clinical Significance*
1. Readiness and ability to learn and retain information	**1.** A client or family failing to achieve learning goals requires a referral for assistance post-discharge.

Interventions

1. Explain the reason for continuous drainage and frequent irrigations postoperatively.

2. If indicated, teach the client intermittent self-catheterization to drain the pouch, covering such measures as the following:

    a. Using a No. 22–26 French red rubber catheter and letting the urine flow by gravity into the toilet

    b. Gradually decreasing the number of intubations to 3 to 4 times/day

    c. Avoiding an interval of more than 6 hours between catheterizations

    d. Irrigating the pouch with normal saline solution after the first morning catheterization

    e. Applying a small gauge over the stoma

3. Instruct the client to notify the physician immediately if he or she is unable to self-catheterize the stoma.

Rationale

1. Continuous drainage is needed to eliminate urine; irrigations help keep the catheter from plugging with mucus.

2. Proper catheterization technique helps maximize pouch capacity, provides complete drainage, and prevents tissue trauma.

3. Inability to catheterize the stoma puts the client at high risk for obstruction.

▲ **Documentation**

Discharge summary record
    Client teaching
    Response to teaching
    Outcome achievement or
      status

References/Bibliography

Broadwell, D.C. (1987). Peristomal skin integrity. *Nursing Clinics of North America, 22*(2), 321–332.

Brogna, L., & Lakaszawski, M.L. (1986). The continent urostomy. *American Journal of Nursing, 86*(2), 160–163.

Carpenito, L.J. (1989). *Nursing diagnosis: Application to clinical practice* (3rd ed.). Philadelphia: J.B. Lippincott.

Coe, M., et al. (1988). Concerns of clients and spouses regarding ostomy surgery. *Journal of Enterostomal Therapy, 15*(6), 84–89.

Gerber, A. (1985). The Kock continent ileal reservoir: An alternative to the conventional urostomy. *Journal of Enterostomal Therapy, 12*(1), 15–17.

Maklebust, J. (1985). United Ostomy Association visits and adjustment following ostomy surgery. *Journal of Enterostomal Therapy, 12*(3), 84–89.

Petillo, M.H. (1987). The patient with a urinary stoma. *Nursing Clinics of North America, 22*(2), 263–279.

Shipes, E. (1987). Psychosocial issues: The person with an ostomy. *Nursing Clinics of North America, 22*(2), 291–302.

Shover, L.R. (1986). Sexual rehabilitation of the ostomy patient. In D.B. Smith & D.E. Johnson (Eds.). *Ostomy care and the cancer patient.* Orlando, FL: Grune and Stratton.

Diagnostic and Therapeutic Procedures

Anticoagulant Therapy

Administration of anticoagulant agents, which disrupt the blood's natural clotting mechanism, aims to prevent thrombus formation or extension. Oral anticoagulants include warfarin (Coumadin) and indandione derivatives; the parenteral agent is heparin sodium.

Diagnostic Cluster

▲ Time Frame
Intratherapy

▲ Discharge Criteria
Before discharge, the client and/ or family will:

1. Describe proper medication use
2. State indications for contacting a health care professional
3. State an intent to wear Medic-alert identification
4. Identify the need for follow-up care

Collaborative Problems

Potential Complication:
Hemorrhage

Nursing Diagnoses

Potential Altered Health Maintenance related to insufficient knowledge of administration schedule, identification card/ band, contraindications, and signs and symptoms of bleeding

Collaborative Problems

▲ Nursing Goal
The nurse will manage and minimize vascular complications.

▲ Documentation
Flow records
    Occult blood test results
      (urine and stool)
Progress notes
    Unusual complaints

Potential Complication: Hemorrhage

Interventions

1. Monitor for signs and symptoms of bleeding:
   a. Bruises
   b. Nosebleeds
   c. Bleeding gums
   d. Hematuria
   e. Severe headaches
   f. Red or black stools

Related Physician-Prescribed Interventions
Medications
  Anticoagulant agents (dosage varies with daily prothrombin time [PT] results)

Intravenous Therapy
  Not applicable

Laboratory Studies
  Prothrombin time
  Partial thromboplastin time (PTT)

Diagnostic Studies
  Not applicable

Therapies
  Not applicable

Rationale

1. The prolonged clotting time caused by anticoagulant therapy can cause spontaneous bleeding anywhere in the body. Hematuria is a common early sign.

Nursing Diagnosis

Potential Altered Health Maintenance related to insufficient knowledge of administration schedule, identification card/band, contraindications, and signs and symptoms of bleeding

Outcome Criteria

The outcome criteria for this diagnosis represent those associated with discharge planning. Refer to the discharge criteria.

1. Knowledge of medication regimen

2. Readiness and ability to learn and retain information

3. Medication history for drugs that can potentiate or inhibit anticoagulant actions.
   a. Substances that can potentiate anticoagulant action include the following:
      - Alcohol
      - Allopurinol
      - Antibiotics
      - Chloral hydrate
      - Chloramphenicol
      - Cimetidine
      - Mineral oil
      - Tolbutamide (Orinase)
      - Phenylbutazone
      - Salicylates
      - Thyroid medications
   b. Substances that can inhibit anticoagulant action include the following:
      - Adrenal corticosteroids
      - Antacids
      - Barbiturates
      - Carbamazepine
      - Colestipol
      - Estrogens
      - Oral contraceptives
      - Rifampin
4. Medical history, for conditions that can increase or decrease
   a. PT Conditions associated with increased PT time include the following:
      - Cachexia
      - Cancer
      - Collagen disease
      - Congestive heart failure
      - Diarrhea
      - Fever
      - Hepatic disorders
      - Malnutrition
      - Pancreatic disorders
      - Radiation therapy
      - Renal insufficiency
      - Thyrotoxicosis
      - Vitamin K deficiency
   b. Conditions associated with decreased PT time include the following:
      - Diabetes mellitus
      - Edema
      - Hereditary resistance to anticoagulants
      - Hypercholesterolemia
      - Hyperlipidemia
      - Hypothyroidism
      - Visceral, carcinoma

1. This assessment identifies learning needs and guides the nurse in planning teaching strategies.
2. A client or family failing to achieve learning goals requires a referral for assistance post-discharge.
3,4. The nurse should identify any medications or conditions that can interfere with anticoagulant therapy before initiation of therapy.

Interventions	*Rationale*
1. Instruct the client to take the medication exactly as prescribed by the physician; provide a written dosage schedule, if possible.	1. Adherence to the prescribed dosage schedule can prevent under- or over-medication.
2. Instruct the client and family to watch for and report signs and symptoms of bleeding: a. Bruises b. Headaches c. Blood in stool or black stools d. Blood in urine e. Nosebleeds f. Bleeding gums g. Coughing or vomiting blood	2. Bleeding can occur if PT is prolonged or if another factor potentiates anticoagulant action.
3. Instruct the client to avoid foods and over-the-counter medications that can affect PT: a. Alcohol b. Antacids c. Aspirin d. Nonsteroidal anti-inflammatory agents e. Vitamin C f. Foods high in vitamin K, including the following: • Turnip greens • Broccoli • Cabbage • Lettuce • Asparagus • Watercress • Beef liver • Green tea	3. Certain substances affect PT by inhibiting anticoagulant metabolism (e.g., alcohol) or inhibiting procoagulant factors (e.g., aspirin and antacids). Increased vitamin K intake decreases anticoagulant action by promoting synthesis of vitamin K-dependent clotting factors.
4. Instruct the client to alert all health care providers of his or her anticoagulant therapy before undergoing any procedures.	4. Precautions may be needed to prevent hemorrhage from routine medical procedures.
5. Instruct the client to avoid potentially hazardous situations while on anticoagulant therapy, e.g., contact sports, pregnancy.	5. Contact sports put the client at risk for bleeding from injury. Anticoagulants cross the placental barrier and can cause fatal fetal hemorrhage.
6. Encourage the client to obtain and wear Medic-alert identification if outpatient therapy is anticipated.	6. In an emergency situation, an ID alerts others that the client is prone to bleeding.
7. Stress the importance of regular follow-up care.	7. Periodic laboratory blood work is needed to evaluate the effects of therapy and risk of bleeding.

▲ **Documentation**

Discharge summary record
  Client and family teaching
  Outcome achievement or
    status

References/Bibliography

Dayle, J.E. (1986). Treatment modalities in peripheral vascular disease. *Nursing Clinics of North America,* *21*(2), 241–253.

Scherer, J.C. (1985). *Lippincott's nurse's drug manual.* Philadelphia: J.B. Lippincott.

Staff. (1987). Hematuria during anticoagulant therapy deserves workup. *Nurses Drug Alert, 11*(10), 77–78.

Walsh, P.N. (1983). Oral anticoagulant therapy. *Hospital Practice, 18*(1), 101–105.

Arteriography

In this diagnostic radiographic procedure, a radiopaque contrast medium is injected by percutaneous catheter to allow visualization of arteries. Arteriography is indicated to help diagnose and monitor the extent of vascular disease.

Diagnostic Cluster

▲ Time Frame
Pre- and postprocedure

▲ Discharge Criteria
Before discharge, the client and/or family will:
1. Relate activity restrictions indicated to reduce postprocedure complications
2. Describe techniques for monitoring the arterial access site
3. State signs and symptoms that must be reported to a health care professional

---

PREPROCEDURE PERIOD
Nursing Diagnoses

Fear related to potential negative findings of arteriogram and insufficient knowledge of routines and expected sensations

POSTPROCEDURE PERIOD
Collaborative Problems

Potential Complications:
Hematoma
Hemorrhage
Paresthesia
Embolism
Thrombosis (arterial site)
Renal Failure
Urinary Retention
Allergic Reaction

Nursing Diagnoses

Potential Altered Health Maintenance related to insufficient knowledge of activity restrictions and signs and symptoms of complications

---

Preprocedure: Nursing Diagnosis

▲ Outcome Criteria
The client will:
1. Express any fears and concerns
2. Relate, if asked, expected routines and postprocedure sensations

Fear related to potential negative findings of arteriogram and insufficient knowledge of routines and expected sensations

Focus Assessment Criteria	*Clinical Significance*
1. Understanding of procedure: equipment, expected sensations, side effects	1–3. This assessment information guides the nurse in planning interventions to help reduce anxiety.
2. Knowledge of the reason for the procedure	
3. Concern about possible arteriogram findings	

Interventions

1. Encourage the client to express his feelings and concerns about the scheduled procedure and possible findings. Reassure him that fear is a normal and common response.
2. Reinforce explanations of the procedure, equipment used, expected sensations, and nursing care that will be provided.

Rationale

1. Sharing can help the client clarify fears and gives the nurse information on the nature and degree of anxiety and fear.

2. The client's understanding of what to expect can help reduce fear associated with the unknown.

▲ Documentation
Teaching record
  Client teaching
  Outcome achievement or status
Progress notes
  Unusual response

Interventions	*Rationale*
3. Correct any misconceptions the client may have.	3. Accurate information may help dispel certain fears.
4. Determine whether the client has a history of allergic response to contrast dye, iodine, or shellfish.	4. The contrast medium is iodine-based. Often, clients who are allergic to shellfish also are allergic to iodine.

Postprocedure: Collaborative Problems

▲ **Nursing Goal**

The nurse will manage and minimize complications post-arteriogram.

Potential Complication: **Hematoma**
Potential Complication: **Hemorrhage**
Potential Complication: **Paresthesias**
Potential Complication: **Embolism**
Potential Complication: **Thrombosis (Arterial Site)**
Potential Complication: **Renal Failure**
Potential Complication: **Urinary Retention**
Potential Complication: **Allergic Reaction**

Interventions

1. Inspect the groin or axilla, depending on the puncture site, for discoloration or hematoma.
2. If hematoma develops, inform the client that it may extend over the next 2 to 3 days.

3. Gently palpate the hematoma to assess its size.
4. Monitor for signs and symptoms of hemorrhage:
   a. Elevated blood pressure
   b. Increased and irregular pulse rate
   c. Abdominal distention
   d. Diminished or absent bowel sounds
   e. Decreased hemoglobin and hematocrit values

5. Monitor for paresthesias by testing the limb distal to the puncture site for numbness and tingling.

6. Evaluate the client's ability to raise the affected leg, if applicable.

7. Report any changes immediately, and restrict the client's movement.
8. Monitor for signs and symptoms of embolism distal to the puncture site:
   a. Dark pink to purple skin
   b. Complaints of localized pain of the toes or foot
9. Monitor for signs and symptoms of thrombosis in the artery used for instillation of contrast medium:
   a. Changes in color, temperature, pulses, and capillary refill time distal to the puncture site
   b. Pain and paresthesias in the affected extremity

Rationale

1. Hematoma typically develops from the trauma of catheter insertion.
2. This can result as gravity causes the blood to shift position along the plane of the muscle fascia when upright or walking.
3. Increasing size may indicate hemorrhage.

4. Atherosclerotic arteries may not seal themselves after puncture, causing blood leakage into the retroperitoneal area. Hematoma or hemorrhage may not be visible. Rarely, a large volume of blood collects, causing life-threatening hypovolemia or dysrhythmias.

5. Paresthesias may result from bleeding into tissue surrounding the puncture site, which can exert increased pressure on the neurovascular bundle.
6. Trauma to or pressure on the nerve can prevent the client from extending or raising the leg.
7. Rapid interventions can help minimize neurovascular damage.
8. Catheter manipulation in an atherosclerotic vessel can dislodge a piece of plaque, which may occlude a small artery and cause tissue ischemia.

9. Acute thrombosis is limb-threatening, but early detection may enable prompt intervention to prevent morbidity. Symptoms reflect disruption of circulation and an inflammatory response.

Interventions

10. Instruct the client to report promptly any changes in sensation.

11. Monitor for signs of renal failure:
    a. Low urine output (< 30 mL/hr)
    b. Increased blood urea nitrogen (BUN) and serum creatinine levels

12. Encourage increased oral fluid intake after the procedure, once nothing-by-mouth (NPO) status has been lifted.

13. Monitor intake and output.

14. Monitor for urinary retention by palpating and percussing the suprapubic area for signs of bladder distention.

15. Monitor for allergic reaction to the contrast medium. Instruct the client to report itching or breathing difficulty.

Rationale

10. Subtle symptoms often are the earliest indicators of a developing problem. Prompt reporting enables further evaluation and, if necessary, immediate intervention to prevent serious complications.

11. Most contrast media are hyperosmotic and typically produce diuresis. A client with renal dysfunction may require a nonionic dye.

12. Adequate fluid intake helps ensure adequate circulating volume and help flush the dye out of the body after the procedure is completed.

13. Accurate intake and output monitoring is necessary to evaluate hydration status.

14. Urinary retention commonly occurs after arteriography. The combination of massive intravenous (IV) fluid infusion and an osmotic contrast medium creates a large volume of urine. Middle-aged and older men requiring arteriography for atherosclerosis also fall into the high-risk group for prostatic hypertrophy; bed rest after the procedure can lead to urinary retention.

15. Early detection enables prompt intervention to prevent serious allergic responses.

▲ **Documentation**

Flow records
   Vital signs
   Intake and output
   Bowel sounds
   Description of hematoma
   Condition of site
   Ability to move limbs
   Temperature, color, sensory
    status distal to site

Related Physician-Prescribed Interventions

Medications
  Not indicated

Intravenous Therapy
  IV line for direct venous access

Laboratory Studies
  Not indicated

Diagnostic Studies
  Not indicated

Therapies
  Activity restrictions
  Site care

Postprocedure: Nursing Diagnosis

▲ **Outcome Criteria**

The outcome criteria for this diagnosis represent those associated with discharge planning. Refer to the discharge criteria.

Potential Altered Health Maintenance related to insufficient knowledge of activity restrictions and signs and symptoms of complications

Focus Assessment Criteria	*Clinical Significance*
1. Readiness and ability to learn and retain information	1. A client or family failing to achieve learning goals requires a referral for assistance postdischarge.

Interventions

1. Reinforce the need for activity restrictions (bed rest).

2. Instruct the client to extend the groin if a transfemoral puncture was performed.

Rationale

1. Restricting activity decreases the risk of thrombus dislodgement and subsequent hemorrhage.

2. Restricting flexion allows the puncture site to clot.

Documentation

Discharge summary record
Client and family teaching
Outcome achievement or
status

3. Stress the need to report promptly any pain, bleeding, dizziness, dyspnea, or altered pulse rate and rhythm.
4. Teach the client to report changes in color or sensation in the distal extremity.

5. Teach the client to palpate the hematoma gently.

3. Increasing pain may result from nerve pressure due to bleeding.

4. Reporting early signs of bleeding enables prompt intervention to prevent serious complications.

5. This enables the client to assess the hematoma for increasing size after discharge.

Guzzetta, C.E., & Dossey, B.M. (1984). *Cardiovascular nursing: Body-mind tapestry.* St. Louis: C.V. Mosby.
Johnson, J.E., & Leventhal, H. (1974). Effects of accurate expectations and behavioral instructions on reactions during a noxious medical examination. *Journal of Personality and Social Psychology, 29,* 710–718.
Mason, R.A., & Arbeit, L.A. (1985). Sexual dysfunction after arteriography. *JAMA, 256*(2), 253–257.

Cardiac Catheterization

This diagnostic procedure assesses the status of the heart and blood vessels by introducing a radiopaque catheter into the right heart or left heart through the brachial, antecubital, or femoral vein. The catheter provides data to measure oxygen concentration, pressure, and cardiac output and to detect shunts.

Diagnostic Cluster

▲ Time Frame
Preprocedure and postprocedure

▲ Discharge Criteria
Before discharge, the client and/or family will:
1. Demonstrate site care
2. Verbalize precautions for activities
3. State signs and symptoms that must be reported to a health care professional

PREPROCEDURE PERIOD
Nursing Diagnoses

Anxiety related to impending cardiac catheterization

POSTPROCEDURE PERIOD
Collaborative Problems

Potential Complications:
Systemic (allergic reaction)
Cardiac (dysrhythmias, myocardial infarction, pulmonary, edema)
Circulatory (hematoma formation or hemorrhage at entry site, hypovolemia, thromboembolic phenomenon)

Nursing Diagnoses

Potential Altered Health Maintenance related to insufficient knowledge of site care, signs and symptoms of complications, and follow-up care

Preprocedure: Nursing Diagnosis

▲ Outcome Criteria
The client will:
1. Demonstrate ability to perform self-care before and after the procedure
2. Verbalize realistic expectations for the procedure
3. Express accurate information about the procedure, anticipated sensations, and postprocedural and home care

Anxiety related to impending cardiac catheterization

Focus Assessment Criteria	*Clinical Significance*
1. Anxiety level (mild, moderate, severe, panic)	1. Anxiety is a normal and expected response to the threat imposed by an invasive cardiac procedure. Mild to moderate anxiety actually helps protect and prepare the client; however, extreme anxiety can interfere with the client's coping ability.
2. Understanding of procedure	2. Modifiable factors that contribute to extreme anxiety include inaccurate or incomplete information about the procedure.
3. Exposure to others who have undergone cardiac catheterization	3. The client may have been positively or negatively influenced by information and insights from others who have undergone the procedure.
4. Desire for additional information	4. The nurse should tailor teaching to the client's desires as well as his needs. Although for many clients, detailed information helps reduce anxiety associated with fear of the unknown, in others, too much detail can increase anxiety.

Interventions	*Rationale*
1. Reinforce the physician's explanations of the procedure and the reason for it; notify the physician if additional information is needed.	1. The physician is legally responsible for providing sufficient explanations to enable informed consent. The nurse may need to supplement or reinforce this information and evaluate whether the physician needs to provide additional information.
2. Describe the preprocedural routine of blood tests, electrocardiogram (ECG), chest x-ray film, food and fluid restrictions, and sedation.	2. Explaining preprocedural routines can help reduce anxiety associated with the unknown and unexpected.

3. Describe the appearance of the catheterization laboratory (use photographs if possible), and explain expected events and sensations during the procedure:
    a. Attachment of telemetry leads for cardiac monitoring
    b. Preparation of catheter insertion site and draping
    c. Positioning of arms and hands
    d. Administration of local anesthesia
    e. Pulling and tickling sensations during catheter insertion
    f. Warmth and flushing as contrast medium is injected
    g. Other possible sensations, e.g., headache, chest pain, shortness of breath
    h. Positioning of x-ray machine over the body
    i. Loud sounds as x-ray films are taken
	3. Descriptions of expected events and sensations can provide familiarity and decrease anxiety associated with the unknown and unexpected.

4. Instruct the client on how he or she can assist with the procedure:
    a. Following physician's instructions, e.g., coughing, deep breathing, moving legs, holding breath, lying still
    b. Communicating sensations during the procedure
	4. The client's cooperation facilitates a successful procedure and enables early detection of problems, both of which can help reduce the risk of complications.

5. Explain the postprocedural routine:
    a. Frequent monitoring of blood pressure, pulse, catheter insertion site, condition of limb distal to the insertion site, fluid intake and output
    b. ECG monitoring
	5. Understanding the reasons for frequent monitoring may reduce anxiety.

6. Instruct the client on his or her role in recovery after the procedure:
    a. Maintaining complete bed rest for the prescribed length of time
    b. Using a bedpan or urinal while on bed rest
    c. Immobilizing the limb used for catheter insertion for the prescribed length of time
    d. Increasing fluid intake to 1 quart/hr or as prescribed, to enhance dye excretion and reduce blood viscosity
	6. The client's understanding of his or her role in recovery may encourage compliance with postprocedure instructions, which can help prevent complications.

7. Instruct the client to report the following:
    a. Chest pain
    b. Pain in the limb used for catheter insertion
    c. Palpitations
    d. Nausea and vomiting
	7. Early detection enables prompt interventions to reduce the seriousness of complications.

▲ **Documentation**

Progress notes
    Understanding of cardiac
        catheterization
    Expectations for cardiac
        catheterization
    Dysfunctional anxiety
Flow records
    Client teaching
    Outcome achievement or
        status

Nursing Goal

The nurse will manage and minimize allergic, cardiac, or circulatory complications.

1. Preprocedure, assess the following:

   a. Allergy or sensitivity to iodine or shellfish

   b. Heart rate and rhythm, blood pressure, respiratory rate and effort
   c. Medication history, for use of angina medication
   d. Medical history, for hypertension, myocardial infarction, congestive heart failure (CHF), or renal dysfunction

   e. Peripheral pulses in all extremities; grade as follows:
      • 2+ = bounding
      • 3+ = full normal
      • 2+ = normal
      • 1+ = diminished
      • 0 = absent
   f. Sensory and motor function of all extremities

2. Notify the physician of the following:
   a. Allergy or hypersensitivity to iodine or shellfish
   b. Abnormal vital signs
   c. Development of angina before the procedure
3. Postprocedure, monitor vital signs at frequent intervals (usually specified by the physician).
4. Monitor the catheter insertion site with each set of vital signs.

5. Monitor the circulatory status in the distal limb nearest the insertion site; note the following:
   a. Peripheral pulse
   b. Color and temperature
6. Monitor intake and output for 8 hours postprocedure.
7. Instruct the client to report the following:
   a. Palpitations
   b. Dyspnea, shortness of breath
   c. Numbness and tingling of face or extremities

1. Preprocedure assessment is necessary to detect any risk factors that could contraindicate or complicate the procedure.
   a. A client with a known allergy to iodine or shellfish is at high risk for developing anaphylactic shock after injection of a contrast medium.
   b–d. Cardiac catheterization can aggravate underlying cardiac conditions. Contrast medium causes myocardial irritability, which can lead to dysrhythmias. A client with a history of CHF is at increased risk for developing postprocedure pulmonary edema owing to the large amounts of fluids given in conjunction with the procedure. A client with renal dysfunction may have difficulty excreting the contrast medium and the large amount of fluids.
   e. Preprocedure assessment identifies whether postprocedure alterations result from the procedure or from underlying arteriosclerotic heart disease.

   f. Again, preprocedure assessment provides a baseline against which to compare postprocedure findings and identify any complications from the procedure.
2. Prompt notification enables the physician to withhold the procedure and conduct further investigations.

3. Vital sign monitoring evaluates circulatory status postprocedure.
4. Frequent monitoring can detect developing bleeding or hematoma formation early, enabling prompt intervention to prevent serious complications.

5. Circulatory status can be impaired by hematomas or thrombosis.

6. Monitoring is needed to ensure optimal hydration and prevent fluid overload.
7. These symptoms may indicate hypoxia due to catheter irritation of the myocardium.

Documentation

Flow records
   Vital signs
   Insertion site status (drainage, edema)
   Peripheral pulse assessment
   Distal extremity status (color, temperature)

Related Physician-Prescribed Interventions

Medications
Sedatives (preprocedure)
Analgesics

Intravenous Therapy
During procedure for direct venous access

Laboratory Studies
Not indicated

Diagnostic Studies
ECG monitoring

Therapies
Catheter insertion site care

Postprocedure: Nursing Diagnosis

▲ Outcome Criteria

The outcome criteria for this diagnosis represent those associated with discharge planning. Refer to the discharge criteria.

Potential Altered Health Maintenance related to insufficient knowledge of site care, signs and symptoms of complications, and follow-up care

Focus Assessment Criteria	*Clinical Significance*
1. Readiness and ability to learn and retain information	1. A client or family failing to achieve learning goals requires a referral for assistance post-discharge.

Interventions

1. Review and reinforce the postprocedural routine as necessary.
2. Reinforce instructions and restrictions for home care.
   a. Cleanse the catheter insertion site with soap and water.
   b. Avoid lifting, pulling, or pushing heavy objects for 48 hours after the procedure.
3. Instruct the client to report the following:
   a. Temperature > 100° F
   b. Swelling and redness in the involved limb
   c. Numbness, acute pain, or coldness in the involved limb

Rationale

1. This review reinforces preoperative teaching and reemphasizes the need for compliance.
2. These instructions and restrictions can help prevent infection and bleeding.

3. These signs and symptoms may indicate complications of infection, phlebitis, or thrombosis. Early detection enables prompt intervention to reduce their seriousness.

▲ Documentation

Discharge summary record
　Client and family teaching
　Outcome achievement or
　　status

References/Bibliography

Armstrong, F., & Finesilver, C. (1983). Cardiac catheterization. *Critical Care Update, 10*(4), 7–13.
Dougles, M.K., & Shinn, J.A. (1985). *Advances in cardiovascular nursing.* Rockville, MD: Aspen Systems.
Hill, N.E., et al. (1988). Evaluating the use of videotape in teaching the precardiac catheterization patient. *Journal of Cardiovascular Nursing, 2*(3), 71–78.

Casts

Composed of dehydrated gypsum that recrystallizes when reconstituted with water, casts are used to immobilize a fractured bone or dislocated joint, to support injured tissues during the healing process, to correct deformities, to prevent movement of joints during healing, and to provide traction force.

Diagnostic Cluster

▲ Time Frame

Intratherapy

▲ Discharge Criteria

Before discharge, the client and/or family will:

1. Describe precautions to take with the cast
2. Identify how to monitor for signs and symptoms of complications
3. Identify barriers in the home environment and relate strategies for overcoming these barriers
4. Identify a plan to meet role responsibilities

Collaborative Problems

Potential Complications:
Compartment Syndrome
Infection

Nursing Diagnoses

Potential Impaired Skin Integrity related to pressure of cast on skin surface
(Specify) Self-Care Deficit related to limitation of movement secondary to cast
Potential Altered Health Maintenance related to insufficient knowledge of cast care, signs and symptoms of complications, use of assistive devices, and hazards
Potential Impaired Home Maintenance Management related to the restrictions imposed by cast on performing activities of daily living (ADLs) and role responsibilities

Collaborative Problems

▲ Nursing Goal

The nurse will detect, manage, and minimize complications after cast application.

Potential Complication: Compartment Syndrome
Potential Complication: Infection

Interventions

1. Instruct the client to report any changes, even if slight. Determine whether these changes are new and different.

2. Monitor for signs and symptoms of compartment syndrome:
   a. Unrelieved or increasing pain
   b. Swelling
   c. Color change (cyanotic or pale)
   d. Cool skin (distal)
   e. Tingling or numbness
   f. Diminished or no pulse
   g. Compromised movement of fingers or toes

3. Warn the client not to mask pain with analgesics until the exact cause has been identified.

4. Investigate any complaints of pain or burning or an offensive odor from inside the cast. Smell the cast to check for odors.

▲ Documentation

Flow records
 Skin color (distal to injury)
 Pulses (distal to injury)
 Sensations (pain, paresthesias, paralysis)
 Odor (under cast)
 Temperature of cast surface
Progress notes
 Unusual complaints

5. Feel the cast surface to identify areas that feel appreciably warmer than other areas ("hot spots"). Particularly evaluate areas over pressure points.

Rationale

1. Neurovascular compromise often begins as minor sensations; early detection can enable prompt intervention to prevent serious complications.

2. These signs and symptoms are indicative of venous or arterial obstruction and nerve compression.

3. Identifying the location and nature of pain assists in differential diagnosis.

4. These signs and symptoms may indicate that a pressure sore is forming or has become infected. Pathological tissue necrosis emits a musty, offensive odor that can easily be detected.

5. Often, areas of tissue necrosis or infection cause the overlying area of the cast to feel warmer.

Related Physician-Prescribed Interventions

Medications
Not applicable

Intravenous Therapy
Not applicable

Laboratory Studies
Not applicable

Diagnostic Studies
X-ray films (pre- and postapplication)

Therapies
Assistive devices
Physical therapy

Nursing Diagnoses

Potential Impaired Skin Integrity related to pressure of cast on skin surface

▲ Outcome Criteria

The client will:

1. Continue to have intact skin
2. Relate instructions to prevent skin breakdown

Focus Assessment Criteria	Clinical Significance
1. Skin condition before cast application	1. Assessment of the skin before cast application is required to identify any lesions or abnormalities that may be aggravated by the cast.
2. Fit and condition of cast	2. An improperly fitted or deteriorating cast can lead to problems with healing.
3. Skin under cast edges	3. Pressure from cast edges can cause skin abrasion or bruising.

Interventions

1. Monitor common pressure sites in relationship to cast application:
   a. Leg: heel, malleoli, dorsal aspect of foot, head of fibula, anterior surface of patella
   b. Arm: medial epicondyle of humerus, ulnar styloid
   c. Plaster jackets or body spica casts: sacrum, anterior and superior iliac spines, vertebral borders of scapulae
   To assess the skin under the cast, pull skin taut and use a flashlight for illumination.
2. Inspect skin of uncasted body areas. Pad elbows and heels of unaffected extremities or the sacrum, if applicable.

3. Apply padding over bony prominences. (When between cast and skin surface, padding should fit smoothly, without wrinkles.) Cover skin surface with stockinette or padding—usually both—before cast application.
4. Use proper technique in handling a cast while it is wet or damp: Support the cast with the open, flat palm of your hand at all times; avoid using fingertips.
5. Avoid rapid cast drying with excessive heat.

Rationale

1. Prolonged pressure of the cast on neurovascular structures and other body parts can cause necrosis, pressure sores, and nerve palsies.

2. The heel on the unaffected side may become sore because the client habitually pushes up in bed with the uninvolved leg. The elbows sometimes become sore because the client braces himself on them to see what is going on around him.
3. Padding over bony prominences is essential to prevent pressure ulcers.

4. Wrinkles or indentations caused by fingers produce pressure points on the skin inder the cast.

5. A cast should dry from the inside out. Too-rapid drying with excessive heat can cause the inner portions of the cast to remain damp and become moldy.

Interventions

Rationale

6. Explain the intense heat sensation that can occur as the cast dries and the need to avoid covering a damp cast.
7. After cast application, clean the skin with a weak solution of vinegar and cloth to remove excess plaster while it is still damp.
8. While the cast is drying, use soft pillows to support it properly; avoid contact with hard surfaces. (Place padding between the cast and plastic-covered pillows.)

9. Keep cast edges smooth and away from skin surfaces.
   a. Petal the edges with moleskin or adhesive; place one side of the material on the inside surface of the cast (1 to 2 inches), then fold over to the outside surface of cast (1 to 2 inches).
   b. Bend cast edges slightly with a duck-billed cast bender.
   c. Elevate the affected limb properly to prevent the cast from pushing against the skin surface.
10. Provide and teach correct skin and cast care:
   a. Bathe only accessible skin, and massage it with emollient lotion. Massage skin underneath the cast with alcohol.
   b. Inspect for loose plaster. Avoid using powder in cast.
   c. Inspect position of padding.

   d. Avoid inserting any foreign object under the cast.
11. Using proper technique, turn a bedridden client every 2 to 4 hours. Turn toward the unaffected limb, and enlist one or more experienced staff members to help. (Number of persons needed depends on the client's size and weight and the type of cast.)

6. Covering the cast can precipitate increased heat, which can cause skin damage.

7. Unless removed, pieces of plaster can dry and get under the cast, causing skin damage.

8. Plastic-covered pillows inhibit evaporation. A wet cast placed on a hard surface can become flattened over bony prominences, with the resulting pressure causing decreased circulation to tissues enclosed in the cast.
9. Rough or improperly bent plaster edges may cause damage to surrounding skin by friction. When an extremity is not elevated properly, cast edges press into the skin and cause pain.

10.
   a. Alcohol helps keep the skin under the cast dry. Lotion or soap under cast creates a film and can irritate skin.
   b. Loose plaster and powder irritate skin under the cast.
   c. Padding that slips down must be pulled up and petaled.
   d. Foreign objects can cause skin injury.

11. Proper technique prevents damage to cast and injury to joints.

▲ **Documentation**

Flow records
   Skin assessment
   Positioning
Discharge summary record
   Client teaching
   Outcome achievement or status

▲ **Outcome Criteria**

The client will:

1. Perform activities of daily living (ADLs) within the limitations of the cast
2. Perform muscle-strengthening exercises on a regular basis as permitted.

(Specify) Self-Care Deficit related to limitation of movement secondary to cast

Focus Assessment Criteria

1. Ability to perform ADLs

2. Available support system

3. Home environment

Clinical Significance

1. This assessment determines the need for and extent of assistance. Any injury requiring immobilization of a part interferes to some degree with the client's ability to perform ADLs.
2. Activities may need to be planned around the availability of assistance.
3. Assessment of the home environment can identify any possible barriers and hazards.

Interventions

1. Teach proper crutch-walking technique, if indicated.

Rationale

1. Proper technique is necessary to prevent injury.

2. Elevate a casted leg when the client is not ambulatory. Elevate a casted arm with a sling when the client is out of bed; teach how to use the sling properly.
3. Instruct the client to use plastic bags to protect the cast during wet weather or while bathing.
4. Teach the client to use a blow dryer at home to dry small areas of a dampened cast.
5. Actively exercise the joints above and below the cast in the following ways:
   a. Raising a casted arm over the head
   b. Moving each finger and thumb or toes
   c. Raising and lowering wrist
   d. Quadricep-setting: tightening and relaxing of muscles
   e. Gluteal-setting
   f. Abdominal tightening
   g. Deep breathing
   h. Opening and closing the hand
6. Teach isometric exercises, starting with the unaffected limb.

7. Teach the client to put unaffected joints through their full range of motion (ROM) four times daily.
8. Consult with a home health coordinator, if indicated.

2. At rest, a dependent extremity develops venous pooling, which causes pain and swelling. Elevation helps prevent this problem.

3. Moisture weakens a cast.

4. Heat speeds drying.

5. Exercise helps prevent complications, promotes healing, and aids the rehabilitation process after cast removal. Moving frequently stimulates circulation and promotes venous return.

6. Isometric exercises produce muscle contraction without bending joints or moving limbs, and they help to maintain muscle strength and mass.
7. Performing full ROM helps maintain muscle tone and mobility.
8. Referral can provide for needed services—e.g., transportation, housekeeping—after discharge.

Documentation

Flow records
   Ability to perform ADLs

Outcome Criteria

The client will demonstrate maximum activity level within the environment.

1. Activity level (pre-injury)

2. Role responsibilities

3. Ability to perform self-care activities

4. Environmental barriers

5. Availability of support persons

1. Assessing preinjury activity level helps the nurse determine realistic expectations and goals for activity after cast application.
2. Impairment of one family member can have a significant impact on the entire family.
3. This assessment evaluates the client's need for assistance.
4. Knowledge of the client's home environment aids the nurse in determining strategies to remove or minimize barriers and hazards.
5. The client may require the assistance of others; if family or friends are not available, referral to a home health agency may be necessary.

1. Identify any barriers or hazards in the home environment and assist in removing or minimizing them.
   a. If the client is bedridden, arrange necessary items within easy reach and arrange for an over-bed trapeze.
   b. Teach the client how to get in and out of bed properly.

1. The cast may make the client feel clumsy; barriers and hazards increase the risk of injury and also can interfere with normal ADLs.

Interventions

    c. Instruct the client to stand up and sit down slowly, to reduce orthostatic hypotension and fainting.

    d. Remove scatter rugs, clutter, exposed cords and wires, low furniture, and other potential hazards, and rearrange the environment to allow more freedom of movement.

2. If the client has an arm cast, do as follows:

    a. Discuss the proper use of a sling.

    b. Instruct the client to take frequent rest periods during the day.

    c. Instruct the client to raise the cast to eye level during periods of rest.

3. Identify a client at risk for unsuccessful adjustment to the home environment owing to cast application.

4. Explore the impact of any necessary role changes or modified patterns on the client or family.

5. Counsel the client and/or family regarding any necessary role changes:

    a. Help identify the client's strengths that can ease adjustment to the role change.

    b. Assist in identifying options.

    c. Encourage the use of coping strategies that have worked in the past.

6. Suggest that the client call the nursing unit for advice and moral support after discharge, when necessary.

Rationale

2. Properly used, a sling relieves the weight of an arm cast and provides proper elevation. Adequate rest is essential to prevent fatigue from carrying the extra burden of the cast. Raising the cast so that the fingers are at eye level reduces swelling in the fingers and also relieves the weight of the cast on the shoulders, neck, and back.

3. To a client whose cast interferes with ADLs (such as an elderly person who lives alone), being discharged with a cast may necessitate a stay in an extended-care facility until he or she regains use of the extremity.

4. Impairment of one family member can have a significant impact on the entire family.

5.

    a. A positive self-concept promotes positive coping behavior, reduces fear, and promotes comfort, growth, and maturity.

    b. Knowledge of options allows informed decision-making and realistic goal-setting.

    c. Reminders of past successes promote positive attitudes toward the role changes.

6. Ready access to information and emotional support can enhance the client's self-care abilities.

▲ **Documentation**

Discharge summary record
   Client teaching
   Outcome achievement or
     status

▲ **Outcome Criteria**

The outcome criteria for this diagnosis represent those associated with discharge planning. Refer to the discharge criteria.

Potential Altered Health Maintenance related to insufficient knowledge of cast care, signs and symptoms of complications, use of assistive devices, and hazards

Focus Assessment Criteria	*Clinical Significance*
1. Readiness and ability to learn and retain information	**1.** A client or family failing to achieve learning goals requires a referral for assistance post-discharge.

Interventions

1. Teach the client and family to watch for and report the following symptoms:

    a. Severe pain

    b. Numbness or tingling

    c. Swelling

    d. Skin discoloration

    e. Paralysis or reduced movement

    f. Cool, white toes or fingertips

    g. Foul odor, warm spots, soft areas, or cracks in the cast

2. Instruct the client never to insert objects down inside edges of the cast.

Rationale

1. Early detection of possible problems enables prompt intervention to prevent serious complications, such as infection or impaired circulation.

2. Sharp objects used for scratching may cause breaks in skin continuity, providing an entry point for infectious microorganisms.

Interventions

3. Teach the client and family to handle a "green" cast with palms of hands only, because fingertips may cause indentations.
4. Instruct to keep the cast *uncovered* until it is completely dry.
5. Instruct to avoid weightbearing or other stress on the cast for at least 24 hours after application.
6. Instruct the client to avoid getting the cast wet; teach how to protect it from moisture.

7. Encourage use of an orthopedic mattress or a mattress with a fracture board placed underneath.
8. Warn against using cast braces or turnbuckles to lift a casted part.

Rationale

3. Cast indentations may lead to pressure sores.

4. A damp, soiled cast can weaken and may cause skin irritation or promote growth of bacteria.
5. Covers restrict escape of heat, especially in a large cast, and prolong the drying process.

6. Ultimate cast strength is obtained after the cast is dry—within 24 to 48 hours, depending on factors such as environmental temperature and humidity.
7. A sagging or soft mattress tends to deform a green cast and may crack a dry cast.

8. These devices are not placed in casts to serve as handles. They may easily be broken, dislocated, or pulled out of casts.

▲ **Documentation**

Discharge summary record
   Client and family teaching
   Response to teaching
   Outcome achievement or
      status

References/Bibliography

American Nurses Association and Orthopedic Nurses Association. (1987). *Standards of orthopedic nursing practice.* Kansas City, MO: American Nurses Association.

Campbell, C. (1984). *Nursing diagnosis and intervention in nursing practice* (2nd ed.). New York: John Wiley & Sons.

Farrell, J. (1982). *Illustrated guide to orthopedic nursing* (2nd ed.). Philadelphia: J.B. Lippincott.

Lancaster, J., & Stanhope, M. (1984). *Community health nursing: Process and practice for promoting health.* St. Louis: C. V. Mosby.

Larson, C., & Gould, M. (1978). *Orthopedic nursing* (9th ed.). St. Louis: C. V. Mosby.

Luckmann, J., & Sorensen, K. (1987). *Medical–surgical nursing* (3rd ed.). Philadelphia: W. B. Saunders.

Mourad, L. (1980). *Nursing care of adults with orthopedic conditions.* New York: John Wiley & Sons.

Powell, M. (1982). *Orthopaedic nursing and rehabilitation* (8th ed.). New York: Churchill Livingstone.

Cesium Implant

Time Frame
Pretherapy, intratherapy, and post-therapy

Discharge Criteria
Before discharge, the client and/ or family will:

1. Describe home care, restrictions, and follow-up care
2. Demonstrate vaginal dilation and explain the required frequency
3. State the signs and symptoms that must be reported to a health care professional
4. Verbalize an intent to share feelings and concerns regarding the condition and treatment with significant others

Outcome Criteria
The client will:

1. Describe the effects of cesium implant therapy
2. Verbalize necessary precautions for both health care staff and visitors
3. Describe the cesium implant procedure

Anxiety related to scheduled internal radiation insertion and the effects of internal radiation and insufficient knowledge of postprocedure restrictions

Potential Complications:
Bleeding
Infection
Pulmonary Complications
Vaginal Stenosis
Radiation Cystitis
Displacement of Radioactive Source
Thrombophlebitis
Bowel Dysfunction

Anxiety related to fear of radiation and its effects, uncertainty of outcome, feelings of isolation, and pain or discomfort
Self-Care Deficit: bathing, toileting related to activity restrictions and isolation
Potential Impaired Skin Integrity related to immobility secondary to prescribed activity restrictions
Social Isolation related to precautions necessitated by cesium implant safety precautions
Potential Altered Health Maintenance related to insufficient knowledge of home care, reportable signs and symptoms, activity restrictions, and follow-up care

1. Understanding of cesium implant therapy, including a history of previous radiation therapy and information obtained from health care professionals, family, friends, and other sources

1–3. During the preoperative period, the client and her family typically experience anxiety related to several factors, including cancer and the possibility of metastasis, the surgical procedure, and the effects of

Focus Assessment Criteria	*Clinical Significance*
2. Feelings and concerns regarding cesium implant surgery and effects of radiation therapy 3. Readiness and ability to learn and retain information	radiation therapy. They also are struggling to maintain a hopeful outlook regarding the outcome of therapy. Nursing interventions to reduce anxiety focus on providing client and family teaching, providing emotional support, and facilitating positive coping strategies.

Interventions

1. Reinforce the physician's explanation of the implant procedure, covering the following:
   a. Enema the evening before the procedure
   b. Betadine douche the morning of the procedure
   c. Shave and preparation of the pubic area
   d. Bladder catheterization
   e. Insertion of the holder into the uterus and vagina
   f. Placement of gauze packing in the vagina, possibly with one or two stitches in the labia, to keep the holder in place
   g. X-ray film to verify proper holder placement
   h. Insertion of the cesium into the holder, either after or before surgical implantation of the holder
2. Emphasize that the cesium implant provides a high dose of ionizing radiation to the cancerous tissue while minimizing effects to normal tissue.
3. Reinforce the principles of radiation safety and explain specific precautions:
   a. Staff and visitors can spend only a limited time with the client at each contact, usually no more than 30 minutes.
   b. Children and pregnant women are denied contact.
   c. Each staff member caring for the client wears a dosimeter.
   d. A lead shield is installed at the foot and side of the bed.
   e. A sign reading "Caution: Radioactive Materials" and including the number of the radiation safety office is posted on the room door.
4. Explain the procedure that would be followed in the event the radiation implant becomes dislodged:
   a. Notify the radiation safety office immediately.
   b. Use long-handled tongs to pick up the implant and place it in a lead-lined container.
   c. Never touch the implant with hands, even when gloved.
5. Discuss postimplantation care measures:

   a. Activity instructions:
      • Complete bed rest with slight head elevation

Rationale

1. The client's understanding of the procedure can help reduce anxiety related to fear of the unknown.

2. This information can eliminate fear of widespread tissue damage from radiation.

3,4. This information can allay anxiety related to radiation exposure and safety of others, and help the client understand why visitation and contact by staff is limited.

5. Preoperative explanations of postoperative activities and events can help reduce anxiety related to the unexpected and may improve compliance.
   a. Bed rest is necessary to keep the holder in place. Log-rolling and exercises provide mobility—promoting circulation and decreasing

Interventions

- Log-rolling technique to move from side to side in bed
- Leg exercises (with feet flat on bed, bend and then straighten legs) 8 to 10 times an hour while awake

b. Fluid and diet instructions: drink 14 to 16 glasses of fluid daily and ingest a low-fiber diet

▲ *Documentation*

Teaching record
  Client teaching
  Outcome achievement or
    status

6. Reassure the client that the implant should not cause severe pain, but that she may experience low backache, dull abdominal cramps, a feeling of pressure from the holder and gauze packing, and slight vaginal discharge.

Rationale

the risk of complications—while minimizing the chance of dislodgement.

b. Increased fluid intake keeps the bladder well-flushed and decreases the risk of bladder infection. A low-fiber diet prevents formation of hard stools, passage of which can disturb the implant.

6. The client's understanding of expected sensations can decrease anxiety associated with the unexpected and also enables the client to identify and report abnormal sensations that could signal complications.

Postprocedure: Collaborative Problems

▲ *Nursing Goal*

The nurse will manage and minimize complications after cesium implant.

Potential Complication: Bleeding
Potential Complication: Infection
Potential Complication: Pulmonary Complications
Potential Complication: Vaginal Stenosis
Potential Complication: Radiation Cystitis
Potential Complication: Displacement of Radioactive Source
Potential Complication: Thrombophlebitis
Potential Complication: Bowel Dysfunction

Interventions

1. Monitor for signs and symptoms of infection:
   a. Increased vaginal redness and swelling
   b. Dark, foul-smelling vaginal discharge
   c. Cloudy urine
   d. Fever
2. Monitor holder placement for proper position.

3. Monitor for complaints of unusual discomfort other than those sensations normally associated with cesium implant.

4. Monitor bladder function by assessing the following:
   a. Urine characteristics: color, odor, presence of blood or mucus
   b. Urine concentration
   c. Bladder distention

▲ *Documentation*

Flow records
  Vital signs
  Circulatory status (peripheral pulses, skin color, temperature)
  Intake and output
  Bowel function (sounds, flatus, type)
  Vaginal appearance
  Vaginal discharge

5. Monitor for signs and symptoms of thrombophlebitis:
   a. Painful leg swelling
   b. Positive Homans' sign
   c. Diminished peripheral pulses

6. Monitor bowel function for diarrhea or constipation.

Rationale

1. A client with cancer has a decreased resistance to infection.

2. Dislodgment of the cesium holder can cause bleeding or, if the holder comes too close to the bladder, radiation cystitis.

3. Expected sensations associated with pressure of the cesium implant include low backache, dull abdominal cramping, and a sensation of rectal fullness. Other complaints—especially of acute pain—may signal complications.

4. Urinary tract infection is a common complication of cesium implant therapy. Radiation cystitis also can occur, particularly if persistent bladder distention occurs.

5. Prolonged postoperative immobilization (complete bed rest for 3 days following cesium implant) carries a risk of thrombophlebitis. Possibly because tumor-induced hypercoagulability, a cancer client is at increased risk, even in the early stages of cancer.

6. Bowel dysfunction—either diarrhea or constipation—could cause cesium holder displacement.

Interventions

7. Monitor fluid loss through these routes:
   a. Vaginal drainage
   b. Urine output
   c. Vomiting or diarrhea

Related Physician-Prescribed Interventions

Medications
Not applicable

Intravenous Therapy
Not applicable

Laboratory Studies
Not applicable

Diagnostic Studies
X-ray films

Therapies
Isolation procedure

Rationale

7. Excessive fluid loss can cause serious problems in an already compromised client.

Postprocedure: Nursing Diagnoses

▲ Outcome Criteria

The client will:

1. Be able to communicate effectively her feelings regarding the cesium implant experience
2. Report only mild to moderate anxiety

Anxiety related to fear of radiation and its effects, uncertainty of outcome, feelings of isolation, and pain or discomfort

Focus Assessment Criteria

1. Anxiety level: mild, moderate, severe, or panic
2. Personal stressors
3. Knowledge of or past experience with radiation therapy and surgery
4. Specific fears and concerns

Clinical Significance

1–4. A client facing cancer and complex therapy may be justifiably afraid of many things, including pain, death, abandonment, dependency, and recurrence. The degree of anxiety a client experiences depends on how the client perceives the threat of cancer and treatment and on her coping ability.

Interventions

1. Assist the client to reduce her anxiety:
   a. Provide reassurance and comfort.
   b. Convey a sense of understanding and empathy.
   c. Encourage the client to verbalize any fears and concerns regarding cancer and cesium implant therapy.
   d. Identify and support effective coping mechanisms.
2. When the client's anxiety is at a mild to moderate level, take the opportunity to teach about procedures, home care, relaxation techniques, and so on.
3. Encourage family and friends to verbalize their fears and concerns to staff members.

4. Provide the client and family with valid reassurance and reinforce positive coping behavior.
5. Encourage the client to use relaxation techniques, such as guided imagery and relaxation breathing.
6. Contact the physician immediately if the client's anxiety is at the severe or panic level.

Rationale

1. An anxious client has a narrowed perceptual field with a diminished ability to learn. The client may experience symptoms caused by increased muscle tension and disrupted sleep patterns. Anxiety tends to feed upon itself, trapping the client in a spiral of increasing anxiety, tension, and emotional and physical pain.

2. Some fears are based on inaccurate information and can be relieved by providing accurate information. A client with severe or panic anxiety does not retain learning.
3. Verbalization allows sharing and provides the nurse with an opportunity to correct misconceptions.
4. Praising the client for effective coping can reinforce future positive coping responses.
5. Relaxation techniques enhance the client's sense of control over her body's response to stress.
6. Severe anxiety interferes with client learning and compliance.

▲ Documentation

Progress notes
Emotional status

▲ **Outcome Criteria**

The client will perform self-care tasks to the limit of her physical ability.

Self-Care Deficit (Bathing, Toileting) related to activity restrictions and isolation

Focus Assessment Criteria

1. Implications of complete bed rest and isolation for self-care
2. Perception of these implications and understanding of their temporary nature
3. Ability to cope and adapt

Clinical Significance

1–3. Cesium implant surgery involves complete bed rest for 3 days after surgery, limited visitation while the radioactive implant is in place, and activity restrictions for some time thereafter. The client needs help in managing some aspects of self-care; careful assessment can guide the nurse in planning appropriate and effective interventions.

Interventions

1. Provide physical care as needed, e.g., partial bathing (normal bathing after holder is removed), regular drawsheet changes.
2. Help the client keep needed items within easy reach.
3. Teach the client new ways to perform tasks that usually involve sitting, e.g., eat while lying on side.
4. Instruct the client to do prescribed leg exercises 8 to 10 times an hour every hour while awake.

▲ **Documentation**

Flow records
   Hygiene provided
   Leg exercises

5. Reassure the client that even though you and other staff members are able to spend only short periods in the room, someone is always immediately available if needed.

Rationale

1. Basic care is essential to maintain good hygiene when the client cannot do so herself.

2. Easy access reduces the need for movements that could cause holder dislodgment.
3. Sitting up in bed is prohibited to minimize the risk of dislodgment.

4. Passive or active muscle movement helps maintain skin integrity, full range of motion (ROM) in joints, and adequate circulation during periods of decreased mobility.
5. Reassurance can allay fears that staff will be unavailable and can ease feelings of isolation.

▲ **Outcome Criteria**

The client will not experience skin breakdown during hospitalization.

Potential Impaired Skin Integrity related to immobility secondary to prescribed activity restrictions

Focus Assessment Criteria

1. Skin, for signs of breakdown

Clinical Significance

1. During cesium implant therapy, complete bed rest with minimal movement is indicated. Immobility puts the client at risk for impaired skin integrity. The elderly, obese, frail, malnourished, or dehydrated, and those with compromised circulation are at high risk.

Interventions

1. Refer to the nursing diagnosis Potential Impaired Skin Integrity in the Immobility care plan, page 243, for specific interventions and rationales.

▲ **Outcome Criteria**

The client will:

1. Interact with staff and visitors to the extent that safety guidelines allow
2. Verbalize feelings of isolation
3. Identify appropriate diversional activities

Social Isolation related to precautions necessitated by cesium implant safety procedures

Focus Assessment Criteria

1. Client's self-perception, including the following:
   a. Feelings of loneliness
   b. Desire for more human contact

Clinical Significance

1. Social isolation can be a very subtle process involving gradual decreases in verbal and nonverbal communication, both in quality as well as in quantity. The client may be aware

Focus Assessment Criteria	*Clinical Significance*
c. Available support systems	of decreased touching and increased distancing, and a lack of feeling-level communication. The number and duration of visits may decrease. Coupled with the seemingly short and hurried visits by staff, this can rapidly lead to feelings of isolation.

Interventions

1. Explain the reasons for limiting visitors and staff (about ½ hour each visit and ½ hour of direct nursing care per nurse per shift) while the radioactive implant is in place.

2. Promote a pleasant environment; e.g., open curtains, keep the room clean, keep a telephone within easy reach.
3. Maintain frequent contact with the client; have someone check hourly on whether she needs anything. Keep a call bell within easy reach.
4. Encourage diversional activities; e.g., reading, talking on the telephone, listening to music, watching TV.

Rationale

1. The radiation safety precautions required during cesium implant therapy automatically put the client in a state of social isolation. Understanding why the precautions are necessary and that they are only temporary can help ease anxiety related to isolation.
2. Enhancing the client's immediate (and only) environment can help combat the negative aspects of isolation.
3. Although isolation cannot be avoided, frequent contact can ease its negative effects and help the client to cope.
4. Diversional activities can help reduce feelings of isolation and loneliness.

▲ **Documentation**

Progress notes
  Interactions
  Activities

▲ **Outcome Criteria**

The outcome criteria for this diagnosis represent those associated with discharge planning. Refer to the discharge criteria.

Potential Altered Health Maintenance related to insufficient knowledge of home care, reportable signs and symptoms, activity restrictions, and follow-up care

Focus Assessment Criteria	*Clinical Significance*
1. Knowledge of the discharge regimen for home care	1. During the postdischarge and follow-up periods, the client comes face to face with the everyday reality of the surgical loss and her ongoing battle with cancer. Nursing interventions call for skill in education, counseling, communication, and locating available community resources.
2. Readiness and ability to learn and retain information	2. A client or family failing to achieve learning goals requires a referral for assistance postdischarge.

Interventions

1. Teach the client that she must continue vaginal dilatation and douching for 1 year after treatment. Explain both methods—sexual intercourse and manual obturator—and the need for dilatation at least three times a week.

2. Elicit a sexual history to determine the feasibility and desirability of engaging in sexual intercourse at least three times a week.

3. If the client chooses to use sexual intercourse for vaginal dilatation, explain that she can resume intercourse 3 weeks after discharge (unless contraindicated) but needs to use a water-based vaginal lubricant (e.g., K-Y jelly). Encourage intercourse at least three times a week.

Rationale

1. Cesium implant, like other pelvic irradiation procedures, may lead to vaginal narrowing or collapse and pelvic fibrosis. Regular vaginal dilatation is essential to minimize these effects, both to maintain normal sexual function and to facilitate follow-up pelvic examinations.
2. Assessing these factors helps the nurse guide the client in choosing the optimum dilatation method: sexual intercourse, mechanical obturation, or a combination of the two.
3. Water-based lubricant is necessary to replace the normal vaginal lubrication lost as a result of radiation therapy and to prevent dyspareunia.

Interventions

4. Reassure the client that she need not be concerned about exposing her partner to radiation.

5. If the client chooses to use an obturator as the sole or a supplemental means of vaginal dilatation, teach proper use:
   a. Inspect the obturator for rough edges or cracks. Do not use an obturator that is not perfectly smooth.
   b. Wash the obturator in hot soapy water and rinse well.
   c. Apply lubricating jelly to the rounded end of the obturator.
   d. Lie on your back with your knees slightly apart, and insert the rounded end of the obturator into the vagina.
   e. Advance the obturator into the vagina as far as you can without causing discomfort. Then withdraw and reinsert the device, again advancing it as deeply as possible. Do this for 5 minutes.
   f. After withdrawing the obturator for the last time, wash it in hot soapy water, rinse and dry it completely, and store it where it will not be dropped or damaged.
   g. Take a vinegar douche (1 tsp of vinegar to 1000 mL of water) after dilatating with the obturator.
   h. Continue to use the obturator at least three times a week (if it is the sole means of dilatation) or as necessary to supplement intercourse to provide dilatation three times a week.

6. Explain that slight vaginal bleeding after intercourse or obturator use, which may persist for a few weeks to a year after treatment, is normal and is no cause for concern.

7. Instruct the client and family on activity restrictions:
   a. Gradually increase activity only as tolerated.
   b. Schedule three or four 15- to 30-minute rest periods each day.

8. Instruct the client to avoid foods that irritate the bowel (e.g., fruits, raw vegetables, other high-fiber foods) if diarrhea becomes a problem.

9. Teach to observe for and promptly report these signs and symptoms:
   a. Unusual, heavy, bright-red, or foul-smelling vaginal discharge
   b. Foul-smelling or cloudy urine

   c. Low-grade fever
   d. Persistent diarrhea or constipation

   e. Difficult or painful vaginal dilatation

Rationale

4. The client may need reassurance that the radiation source is eliminated after removal of the cesium implant and that intercourse is perfectly safe.

5. Careful, thorough teaching about obturator use, emphasizing the need for long-term regular dilatation, can help promote compliance with dilatation therapy after discharge. Many clients—particularly many elderly women—find the obturation procedure degrading and repulsive, and need extra encouragement and attention.

6. Understanding that slight bleeding is normal helps reduce anxiety.

7. Regular activity within tolerance limits is necessary to minimize the complications associated with immobility.

8. Bowel upset and diarrhea commonly persist for 3 weeks to 3 months after cesium implant therapy.

9. Early detection of complications enables prompt intervention to decrease their severity.
   a. Changes in discharge may signal bleeding or infection.
   b. Urine changes may indicate urinary tract infection.
   c. Fever is a cardinal sign of infection.
   d. Diarrhea or constipation may be an inflammatory bowel response.
   e. Problems with dilatation reflect vaginal stenosis.

▲ **Documentation**

Discharge summary record
  Status at discharge
  Client teaching
  Outcome achievement or
    status
  Referrals, if indicated

Interventions	*Rationale*
10. Provide a list of available community resources or refer to social services for other referrals.	**10.** The client and family may need assistance to cope with the varied demands cancer places on roles, relationships, financial status, and other aspects of life.

References/Bibliography

Burns, N. (1982). *Nursing and cancer.* Philadelphia: W.B. Saunders.

Hassey, K. (1985). Demystifying care of patients with radioactive implants. *American Journal of Nursing, 85*(3), 788–792.

McNally, J.C., et al. (1985). *Guidelines for cancer nursing practice.* Orlando, FL: Grune and Stratton.

Richards, S., & Hiratzka, S. (1986). Vaginal dilatation post-pelvic irradiation: A patient education tool. *Oncology Nursing Forum, 13*(4), 89–91.

Vredevor, D.L. (1981). *Concepts of oncology nursing.* Englewood Cliffs, NJ: Prentice-Hall.

Chemotherapy

This systemic cancer treatment modality aims to safely eradicate or control the growth of cancerous cells by producing maximum cancer cell death with minimum toxicity. Chemotherapy may be the sole treatment provided, as with leukemia, or it may be used in combination with surgery, radiation, or biological response therapy. Chemotherapeutic agents may be given alone or in combination and may be administered either continuously or intermittently using various routes, techniques, and special equipment. Most agents affect proliferating cells and thus are most effective against rapidly dividing cancer cells. However, they also can damage rapidly dividing normal cells, such as blood cells and cells of the gastrointestinal (GI) epithelium and hair follicles, producing adverse effects that require careful management.

Diagnostic Cluster

▲ Time Frame
Pretherapy and intratherapy

▲ Discharge Planning
Before discharge, the client and/or family will:

1. Relate home care requirements (rest, oral care, nutrition)
2. Describe signs and symptoms that must be reported to a health care professional
3. Relate an intent to share feelings with significant others
4. Identify available community resources

Collaborative Problems

Potential Complications:
Anaphylactic Reaction
Congestive Heart Failure
Electrolyte Imbalance
Extravasation of Vesicant Drugs
Hemorrhagic Cystitis
Myelosuppression
Renal Insufficiency
Lung Fibrosis
Neurotoxicity
Renal Calculi

Nursing Diagnoses

Anxiety related to prescribed chemotherapy, insufficient knowledge of chemotherapy, and self-care measures

Altered Comfort related to gastrointestinal cell damage, stimulation of vomiting center, fear, and anxiety

Altered Nutrition: Less Than Body Requirements, related to anorexia, taste changes, persistent nausea/vomiting, and increased metabolic rate

Altered Oral Mucous Membrane related to dryness and epithelial cell damage secondary to chemotherapy

Fatigue related to effects of anemia, malnutrition, persistent vomiting, and sleep pattern disturbance

Potential Colonic Constipation related to autonomic nerve dysfunction secondary to *Vinca* alkaloid administration and inactivity

Diarrhea related to intestinal cell damage, inflammation, and increased intestinal mobility

Potential Impaired Skin Integrity related to persistent diarrhea, malnutrition, prolonged sedation, and fatigue

Self-Concept Disturbance related to change in life style, role, alopecia, and weight loss or gain

Refer to:

Inflammatory Joint Disease
Immobility or Unconsciousness

Inflammatory Intestinal Disease
Immobility or Unconsciousness
Cancer (Initial Diagnosis)

Collaborative Problems

▲ *Nursing Goal*
The nurse will manage and mini-mize complications of chemo-therapy.

Potential Complication: Anaphylactic Reaction
Potential Complication: Congestive Heart Failure
Potential Complication: Electrolyte Imbalance
Potential Complication: Extravasation of Vesicant Drugs
Potential Complication: Hemorrhagic Cystitis
Potential Complication: Myelosuppression
Potential Complication: Renal Insufficiency
Potential Complication: Lung Fibrosis
Potential Complication: Neurotoxicity
Potential Complication: Renal Calculi

Interventions

1. Inquire about previous drug reactions and record baseline vital signs and mental status before administering chemotherapy.

2. Monitor for symptoms of anaphylactic reaction:
   a. Urticaria, pruritus
   b. Sensation of lump in throat
   c. Shortness of breath

3. If symptoms develop, discontinue chemotherapy and apply a tourniquet proximal to the injection site.

4. Monitor vital signs every 15 minutes until stable.

5. Monitor for signs and symptoms of congestive heart failure (CHF):
   a. Gradual increase in heart rate
   b. Increased shortness of breath
   c. Diminished breath sound, rales
   d. Decreased systolic blood pressure
   e. Presence of or increase in S3 or S4 gallop
   f. Peripheral edema
   g. Distended neck veins

6. Monitor for electrolyte imbalances:

   a. Hyponatremia or hypernatremia

   b. Hypokalemia or hyperkalemia

   c. Hypomagnesemia

Rationale

1. Any cytotoxic drug—including cisplatin, teniposide, nitrogen mustard, doxorubicin, bleomycin, and methotrexate—can precipitate anaphylaxis. Release of histamine in an antigen–antibody reaction results in cutaneous symptoms (urticaria, pruritus) and systemic symptoms (laryngeal edema, bronchospasm, and dyspnea).

2. These assessment steps help determine the risk of complications and provide a baseline against which to compare subsequent findings.

3. Prompt discontinuation prevents possible serious response; tourniquet application retards drug absorption.

4. Careful monitoring can detect early signs of hypotension and shock.

5. CHF is associated with cardiotoxic effects and dysrhythmias precipitated by cardiotoxic drugs such as daunorubicin and doxorubicin, especially in high-dose therapy.

6. Chemotherapeutic agents often precipitate electrolyte imbalance.
   a. Hyponatremia is caused by secretion of antidiuretic hormone secondary to vincristine or cyclophosphamide therapy, excessive hydration, or decrease in peripheral blast count secondary to daunorubicin or cytosine therapy. Hypernatremia may result from renal failure secondary to drug nephrotoxicity.

   b. Hypokalemia may be due to intercellular shift, excessive diarrhea, or renal tubular injury. Hyperkalemia is caused by cell lysis and renal damage.

   c. Hypomagnesemia can result from vomiting, diarrhea, or cisplatin therapy, which causes excretion of divalent ions.

Interventions

    d. Hypophosphatemia

    e. Hypocalcemia or hypercalcemia
      (Refer to the Collaborative Problems section of the Chronic Renal Failure care plan for specific signs and symptoms of each electrolyte imbalance.)

7. Monitor and teach the client and family to monitor for and report the following:
   a. Excessive fluid loss or gain
   b. Change in orientation or level of consciousness
   c. Changes in vital signs
   d. Weakness or ataxia
   e. Paresthesias
   f. Seizure activity
   g. Persistent headache
   h. Muscle cramps, twitching, or tetany
   i. Nausea and vomiting
   j. Diarrhea

8. Take steps to reduce extravasation of vesicant medications—agents that cause severe necrosis if they leak from blood vessels into tissue. Examples of vesicant medications are the following: amsacrine, bisantrene, dactinomycin, dacarbazine, daunomycin, daunorubicin, estramustine, maytansine, mithramycin, mitomycin, nitrogen mustard, pyrazofurin, vinblastine, vincristine, and vindesine.
   a. Preventive measures are as follows:
      • Avoid using the antecubital fossa, wrist, and hand when administering vesicants.
      • Avoid multiple punctures of the same vein.
      • Administer the drug through a long-term venous catheter.
      • Do not administer the drug if edema is present.

9. Monitor during drug infusion:
   a. Assess patency of intravenous (IV) infusion line.
   b. Observe tissue at the IV site every 30 minutes for the following:
      • Leakage
      • Burning
      • Swelling
      • Inflammation
      • Erythema
      • Hyperpigmentation
      • Ulceration
      • Necrosis

10. If extravasation occurs, take the following steps, depending on the agent.
    a. With doxorubicin:
       • Remove the IV line immediately.
       • Apply ice.
    b. With nitrogen mustard:
       • Remove the IV line immediately.

Rationale

    d. Hypophosphatemia is associated with hypercalcemia, hypokalemia, and hypomagnesemia.

    e. Hypercalcemia is secondary to hypophosphatemia, renal failure, or mithramycin therapy; hypocalcemia, to hyperphosphatemia or renal failure.

7. Electrolyte imbalances affect neurotransmission, muscle activity, and fluid balance.

8. Extravasation may occur secondary to improper placement, damaged vein, or obstructed venous drainage secondary to superior vena cava syndrome, edema, or tumor.

9,10. Detecting signs of extravasation early enables prompt intervention to prevent serious complications, including tissue necrosis.

Interventions

    c. With *Vinca* alkaloids (vinblastine, vincristine, vendesine):
- Remove the IV line immediately.
- Do not apply ice, because it increases skin toxicity of *Vinca* alkaloids.

11. When administering cyclophosphamide, monitor for signs and symptoms of hemorrhagic cystitis:
    a. Dysuria
    b. Frequency
    c. Urgency
    d. Hematuria
12. Administer cyclophosphamide early in the day.

13. Teach the client to do the following:
    a. Void every 2 hours
    b. Increase fluid intake to 2500 to 3000 mL/day, unless contraindicated.
14. Monitor for signs of myelosuppression:
    a. Decreased white blood cell (WBC) and red blood cell (RBC) counts
    b. Decreased platelet count

15. Explain the risks of bleeding and infection. (Refer to the Corticosteroid Therapy care plan, page 542, for strategies to reduce these risks.)

16. Monitor for signs of renal insufficiency:

    a. Sustained elevated urine specific gravity
    b. Elevated urine sodium levels

    c. Sustained insufficient urine output (< 30 mL/hr)
    d. Elevated blood pressure

    e. Increasing blood urea nitrogen (BUN) and serum creatinine, potassium, phosphorus, and ammonia, and decreased creatinine clearance
17. When administering bleomycin and nitrosoureas, monitor for signs and symptoms of lung fibrosis:
    a. Cough
    b. Fever
    c. Tachycardia
    d. Dyspnea
    e. Weakness
    f. Cyanosis
    g. Abnormal arterial blood gas analysis
    h. Abnormal chest x-ray film
    i. Abnormal pulmonary function tests
18. Instruct the client to cough and do deep breathing every 2 hours.

Rationale

11. Cyclophosphamide administration is associated with the development of hemorrhagic cystitis.

12. Administration early in the day reduces the high drug concentration that can occur during the night secondary to reduced intake.
13. Frequent voiding and optimal hydration reduce drug concentration in the bladder.

14. Chemotherapeutic agents act primarily on rapidly dividing cells, such as bone marrow cells, WBCs, and platelets. Although RBCs are less affected because they divide more slowly, anemia still may develop.
15. Decreased or nonfunctioning WBCs impair the body's phagocytic defense against microorganisms. Platelets form a temporary plug to stop bleeding and activate clotting factors; decreased platelets can interfere with clotting.
16. Cisplatin, methotrexate, and mitomycin are nephrotoxic drugs, producing possibly toxic effects on the renal glomeruli and tubules.
    a,b. Decreased ability of the renal tubules to reabsorb electrolytes causes increased urine sodium levels and increased urine specific gravity.
    c,d. Decreased glomerular filtration rate eventually causes insufficient urine output and stimulates renin production, leading to blood pressure elevation in an attempt to increase blood flow to the kidneys.
    e. Decreased excretion of urea and creatinine in the urine results in elevated BUN and creatinine, triggering the other changes.
17. Lung inflammation and fibrosis are associated with administration of bleomycin and nitrosoureas. The extent of fibrosis determines the severity of respiratory dysfunction.

18. These activities help reduce retention of secretions and dilate alveoli.

Interventions

19. When administering *Vinca* alkaloids and L-asparaginase, monitor for signs and symptoms of neurotoxicity:
    a. Paresthesias
    b. Gait disturbance
    c. Altered fine motor activity
    d. Constipation
    e. Lethargy
    f. Numbness
    g. Muscle weakness
    h. Foot or wrist drop
    i. Somnolence
    j. Disorientation
    k. Impotence
    l. Confusion
20. If dysfunction results from neurotoxicity, refer to the Immobility care plan, page 243, for interventions to prevent complications.
21. Monitor for signs and symptoms of renal calculi:
    a. Flank pain
    b. Nausea and vomiting
    c. Abdominal pain

22. Refer to the Urolithiasis care plan, page 195, for specific interventions to reduce the risk of renal calculi.

Rationale

19. High or cumulative doses of *Vinca* alkaloids can impair neural conduction. L-Asparaginase has been linked to cerebral dysfunction.

20. Prompt intervention is necessary to prevent serious complications.

21. Renal calculi may result from chemotherapy as rapid cell lysis of tumor cells produces hyperuricemia. Pain is caused by the pressure of calculi on the renal tubules. Afferent stimuli in renal capsule may cause pylorospasm of the smooth muscle of the enteric tract and adjacent structures.

▲ **Documentation**

Flow records
    Vital signs
    Abnormal laboratory values
    (electrolytes, CBC, platelets, BUN)
    Condition of injection sites
    Intake and output
    Urine specific gravity
    Client teaching
    Progress notes
    Complaints of rashes, unusual sensations

Related Physician-Prescribed Interventions
Medications
    Antiemetics
Intravenous Therapy
    Not indicated
Laboratory Studies
    Complete blood count   BUN
    Urinalysis   Serum albumin
    Electrolytes
Diagnostic Studies
    Not indicated
Therapies
    Not indicated

Nursing Diagnoses

▲ **Outcome Criteria**

The client will:

1. Share feelings regarding scheduled chemotherapy
2. Describe the anticipated effects of chemotherapy
3. Relate signs and symptoms of toxicity
4. Identify important self-care measures

Anxiety related to prescribed chemotherapy, insufficient knowledge of chemotherapy, and self-care measures

Focus Assessment Criteria

1. Attitude and experiences with chemotherapy

Clinical Significance

1. Chemotherapy is poorly understood and feared by the general public. Personal experiences with friends and relatives influence the client's emotional response.

Focus Assessment Criteria	*Clinical Significance*
2. Knowledge of treatment plan 3. Knowledge of the effects and management of chemotherapy effects 4. Knowledge of signs and symptoms of toxicity	2,3. The client's understanding of the chemotherapeutic regimen and side effects and their management enhances his or her sense of control and can reduce anxiety. 4. This information enables the client to detect problems early and promotes involvement in the care regimen.

Interventions	*Rationale*

1. Encourage the client to share feelings and beliefs regarding chemotherapy. Delay teaching if high levels of anxiety are present.
2. Reinforce the physician's explanations of the chemotherapeutic regimen—the drugs, dosage schedules, actions, and side effects.
3. Explain the therapeutic effects of cytotoxic drugs; provide written information. (*Note:* Client education booklets are available from the National Cancer Institute and the American Cancer Society.)
4. Explain the common side effects and toxicities of chemotherapy:
  a. Decreased WBC count
  b. Decreased platelet count
  c. Infection
  d. Gastrointestinal (GI) alterations
  e. Hair loss
  f. Fatigue
  g. Emotional responses
5. Discuss self-care measures to reduce the risk of toxicities:
  a. Nutrition
  b. Hygiene
  c. Rest
  d. Activity
6. Refer also to the Cancer (Initial Diagnosis) care plan, page 322, for additional information.
	1. Verbalization can identify sources of anxiety and allow the nurse to correct misinformation. High anxiety impairs learning.
	2–5. Specific explanations provide information to help reduce anxiety associated with fear of the unknown and loss of control.

▲ **Documentation**

Discharge summary record or teaching record
  Client teaching
  Outcome achievement or status
Progress notes
  Dialogues

▲ **Outcome Criteria**

The client will:

1. Report decreased nausea and vomiting
2. Report increasing ability to tolerate food and fluids

Altered Comfort related to gastrointestinal cell damage, stimulation of vomiting center, and fear and anxiety

Focus Assessment Criteria	*Clinical Significance*

1. Factors contributing to or promoting nausea and vomiting:
  a. Chemotherapeutic agents
  b. Antiemetic therapy
  c. Activity
  d. Fear and anxiety
  e. Food or fluid ingestion
  f. Changes in taste sensation
  g. Environmental conditions (e.g., odors)
2. Frequency and severity of vomiting episodes
3. Signs and symptoms of fluid and electrolyte imbalance
	1. Chemotherapy-induced nausea and vomiting result from both physiological and psychological factors. Cytotoxic drugs damage GI cells, which can produce a vagal response. They can also stimulate the vomiting center in the brain. Anxiety and fear contribute to the problem.
	
	2,3. Severe or prolonged vomiting can cause fluid and electrolyte imbalances.

Interventions

1. Promote a positive attitude about chemotherapy; reinforce its cancer cell-killing effects.
2. Explain the possible reasons for nausea and vomiting.

3. Explain the rationale for antiemetic agents, and administer them before initiating chemotherapy.
4. Infuse cytotoxic drugs slowly.

5. Administer cytotoxic drugs at night (during sleep if possible), or have the client lie quietly for 2 hours after administration.
6. Suggest that the client suck on hard candy during chemotherapy.

7. Encourage the client to eat small, frequent meals and to eat slowly.
8. Eliminate unpleasant sights and odors from the eating area.
9. Instruct the client to avoid the following:

    a. Hot or cold liquids

    b. Foods containing fat and fiber

    c. Caffeine
10. Encourage the client to rest in semi-Fowler's position after eating and to change position slowly.
11. Teach stress reduction techniques, such as these:
    a. Relaxation exercises
    b. Visual imagery

Rationale

1. Frank discussions can increase motivation to reduce and tolerate nausea.
2. Helping the client understand the reason for nausea and vomiting can reduce fear associated with the unexpected.
3. Antiemetics are given before chemotherapy to reduce nausea.

4. Slow infusion can decrease stimulation of the vomiting center.
5. Activity stimulates the GI tract, which can increase nausea and vomiting.

6. Hard candy can reduce the metallic or bitter taste that a client commonly experiences during chemotherapy.
7. Intake of small amounts prevents gastric distention from stimulating vomiting.
8. Eliminating noxious stimuli can decrease stimulation of the vomiting center.
9. Certain foods increase peristalsis and provoke nausea and vomiting.
    a. Cold liquids can induce cramping; hot liquids can stimulate peristalsis.
    b. High-fat and high-fiber food and drinks increase peristalsis.
    c. Caffeine stimulates intestinal motility.
10. Muscle relaxation can reduce peristalsis.

11. These techniques reduce muscle tension and decrease the client's focus on nausea.

▲ **Documentation**

Flow records
    Intake and output
    Tolerance of intake

▲ **Outcome Criteria**

The client will:
1. Maintain ideal weight with no further weight loss
2. Exhibit normal BUN and serum albumin and protein laboratory values

Altered Nutrition: Less Than Body Requirements related to anorexia, taste changes, persistent nausea/vomiting, and increased metabolic rate

Focus Assessment Criteria

1. Actual weight versus ideal weight
2. History of weight loss
3. Dietary intake
4. Reports of the following:
    a. Fatigue
    b. Anorexia
    c. Taste changes
    d. Nausea and vomiting
    e. Chemotherapy
    f. Stress and anxiety
5. Laboratory findings: serum albumin and protein

Clinical Significance

1–3. A baseline is needed to assess quality and amount of intake and to monitor for negative nitrogen balance.
4. This assessment identifies factors that may be interfering with intake.

5. Decreased protein intake results in decreased plasma proteins.

Interventions

1. Help the client identify reasons for inadequate nutrition and explain possible causes:
    a. Increased metabolic rate

Rationale

1. Nutritional deficits associated with chemotherapy can have many causes. Cytotoxic drugs can stimulate the vomiting center in the brain.

Interventions

    b. GI tract injury
    c. Stimulation of vomiting
    d. Decreased appetite
    e. Taste changes
    f. Anxiety and fear

  2. Stress the need to increase caloric intake.

  3. Encourage resting before meals.
  4. Offer small, frequent meals (optimally, six per day plus snacks).

  5. Restrict liquids with meals and avoid fluids 1 hour before and after meals.

  6. Maintain good oral hygiene before and after eating.
  7. Arrange to have the foods with the greatest protein and caloric value served at the times the client feels most like eating.
  8. Teach techniques to reduce nausea:
    a. Avoid the smell of food preparation and other noxious stimuli.
    b. Loosen clothing before eating.
    c. Sit in fresh air.
    d. Avoid lying flat for at least 2 hours after eating. (A client who must rest should sit or recline with the head elevated at least 4 inches higher than the feet.)
  9. Instruct the client to limit foods and fluids high in fat.
10. Suggest dietary modifications such as these:
    a. Eating fish, chicken, eggs, and cheese if pork and beef taste bitter
    b. Eating meat for breakfast rather than later in the day
    c. Experimenting with different flavorings and seasonings
11. Teach techniques to enhance protein and calorie content when preparing meals at home:
    a. Add powdered milk or egg to milkshakes, gravies, sauces, puddings, cereals, meatballs, or milk to increase protein and calorie content.
    b. Add blenderized or baby foods to meat juices or soups.
    c. Use fortified milk (i.e., 1 cup instant nonfat milk added to 1 quart fresh milk).

Rationale

    (See the nursing diagnosis Altered Comfort: Nausea/Vomiting in this entry for more information.) They also can alter GI cells, causing anorexia, taste changes, nausea and vomiting, and altered protein metabolism. Damage to the absorptive surface of the GI mucosa can lead to nutrient malabsorption. Chemotherapy-induced mucositis also inhibits intake and absorption of nutrients. Finally, anxiety and stress can inhibit appetite and lead to decreased intake.

  2. Cytotoxic drugs raise the metabolic rate through destruction of rapidly proliferating cells. This factor, coupled with the body's increased nutritional needs resulting from GI damage or other factors, necessitates increased caloric intake to maintain adequate nutritional status.

  3. Fatigue further decreases appetite.
  4. Increased intra-abdominal pressure from fluid accumulation (ascites) compresses the GI tract and decreases capacity.

  5. Fluid restrictions at meals can help prevent gastric overdistention and can enhance appetite.

  6. Poor oral hygiene can result in foul odors or taste, which diminishes appetite.
  7. This strategy increases the client's chance of consuming more protein and calories.

  8. Nausea can be reduced by controlling environmental conditions and promoting positions that minimize abdominal pressure.

  9. Fatty foods are difficult to absorb.

10. These measures can help make food more palatable and encourage increased intake.

11. These simple measures can increase the nutritional content of foods even when intake is limited.

Interventions

    d. Use milk or half-and-half instead of water when making soups and sauces: soy formulas can also be used.

    e. Add cheese or diced meat whenever able.

    f. Add cream cheese or peanut butter to toast, crackers, celery sticks.

    g. Add extra butter or margarine to soups, sauces, vegetables.

    h. Use mayonnaise (100 cal/T) instead of salad dressing.

    i. Add sour cream or yogurt to vegetables or as dip.

    j. Use whipped cream (60 cal/T) as much as possible.

    k. Add raisins, dates, nuts, and brown sugar to hot or cold cereals.

    l. Have snacks readily available.

12. Refer the client to a dietitian for further nutritional information.

Rationale

12. Additional nutritional information can be acquired from an expert

▲ **Documentation**

Flow records
    Weight
    Intake (type, amount)
Progress notes
    Complaints of nausea
    and vomiting

▲ **Outcome Criteria**

The client will:

1. Relate the need for optimal oral hygiene
2. Report decreased discomfort

Altered Oral Mucous Membrane related to dryness and epithelial cell damage secondary to chemotherapy

Focus Assessment Criteria	*Clinical Significance*
1. Oral mucosa for redness, swelling, dryness, lesions, ulcerations, viscous saliva, and infection 2. Difficulty swallowing 3. Pain or discomfort in oral mucosa	1–3. Cytotoxic drugs damage the rapidly dividing epithelial cells lining the oral mucosa. They also decrease WBC count, predisposing to stomatitis, a condition that interferes with salivation. The resulting mucosal dryness increases the risk of damage. Difficulty swallowing inhibits oral fluid intake, also enhancing oral dryness and discomfort.

Interventions

1. Explain the need for regular, meticulous oral hygiene.

2. Instruct the client to do the following:

    a. Perform the oral care regimen after meals and before bedtime (and, if necessary, before breakfast).

    b. Avoid mouthwashes high in alcohol, lemon/glycerine swabs, and prolonged use of hydrogen peroxide.

    c. Use an oxidizing agent to loosen thick, tenacious mucus; gargle and expectorate. For example, use hydrogen peroxide and water ¼ strength (avoid prolonged use) or 1 T sodium bicarbonate mixed in 8 oz warm water (flavored, if desired, with mouthwash, oil of wintergreen, etc.).

    d. Rinse the mouth with saline solution after gargling.

    e. Apply a lubricant to lips every 2 hours and as needed (e.g., lanolin, A & D ointment, petroleum jelly).

Rationale

1. Chemotherapy increases the mucosal cells' susceptibility to infection. Frequent oral hygiene removes microorganisms and reduces the risk.

2. These practices can eliminate sources of microorganism growth and prevent mucosal drying and damage.

Interventions

    f. Inspect the mouth daily for lesions and inflammation, and report any alterations.

3. If the client cannot tolerate brushing or swabbing, teach mouth irrigation:

    a. Use a baking soda solution (4 T in 1 liter warm water) in an enema bag (labeled for oral use only) with a soft irrigation catheter tip.

    b. Place the catheter in the mouth and slowly increase the flow while standing over a basin or having someone hold a basin under the chin.

    c. Remove dentures before irrigation; do not replace them if the client has severe stomatitis.

    d. Perform irrigation every 2 hours or as needed.

4. Teach precautionary measures:

    a. Breathe through the nose rather than the mouth.

    b. Consume cool, soothing liquids and semisolids, such as gelatin.

    c. Avoid smoking.

    d. Avoid hot and spicy or acidic food and fluids.

    e. Omit flossing if excessive bleeding occurs.

5. Consult with the physician for an oral pain relief solution; e.g., lidocaine (xylocaine), diphenhydramine.

Rationale

3. Brushing can further damage irritated mucosa; these measures enable maintenance of good hygiene in clients who cannot brush.

4. These practices can reduce oral irritation.

5. Medications may be needed to reduce pain and enable adequate nutritional intake.

▲ **Documentation**

Flow records
    Oral assessments
    Treatments

References/Bibliography

Carpenito, L.J. (1989). *Nursing diagnoses: Application to clinical practice* (3rd ed.). Philadelphia: J.B. Lippincott.

Chennecky, C.C., & Ramsey, P.W. (1984). *Critical nursing care of the client with cancer.* E. Norwalk, CT: Appleton-Century-Crofts.

Groenwald, S.L. (1987). *Cancer nursing principles and practice.* Boston, MA: Jones and Bartlett Publishers.

Love, R.R., et al. (1989). Side effects and emotional distress during cancer chemotherapy. *Cancer, 63*(3), 604–612.

Lydon, J. (1989). Assessment of renal function in the patient receiving chemotherapy. *Cancer Nursing, 12*(3), 133–143.

Mariono, L.B. (1981). *Cancer nursing.* St. Louis: C.V. Mosby.

McNally, J.C., Stair, J.C., & Somerville, E. (1985). *Guidelines for cancer nursing practice.* Orlando, FL: Grune & Stratton.

Morrow, G.R. (1989). Chemotherapy-related nausea and vomiting: Etiology and management. *CA, 39*(2), 89–104.

Rhodes, V.A., et al. (1988). Patterns of nausea and vomiting in antineoplastic postchemotherapy patients. *Applied Nursing Research, 1*(3), 143–144.

Ulrick, C.P., Canale, S.W., & Wendell, S.A. (1986). *Nursing care planning guides: A nursing diagnosis approach.* Philadelphia: W.B. Saunders.

Corticosteroid Therapy

Corticosteroids are indicated as replacement therapy for adrenal insufficiency, for inflammation suppression, for control of allergic reactions, and for reducing the risk of graft rejection in transplantation. A client on long-term corticosteroid therapy has suppressed pituitary and adrenal function.

Diagnostic Cluster

▲ **Time Frame**

Pretherapy and intratherapy

▲ **Discharge Criteria**

Before discharge, the client and/or family will:

1. Relate proper use of the medication
2. Identify circumstances that require notification of a health care professional
3. Relate dietary sodium restrictions
4. Identify signs and symptoms of side effects and adverse reactions
5. Describe practices that can reduce the side effects of corticosteroid therapy
6. Verbalize an intent to seek ongoing follow-up care
7. Verbalize an intent to wear Medic-alert identification

Collaborative Problems

Potential Complications:
Diabetes Mellitus
Hypertension
Osteoporosis
Peptic Ulcer
Thromboembolism
Hypokalemia
Avascular Necrosis

Nursing Diagnoses

Potential Fluid Volume Excess related to sodium and water retention
Potential Altered Nutrition: more than body requirements related to increased appetite
Potential for Infection related to immunosuppression
Potential Self-Concept Disturbance related to changes in appearance
Potential Altered Health Maintenance related to insufficient knowledge of administration schedule, adverse reactions, signs and symptoms of complications, hazards of adrenal insufficiency, and potential causes of adrenal insufficiency

Collaborative Problems

▲ **Nursing Goal**

The nurse will manage and minimize complications of corticosteroid therapy.

Potential Complication: **Diabetes Mellitus**
Potential Complication: **Hypertension**
Potential Complication: **Osteoporosis**
Potential Complication: **Peptic Ulcer Disease**
Potential Complication: **Thromboembolism**
Potential Complication: **Hypokalemia**
Potential Complication: **Avascular Necrosis**

Interventions

1. Monitor for signs and symptoms of diabetes mellitus:
   a. Polyuria, polydipsia
   b. Glycosuria
   c. Proteinuria
2. Monitor for hypertension.

3. Monitor for signs and symptoms of osteoporosis:
   a. Pain
   b. Localized tenderness

Rationale

1. Excessive glucocorticoid level antagonizes insulin and promotes glyconeogenesis, resulting in increased urine excretion and thirst.

2. Mineralocorticoids increase sodium reabsorption, with resulting fluid retention.
3. Corticosteroids increase calcium and phosphorus excretion and bone wasting.

Interventions

4. Teach the client measures to reduce the risk of pathological fractures. (Refer to the Osteoporosis care plan, page 291, for more details.)
5. Teach the relationship of increased calcium and vitamin D intake and weightbearing exercise to reduced risk of osteoporosis.

6. Monitor for signs and symptoms of peptic ulcer:
   a. Positive guaiac stool test
   b. Gastric pain
7. Teach the client to take prescribed medication with food or milk.
8. Monitor for signs and symptoms of thromboembolism:
   a. Edema
   b. Decreased capillary refill time
   c. Pain
   d. Paresthesias
   e. Redness, pallor, or cyanosis
9. Monitor for signs and symptoms of hypokalemia:
   a. Weakness
   b. Lethargy
   c. Serum potassium level < 3.5 mEq/L
   d. Nausea and vomiting
   e. Characteristic electrocardiographic (ECG) changes

Related Physician-Prescribed Interventions

Symptom-specific

Rationale

4. A client on long-term corticosteroid therapy—especially an elderly client—is at increased risk for fractures owing to loss of bone density.
5. Increase in vitamin D and calcium intake increases their availability to bone. Weightbearing exercise (e.g., walking) slows the rate of calcium loss from bone.
6. Corticosteroid therapy causes increased secretion of gastric hydrochloric acid (an irritant) and decreased secretion of gastric mucus (a protectant).
7. Food or milk can help neutralize the gastric hydrochloric acid, minimizing gastric upset.
8. Corticosteroids stimulate red blood cell production, increasing blood viscosity and increasing the risk of thrombophlebitis.

9. Excessive mineralocorticoids increase sodium retention and potassium excretion.

▲ *Documentation*

Flow records
    Vital signs
    Urine glucose and other laboratory values
    Pain and numbness in extremities
    Gastric pain
    Intake and output
    Stool guaiac results

Nursing Diagnoses

▲ *Outcome Criteria*

The client will:
1. Relate causative factors of edema
2. State controllable factors for edema prevention

Potential Fluid Volume Excess related to sodium and water retention

Focus Assessment Criteria

1. Current daily corticosteroid dosage
2. Recent weight gain
3. Presence and extent of edema
4. Dietary sodium intake
5. Blood pressure readings

Clinical Significance

1–5. These assessment data help the nurse identify risks for and the presence of edema.

Interventions

1. Encourage the client to decrease sodium intake, and provide some strategies:
   a. Review foods high in sodium.
   b. Discuss changes in food preparation methods that decrease overall sodium intake.

2. Identify strategies to decrease dependent edema:
   a. Frequent position changes
   b. Avoiding constrictive clothing
   c. Elevating the legs when sitting
   d. Wearing elastic support stockings

Rationale

1. Corticosteroids contain both glucocorticoid and mineralocorticoid elements. The mineralocorticoid element promotes sodium reabsorption and potassium excretion from distal renal tubules. Resultant sodium retention expands extracellular fluid volume by preventing water excretion.
2. Edema develops as increased extracellular fluid enters interstitial spaces and the blood, increasing interstitial fluid and blood volume.

Flow records
  Weight
  Presence and degree of
    edema

▲ **Outcome Criteria**

The client will:

1. Relate factors that contribute to weight gain
2. Identify behaviors that remain under his or her control

Interventions

3. Explain measures to protect the skin from injury:
   a. Avoid walking barefoot
   b. Breaking in new shoes slowly
   c. Avoiding contact sports

Rationale

3. Besides the increased risk of skin injury due to edema, the loss of perivascular collagen in the small vessels of the skin makes them more susceptible to damage.

Potential Altered Nutrition: More than Body Requirements related to increased appetite

Focus Assessment Criteria	Clinical Significance
1. Current corticosteroid dosage 2. Knowledge of nutritional concepts 3. Current eating patterns 4. Willingness to comply with dietary modifications	1–3. The weight gain associated with corticosteroid therapy is related to both fluid retention and the drug's appetite-enhancing effects. 4. The client's cooperation is essential to prevent weight gain or to promote weight loss.

Interventions

1. Increase the client's awareness of actions that contribute to excessive food intake:
   a. Request that he write down all the food he ate in the past 24 hours.
   b. Instruct him to keep a diet diary for 1 week that specifies the following:
      • What, when, where, and why eaten
      • Whether he was doing anything else (e.g., watching TV, cooking) while eating
      • Emotions before eating
      • Others present (e.g., snacking with spouse, children)
   c. Review the diet diary to point out patterns (e.g., time, place, emotions, foods, persons) that affect food intake.
   d. Review high- and low-calorie food items.
2. Teach behavior modification techniques to decrease caloric intake:
   a. Eat only at a specific spot at home (e.g., the kitchen table).
   b. Do not eat while performing other activities.
   c. Drink an 8-oz glass of water immediately before a meal.
   d. Decrease second helpings, fatty foods, sweets, and alcohol.
   e. Prepare small portions, just enough for one meal, and discard leftovers.
   f. Use small plates to make portions look bigger.
   g. Never eat from another person's plate.
   h. Eat slowly and chew food thoroughly.
   i. Put down utensils and wait 15 seconds between bites.
   j. Eat low-calorie snacks that must be chewed to satisfy oral needs (e.g., carrots, celery, apples).
   k. Decrease liquid calories by drinking diet soda or water.

Rationale

1. The ability to lose weight while on corticosteroid therapy likely depends on limiting sodium intake and maintaining a reasonable caloric intake.

2. These measures can help control caloric intake. Often, obesity is promoted by an inappropriate response to external cues—most often, stressors. This response triggers an ineffective coping mechanism in which the client eats in response to stress rather than physiological hunger.

Interventions

   1. Plan eating splurges (save a number of calories each day and have a treat once a week), but eat only a small amount of "splurge" foods.

   3. Instruct the client to increase activity level to burn calories; encourage him to do the following:

     a. Use the stairs instead of elevators

     b. Park at the farthest point in parking lots and walk to buildings

     c. Plan a daily walking program with a progressive increase in distance and pace

   Urge him to consult with a physician before beginning any exercise program.

Rationale

   3. Increased activity can promote weight loss. Keep in mind, however, that the client's ability to exercise may be limited by the pathological condition that necessitates corticosteroid therapy, as well as by the adverse effects of the drug (e.g., osteoporosis, muscle wasting).

▲ **Documentation**

Flow records
   Weight
   Intake
   Activity level

Potential for Infection related to immunosuppression

▲ **Outcome Criteria**

The client will:

1. Relate risk factors associated with potential for infection
2. Practice appropriate precautions to prevent infection

Focus Assessment Criteria

1. Current corticosteroid dosage
2. Changes in overall health status, e.g., fatigue, decreased appetite
3. Evidence of infection with opportunistic organisms

Clinical Significance

1–3. Corticosteroid therapy decreases the ability of T lymphocytes to fight infection and increases the client's susceptibility to infection from opportunistic organisms, e.g., *Candida.*

Interventions

1. Explain the increased risk of infection, and stress the importance of reporting promptly any change in status.

2. Instruct the client to avoid persons with infections and large crowds in close quarters.

Rationale

1. Corticosteroids can mask the usual signs and symptoms of infection, such as fever and increased WBC count, necessitating increased vigilance for subtle changes.
2. These precautions can help limit exposure to infectious microorganisms.

▲ **Documentation**

Flow records
   Temperature
Progress notes
   Change in health status

Potential Self-Concept Disturbance related to changes in appearance

▲ **Outcome Criteria**

The client will:

1. Relate factors contributing to altered body image
2. Demonstrate movement toward reconstruction of an altered body image

Focus Assessment Criteria

1. Signs of iatrogenic Cushing's syndrome:
   a. Weight gain
   b. Abnormal fat distribution
   c. Hirsutism
   d. Fluid retention
   e. Skin changes
   f. Extremity muscle wasting
   g. Moon face
2. Response to appearance changes

Clinical Significance

1. Excessive corticosteroid levels can cause virilism, protein tissue wasting, some matrix wasting, and abnormal fat distribution.

2. This assessment can provide a starting point at which to begin dialogue.

Interventions

1. Explain that appearance changes are drug-induced and diminish or resolve with discontinuation or dosage reduction.
2. Encourage the client to express feelings about appearance changes.
3. Promote social interaction.

Rationale

1. This explanation can reduce the fear of permanent appearance changes and help preserve a positive self-concept.
2. Sharing concerns promotes trust and enables clarification of misconceptions.
3. Social isolation can promote fear and unrealistic perceptions.

▲ **Documentation**

Progress notes
   Interactions

▲ **Outcome Criteria**

The outcome criteria for this diagnosis represent those associated with discharge planning. Refer to the discharge criteria.

Potential Altered Health Maintenance related to insufficient knowledge of administration schedule, adverse reactions, signs and symptoms of complications, hazards of adrenal insufficiency, and potential causes of adrenal insufficiency

Focus Assessment Criteria	*Clinical Significance*
1. Knowledge of corticosteroid therapy	1. Assessing knowledge level identifies learning needs and guides the nurse in planning effective teaching strategies.
2. Readiness and ability to learn and retain information	2. A client or family failing to achieve learning goals requires a referral for assistance post-discharge.

Interventions

1. Instruct the client to take his drug dose exactly as prescribed, keeping in mind these considerations:
   a. Do not discontinue administration because of adverse effects; if unable to tolerate oral medication, contact the physician for instructions.
   b. If possible, take the daily dose in the morning.
   c. Take the daily B_{12} dose before 4 PM.
2. Provide written instructions on dosage schedule, if appropriate.
3. Teach the client to watch for and report serious adverse effects, such as the following:
   a. Altered mood, such as euphoria or even psychosis
   b. Increased susceptibility to skin injury
   c. Weight gain
   d. Hypertension
   e. Diabetes
   f. Severe edema
   g. Cataracts
   h. Hypokalemia
   i. Thromboembolism
   j. Peptic ulcer
   k. Osteoporosis
   l. Increased susceptibility to infection
4. Teach the client to recognize and report signs and symptoms of adrenal insufficiency:
   a. Hypoglycemia
   b. Nausea and vomiting
   c. Diarrhea
   d. Decreased mental acuity
   e. Fatigue, weakness, malaise
   f. Hyponatremia
   g. Orthostatic hypotension
   h. Palpitations
5. Encourage the client scheduled for long-term corticosteroid therapy to obtain and wear Medic-alert identification.
6. Inform the client that he should notify his physician before undergoing invasive procedures or when experiencing infection, for a possible increase in corticosteroid dosage.

Rationale

1. Abrupt cessation of medication in the presence of adrenal insufficiency may precipitate an adrenal crisis. Early morning doses stimulate the body's natural peak excretion.

2. A printed schedule may help improve compliance.
3. The client's vigilance can aid early detection of serious side effects.

4. Corticosteroid therapy inhibits pituitary function, resulting in inhibited adrenal function. Early detection enables prompt intervention to prevent serious complications.

5. A visible identification bracelet or necklace can aid early detection of adrenal insufficiency.

6. Additional stress normally triggers an increased adrenal response; however, corticosteroid therapy interferes with adrenal function, possibly necessitating increased corticosteroid dosage to maintain homeostasis.

▲ **Documentation**

Discharge summary record
    Client teaching
    Outcome achievement or
        status

References/Bibliography

Donham, J. (1986). The weakness of steroids. *American Journal of Nursing, 86*(8), 917–919.

Grady, C. (1988). Host defense mechanisms: An overview. *Seminars of Oncologic Nursing, 4*(2), 86–94.

Gurevich, I., et al. (1986). The compromised host, deficit-specific infection and the spectrum of prevention. *Cancer Nursing, 9*(5), 263–275.

Harper, J. (1988). Use of steroids in cerebral edema: Therapeutic implications. *Heart & Lung, 17*(1), 70–75.

Vernoski, B., & Chernow, B. (1983). Steroids: Use and abuse. *Critical Care Quarterly, 6*(3), 28–38.

Enteral Nutrition

Administration of an elemental liquid diet (calories, minerals, vitamins) to the gastrointestinal (GI) tract through a feeding tube, enteral nutrition is indicated when oral intake is impossible or inadequate. Enteral tube feedings may be delivered through various routes, including nasoduodenal, esophagostomy, gastrostomy, and needle jejunostomy.

Diagnostic Cluster

▲ **Time Frame**

Preprocedure and postprocedure

▲ **Discharge Criteria**

Before discharge, the client and/or family will:

1. Identify therapeutic indications and nutritional requirements
2. Demonstrate tube feeding administration and management
3. Discuss strategies for incorporating enteral management into activities of daily living (ADLs)
4. State signs and symptoms that must be reported to a health care professional

Collaborative Problems

Potential Complications:
Hypoglycemia/Hyperglycemia
Hypervolemia
Hypertonic Dehydration
Electrolyte and Trace Mineral Imbalances
Mucosal Erosion

Nursing Diagnoses

Potential for Infection related to gastrostomy incision and enzymatic action of gastric juices on skin
Altered Comfort: Cramping, Distention, Nausea, Vomiting related to type of formula, rate, or temperature
Diarrhea related to adverse response to formula, rate, or temperature
Potential for Aspiration related to position of tube and individual
Potential Self-Concept Disturbance related to inability to taste or swallow food and fluids
Potential Altered Health Maintenance related to lack of knowledge of nutritional indications/requirements, home care, and signs and symptoms of complications

Collaborative Problems

▲ **Nursing Goal**

The nurse will manage and minimize complications of enteral therapy.

Potential Complication: Hypoglycemia or Hyperglycemia
Potential Complication: Hypervolemia
Potential Complication: Hypertonic Dehydration
Potential Complication: Electrolyte and Trace Mineral Imbalance
Potential Complication: Mucosal Erosion

Interventions	*Rationale*
1. Monitor for symptoms of hypoglycemia after completion of tube feeding: a. Tachycardia b. Diaphoresis c. Confusion d. Dizziness e. Generalized weakness	1. Sudden cessation of enteral feedings in a physiologically stressed client may trigger a hypoglycemic reaction.
2. Monitor for symptoms of hyperglycemia during formula administration: a. Thirst b. Increased urination c. Fatigue	2. Hyperglycemia most commonly occurs in clients with inadequate insulin reserves. Enteral formulas with a higher fat percentage are less likely to contribute to hyperglycemic reaction.

Interventions

    d. Generalized weakness

    e. Increased respirations

    f. Increased pulse

    g. Nausea

3. Monitor for signs and symptoms of overhydration during formula administration:

    a. Tachycardia

    b. Elevated blood pressure

    c. Pulmonary edema

    d. Shortness of breath

    e. Peripheral edema

4. Monitor for signs and symptoms of hypertonic dehydration during formula administration:

    a. Dry mucous membranes

    b. Thirst

    c. Rising serum electrolytes

    d. Decreasing urine output

    e. Concentrated urine

5. Monitor tube exit and entrance sites for the following:

    a. Mucosal erosion

    b. Pain and tenderness

    c. Bleeding

    d. Ulceration

6. Take steps to reduce tube irritation:

    a. Tape tubes securely without causing pressure or tension.

    b. Prepare skin prior to taping with a skin protective agent.

    c. Use small-bore silicone tubes for enteral feedings administered by the nasogastric route.

Rationale

3. Hypervolemia usually is associated with the high water and sodium content of the enteral formula. This complication most often occurs as feeding is initiated or reintroduced in a client with compromised cardiac, renal, or hepatic function.

4. Hypertonic dehydration most often results when a formula of high osmolarity and protein content is administered to a client unable to recognize or respond to thirst.

5,6. External pressure or tension on delicate structures can produce mucosal erosion. Prolonged use of large-bore polyvinyl chloride (PVC) catheters has been linked to nasal cartilage destruction.

▲ **Documentation**

Flow records
  Vital signs
  Intake and output
  Urine specific gravity
  Serum glucose
  Tube site condition

Related Physician-Prescribed Interventions

Medications
  Formula (frequency, dilution)

Intravenous Therapy
  Not applicable

Laboratory Studies
  Not applicable

Diagnostic Studies
  Not applicable

Therapies
  Dependent on the type of tube used

Nursing Diagnoses

▲ **Outcome Criteria**

The client will:

1. Describe measures for infection prevention
2. Report any discomfort around the gastrostomy site

Potential for Infection related to gastrostomy incision and enzymatic action of gastric juices on skin

Focus Assessment Criteria

1. Temperature
2. Gastrostomy incision and tube insertion site
3. Drainage characteristics
4. Complaints of discomfort

Clinical Significance

1–5. Leaking of gastric or intestinal digestive juices to skin surface can cause subsequent excoriation and ulceration. The gastrostomy tube provides an entry site for microorganisms.

Interventions

1. Cleanse the incision and tube insertion site regularly following standard protocol.
2. Protect the skin around the external feeding tube with a protective barrier film. Apply a loose dressing cover, and change it when moist. For excessive drainage, protect skin with an adhesive barrier square and ostomy pouch to capture drainage; change the barrier when nonadherent or soiled.
3. For a temporary gastrostomy or jejunostomy tube, anchor the tube to an external surface to minimize tube migration and retraction.
4. Teach the client to report discomfort around the incision or tube promptly.
5. If skin problems persist, consult a clinical nurse specialist or enterostomal therapist for assistance.

Rationale

1. Cleaning removes microorganisms and reduces the risk of infection.
2. The catheter can irritate skin and mucosa. Gastric juices can cause severe skin breakdown.

3. Movement can cause tissue trauma and create entry points for opportunistic microorganisms.
4. Early detection and reporting enables prompt intervention to prevent serious inflammation.
5. The expertise of a skin care specialist may be needed.

▲ **Documentation**

Flow records
　Vital signs
　Drainage (characteristics, amount)
　Site condition

▲ **Outcome Criteria**

The client will tolerate enteral feedings without episodes of cramping, distention, nausea, or vomiting.

Altered Comfort: Cramping, Distention, Nausea, Vomiting related to type of formula, administration rate, or formula temperature

Focus Assessment Criteria	Clinical Significance
1. History of lactose or fat intolerance 2. Residual contents (gastric feedings only) 3. Complaints of cramping, nausea, vomiting, abdominal distention 4. Complaints of foul formula odor	1–3. A high-osmolarity formula administered rapidly can cause retention, nausea, and vomiting. These complications also may occur after administration to a client with lactose intolerance. 4. The odor of enteral formula seems to provoke nausea and vomiting in some clients.

Interventions

1. Initiate feedings slowly, and increase the rate gradually based on tolerance. Begin with an isotonic, lactose-free formula or, alternately, dilute other types of feedings with water to decrease osmolarity.
2. Instill the formula at room temperature directly from the can, whenever possible.

3. Discard unused portions or store in a tightly sealed container.
4. For continuous feeding, fill the container with enough formula for a 4-hour feeding. Do not overfill or allow the formula to stand for a longer period.
5. For intermittent feeding, instill the formula gradually over a 15- to 45-minute period. Do not administer as a bolus or at a rapid rate.

Rationale

1,2. The feeding regimen itself may cause problems. For example, a bolus feeding of high osmolarity and at cold temperature can provoke gastric and digestive problems. Uncontrolled feedings by the jejunal route are particularly prone to these complications, because the feeding is not processed in the stomach before it reaches the intestines.
3,4. Extended exposure of a feeding to room temperature promotes microorganism growth.

5. Slow administration can reduce cramping, nausea, and vomiting.

▲ **Documentation**

Flow records
　Intake and output
Progress notes
　Unusual events or problems

▲ **Outcome Criteria**

The client will demonstrate a tolerable, consistent bowel pattern with no episodes of diarrhea.

Diarrhea related to adverse response to formula contents, administration rate, or formula temperature

Focus Assessment Criteria	Clinical Significance
1. Bowel pattern before initiation of enteral feedings 2. Current bowel pattern: amount, nature, consistency	1–4. Diarrhea results from altered intestinal absorptive capacity. Severe malnutrition and protein depletion can precipitate this reaction because of impaired ability of the

Focus Assessment Criteria
3. Elimination pattern in relation to feedings
4. Formula characteristics (osmolarity, lactose, fiber, and protein) content and feeding regimen (amount, rate, times)

Clinical Significance
osmotic transport mechanism to transfer nutrients to the intestinal capillary network.

Interventions
1. Initiate feedings slowly, progressing gradually as tolerated. Begin with an isotonic, lactose-free supplement.
2. Instill the formula at room temperature directly from the can when possible.
3. Discard unused portions or store in a tightly sealed container.
4. For continuous feeding, fill the container with enough formula for a 4-hour feeding. Do not overfill or allow the formula to stand for a longer period.

5. For intermittent feeding, instill the formula gradually over a 15- to 45-minute period. Do not administer as a bolus or at a rapid rate.
6. Consult with the physician for antidiarrheal medications, as necessary.

Rationale
1. Diminished intestinal absorption must be compensated for through gradual, progressive introduction of enteral supplements.
2. Administering cold formula can cause cramping and possibly lead to elimination problems.
3. These precautions can minimize growth of microorganisms.
4. Each type of formula has an individual shelf-life after opening. Formula should be protected from environmental contaminants, to prevent bacterial growth and possible resultant diarrhea.
5. Contaminated intestinal feedings are particularly likely to induce diarrhea because of their lack of hydrochloric acid.
6. Medications may be needed to control severe diarrhea.

▲*Documentation*
Flow records
   Intake and output

▲*Outcome Criteria*
The client will digest feedings without aspiration.

Potential for Aspiration related to position of tube and client

Focus Assessment Criteria
1. Vital signs
2. Breath sounds
3. Position of tube
4. History of aspiration, swallowing difficulty
5. Abdominal distention, bloating, bowel sounds

Clinical Significance
1–5. Aspiration pneumonia is a potential complication for all tube-fed clients. Most commonly, it is marked by sudden onset of respiratory distress or failure following an episode of vomiting. Sometimes the presence of aspiration is insidious and occurs without overt evidence of vomiting. This type of aspiration occurs most commonly in a client with impaired mentation, glottic stenosis, swallowing difficulty, or tracheostomy.

Interventions
1. Elevate the head of the bed 30 to 45 degrees during feedings and for 1 hour afterwards.
2. Add a few drops of blue food coloring to the formula.

3. For a nasogastric or nasojejunal tube, verify proper tube placement by air auscultation.
4. For a tube positioned gastrically, verify placement by aspirating for residual contents.
5. Administer a scheduled intermittent tube feeding only if residual contents are less than 150 mL; administer continuous feedings only if residual contents are not more than 20% of the hourly administration rate.
6. Regulate intermittent gastric feedings to allow gastric emptying between feedings.

Rationale
1. Upper body elevation can prevent reflux through use of reverse gravity.
2. Blue is a nonphysiological color that allows easy visualization of regurgitated gastric contents and their differentiation from tracheal secretions.
3,4. Proper tube position must be verified before feeding to prevent introducing formula into the respiratory tract.

5. Administering feedings in the presence of excessive residual contents increases the risk of reflux and aspiration.

6,7. Such regulation is necessary to prevent overfeeding and increased risk of reflux and aspi-

Interventions

7. Regulate continuous feedings to allow periods of rest so the client can ambulate unencumbered by the feeding apparatus.

8. Flush the feeding tube with water after completion of feeding.

Rationale

ration. Gastric feedings should be administered intermittently when the potential for aspiration is high. Continuous feedings increase the risk of aspiration because the stomach contains a constant supply of formula.

8. Flushing is necessary to remove formula, which can provide a medium for microorganism growth.

▲ **Outcome Criteria**

The client will:

1. Share feelings related to lack of oral ingestion
2. Verbalize the necessity of continued enteral feedings

Potential Self-Concept Disturbance related to inability to taste or swallow food and fluids

Focus Assessment Criteria

1. Feelings and concerns related to the inability to ingest food orally

Clinical Significance

1. Food and eating have many social and cultural implications besides nutritional intake. Prolonged or permanent NPO status can interfere with socialization and create isolation.

Interventions

1. Encourage the client to verbalize concerns related to lack of oral ingestion.

2. Explore possible alternatives to oral ingestion, or substitute diversional activities.

3. Provide regular feedback on progress and positive reinforcement on appearance and weight gain.

4. Arrange for visits from others on enteral nutrition, if feasible.

5. If permitted, allow the client to taste—but not swallow—desired foods.

Rationale

1. Sharing helps identify and clarify the client's concerns and problems, guiding the nurse in planning effective interventions.

2. Substituting activities for meals may help reduce the sense of loss related to lack of oral intake.

3. Feedback and reinforcement promote self-esteem and encourage continued compliance.

4. Sharing with others in the same situation allows opportunities for mutual validation and support.

5. Placing food in the mouth without swallowing may help satisfy the need to taste and smell food.

▲ **Outcome Criteria**

The outcome criteria for this diagnosis represent those associated with discharge planning. Refer to the discharge criteria.

Potential Altered Health Maintenance related to lack of knowledge of nutritional indications/requirements, home care, and signs and symptoms of complications

Focus Assessment Criteria

1. Understanding of therapeutic indications and requirements
2. Available support persons to assist with home therapy
3. Readiness and ability to learn and retain information

Clinical Significance

1. Assessment establishes a baseline for teaching
2. Assistance is often needed for at-home treatment
3. A client or family failing to achieve learning goals requires a referral for assistance postdischarge.

Interventions

1. Explain the rationale for and aspects of enteral nutrition therapy. Discuss the client's specific nutritional requirements and specific indications for therapy.

Rationale

1. Explaining the need for optimal nutrition and the advantages of enteral feedings can reduce misconceptions and encourage compliance.

Interventions

2. Explain the rationale for continued diagnostic tests, e.g., daily weighing, intake and output measurements, urine tests, serum evaluation.

3. Review potential problems and complications, such as these:
   a. Vomiting
   b. Improper tube placement
   c. Aspiration

4. Refer to a home care agency for follow-up home visits.

5. Teach insertion and care of a nasogastric tube for home care, including the following:
   a. Preparation
   b. Hygiene
   c. Position check
   d. Taping
   e. Removal
   f. Care of equipment

6. Teach aspects of the enteral feeding regimen, covering these elements:
   a. Hand washing
   b. Work surface preparation
   c. Formula preparation
   d. Administration procedure
   e. Completion of feeding
   f. Dressing changes and skin protection measures
   g. Equipment operation and care

7. Have the client or support person perform return demonstration of selected care measures.

8. Explain measures to prevent aspiration. (Refer to the nursing diagnosis Potential for Aspiration in this entry for more information.)

9. Teach other self-care measures, including these:
   a. Use tap water to irrigate the feeding tube before and after instilling formula.

   b. Chew gum—sugar-free, if indicated.
   c. Brush teeth and use mouthwash 3 to 4 times a day.

   d. Do not mix medication with formula.

   e. Mark the tube when it is in the correct position.

10. Provide a written list of required equipment and supplies and sources for these items.

Rationale

2. Careful monitoring is needed to evaluate the effectiveness and safety of enteral therapy and enable early detection of problems or complications.

3. The client's and family's understanding of potential complications enables them to detect and report signs and symptoms soon after they develop.

4. A home health agency can provide ongoing assistance and support.

5. Some clients and families can be taught insertion of feeding tubes.

6. Certain knowledge is needed for proper administration and prevention of complications.

7. Return demonstration lets the nurse evaluate the client's and family's ability to perform feedings safely.

8. Aspiration is a potential complication of all types of tube feedings.

9.

   a. Irrigation allows evaluation of tube patency, clears the tubes, and ensures delivery of a full dose of formula.
   b. Gum can help keep the mouth moist.
   c. Frequent mouth care can maintain moist mucous membranes and remove microorganisms.
   d. Mixing can increase the likelihood of inaccurate dosage.
   e. Markings provide a visible cue of a tube position change.

10. Advance planning can prevent shortages and improper substitutions.

▲ **Documentation**

Discharge summary record
  Client and family teaching
  Outcome achievement or status
  Referrals, if indicated

References/Bibliography

Allen, T.M. (1982). An enteral feeding protocol. *Nutritional Support Services, 2*(3), 27.

Breach, C., & Saldanha, L. (1988). Tube feeding complications: Part 1. *Nutritional Support Systems, 8*(3), 15–17.

Breach, C., & Saldanha, L. (1988). Tube feeding complications: Part 2. *Nutritional Support Systems, 8*(5), 28–32.

Breach, C., & Saldanha, L. (1988). Tube feeding complications: Part 3. *Nutritional Support Systems, 8*(6), 16–19.

Kaminski, M.V. (1981). Enteral hyperalimentation: Prevention and treatment of complications. *Nutritional Support Services, 1*(4), 29.

Konstantinides, N.N., & Shronts, E. (1983). Tube feedings: Managing the basics. *American Journal of Nursing, 83*(9), 1312.

Loewenhardt, P.M. (1989). Assuring successful home enteral feedings. *Home Healthcare Nurse, 7*(5), 16–20.

McGee, L. (1987). Feeding gastrostomy: Nursing care, Part 2. *Journal of Enterostomy Therapy, 14*(5), 201–211.

Randall, H.T. (1984). Enteral nutrition: Tube feeding in acute and chronic illness. *Journal of Parenteral Enteral Nutrition, 8*(2), 113.

Rombeau, J.L., & Caldwell, M.D. (1984). *Enteral and tube feeding: Volume 1.* Philadelphia: W.B. Saunders.

External Arteriovenous Shunting

In external arteriovenous (A–V) shunting, an external connection of an artery and vein created to provide easy access for repeated dialysis, two flexible silastic tubes are surgically inserted—one into an artery, the other into a vein, usually in the forearm. A removable connector joins the tubes. For dialysis, the connector is removed and the tubes are attached to the artificial kidney machine. The major advantage of A–V shunting is that it can be used immediately after surgical implantation, which usually takes less than 1 hour.

Diagnostic Cluster

▲ **Time Frame**

Pretherapy, intratherapy, and post-therapy

▲ **Discharge Criteria**

Before discharge, the client and/or family will:

1. Demonstrate site care and identify precautions
2. Demonstrate how to evaluate thrills and bruits
3. Relate prescribed activity restrictions
4. Describe emergency measures for disconnections and clots
5. State signs and symptoms that must be reported to a health care professional
6. Identify available community resources

Collaborative Problems

Potential Complications: *Refer to:*
Thrombosis
Bleeding

Nursing Diagnoses

Potential Altered Health Maintenance related to insufficient knowledge of catheter care, precautions, emergency measures, prevention of infection, and activity limitations
Anxiety related to upcoming shunt insertion   General Surgery

Collaborative Problems

▲ **Nursing Goal**

The nurse will manage and minimize vascular complications.

Potential Complication: Thrombosis
Potential Complication: Bleeding

Interventions	*Rationale*

1. Monitor for thrombosis of shunt:
  a. No palpable thrill or audible bruit with stethoscope
  b. Dark or separated blood present in the tubing
  c. Blood in cannula cool to touch
  d. Slow, sluggish flow noted during dialysis procedure
	1. Straight connectors carry a lower risk of clotting than do cannulas. Detection of clotting in its early stages may prevent permanent loss as an access site.

2. Monitor patency by palpating for a thrill or auscultating for a bruit every hour for the first 24 hours postinsertion, then every 4 hours. Report findings to the physician immediately.	2. Early detection of a thrill (a "ripping" sensation palpable over the venous site of the fistula) or a bruit (a "rushing" noise auscultated and timed with each heartbeat) enables prompt declotting to improve the chances for shunt survival.

3. Teach the client to do the following:
  a. Avoid excessive activity of cannulated limb
  b. Monitor blood pressure and report abnormalities
	3.
	  a. The fistula is highly vulnerable to injury.
	  b. This strategy prevents reduced blood flow to the shunt, which can increase the risk of clotting.

Interventions

   c. Avoid any punctures in the cannulated extremity
   d. Apply no constricting devices over or above the cannulas, e.g., blood pressure cuff, tourniquets, tight dressings, and watches
   e. Avoid abnormal or cramped positions of the cannulated limb for prolonged periods (special attention should be given during resting or sleeping)
   f. If the shunt is in the leg, avoid crossing the cannulated leg over the opposite leg
   g. Be sure that cannulas are in a straight line and are not twisted in any abnormal fashion
   h. Avoid extremes of hot or cold applied to the exposed cannulas

   i. Notify the physician if you note fibrin (whitish protein)

4. Place an overhead sign on the bed to indicate that the client should have no venipunctures or blood pressure readings on the affected extremity.
5. When the cannulas are connected, ensure that both Silastic limbs cover the Teflon connector adequately and equally. Further secure with tape bridges, and check the Teflon connector every 4 hours for security.
6. Ensure that both cannulas extend beyond the skin exit equally.

7. Take care not to puncture the cannula tubing by needles.
8. If separation of Teflon connector occurs, do as follows:
   a. Immediately place a clamp on each limb approximately ½ inch from the exit site. (Use fingers to pinch the tubing if clamps are not available).

   b. Cleanse the cannula and connector ends with antiseptic agent and reconnect after the tubing fills sufficiently with blood.
9. If Teflon tip is incorrectly positioned in artery or vein, do the following:
   a. Immediately clamp the cannula.
   b. If bleeding continues, apply three-finger pressure over the bleeding exit site and vessel proximally and notify physician immediately.
10. Monitor for bleeding at the site every 2 to 4 hours; check for bruit or thrill.

11. Reassure the client and family that slight bleeding from a new shunt is expected, but instruct them to report any excessive bleeding.

Rationale

   c. Entering the fistula increases the risk of introducing microorganisms.
   d–g. This strategy prevents reduced blood flow to the shunt, which can increase the risk of clotting.

   h. Cold decreases blood flow: heat increases blood flow initially, followed by rebound constriction.
   i. Fibrin is released during the clotting process; its presence indicates an impending clot that can cause shunt occlusion.

4. This measure can help protect against accidental injury.

5. These measures help prevent accidental disconnection.

6. If either cannula seems to be extended beyond the skin exit site abnormally, the cannula could be slipping out.
7. The tubing cannot reseal punctures; surgical replacement is required.
8.

   a. The Teflon connector may separate from either the arterial or the venous Silastic limb, resulting in major blood loss in a very short time. Rapid determination of the cause is of utmost importance.
   b. Filling the tube with blood prevents air embolism after reconnection.
9. Although the Teflon vessel tips are sutured in, they may slip out of the artery or vein.
   a. Clamping prevents further blood loss.
   b. Pressure over site and proximally decreases bleeding.

10. Persistent bleeding around the exit site may indicate infection or other complications. Adequate blood flow can be determined by assessing for a bruit or thrill.

11. A small amount of bleeding may occur around the exit site, particularly in the immediate post-cannulation period. This usually subsides

▲ **Documentation**

Progress notes
   Assessment of bruit or thrill
   Patency of cannula
   Assessment of site (patency, temperature, bleeding, drainage)

Interventions

If bleeding occurs around the exit site, loosely reapply dry sterile dressing.

Related Physician-Prescribed Interventions

Refer to the Peritoneal Dialysis care plan, page 597.

Rationale

spontaneously. A loose dressing does not occlude the blood flow. A new dressing facilitates assessment of continued bleeding.

Nursing Diagnosis

▲ **Outcome Criteria**

The outcome criteria for this diagnosis represent those associated with discharge planning. Refer to the discharge criteria.

Potential Altered Health Maintenance related to insufficient knowledge of catheter care, precautions, emergency measures, prevention of infection, and activity limitations

Focus Assessment Criteria	*Clinical Significance*
1. Readiness and ability to learn and retain information	1. A client or family failing to achieve goals for learning requires a referral for assistance postdischarge.
2. Previous shunt experience	2. A client with previous shunt experience requires careful evaluation of knowledge and any misconceptions.

Interventions

1. Teach shunt care measures, covering the following:
   a. Maintaining a clean work area away from open windows
   b. Site cleaning using aseptic technique
   c. Dressing and elastic bandage application
   d. Shunt clamp attachment
   e. Heparinization, if ordered

2. Calmly explain what accidents can occur and teach how to manage; cover the following:
   a. Shunt bleeding
   b. Clotting
   c. Crusting
   d. Disconnection
3. Instruct the client to change dressings three times a week in conjunction with dialysis treatments, and as needed whenever dressing is wet or soiled. Stress the importance of washing hands well before and after a dressing change.
4. Teach the client to protect shunt dressing from water with Saran wrap or a plastic bag.
5. Teach how to evaluate a thrill or bruit and to report abnormalities immediately to the physician.

Rationale

1.
   a. The work area should be as free of dust as possible.
   b. The risk of infection can be reduced by controlling microorganisms at the site.
   c. This measure protects the shunt but allows access to check patency.
   d. Shunt clamps are clipped to the dressing for ready access in the event of accidental disconnection.
   e. Systemic heparinization is sometimes used to prevent clotting in the extracorporeal system. (Refer to the Anticoagulant Therapy care plan, page 507, for more information.)

2. Specific instructions for emergencies or complications can reduce the anxiety if they occur.

3. Sterile, dry dressings are needed to prevent microorganisms from entering the shunt site. Washing hands before reduces the possibility of contaminating the site with microorganisms. Washing after reduces exposure to infections transmitted by blood, e.g., hepatitis.
4. Water can transmit microorganisms to the shunt site.
5. Early detection of a thrill (a "ripping" sensation palpable over the venous site of the fistula) or a bruit (a "rushing" noise auscultated and timed with each heartbeat) enables prompt declotting to improve the chances for shunt survival.

Interventions	Rationale
6. Teach the client to protect the shunt from injury. (Refer to the Collaborative Problems section of this entry for more information.)	6. The shunt is highly vulnerable to injury.
7. Teach the client and family to watch for and report the following:	7. Early detection and reporting enables prompt intervention to prevent serious complications.
a. Absence of thrill or bruit	a. Absence of bruits or thrill may indicate obstruction or thrombosis.
b. Skin abnormalities in affected limbs	b. Skin changes may point to insufficient circulation.
c. Presence of dark, separated blood in tubing	c. Dark, separate blood in tubes indicates clotting.
d. Redness, drainage at site	d. Redness and drainage at the site indicate inflammation or infection.
8. Teach precautions, including these:	8.
a. Avoid bending the shunted extremity (knee or elbow) for the specified period.	a. Prolonged bending can kink the tubing.
b. Avoid strenuous exercise, heavy lifting, or excessive motion of the shunted arm or leg.	b. Increased muscle tension in the shunted arm or leg can dislodge the tubing.
9. Provide names and phone numbers of health care professionals to contact for information or an emergency.	9. Knowledge of whom to contact can reduce the fears associated with anticipated problems.
10. Refer to a home care agency for follow-up, as indicated.	10. A home care nurse can evaluate the client's and family's ability to manage shunt care.

▲ **Documentation**

Discharge summary record
  Client and family teaching
  Outcome achievement or
    status
  Referrals, if indicated

References/Bibliography

Cleo, R.J. (1985). *Comprehensive nephrology nursing.* Boston: Bozeman, Little, Bunn and Co.

Kee, J.L. (1982). *Fluids and electrolytes and clinical applications: A programmed approach* (3rd ed.). New York: John Wiley and Sons.

Lancaster, L.E. (1987). *American Nephrology Nurses' Association core curriculum for nephrology nursing.* Pitman, NJ: Anthony J. Jannette.

Larsen, E., Lindbloom, L., & Davis, K.B. (1986). *Development of the clinical nephrology practitioner: A focus on independent learning.* Seattle: University of Washington Hospital.

Massry, S.G., & Sellers, A.L. (1979). *Clinical aspects of uremia and dialysis* (2nd ed.). Springfield, IL: Charles C Thomas.

Walsh, J., Persons, C.B., & Wieck, L. (1987). *Manual of home health care nursing.* Philadelphia: J.B. Lippincott.

Hemodialysis

Hemodialysis is the removal of metabolic wastes and excess electrolytes and fluids from the blood to treat acute or chronic renal failure. The procedure uses the principles of diffusion, osmosis, and filtration. Blood is pumped into an artificial kidney through a semipermeable, cellophane-like membrane surrounded by a flow of dialysate, a solution composed of water, glucose, sodium, chloride, potassium, calcium, and acetate or bicarbonate. The amounts of these constituents vary depending on the amount of water, waste products, or electrolytes to be removed.

Diagnostic Cluster

▲ **Time Frame**

Pretherapy, intratherapy, and post-therapy

Collaborative Problems

Potential Complications: *Refer to:*
Electrolyte Imbalance (Potassium, Sodium)
Nausea/Vomiting
Transfusion Reaction
Hemorrhage
Hemolysis
Seizures
Dialysis Disequilibrium Syndrome
Dialysate Leakage
Clotting
Air Embolism
Sepsis
Hyperthermia
Fluid Imbalances   Peritoneal Dialysis
Hypertension/Hypotension   Peritoneal Dialysis

Nursing Diagnoses

▲ **Discharge Criteria**

Before discharge, the client and/or family will:

1. Describe the purpose of hemodialysis
2. Discuss feelings and concerns regarding the effects of long-term therapy on self and family
3. State signs and symptoms that must be reported to a health care professional

Potential for Infection Transmission related to frequent contacts with blood and high risk of hepatitis B
Powerlessness related to need for treatments to live despite effects on life style   Chronic Renal Failure
Altered Family Processes related to the interruption of role responsibilities caused by the treatment schedule   Chronic Renal Failure

Related Care Plans

Chronic or Acute Renal Failure
External Arteriovenous Shunting

Collaborative Problems

▲ **Nursing Goal**

The nurse will manage and minimize complications of hemodialysis.

Potential Complication: Electrolyte Imbalance (Potassium, Sodium)
Potential Complication: Nausea/Vomiting
Potential Complication: Transfusion Reaction
Potential Complication: Hemorrhage
Potential Complication: Hemolysis
Potential Complication: Seizures
Potential Complication: Dialysis Disequilibrium Syndrome
Potential Complication: Dialysate Leakage
Potential Complication: Clotting
Potential Complication: Air Embolism
Potential Complication: Sepsis
Potential Complication: Hyperthermia

Interventions	*Rationale*
1. Assess the following:	1. Predialysis assessment and documentation of the client's status is mandatory before initiation of the hemodialysis procedure to establish a baseline and to identify problems.
a. Skin (color, turgor, temperature, moisture, edema)	a. Skin assessment can provide data to evaluate circulation, level of hydration, fluid retention, and uremia.
b. Blood pressure (lying and sitting)	b. Low blood pressure may indicate intolerance to transmembrane pressure, hypovolemia, or the effects of antihypertensive medication given predialysis. High blood pressure may indicate overhydration, increased renin production, or dietary and fluid indiscretion.
c. Apical pulse (rhythm, rate)	c. Cardiac assessment evaluates the heart's ability to compensate for changes in fluid volume.
d. Respirations (rate, effort, abnormal sounds)	d. Respiratory assessment evaluates compensatory ability of the system and presence of infection.
e. Weight (gain, loss)	e. Predialysis weight indicating gain or loss may necessitate a need to reevaluate dry weight.
f. Vascular access (site, patency)	f. The vascular access site is assessed for signs of infection or abnormal drainage. Patency is evaluated by assessment of bruits and thrills.
2. Assess the client's complaints of the following symptoms: a. Chest pain b. Shortness of breath c. Cramps d. Headache e. Dizziness f. Blurred vision g. Nausea and vomiting h. Change in mentation or speech.	2. These assessment data help determine if there has been a change in the client's condition since last treatment or if a change in treatment is indicated. When a client presents with problems predialysis, underlying etiology needs to be determined before initiation of treatment.
3. Check the dialysis machine set-up for the following: a. Evidence of air in line b. Secure connections c. Armed air detector d. Poor connection or crack around the hub of the vascular needles e. Fluid in normal saline bag f. Arterial needle site collapse, allowing air to enter around the needle	3. Careful checking can detect air or leaks.
4. Intradialysis, monitor for signs and symptoms of potassium and sodium imbalance. (Refer to the Peritoneal Dialysis care plan, page 597, for more information.)	4. Dialysate fluid composition and rates of inflow and outflow determine the presence or absence of electrolyte imbalances.
5. Monitor for causes of nausea and vomiting, such as these: a. Hypotension b. Hypertension c. Electrolyte imbalances (potassium and sodium) d. Elevated acetate levels	5. Excessive ultrafiltration during hemodialysis may cause a hypovolemic state demonstrated by hypotension, nausea, and vomiting. Potassium and sodium imbalance also may contribute to nausea and vomiting. Acetate, used as a buffer in dialysate, is metabolized in the liver to bicarbonate. If not readily metabolized, acetate can cause myocardial depression and va-

Interventions

6. Monitor for signs and symptoms of transfusion reaction:
   a. Fever
   b. Chills
   c. Dyspnea
   d. Cyanosis
   e. Chest pain
   f. Back pain
   g. Arm pain
   h. Nausea
   i. Hives or skin rash
7. Take steps to reduce the risk of hemorrhage:
   a. Ensure that all connections are tightly secured and needles are taped securely to the patient.
   b. If separation occurs, clamp both blood lines and turn off the blood pump.
   c. Check that blood lines are properly threaded into the blood pump.
   d. Ensure that the blood leak detector is turned on and operating properly.
   e. Observe for pink- to red-tinged dialysate; check the arterial dialysate line with Hemastix to confirm positive result.
8. Do not leave the client unattended at any time during dialysis.

9. Alternate puncture sites with every treatment and question the client regarding pain in the area of access.
10. Apply pinpoint pressure to fistula sticks post-dialysis to control bleeding. When cannulating a new gortex, maintain pressure for 20 minutes, then apply pressure dressings after bleeding is controlled.
11. Check the shunt dressing every 2 hours for bleeding or disconnection.
12. Monitor for manifestations of hemolysis:
    a. Bright red blood in venous line
    b. Burning at the circulatory return site
    c. Pink- to red-tinged dialysate
13. Monitor for seizure activity.

14. Monitor for signs and symptoms of dialysis/disequilibrium syndrome:
    a. Headache
    b. Nausea
    c. Vomiting
    d. Restlessness
    e. Hypertension
    f. Increased pulse pressures
    g. Altered sensorium
    h. Convulsions
    i. Coma

Rationale

sodilatation, which can stimulate nausea and vomiting, among other effects.

6. Because of decreased erythropoietin production, chronic hemodialysis clients require frequent transfusions. Transfusions are administered during hemodialysis in conjunction with ultrafiltration (fluid removal to prevent fluid overload). Blood reactions are most commonly seen in clients who are repeatedly transfused and have some blood dyscrasias. Signs and symptoms are caused by the blockage of blood vessels by hemolyzed or agglutinated cells and the body's inflammatory response.

7. Hemorrhage may occur because of accidental separation of blood line, needles accidentally dislodged from circulatory access site, ruptured blood lines, ruptured dialyzer membrane, and separation of external cannula from itself or from the vessel. Underlying coagulopathy or blood dyscrasia complicated by heparin administration during hemodialysis can increase the risk of hemorrhage.

8. A complication such as hemorrhage, transfusion reaction, or clotting can quickly become serious if not detected and treated promptly. Early detection can prevent substantial blood loss.

9. Repeated needle punctures at the same site can cause an aneurysm.

10. These measures can help prevent exsanguination from the access site.

11. Bleeding can be a sign of disconnected or clotted shunt tubing.
12. Rupture of red blood cells can result from the hypotonic dialysate, high dialysate temperature, or the presence of chloramines, nitrates, copper, zinc, or formaldehyde in the dialysate.

13. Hypotension caused by rapid fluid loss can precipitate a seizure.
14. As a result of hemodialysis, the concentration of blood urea nitrogen (BUN) is reduced more rapidly than the urea nitrogen level in cerebrospinal fluid and brain tissue because of the slow transport of urea across the blood–brain barrier. Urea acts as an osmotic agent, drawing water from the plasma and extracellular fluid into the cerebral cells and producing cerebral edema. Other factors, such as rapid *p*H changes and electrolyte shifts, also can cause cerebral edema.

Interventions	*Rationale*

15. Monitor for manifestations of dialysate leakage:
  a. Activated blood leak detector alarm
  b. Positive Hemastix results
  c. Pink- or red-tinged outflow
	15. A blood leak can result from rupture of the dialyzer fibers, which causes blood to cross the semipermeable membrane into the dialysate compartment. The blood leak monitor can detect blood losses of less than 0.45 mL/min, activating audible and visible alarms and stopping the pump. A leak of 0.45 mL/min is considered major, necessitating changing the dialysate. Causes of dialyzer fiber rupture can result from defective dialyzer membrane, transmembrane pressure beyond the membrane's ability to tolerate, or pumping of blood pump against an obstruction, causing an excessive positive pressure in the dialyzer.

16. Monitor for clotting:
  a. Observe for clot formation in kidney and drip chambers.
  b. Monitor pressure readings every 15 minutes.
  c. Observe for clots when aspirating fistula needles, arteriovenous shunt, or subclavian catheter.
	16. Blood contacting the nonvascular surface of the extracorporeal circuit activates the normal clotting mechanism. During dialysis, fibrin formation within the venous trap and a gradual increase in the circuit's venous pressure (resulting from clotting in the venous trap or needle) may indicate inadequate heparinization. Clot formation elevates blood pressure readings.

17. Monitor for signs and symptoms of air embolism:
  a. Cyanosis
  b. Shortness of breath
  c. Chest pain
  d. Visual changes: diplopia, "seeing stars," blindness
  e. Anxiety
  f. Persistent cough
	17. As little as 10 mL of air introduced into the venous circulation is clinically significant. Large air bubbles are changed to foam as they enter the heart. Foam can decrease the volume of blood entering the lungs, decreasing left heart blood flow and cardiac output.

18. If signs and symptoms of air embolism occur, take these steps:
  a. Clamp the venous line and stop the blood pump.
  b. Position the client on his left side with feet elevated for 30 minutes.
	18.
	  a. Clamping the line and stopping the pump can stop infusion of air.
	  b. This prevents air from going to the head, and traps the air in the right atrium and in the right ventricle, away from the pulmonic valve.

19. Monitor for signs and symptoms of sepsis:
  a. Fever
  b. Chills
  c. Nausea and vomiting
  d. Tachycardia
  e. Chest pain
	19. Sepsis can result from a pyrogenic reaction due to diffusion of bacterial toxins across membranes into the blood, or transfusion reaction. Negative cultures and the absence of other possible causes usually indicate a pyrogenic reaction.

20. Maintain dialysate temperature at 100°. Assess for hyperthermia:
  a. Complaints of feeling hot
  b. Skin hot to touch
  c. Possible cessation of perspiration, with abnormally dry skin
  d. Headache, delirium
  e. Rapid, shallow respirations
  f. Tachycardia
  g. Dark-red blood
	20. Hyperthermia can be due to overheated dialysate. Possible causes of overheated dialysate include these:
	  a. Failure of thermostat
	  b. Thermostat set inappropriately
	  c. Failure of dialysate high temperature sensor
	  d. Failure of machine to go into bypass mode

▲ **Documentation**

Flow records
    Vital signs
    Weight
    Vascular access site
    Dialysis (time, solution)
Progress notes
    Predialysis complaints
    Intradialysis complaints

Related Physician-Prescribed Interventions

Medications
Refer to the Chronic Renal Failure care plan.

Intravenous Therapy
Not indicated

Laboratory Studies
Refer to the Chronic Renal Failure care plan.

Diagnostic Studies
Refer to the Chronic Renal Failure care plan.

Therapies
Dialysate solution

Nursing Diagnosis

▲ Outcome Criteria

The client will:

1. Be free of hepatitis B virus (HBV)
2. Take precautions to prevent transmission of HBV

Potential for Infection Transmission related to frequent contacts with blood and individuals at high risk for hepatitis B

Focus Assessment Criteria	*Clinical Significance*
1. Monthly screening for HBV	1. Clients and personnel are at high risk for HBV because of many contacts with blood or blood products.

Interventions

1. Check the HBV core antibody—and antigen if the core antibody is positive—on all new dialysis clients before hemodialysis is initiated. Monthly screening for HBV in regular clients, transient clients, and staff also is recommended.
2. Observe strict isolation procedure:
   a. Wear an isolation gown and mask during dialysis treatment.
   b. Dialysis should be performed in client's private room or a Dialysis Unit isolation area.
   c. All blood or dialysis effluent spills must be cleaned up immediately with antimicrobial soap and water.
   d. Observe isolation disposal procedure for all needles, syringes, and effluent.
   e. Do not permit nurses and other personnel or visitors to eat or drink anything in the client's room or isolation area.
   f. Ensure that all specimens for laboratory analysis are labeled "Isolation" and placed in bags also labeled "Isolation."
   g. Use special disposable thermometers to assess temperature.
   h. Avoid contact with other dialysis clients, if staffing level permits. If contact is necessary, change isolation gowns and wash hands carefully.
   i. Avoid any skin contact with the client's blood.
   j. Follow isolation procedure for waste and linen disposal per institutional protocol.
   k. Follow the recommended sterilization procedure for the hemodialysis machine after use.

Rationale

1. Each dialysis unit needs clearly defined procedures to protect staff and clients by controlling the spread of hepatitis.

2. HBV is found in the blood, saliva, semen, and vaginal secretions. Transmission is usually through blood (percutaneous or permucosal). Protection is provided by regularly practicing certain precautions.

Interventions

3. Discuss the need for prophylaxis for HBV passive immunity with hepatitis B immunoglobin (HBIG) or active HBV immunity vaccine (Heptavax B) with the client, family, and other close support persons.

4. Assess for signs and symptoms of hepatitis (*note:* keep in mind that a client receiving dialysis often is asymptomatic):
   a. Jaundice
   b. Nausea and vomiting, anorexia
   c. Fatigue
   d. Photophobia
   e. Itching
   f. Positive serum HbsAg, hepatitis B core antigen (HbcAg).

5. Reinforce to the client and family the serious nature of HBV and precautions and risks.

Rationale

3. High-risk clients and others should be immunized.

4. Incubation of HBV ranges from two to six months. Circulatory toxins from inadequate liver detoxification cause symptoms.

5. Reiterating the seriousness of HBV and its possible sequelae may encourage compliance with instructions and precautions.

▲ **Documentation**

Teaching record
    Client and family teaching
Flow records
    Monthly HBV screening results

References/Bibliography

Bihl, M.A. et al. (1988). Comparing stressors and quality of life of dialysis patients. *ANNA Journal, 15*(1), 27–36.

Cleo, R.J. (1985). *Comprehensive nephrology nursing.* Boston: Bozeman, Little, Bunn and Co.

Fuchs, J., et al. (1988). Patients' perceptions of CAPD and hemodialysis stressors. *ANNA Journal, 15*(5), 282–300.

Gurklis, J.A., et al. (1988). Identification of stressors and use of coping methods in chronic hemodialysis patients. *Nursing Research, 37*(4), 236–239.

Kee, J.L. (1982). *Fluids and electrolytes and clinical applications: A programmed approach* (3rd ed.). New York: John Wiley & Sons.

Lancaster, L.E. (1987). *Core curriculum for nephrology nursing, American Nephrology Nurses' Association.* Pitman, NJ: Anthony J. Jannette, Inc.

Larsen, E., Lindbloom, L., Davis, K.B. (1986). *Development of the clinical nephrology practitioner: A focus on independent learning.* Seattle: University of Washington Hospital.

Nyamathi, A. (1989). Coping responses of spouses of MI patients and of hemodialysis patients as measured by the Jalowiec coping scale. *Journal of Cardiovascular Nursing, 2*(1), 67–74.

Massry, S.G., Sellers, A.L. (1979). *Clinical aspects of uremia and dialysis* (2nd ed.). Springfield, IL: Charles C Thomas.

Plawecki, H.M., et al. (1987). Chronic renal failure. *Journal of Gerontologic Nursing, 13*(12), 14–17.

Hemodynamic Monitoring

In hemodynamic monitoring, cardiovascular pressures are measured and monitored through catheter tips placed in the atria, pulmonary artery, or systemic arteries. These measurements assist the nurse in monitoring cardiac output, fluid volume, and myocardial function.

Diagnostic Cluster

▲ **Time Frame**

Intramonitoring

▲ **Discharge Criteria**

Because hemodynamic monitoring is discontinued before discharge, no discharge criteria are indicated.

Collaborative Problems

Potential Complications: *Refer to:*
System Interference
Hemorrhage
Thrombosis/Thrombophlebitis
Pulmonary Embolism, Air Embolism
Arterial Spasm

Nursing Diagnoses

Potential for Infection related to invasive lines
Impaired Physical Mobility related to position restrictions
  secondary to hemodynamic monitoring
Anxiety related to impending procedure, loss of control, and   General Surgery
  unpredictable outcome

Collaborative Problems

▲ **Nursing Goal**

The nurse will manage and minimize vascular complications.

Potential Complication: System Interference
Potential Complication: Hemorrhage
Potential Complication: Thrombosis/Thrombophlebitis
Potential Complication: Pulmonary Embolism, Air Embolism
Potential Complication: Arterial Spasm

Interventions	*Rationale*

1. Monitor and intervene for the following:
  a. Damped waveform (decreased amplitude)
	1.
	  a. Damped waveform results from interference in the system, as from air, blood, kinks, loose connections, or occluded catheter tip.

1) Compare to previous waveform.	**1)** Comparison provides baseline assessment.
2) Monitor blood pressure and assess client.	**2)** Blood pressure and other assessment can determine actual hemodynamic function.
3) Check set-up of monitoring system.	**3)** Long lengths of tubing or overly compliant tubing can cause damped waveforms.
4) Check calibration.	**4)** Carefully checking the equipment can help ensure its accuracy.
5) Make sure pressure transducer system is inflated to 300 mm Hg and that all connections are tight.	**5)** This pressure setting helps prevent blood back-up.
6) Check system for air bubbles.	**6)** Air bubbles can enter the system through loose connections, damage, or too-vigorous flushing.

Interventions

    7) Check catheter for kinking.
    8) Aspirate any blood.
    9) Flush the system for less than 2 seconds.
  10) For a pulmonary arterial line, make sure the balloon is deflated.
  11) For a pulmonary arterial line, have the client cough or stimulate cough.
  12) For an arterial line, manipulate the extremity.

b. No waveform
    1) Make sure the monitor is turned on.
    2) Check the transducer cable at the monitoring insertion site.
    3) Check calibration.
    4) Make sure all connections are tight.
    5) Make sure all stopcocks are open to the client.
    6) Make sure the proper scale is set.
    7) Change the transducer or monitor.
    8) Aspirate any blood from the catheter.

    9) For a pulmonary arterial line, make sure the transducer is attached to the distal lumen.

c. Inaccurate data
    1) Check transducer level.
    2) Recalibrate, making sure the zero point on the tracing paper is accurate.

    3) Check for air bubbles.
    4) Change the transducer or monitor.

    5) Check the infusion rate of flushing solution.
    6) For an atrial line, compare cuff blood pressure measurements to invasive blood pressure readings. If they differ by more than 20 mm Hg, recheck the monitoring system.

d. Misinterpreted data
    1) For a pulmonary arterial line, measure pulmonary wedge pressure at end expiration.

    2) For a pulmonary arterial line, if the client is on mechanical ventilation, take all readings during therapy.

e. Artifact
    1) Make sure the waveform is free from catheter fling.

    2) Check the transducer and cable for cracks or moisture.

Rationale

    7) Kinking can cause damped waveform.

  9,10) In a pulmonary artery line, the catheter tip is prone to occlusion by the inflated balloon.
 11,12) Coughing and manipulation may help dislodge the catheter tip from the arterial wall and return it to its correct position.

b.
 1–7) No waveform indicates disruption of the monitoring system.

    8) Ability to aspirate blood may indicate that the catheter tip is occluded or lodged against an arterial wall.

c.
 1,2) The transducer's air–fluid interface must be at the level of the plebostatic axis. A lower position results in falsely high readings; a higher position, in false low readings.
    3) Air bubbles can amplify readings.
    4) Malfunctioning equipment must be replaced promptly.
    5) Improper infusion rate can skew readings.
    6) Invasive pressure 5 to 20 mm Hg over cuff pressure is considered normal; discrepancies beyond this range call for careful evaluation of the entire monitoring system.

d.
    1) End expiration is measured on the wedge tracing. In a client receiving mechanical ventilation, end expiration is manifested as the end of the negative slope. In a client with spontaneous respirations, and expiration is at the end of the positive slope.
    2) This allows accurate tracking of any trend.

e.
    1) Improper catheter placement and excessive catheter movement may cause fling.
    2) Erratic or noisy tracings may result from electrical interference.

Interventions

    3) Take readings while the client is lying quietly.
    4) Check the length of tubing in the monitoring system.
    5) Notify the physician.

  f. Continuous wedge
    1) Check the balloon for complete deflation.

    2) Do not flush the catheter.
    3) Have the client cough.

    4) Reposition the client from side to side.

    5) Aspirate from the distal port.

    6) Notify the physician.

  g. No wedge
    1) Deflate the balloon and compare the waveform with previous wedge waveforms.
    2) Inflate the balloon with the recommended amount of air.
    3) If you feel no resistance during inflation, stop inflating.
    4) Notify the physician.

  h. Overwedge waveform
    1) Make sure the balloon is deflated at initiation of the wedge procedure.

    2) Stop balloon inflation when wedge waveform appears.

    3) Record the amount of air used to obtain a waveform.
    4) Allow the balloon to remain inflated for only a few seconds, and limit the frequency of wedging.

  i. Right ventricular waveform
    1) Compare current waveform with previous findings.

    2) Monitor for ventricular dysrhythmias.
    3) Inflate the balloon.

    4) Notify the physician.

  j. Blood backup
    1) Make sure all connections are tight.
    2) Check the transducer system for cracks.
    3) Make sure all stopcocks are open to the client.

Rationale

    3) Having the client lie quietly reduces interference.
    4) Tubing more than 3 feet long may cause artifact.
    5) The physician may need to reposition the catheter.

  f.
    1) Incomplete balloon deflation may lead to pulmonary hemorrhage or infarction.
    2) Flushing can cause tissue damage.
    3) Coughing may help move the catheter tip away from the vessel wall.
    4) Repositioning may help move the catheter into proper position.
    5) An arterial sample is necessary for arterial blood gas (ABG) analysis.
    6) The physician may have to reposition the catheter and suture it into place.

  g.
    1) This step identifies whether or not the catheter is already wedged.

    2) Insufficient air volume may cause no wedge.
    3) Lack of resistance may indicate balloon rupture.
    4) The physician may need to reposition or replace the catheter to ensure balloon integrity and the ability to wedge properly.

  h.
    1) Passive deflation is used to avoid possible balloon rupture by aspiration of air.
    2) Overinflation causes overwedge waveform and may rupture the balloon or cause pulmonary infarction.
    3) This measure helps prevent overwedging from excessive inflation.
    4) Limiting balloon inflation and wedging reduces the risk of balloon rupture and circulatory interruptions.

  i.
    1) Dissimilar waveforms may indicate that the catheter has moved back into the right ventricle.
    2) Evaluation can rule out dysrhythmias.
    3) Inflation may help the catheter migrate into the pulmonary artery.
    4) The physician may need to reposition the catheter.

  j.
    1,2,3) These measures can help prevent blood back-up.

Interventions

Rationale

    4) Make sure the pressure system is inflated to 300 mm Hg.

    5) Flush the system.

2. Monitor for signs and symptoms of hemorrhage/shock:
   a. Increased pulse rate with normal or slightly decreased blood pressure
   b. Urine output < 30 mL/hr
   c. Restlessness, agitation, altered mentation
   d. Increased respiratory rate
   e. Diminished peripheral pulses
   f. Cool, pale, or cyanotic skin
   g. Thirst
3. Monitor all pressure system connections for tightness.
4. Apply secure dressings; recheck periodically.

5. If a femoral catheter is in place, minimize leg movement on the affected side.
6. Restrain the extremity of a disoriented client.
7. Instruct the client to report any bleeding immediately.
8. Apply firm pressure above the insertion site while removing the catheter. Apply direct pressure for at least 5 minutes or until bleeding stops. Then apply a pressure dressing for 20 minutes, making sure distal circulation is not obstructed.
9. Use a sandbag on a femoral insertion site for 1 hour after catheter removal.
10. Monitor for signs and symptoms of thrombophlebitis:
    a. Positive Homans' sign (pain on dorsiflexion of foot)
    b. Calf tenderness, unusual warmth, redness
11. Encourage leg exercises; discourage placing pillows under the knees, using a knee gatch, crossing the legs, and prolonged sitting.
12. Elevate the extremity and apply a warm compress if signs of ischemia develop.
13. Flush only 2 to 3 mL of fluid at one time.

14. Monitor for signs and symptoms of pulmonary embolism:
    a. Acute chest pain
    b. Tachycardia
    c. Dyspnea
    d. Pallor
    e. Agitation
    f. Decreased pO_2
15. Instruct the client to report any chest pain immediately.
16. Ensure the client that all connections are tight and stopcocks are in correct position.
17. Flush all lumina before insertion and check the system for air bubbles.

4) System pressure lower than the client's blood pressure can result in blood back-up.
5) The system always must be flushed after drawing blood samples.
2. The compensatory response to decreased circulatory volume aims to increase blood oxygen levels by increasing heart and respiratory rates and decreasing circulation to peripheral areas.

3. Disconnection can cause rapid exsanguination.

4. A secure dressing can prevent dislodgment from bumping.
5,6. Movement of the extremity can disconnect or dislodge the catheter.

7. Massive blood loss can occur in only a few seconds.
8. Direct pressure decreases the likelihood of hematoma.

9. External pressure promotes clotting.

10. Catheters can irritate the vessel, predisposing to thrombophlebitis.

11. Exercise increases venous return and prevents venous stasis.

12. Warmth and elevation promote venous return.

13. Larger volumes may cause backflow of blood and thrombus formation.
14. Signs can indicate a blockage of a portion of the pulmonary arterial system due to a clot originating in the system. Air emboli result from leaks or disruptions in the system.

15. Prompt reporting enables timely evaluation and treatment.
16. Correct position prevents air from entering the system.
17. Flushing removes air from the system.

▲ Documentation

Flow records
  Waveform, measurements
  System maintenance
  Vital signs
  Insertion site
  Heart rhythm
  Circulation distal to inser-
    tion site (color, tempera-
    ture, capillary refill, move-
    ment, sensation, edema)
Progress notes
  System troubleshooting
  Unusual events

Interventions

18. If you suspect air embolus, have the client perform Valsalva's maneuver, then place him in Trendelenburg's position.
19. Monitor for signs and symptoms of arterial spasm:
    a. Decreased or absent pulse distal to site

    b. Pain
20. Manipulate the catheter and extremity as little as possible.
21. Flush or aspirate the catheter using gentle technique.

Related Physician-Prescribed Interventions

Medications
  Heparin flush
Intravenous Therapy
  Saline intravenous flush
Laboratory Studies
  Hemoglobin, hematocrit   Arterial blood gas analysis
  Coagulation studies
Diagnostic Studies
  Chest x-ray film
  Lung scan
Therapy
  Oxygen therapy
  Protocols for system interference

Rationale

18. Movement of emboli is deterred by increasing intrathoracic pressure and decreasing venous return.
19. The catheter can irritate the vessel, causing a spasm
    a. A vessel in spasm provides diminished or no circulation to the distal area.
    b. Tissue ischemia produces pain.
20. Limited movement helps prevent irritation and trauma.
21. Forceful flushing or aspiration may cause arterial spasms.

Nursing Diagnoses

▲ Outcome Criteria

The client will remain free of infection at insertion sites.

Potential for Infection related to invasive lines

Focus Assessment Criteria

1. Site, for redness, inflammation, purulent drainage, tenderness, and warmth
2. Temperature
3. Chills, diaphoresis

Clinical Significance

1–3. This assessment focuses on detecting signs of the body's response to pyrogens.

Interventions

1. Use sterile technique when assisting with catheter insertion and removal and when maintaining the system and providing insertion site care.
2. Ensure complete skin preparation before insertion.
3. Coordinate changes of pressure system and catheter site dressing every 48 hours.
4. Change the flushing solution every 24 hours.

5. Use only the necessary stopcocks. Ensure that a Luer-lok cap is applied to each open port.
6. Flush the stopcock and system after all blood sampling.

7. Ensure catheter removal within 72 hours of insertion.

Rationale

1,2. Aseptic technique reduces microorganisms on equipment and insertion site.

3. Proper coordination minimizes opening of the system.
4. Discarding solution every 24 hours reduces microorganism growth.
5. The fewer stopcocks used, the fewer portals of entry for microorganisms are available.
6. Flushing removes all blood—an excellent medium for bacterial growth—and reduces the risk of infection.
7. Reducing the length of catheter insertion time can decrease the risk of nosocomial infection.

▲ **Documentation**

Flow records
  System maintenance
  Condition of site

▲ **Outcome Criteria**

The client will not experience complications of immobility.

Interventions

8. If blood backs up into the pressure system, change the system.

Rationale

8. Blood is an excellent culture medium; contamination of the pressure system necessitates changing the system to eliminate a potential source of infectious microorganisms.

Impaired Physical Mobility related to position restrictions secondary to hemodynamic monitoring

Focus Assessment Criteria	*Clinical Significance*
1. Motor function 2. Dominant hand 3. Restrictiveness of pressure system and dressings 4. Range of motion (ROM)	1–4. Assessment can determine the client's mobility and ability to perform activities of daily living (ADLs).

Interventions

1. Position the client so that the transducer is level with the phlebostatic axis when recording values.
2. Increase activity in correlation with hemodynamic stability.
3. Provide a pressure relief device on the bed.

4. Reposition the client with the extremities, head, and neck in natural positions every 2 hours using pillows, towels, and blanket rolls.
5. Develop a turning schedule to correlate with hemodynamic measurements and client preferences, if possible.
6. Encourage active ROM exercises or, if the client cannot comply, perform passive ROM every 6 hours.
7. If a radial arterial catheter restricts the client's use of his dominant hand, teach strategies to improve function of his nondominant hand.
8. Limit ROM to extremities distal to catheter insertion sites, e.g., radial, femoral, brachial.
9. Allow a client with a pulmonary artery catheter to dangle legs or sit in a chair only with the physician's consent.
10. Teach that impaired movement is a temporary state persisting only for the duration of hemodynamic monitoring.
11. Teach isometric exercises.

Rationale

1. This position increases the accuracy of readings.

2. Optimal mobility preserves function and helps prevent complications.
3. If immobility is prolonged, such a device can help prevent pressure ulcers.
4. Regular repositioning alternates pressure on tissues and helps prevent skin breakdown.

5. Establishing a schedule can reduce unnecessary movement to prevent catheter dislodgment.
6. ROM can promote muscle strength, improve circulation, and reduce contractures.

7. Adaptations may be needed to enhance self-care ability.

8. These restrictions are needed to prevent possible catheter dislodgment.
9. Excessive movement may cause catheter migration.

10. Explanation can reduce anxiety associated with fear of disability.

11. Isometric exercises can be done without bending or moving the extremity.

▲ **Documentation**

Flow records
  Position changes
Progress notes
  Ability to perform ROM exercises

References/Bibliography

Bolten, E. (1981). Procedural guidelines for the use of balloon-tipped, flow-directed catheters. *Critical Care Nurse, 1*(2), 33–40.

Daily, E.K., & Schroeder, J.S. (1981). *Techniques in bedside hemodynamic monitoring.* St. Louis: C.V. Mosby.

DeGroot, K., & Damato, M. (1986). Monitoring intra-arterial pressure. *Critical Care Nurse, 6*(1), 74–78.

Gardner, R.M., et al. (1988). Technologic advances in invasive pressure monitoring. *Journal of Cardiovascular Nursing, 2*(3), 52–55.

Gibbs, N.C., et al. (1988). Dynamics of invasive pressure monitoring systems: Clinical and laboratory evaluation. *Heart & Lung, 17*(1), 43–51.

Hirsch, J., & Hancock, L. (Eds.). (1981). *Clinical nursing procedures.* St. Louis: C.V. Mosby.

Johanson, B.C., Dungea, C.U., Hoffmeister, D., & Wells, S.J. (1985). *Standards for critical care* (2nd ed.). St. Louis: C.V. Mosby.

Kaye, W. (1983). Invasive monitoring techniques: Arterial cannulation, bedside pulmonary artery catheterization, and arterial puncture. *Heart & Lung, 12*(4), 395–427.

Kinney, M., Dear, C.B., Packa, D.R., & Voorman, D.N. (1981). *AACN's clinical reference for critical care nursing.* New York: McGraw-Hill.

Kirchoff, K., Rebenson-Piano, M., & Patel, M. (1984). Mean arterial pressure reading: Variations with positions and transducer level. *Nursing Research, 33*(6), 343–345.

Lough, M.E. (1987). Introduction to hemodynamic monitoring. *Nursing Clinics of North America, 22*(1), 89–110.

McIntyre, K., & Lewis, J.A. (Eds.). (1983). *Textbook of advanced cardiac life support.* Dallas: American Heart Association.

Meehan, P. (1986). Hemodynamic assessment using the automated physiologic profile. *Critical Care Nurse, 6*(1), 29–46.

Millar, S., Sampson, L.K., & Soukup, M. (Eds.). (1985). *AACN's procedure manual for critical care nursing.* Philadelphia: W.B. Saunders.

Santolla, A., & Weckel, C. (1983). A new closed system for arterial lines. *RN, 46*(6), 49–52.

Zorb, S. (1988). Care of the cardiac patient: Assessment, evaluation and nursing implications. Interpretation of laboratory data and hemodynamic monitoring, Part 2. *Journal of Intravenous Nursing, 11*(2), 113–118.

Long-Term Venous Access Devices

Long-term venous access devices (VADs) are used for clients who have need for frequent venous access to deliver chemotherapy, intravenous fluids, and blood products. They can also be used for blood sampling. The three types of VADs are *open atrial catheters* (e.g., Hickman catheter, Broviac catheter), *closed atrial catheters* (e.g., Groshong catheter), and *vascular access ports* (e.g., Porta-cath, Infusa-port, Med-a-port).

Diagnostic Cluster

▲ Time Frame
Preprocedure and postprocedure

▲ Discharge Criteria
Before discharge, the client and/or family will:
1. Demonstrate procedure and discuss conditions of catheter care and administration at home
2. Discuss strategies for incorporating catheter management in activities of daily living (ADLs)
3. Verbalize necessary precautions
4. State signs and symptoms that must be reported to a health care professional
5. Identify available community resources

Collaborative Problems

Potential Complications:
Pneumothorax
Hemorrhage
Embolism/Thrombosis
Sepsis

Nursing Diagnoses

Anxiety related to upcoming insertion of catheter and insufficient knowledge of procedure
Potential Altered Health Maintenance related to insufficient knowledge of home care, signs and symptoms of complications, and community resources
Potential for Infection related to catheter's direct access to bloodstream

Related Care Plans

Cancer (Initial Diagnosis)
Chemotherapy

Refer to:

Total Parenteral Nutrition

Collaborative Problems

▲ Nursing Goal
The nurse will manage and minimize vascular and respiratory complications.

Potential Complication: Pneumothorax
Potential Complication: Hemorrhage
Potential Complication: Embolism/Thrombosis
Potential Complication: Sepsis

Interventions

1. Monitor for signs and symptoms of pneumothorax:
   a. Sudden, stabbing chest pain
   b. Shortness of breath (SOB)
   c. Decreased or absent breath sounds
   d. Asymmetrical chest movement
2. Monitor for signs and symptoms of hemorrhage:
   a. Hypotension
   b. Tachycardia
   c. Evidence of bleeding

Rationale

1. Placement of a long-term venous catheter can result in laceration of the subclavian artery and fluid leakage into the pleural cavity, leading to alveolar rupture.

2. Hemorrhage is a serious surgical complication of long-term venous access catheter placement. It can occur within several hours of insertion, after blood pressure returns to preinsertion levels and put increased pressure on a newly formed clot. It also can develop later, secondary to vascular erosion due to infection.

Interventions

3. Monitor for signs and symptoms of embolism:
   a. Anxiety, restlessness
   b. Altered level of consciousness
   c. SOB
   d. Tachycardia

4. Monitor for signs and symptoms of hematoma:
   a. Tenderness and swelling at the insertion site
   b. Discoloration at the insertion site

5. Monitor for signs of septicemia:
   a. Temperature >101° F or < 98.6° F
   b. Decreased urine output
   c. Tachycardia, tachypnea
   d. Pale, cool skin
   e. WBCs and bacteria in urine
   f. Positive blood culture

6. Institute VAD care procedures as dictated by institutional policy and procedure. Keep the dressing intact, and tape the external catheter to the skin to prevent pulling.

7. Monitor for catheter displacement, damage, and obstruction:
   a. Superior vena cava syndrome (facial edema, distention of thoracic and neck veins)
   b. Swelling, redness, tenderness or drainage from insertion site
   c. Leakage of fluid from catheter
   d. Inaccurate infusion rate
   e. Inability to infuse or draw blood
   f. Bulging of catheter during infusion

Rationale

3. A client with a long-term VAD is at increased risk for embolism. Accidental leakage of air from the catheter can occlude a major pulmonary artery; obstruction of blood flow to the alveoli decreases alveolar perfusion, shunts air to patent alveoli, and leads to bronchial constriction and possible collapse of pulmonary tissue.

4. Long-term VAD placement can cause soft tissue injury resulting in rupture of small vessels. As blood collects at the insertion site, hematoma forms.

5. The invasive nature of a VAD puts the client at risk for opportunistic infection and septicemia. If the VAD is used to instill chemotherapy, the possibility of chemotherapy-induced leukopenia further increases the risk. Sepsis causes massive vasodilatation and resultant hypovolemia, leading to tissue hypoxia and decreased renal and cardiac function. The body's compensatory response increases respiratory and heart rates in an attempt to correct hypoxia and acidosis.

6. Precautions and preventive care measures are necessary to reduce the risk of infection.

7. Catheters can malfunction, obstruct, or displace from misuse or defects.

▲ *Documentation*

Flow records
  Vital signs
  Respiratory assessment
  Catheter site/patency
    assessment

Related Physician-Prescribed Interventions

Refer to the care plan for the underlying condition necessitating VAD use, e.g., Cancer (Initial Diagnosis).

Nursing Diagnoses

▲ *Outcome Criteria*

The client will:

1. Share feelings regarding scheduled catheter insertion
2. Relate what to expect during insertion

Anxiety related to upcoming insertion of catheter and insufficient knowledge of procedure

Focus Assessment Criteria	*Clinical Significance*
1. Knowledge of procedure 2. Knowledge of therapy	1,2. Knowledge about therapy and its effects enhances the client's sense of control and can reduce anxiety associated with fear of the unknown. Assessing the client's knowledge level guides the nurse in planning effective teaching strategies to address learning needs.
3. Anxiety level (mild, moderate, severe, panic)	3. Extreme anxiety can interfere with the client's coping ability. Modifiable factors that contribute to extreme anxiety include inaccurate or incomplete information about the threatening event.

Interventions

1. Reinforce the physician's explanation of the surgical diagnostic procedure. Notify the physician if additional explanations are indicated.

2. Provide an opportunity for the client to share fears and beliefs regarding chemotherapy. Delay teaching if high levels of anxiety are present.
3. Explain what to expect:
   a. Preprocedure (e.g., site preparation, draping)
   b. During insertion (e.g., positioning, sensations)
4. Instruct the client on how he or she can assist during the procedure:
   a. Communicating any sensations felt to the physician
   b. Following physician's instructions (e.g., holding breath and lying still during insertion; coughing, deep breathing, exercising legs postprocedure
5. Explain that nursing staff monitors the following at frequent intervals:
   a. Blood pressure
   b. Pulse rate and rhythm
   c. Condition of the catheter insertion site
   d. Condition of the limb distal to the insertion site

   Also explain that a chest x-ray film will be obtained.

6. Instruct on the need to immobilize the limb used for the procedure for the prescribed length of time.
7. Refer to the Cancer (Initial Diagnosis) care plan, page 322, for additional specific strategies to reduce anxiety.

Rationale

1. The physician is legally responsible for explanations for an informed consent; the nurse, for clarifying information, evaluating understanding, and notifying the physician if more information is necessary.
2. Sharing helps the nurse identify sources of anxiety and correct misinformation. High anxiety prevents retention of information.
3. Perception of an event is gained through all senses. Providing sensory information along with procedural information gives the client more data to use to accurately interpret and master the event.
4. Eliciting the client's cooperation with the procedure can help improve compliance and reduce the risk of complications.

5. Instructions about specific procedures can help reduce anxiety associated with the unknown and the unexpected.

6. Immobilization helps reduce complications of hemorrhage or thrombosis.

▲ *Documentation*

Teaching record
  Client teaching
  Outcome achievement or
    status

▲ *Outcome Criteria*

The outcome criteria for this diagnosis represent those associated with discharge planning. Refer to the discharge criteria.

Potential Altered Health Maintenance related to insufficient knowledge of home care, signs and symptoms of complications, and community resources

Focus Assessment Criteria

1. Knowledge of the procedure and perception of why it is needed

2. Available support systems to assist with home therapy
3. Readiness and ability to learn and retain information

Clinical Significance

1. Assessing knowledge level identifies learning needs and guides the nurse in planning effective teaching strategies.
2. Successful home management often hinges on availability of needed support systems.
3. A client or family failing to achieve learning goals requires a referral for assistance postdischarge.

Interventions

1. Reinforce the physician's explanation of the catheterization procedure, including line placement, incorporating individually oriented media when possible.
2. Explain the advantages and disadvantages of the atrial catheters and vascular access ports.

Rationale

1. Explanations can reduce misconceptions and increase participation.

2. Discussing the different devices can help the client better understand how the decision on

Interventions

a. Atrial catheters (open and closed)—advantages
   - Provide unlimited venous access
   - Eliminate the need for painful needle sticks
   - Can be used for continuous infusion in both the hospital and the home
   - Carry a reduced risk of extravasation
   - Cause little discomfort
b. Atrial catheters (open and closed)—disadvantages
   - Require dressing changes
   - Require heparin (open) or saline (closed) flushes
   - Require cap changes (usually weekly)

c. Vascular access ports—advantages
   - Free client from most responsibility for routine dressing changes and flushing
   - Carry a lower risk of infection
d. Vascular access ports—disadvantages
   - Require needle sticks through the skin to gain access
   - Allow a limited number of accesses, depending on needle size (typically 1000–2000)
   - Require surgery to implant and remove
3. Explain the reasons for continued assessment procedures and diagnostic tests, e.g., daily weights, intake and output monitoring, urine and serum evaluations.
4. Explain aseptic technique; obtain return demonstration of handwashing and preparation of work surface.
5. Explain home care measures and discuss the roles and expectations of all concerned—the client, family members, visiting nurse, and others as appropriate.
6. Teach manipulation of syringe and needle and method of drawing up solution. Obtain return demonstrations from the client and family members to demonstrate understanding and mastery.
7. Teach catheter care according to protocols; obtain return demonstrations of care measures, as necessary. Provide written material for the following:
   a. Dressing change
   b. Site care
   c. Emergency measures
   d. Heparinizing the catheter
   e. Changing injection cap
   f. Managing a clotted catheter
   g. Catheter repair

Rationale

which type to use was made. Seeing the logic behind the decision may encourage compliance.
a. Open catheter method provides a catheter at the skin surface for medication administration. Single- and double-lumen catheters are available. Double-lumen catheters provide greater flexibility with treatment; e.g., chemotherapy and total parenteral nutrition (TPN) can be administered simultaneously. Both the open and closed catheters require surgical insertion.
b. Vascular access ports consist of a chamber with a septum that is attached to a catheter. The chamber and the catheter are surgically implanted under the skin. Drugs and fluids are administered by injecting a noncoring needle through the skin and into the chamber. The fluid flows through the needle into the chamber and through the catheter into the right atrium.

3. The client's understanding that careful monitoring is needed to assess status and to detect problems early promotes his cooperation with procedures.
4. Understanding enables compliance with measures to prevent infection.

5. Expectations should be clear to prevent misunderstanding.

6. These skills are needed for home management.

7. Understanding the protocols and techniques for home care is critical to prevent infection and clotting and to manage problems or emergencies.

Interventions

8. Discuss strategies for keeping the home environment safe and conducive to good care:
   a. Store supplies in a clean, dry place.
   b. Do not tell others that syringes are stored in the home.
   c. Use a shoebox with a small hole in the top for discarding used syringes.
   d. Tape and discard the box when filled.
   e. Keep clean syringes, the used syringe box, and heparin out of reach and sight of children and confused adults.
   f. Perform catheter care in the bathroom or kitchen, where a sink is available for handwashing.
   g. Thoroughly clean the work area before laying out supplies.

9. Explain signs and symptoms of VAD complications:

   a. Fever
   b. Tenderness, swelling, drainage at site
   c. Inaccurate infusion rate
   d. Inability to infuse

   e. Facial edema, distended neck veins

10. Provide a list of required equipment and supplies.
11. Instruct on who the client or family can call with questions day or night, e.g., nurses' station, physician.

Rationale

8. These measures help reduce the risk of injury and infection transmission.

9. Understanding the signs and symptoms of complications enables early detection and reporting to a health care professional for timely intervention.
   a,b. Fever and changes at the insertion site may indicate infection.
   c,d. Inaccurate infusion rate or inability to infuse points to obstruction or catheter damage.
   e. Facial edema and neck vein distention may indicate superior vena caval syndrome.

10. Planning can prevent shortages and improper substitutions.
11. Questions are likely to arise after discharge.

▲ **Documentation**

Discharge summary record
  Client and family teaching
  Outcome achievement or
    status

References/Bibliography

Bejletich, J. (1980). The Hickman indwelling catheter. *American Journal of Nursing, 80*(1), 62–65.
Carelli, R.M., & Herink, E. (1984). Hickman/Broviac catheters: Results of survey and patient care consideration. *NITA, 7*(4), 287–289.
Duval, A. (1984). The multi-lumen catheter: A new concept in infusion therapy. *Nutrition Support Services, 4*(2), 22–26.
Goodman, M.S., & Wickham, R. (1984). Venous access devices: An overview. *Oncology Nursing Forum, 11*(5), 16–23.
Handy, C.M. (1989). Vascular access devices: Hospital to home care. *Journal of Intravenous Nursing, 12*(1), S10–S18.
Winters, V. (1984). Implantable vascular access devices. *Oncology Nursing Forum, 11*(6), 25–30.

Mechanical Ventilation

Indicated for continuous control of ventilation and oxygen administration, continuous mechanical ventilation uses a positive or negative pressure breathing device that can automatically maintain respirations. Negative pressure ventilators include the iron lung, portalung, body wrap, and chest cuirass. Positive pressure ventilators are either pressure-cycled, time-cycled, or volume-cycled. For continuous use, endotracheal intubation or tracheostomy is required. Conditions that necessitate continuous mechanical ventilation include CNS disorders that compromise the respiratory center in the medulla, musculoskeletal conditions that limit chest expansion, neuromuscular disorders, heart failure, respiratory disorders, and upper airway obstruction.

Diagnostic Cluster

▲ **Time Frame**

During therapy in facility

Collaborative Problems

Potential Complications:
Respiratory Insufficiency
Atelectasis
Oxygen Toxicity
Decreased Cardiac Output
Gastrointestinal (GI) Bleeding

Nursing Diagnoses

	Refer to:
Potential Ineffective Breathing Pattern related to weaning attempts, respiratory muscle fatigue secondary to mechanical ventilation, increased work of breathing, supine position, protein-calorie malnutrition, inactivity, and fatigue	
Potential for Disuse Syndrome related to imposed immobility	Immobility or Unconsciousness
Fear related to the nature of the situation, uncertain prognosis of ventilator dependence, or weaning	Chronic Obstructive Pulmonary Disease
Impaired Verbal Communication related to effects of intubation on ability to speak	Tracheostomy
Potential for Infection related to disruption of skin layer secondary to tracheostomy	Tracheostomy
Potential Ineffective Airway Clearance related to increased secretions secondary to tracheostomy, obstruction of inner cannula, or displacement of tracheostomy tube	Tracheostomy
Powerlessness related to dependency on respirator, inability to talk, and loss of mobility	Chronic Obstructive Pulmonary Disease

▲ **Discharge Criteria**

Because mechanical ventilation is discontinued before discharge, no discharge criteria are applicable.

Collaborative Problems

▲ **Nursing Goal**

The nurse will manage and minimize complications of mechanical ventilation.

Potential Complication: **Respiratory Insufficiency**
Potential Complication: **Atelectasis**
Potential Complication: **Oxygen Toxicity**
Potential Complication: **Decreased Cardiac Output**
Potential Complication: **GI Bleeding**

Interventions

1. Assess respiratory status: auscultate breath sounds and observe symmetry of chest movements.

Rationale

1. Auscultating breath sounds assesses adequacy of airflow and detects the presence of adventitious sounds. Asymmetrical chest movements can indicate improper tube placement.

577

Interventions

2. Monitor for signs of respiratory insufficiency:
   a. Increased respiratory rate
   b. Labored respirations
   c. Restlessness, agitation, confusion
   d. Unstable vital signs
   e. Abnormal arterial blood gas (ABG) analysis values

3. Monitor for signs of atelectasis:
   a. Marked dyspnea
   b. Anxiety
   c. Cyanosis
   d. Tachycardia

4. Maintain a patent airway; suction as needed.

5. Maintain proper cuff inflation.

6. Monitor for signs and symptoms of oxygen toxicity:
   a. Substernal distress
   b. Paresthesias in extremities
   c. Progressive dyspnea
   d. Restlessness

7. Monitor for signs of decreased cardiac output:
   a. Dysrhythmias
   b. Diminished peripheral pulses
   c. Altered vital signs
   d. Cold, clammy skin
   e. Dyspnea

8. Monitor for GI bleeding: evaluate stool for occult blood, and gastric pH (if the client is receiving nothing by mouth [NPO]).

Rationale

2. Respiratory insufficiency can result from airway obstruction, ventilator problems, atelectasis, bronchospasm, or pneumothorax.

3. Atelectasis can result from bronchial obstruction due to a mucous plug or from upward diaphragmatic displacement due to increased intra-abdominal pressure. The resulting signs and symptoms reflect decreased alveolar exchange and circulating oxygen.

4. Airway obstruction causes respiratory insufficiency. An intubated client is dependent on suctioning to remove secretions, because of ineffective cough reflex or fatigue.

5. Underinflation allows aspiration of gastric or respiratory secretions. Overinflation can cause tracheal tissue compression, resulting in ulceration.

6. Oxygen toxicity, resulting from prolonged administration of excessive oxygen concentrations, leads to decreased surfactant secretion, causing decreased lung compliance, and colloid degeneration, causing hyaline membrane formation in the lung lining and the development of pulmonary edema.

7. Positive-pressure ventilation increases intrathoracic pressure, which can reduce venous return and cardiac output. The resulting signs reflect decreased venous return and hypoxemia.

8. Profound stimulation of the vagus nerve causes hypersecretion of gastric secretions and possible ulcer formation.

▲ **Documentation**

Flow records
  Vital signs
  Respiratory assessment
  Cuff pressure

Related Physician-Prescribed Interventions

Medications
  Bronchodilators
  Antacids
  Short-acting hypnotics

Intravenous Therapy
  Total parenteral nutrition
  Fluid/electrolyte replacement

Laboratory Studies
  Arterial blood gases
  Serum protein, creatinine
  Serum electrolytes

Diagnostic Studies
  Chest x-ray film

Therapies
  Type and operation of ventilator (volume, pressure, rate, control mode, percentage of oxygen)
  Type and size of tube

Nursing Diagnoses

▲ **Outcome Criteria**

The client will:

1. Demonstrate required protein and calorie intake
2. Participate in activities to reduce inactivity
3. Demonstrate required fluid intake

Potential Ineffective Breathing Pattern related to weaning attempts, respiratory muscle fatigue secondary to mechanical ventilation, increased work of breathing, supine position, protein-calorie malnutrition, inactivity, and fatigue

Focus Assessment Criteria	*Clinical Significance*

1. Respiratory function
2. Laboratory studies:
  a. Hemoglobin and hematocrit
  b. ABG analysis
  c. Serum protein and electrolytes
3. Intake (oral and parenteral)
4. Urine output
5. GI function (bowel sounds, bowel movements)
6. Daily weights
7. Sleep (quality and quantity)
8. Activity level
	1–8. Continuous assessment is needed to detect factors that could impair weaning.

Interventions

1. Removal secretions, as necessary.

2. Promote chest expansion.

3. Assess for tube-related causes of resistance to flow, such as these:
   a. Too-small endotracheal tube
   b. Too-long endotracheal tube
   c. Inflated cuff
   d. T-piece weaning
4. Assess for dyspnea.

5. Position the client upright, sitting, or in bed with legs dangling.

6. Plan adequate rest periods before and after activity and during weaning efforts.

7. Take precautions to prevent infection:
   a. Change tubing every 24 to 48 hours.
   b. Remove lines early.
   c. Reduce endogenous organisms through frequent handwashing, careful housekeeping, and other measures.
8. Promote optimal nutrition:

Rationale

1. A tube partially obstructed with secretions increases resistance to flow, increasing the work of breathing.
2. Any impediment to chest expansion increases the work of breathing.
3. An endotracheal tube's caliber and length influence the resistance to flow. If risk of aspiration is minimal, a deflated cuff reduces resistance. Continuous positive airway pressure decreases the work of breathing, as compared to T-piece weaning.
4. Dyspnea interferes with successful weaning. A weaning schedule that reduces tidal volume slowly and increases endurance is recommended.
5. An upright position maximizes diaphragm excursion, increasing lung volume and gas exchange.
6. Respiratory muscle fatigue can result from prolonged artificial ventilation, increased work of breathing, and reduction in energy reserves.
   a. Rest periods help replenish energy expended in activity.
   b. Alternating weaning with rest periods on mechanical ventilation rests fatigued muscles.
7. A client on long-term ventilation is at increased risk of infection owing to microorganisms on equipment and in the environment and altered defense mechanisms.

8. Malnutrition has a negative effect on respiratory function, which depends on adequate muscle function and uses energy continu-

Interventions

Rationale

ously. A malnourished client has a decreased response to hypoxia, expiratory muscle weakness, reduced muscle endurance, decrease surfactant, impaired immune responses, and fluid imbalances from electrolyte changes.

   a. Consult a nutritionist to calculate specific protein and calorie needs.

   a. The nurse may need assistance to calculate the client's specific nutritional requirements according to metabolic demands. Underfeeding can increase the risk of pulmonary complications; overfeeding can increase metabolic rate and carbon dioxide production.

   b. Weigh the client daily.

   b. Actual weight on a properly calibrated scale can provide a reflection of overall nutritional status. Weekly weight loss of 1% to 2% of total body weight is significant.

   c. Monitor laboratory study results:
     • Serum albumin and transferrin
     • Total white blood cell (WBC) count
     • Creatinine index

   c. Laboratory data can provide information on nutritional status, especially when weight fluctuates with fluid retention or loss.

9. Consult with the physician regarding enteral or parenteral nutrition, as appropriate.

9. In most cases, a client with an artificial airway is unable to meet his or her nutritional needs solely through oral ingestion. When supplemental feeding is required, the enteral route is preferred over the parenteral route because of the latter's greater risk of catheter-related sepsis.

10. Take steps to prevent constipation:
   a. Ensure adequate fluid and fiber intake.
   b. Establish a regular time for defecation and promote a close-to-normal (semi-squatting) position on the bedpan, commode, or toilet.

10. Abdominal distention from gas, ileus, or constipation prevents adequate diaphragm function.

11. Promote optimal activity:
   a. Encourage active or perform passive range-of-motion (ROM) exercises, as the client's ability permits.
   b. Provide a wheelchair for a client with a portable ventilator.

11. Inactivity decreases respiratory muscle size and strength, interfering with optimal respiratory effort.

12. Institute measures to ensure uninterrupted rapid-eye-movement (REM) sleep (4 to 5 cycles of 70 to 100 minutes):
   a. Reduce noise.
   b. Teach relaxation techniques.
   c. Consult with the physician for a short-acting hypnotic agent, if needed.

12. Deprivation of REM sleep frequently occurs in the hospital. Prolonged inadequate REM sleep results in sluggish thought processes and anxiety.

13. Take steps to reduce pain to tolerable levels, e.g., analgesics or nonpharmacological pain relief measures such as relaxation, distraction, and guided imagery.

13. Pain can contribute to anxiety, inhibit chest excursion on respiration, and restrict coughing.

14. Consult with the physician to delay weaning if any of these factors occurs:
   a. Irreversible underlying disease
   b. Metabolic alkalosis or acidosis
   c. Multisystem failure
   d. Clinical instability
   e. Protein-calorie malnutrition

14.

   a–d. A client who is not improving or is not clinically stable does not have the reserves to accommodate successfully to weaning.

   e. A malnourished client is unable to produce sufficient energy supplies to allow weaning.

Interventions

f. Decreased maximal inspiratory pressure (MIP) during weaning
g. Rapid, shallow breathing during weaning
15. Before weaning, discuss the process with the client and family.

16. Before, during, and after weaning attempts, assess the following factors:
a. Vital capacity
b. Inspiratory force
c. Vital signs
d. Arterial blood gas values

Rationale

f,g. A decrease in MIP or rapid, shallow breathing in response to weaning indicates poor respiratory muscle strength.
15. Adequate preparation is needed to reduce fears. Emphasizing that the client is improving, explaining the procedure, and providing constant supervision can improve motivation and decrease anxiety.
16. The client's ventilator capacities and perfusion serve as criteria for evaluating whether or not to progress weaning.

▲ **Documentation**

Flow records
  Vital signs
  Ventilator settings
  Type of tube (inflation)
  Respiratory assessment
  Intake and output
  Bowel sounds
  Rest and activity patterns
  Suctioning provided
  Pre-, intra-, and postweaning
    assessments
  Client teaching
Progress notes
  Psychological status

References/Bibliography

Celentano-Norton, L., & Neureuter, A. (1989). Weaning the long-term ventilator-dependent patient: Common problems and management. *Critical Care Nurse, 9*(1), 42–52.

Craven, D.E., Connolly, M.G., & Lichtenberg, D.A. (1976). Contamination of mechanical ventilators with tubing change every 24 or 48 hours. *New England Journal of Medicine, 306*(9), 1505–1509.

Hagarty, E. (1984). Weaning your COPD patient from the ventilator. *Nursing Research, 47*(8), 36–40.

Helton, M., Gordon, S., & Nunnery, S. (1980). The correlation between sleep deprivation and intensive care unit syndrome. *Heart & Lung, 9*(5), 464–468.

Hess, D. (1988). Controversies in respiratory critical care. *Critical Care Nurse Quarterly, 11*(3), 62–78.

Irwin, M.M., & Openbrier, D.R. (1985). A delicate balance: Strategies for feeding ventilated COPD patients. *American Journal of Nursing, 85*(3), 274–280.

Majors, M. (1988). Nutritional support of the mechanically ventilated patient. *Critical Care Nurse Quarterly, 11*(3), 50–61.

Nett, L.M., Morganroth, M., & Petty, T.L. (1987). Weaning from the ventilator. *American Journal of Nursing, 87*(9), 1173–1184.

Vasbinda-Dillon, D. (1988). Understanding mechanical ventilation. *Critical Care Nurse, 8*(7), 42–43.

Weissman, C., Kemper, M.C., & Askanazi, J. (1986). Resting metabolic rate of critically ill patients: Measured vs predicted. *Anesthesiology, 64*(6), 673–679.

Pacemaker Insertion

A pacemaker is an electrical device implanted to help maintain normal cardiac rhythm in the presence of SA–AV node conduction disturbances, e.g., bradycardia, heart block, and certain tachydysrhythmias. In the implantation procedure, a bipolar or unipolar electrode is inserted through the subclavian vein into the right atrium or ventricle under fluoroscopy. Permanent pacemakers have a pulse generator, which requires periodic recharging, implanted in a subcutaneous pouch in the chest or abdomen. The pacemaker can be set on a demand or fixed rate.

Diagnostic Cluster

▲ Time Frame
Preprocedure and postprocedure

▲ Discharge Criteria
Before discharge, the client and/or family will:

1. Demonstrate accuracy in counting a pulse
2. Verbalize precautions to take with regard to the pacemaker
3. State signs and symptoms that must be reported to a health care professional
4. Verbalize an intent to share feelings and concerns related to the pacemaker with significant others

---

PREPROCEDURE PERIOD
Nursing Diagnoses

Anxiety related to impending pacemaker insertion and prognosis

POSTPROCEDURE PERIOD
Collaborative Problems

Potential Complications:
Cardiac
Pacemaker Malfunction
Rejection of Unit
Necrosis over Pulse Generator

Nursing Diagnoses

Impaired Physical Mobility related to incisional site pain, activity restrictions, and fear of lead displacements
Self-Concept Disturbance related to perceived loss of health and dependence on pacemaker
Potential Altered Health Maintenance related to insufficient knowledge of activity restrictions, precautions, signs and symptoms of complications, and follow-up care

---

Preprocedure: Nursing Diagnosis

▲ Outcome Criteria
The client will:

1. Verbalize the goal of pacemaker implantation as treatment, not cure
2. Verbalize accurate information about the procedure and postprocedure care

Anxiety related to impending pacemaker insertion and prognosis

Focus Assessment Criteria	*Clinical Significance*
1. Understanding of symptoms, the need for a pacemaker, and preprocedure and postprocedure care measures	1. Assessment is needed to determine if additional information is needed.
2. Method of implantation (transvenous versus transthoracic)	2. Preprocedure and postprocedure nursing care varies depending on the implantation method.

Interventions

1. Reinforce the physician's explanation of the surgical procedure.

2. Assess understanding and notify the physician if additional explanations are needed.

Rationale

1. If anxiety impedes the client's ability to assimilate information, repeated exposure to this or any other information may be helpful.

2. The physician is responsible for explaining the surgery to the client and family; the

582

Interventions

Rationale

nurse, for determining the level of understanding and notifying the physician if they require additional explanations.

3. Have the client recall symptoms leading up to the present point. Explain that symptoms are the manifestation of a heart rhythm disturbance.

3. Recognition of the symptoms as a manifestation of an underlying problem helps the client understand and accept the need for a pacemaker.

4. Show the client a pulse generator, if available.

4. Handling actual equipment provides visual and tactile information and helps the client better understand the device and its operation.

5. Describe the preprocedural routine (as appropriate for the client) of blood tests, electrocardiogram (ECG), chest x-ray film, and food and fluid restriction.

5–8. Explaining what to expect may help reduce the client's anxiety related to fear of the unknown and unexpected and may enhance his sense of control over the situation.

6. Explain that the client will be awake during the insertion but that a sedative will be given to aid relaxation.

7. Explain the physical appearance of the catheterization laboratory or operating room, wherever the procedure will be done.

8. Instruct concerning pacemaker insertion and associated sensations, covering the following:
   a. Attachment of telemetry leads to monitor cardiac function
   b. Insertion of intravenous lines to provide direct IV access if needed
   c. Preparation of the skin where the incision is to be made
   d. Injection of local anesthetic into the entire area
   e. Expected sensations of pressure and pulling during lead insertion, with no sensation after insertion is complete
   f. The need to notify the physician of pain experienced during the procedure
   g. Positioning of the x-ray machine over the body and loud sounds from the x-ray machine
   h. Possibility of palpitations during assessment of lead placement
   i. Creation of a small pocket underneath the skin and closure with sutures
   j. Return to the recovery room or unit on telemetry
   k. Possibility that the client may be able to feel the pacemaker turn on and off for the first month or so after implantation
   l. Likelihood that he or she will notice the pulse generator under the skin for about 6 months, at which point conscious awareness of the implant should diminish
   m. When the client will be able to see family and other support persons

9. Instruct on the postprocedure routine, covering these factors:
   a. Frequent monitoring of blood pressure and pulse
   b. Telemetry ECG
   c. Frequent assessment of the insertion site

9. The client's understanding that careful monitoring is necessary to evaluate his response to the pacemaker can ease anxiety and encourage cooperation.

Interventions

10. Instruct the client not to use the affected arm while transferring from or to the bed or pushing himself up in bed for the first 24 to 48 hours.

11. Instruct the client to report the following immediately:
    a. Pain at the insertion site

    b. Palpitations

    c. Dizziness

    d. Rapid hiccups or chest muscle twitching

12. Provide written materials that reinforce teaching.

▲ *Documentation*

Teaching record
   Client teaching
   Outcome achievement or
     status
Progress notes
   Unusual responses

13. If possible, arrange for the client to talk with a person who has successfully gone through pacemaker implantation.

14. Refer to a clinical nurse specialist, social worker, or clergy if anxiety is dysfunctional.

Rationale

10. Movement restrictions aim to prevent displacement of leads.

11. Early detection enables prompt intervention to reduce the severity of complications.
    a. Pain at the site may indicate compression from hemorrhage or edema.
    b. Palpitations can indicate failure of the pacemaker to control the heart rate.
    c. Dizziness may result from decreased cardiac output with resultant cerebral hypoxia.
    d. Hiccups or chest muscle twitching may point to perforation of the ventricle and stimulation of the diaphragm or intercostal muscle by the lead.

12. The client and family can retain and refer to written materials after discharge. Such materials also can provide information to support persons not accompanying the client for teaching.

13. A person who has had a pacemaker implanted successfully can provide a role model for the client and promote a relaxed, healthy attitude toward the procedure.

14. For some clients, referrals may be necessary for intensive interventions and consultation.

Postprocedure: Collaborative Problems

▲ *Nursing Goal*

The nurse will manage and minimize complications after pacemaker implantation.

Potential Complication: Cardiac Problem
Potential Complication: Pacemaker Malfunction
Potential Complication: Rejection of Unit
Potential Complication: Necrosis over Pulse Generator

Interventions

1. Monitor for signs of perforation of the right or left ventricle:
   a. Distended neck veins
   b. Hepatic engorgement
   c. Narrow pulse pressure
   d. Decreased blood pressure
2. Monitor for dysrhythmias.

3. Monitor for pacemaker failure, marked by no pacemaker activation visible on the ECG with a heart rate below the preset limit. If it occurs, notify the physician and monitor for hemodynamic compromise.
4. Monitor for electromagnetic interference, marked by onset of prepacemaker symptoms when near a source of electromagnetic interference (e.g., transcutaneous electrical nerve stimulation [TENS] units, electromagnets) or by intermittent failure to pace with an artifact absent. If it occurs, move the client away from the source of interference.

Rationale

1. Perforation of the right or left ventricle results in decreased cardiac output, circulatory congestion (particularly in the hepatic and neck areas), and shock.

2. Rhythm disturbances are common for 48 to 72 hours after implantation owing to myocardial irritability and injury from lead insertion.
3. Pacemaker failure may result from battery failure, complete lead fracture, or a broken connection between the lead and pulse generator.

4. Electromagnetic interference can inhibit pacemaker function or cause it to revert to a fixed mode of pacing.

Interventions

5. Monitor for undersensing—no recycling of the pacemaker by intrinsic beats. If it occurs, monitor for pacemaker-initiated dysrhythmias.

6. Monitor for oversensing, marked by a distance from the oversensed wave or complex to the next pacemaker artifact equal to that of a normal escape interval. If it occurs, monitor for hemodynamic compromise.

7. Monitor for partial or improper sensing, characterized by inconsistent escape intervals; if it occurs, monitor for hemodynamic compromise.

8. Monitor for noncaptured pacemaker artifact—visible pacemaker artifact without resultant depolarization. If it occurs, monitor for hemodynamic compromise.

9. Monitor for runaway pacemaker, marked by a paced rate accelerating to the upper limit of the pulse generator (can be intermittent) and palpitations. If it occurs, monitor for hemodynamic compromise.

10. Monitor for diaphragmatic or phrenic nerve pacing—diaphragmatic contractions or hiccups at the pacemaker rate, with pacemaker artifact.

11. Monitor for chest muscle stimulation around the pulse generator; if it occurs, verify that the client is not moving the pulse generator.

12. Monitor the pulse generator implantation site for the following:
    a. Hemorrhage
    b. Signs and symptoms of infection
    c. Skin inflammation or necrosis over and around the pulse generator

Rationale

5. Undersensing may result from the pacemaker electrodes' failure to sense the vector of a spontaneous beat (PVC) as greater than 2 mV and subsequent failure to trigger the sensing mechanism. It can also occur if the size of the intrinsic R or P wave is less than the millivolt sensitivity of the pacemaker.

6. The pulse generator may be sensitive enough to interpret other waves (e.g., T waves) as a QRS.

7. Poor positioning of catheter electrodes or low voltage of intracavitary signals may cause incomplete recycling of the sensing mechanisms, resulting in short escape intervals. Partial sensing also may be due to incomplete lead fracture. A faulty sensing mechanism can cause pacer spike to fall during a vulnerable period of the T wave if competitive rhythm develops.

8. Noncaptured beats may be due to lead displacement or high threshold of the myocardium from fibrosis or ischemia at the lead tip.

9. Component failure may cause runaway pacemaker.

10. Lead placement near the diaphragmatic portion of the right ventricle or the tip of the atrial lead may be too close to the phrenic nerve, leading to stimulation of these nerves.

11. Chest muscle stimulation may result from high pacemaker output, high current density, lead fracture, flipped pulse generator, or low threshold to muscle pacing.

12. The surgical implantation and the presence of a foreign body increases the risk of hemorrhage, necrosis, and infection. Careful monitoring can help ensure early detection of problems.

▲ **Documentation**

Flow records
    Vital signs
    Rhythm strips
    Wound and dressing status

Related Physician-Prescribed Interventions

Medications
  Antibiotics

Intravenous Therapy
  Intravenous line for direct venous access

Laboratory Studies
  Electrolytes

Diagnostic Studies
  ECG   Electrophysiology studies
  Chest x-ray film

Therapies
  Pacemaker setting   Site care

Postprocedure: Nursing Diagnoses

▲ Outcome Criteria

The client will:

1. Demonstrate the ability to raise the affected arm over the head after 48 hours of immobilization
2. Demonstrate the ability to perform activities of daily living (ADLs)
3. Verbalize prescribed restrictions

Impaired Physical Mobility related to incisional site pain, activity restrictions, and fear of lead displacement

Focus Assessment Criteria	*Clinical Significance*
1. Range of motion (ROM) of affected extremity	1,2. Pain and activity restrictions serve as signals to the client to immobilize the affected extremity.
2. Pain at incision site	3. Fear of lead displacement may magnify the significance of these signals to such a degree that the client inappropriately immobilizes the arm.
3. Understanding of activity restrictions, fears regarding movement	

Interventions	*Rationale*
1. Explain the need to remain on bed rest with the head elevated no more than 30 degrees for 48 to 72 hours after implantation.	1. Complete bed rest is prescribed to allow fibrosis to occur around the pacemaker and electrodes, which helps prevent dislodgment.
2. Medicate with prescribed analgesics before the client engages in any activity.	2. Judicious use of pain medication keeps pain signals from discouraging use of the affected arm.
3. Explain that the incision and subcutaneous pocket should feel sore for 3 to 4 weeks, but that discomfort eventually does disappear.	3. Understanding that discomfort is temporary encourages the client to accept the pacemaker and participate in activity.
4. Encourage the client to perform active ROM exercises in the affected arm following the physician's instructions.	4. Regular ROM exercise maintains joint function and prevents muscle contractures.
5. Encourage early and complete participation in ADLs.	5. Self-care increases independence and a sense of well-being.
6. Reinforce physician-prescribed postoperative activity restrictions; these may include no driving, no lifting, no golfing, no bowling, etc., for 4 to 6 weeks after surgery.	6. Activity restrictions allow continued fibrosis around the pacemaker and electrodes to provide increased stabilization.
7. Provide written information on activity instructions and restrictions.	7. Written materials can serve as a valuable resource for postdischarge care at home.

▲ Documentation

Discharge summary record
Level of activity
Client teaching
Outcome achievement or status
Referrals, if indicated

▲ Outcome Criteria

The client will:

1. Verbalize an intent to follow the prescribed medical regimen
2. Verbalize recognition that despite the physical loss, he or she remains much the same person
3. Verbalize recognition that he or she is a unique individual not to be compared with others
4. Verbalize the value of other personal attributes besides physical ability and appearance

Self-Concept Disturbance related to perceived loss of health and dependence on pacemaker

Focus Assessment Criteria	*Clinical Significance*
1. Accuracy of the client's perceptions regarding pacemaker	1. Pacemaker implantation can cause a sense of loss, which can negatively affect self-concept.
2. Client's self-concept before pacemaker implantation	2. Acceptance of the pacemaker can be affected by many factors; however, a person's ability to adjust depends on his or her ability to identify personal strengths still present, compensate for what is lost, and view himself or herself as a unique person.
3. Length of preoperative illness	3. A client with longstanding symptoms before pacemaker implantation generally adjusts better than one with an acute preoperative illness.
4. Availability of support	4. A strong support system can greatly aid the client's adjustment.

Interventions

1. Identify and correct any misinformation the patient may have regarding pacemakers.

2. Encourage the client to share feelings and concerns about living with a pacemaker.

3. Assist the client in distinguishing areas of life in which he or she is not dependent on others.

4. Help the client identify personal strengths that might aid coping.

Rationale

1. Incorrect assumptions can cause doubt and uncertainty and contribute to poor self-concept. Many times, a client and family have information related to old pacemakers. Today's pacemakers can be self-adjusting (versus fixed rate) and require less frequent battery changes, e.g., 3 to 4, 10, or even 20 years.

2. Sharing gives the nurse the opportunity to identify and clarify misconceptions and address areas of concern.

3. This measure emphasizes areas for control and self-determination in learning to accept the pacemaker and altered body image.

4. Discussing strengths encourages the client to deemphasize the disability.

▲ **Documentation**

Progress notes
   Emotional status
   Dialogues

▲ **Outcome Criteria**

The outcome criteria for this diagnosis represent those associated with discharge planning. Refer to the discharge criteria.

Potential Altered Health Maintenance related to insufficient knowledge of activity restrictions, precautions, signs and symptoms of complications, and follow-up care

Focus Assessment Criteria	Clinical Significance
1. Readiness and ability to learn and retain information	1. A client or family failing to achieve learning goals requires a referral for assistance post-discharge.

Interventions

1. Review the postprocedural routine, as needed.

2. Instruct on incisional care, including the following:
   a. Wound cleansing
   b. Suture removal (usually after 7 days)
   c. Expected swelling for 2 to 4 weeks
   d. Recognizing signs and symptoms of infection
   e. For a woman, wearing a brassiere for support, with a gauze pad over the pulse generator to decrease rubbing over the suture line.

3. Instruct on home care measures:

   a. Keep the affected arm immobile for 24 to 48 hours postprocedure.
   b. Continue taking prescribed cardiac medication until otherwise instructed by the physician.

4. Teach the client and family to watch for and promptly report the following:
   a. Redness, swelling, and pain at the surgical wound
   b. Joint stiffness, pain, and muscle weakness in affected arm
   c. Light-headedness, fainting, or dizzy spells

   d. Very rapid or very slow pulse

Rationale

1. Reviewing enables the nurse to evaluate whether the client needs additional teaching.

2. Proper incision care helps prevent infection and other complications.

3. Understanding home care enables the client to comply with the regimen.
   a. Arm movement could cause traction on the lead and possible lead displacement.
   b. Pacemaker implantation does not preclude the need for medication.

4. Early detection enables prompt treatment to prevent serious complications.
   a. These signs and symptoms point to wound infection.
   b. Joint stiffness, pain, and muscle weakness may indicate neurovascular compression.
   c. Light-headedness, fainting, or dizzy spells may result from cerebral hypoxia owing to insufficient cardiac output.
   d. Pulse changes may indicate pacemaker failure.

Interventions

    e. Chronic hiccups or chest muscle twitching

    f. Swelling of ankles or hands

5. Instruct the client to avoid these activities permanently:
   a. Mowing the lawn
   b. Lifting anything weighing more than 25 pounds
   c. Using an axe by lifting it over the head and dropping it to cut
   d. Participating in contact sports
   e. Using an air hammer
   f. Firing a rifle from the affected side
   g. Serving overhead-style when playing tennis
   h. Diving head first into water
6. Reassure that the pacemaker should not interfere with sexual activity.
7. Instruct the client to carry a pacemaker identification card at all times. (He or she will receive a temporary card before going home; the pacemaker manufacturer will mail a permanent card later.)
8. Instruct the client to notify physicians, nurses, and dentists about his or her pacemaker so that prophylactic antibiotics may be given before invasive procedures, if needed.
9. Instruct the client to avoid strong electromagnetic fields, including magnetic resonance imaging equipment, heliart welding equipment, dental ultrasonic cleaners, drills, internal combustion engines, and poorly shielded microwave ovens.
10. Warn that the pacemaker triggers magnetic detection alarms, such as those found at airports.
11. Emphasize the necessity of long-term follow-up care; reinforce the physician's instructions.
12. Explain that the battery is not lifelong, and replacement might be necessary. (Average battery life is 5 to 10 years; 20 years, if nuclear-powered.)
13. Teach pulse-taking, if appropriate, and instruct the client to notify the physician if the pulse rate falls below the pacemaker set rate.
14. Provide written instructional materials at discharge.
15. Provide names and phone numbers of persons the client can call should questions or an emergency arise (day or night).

Rationale

    e. Chronic hiccups or chest muscle twitching may indicate lead displacement and electrical stimulation of diaphragm or intercostal muscles.

    f. Swelling of ankles or hands may indicate congestive heart failure related to insufficient cardiac output.

5. These activities could damage either the pulse generator or leads.

6. Specifically discussing sexual activity can reduce fears and let the client share concerns.
7. A pacemaker identification card provides important information to caregivers in emergency situations.

8. Because the pulse generator increases tissue susceptibility to infection, prophylactic therapy is indicated before many invasive procedures.
9. Electromagnetic fields can interfere with pacemaker function.

10. This information allows the client to inform airport security personnel at detectors to avoid misunderstanding and embarrassment.
11. Regular follow-up care is essential for ongoing evaluation.
12. Understanding the need for battery replacement assists with coping should replacement be needed.
13. Pulse-taking may help enhance the client's sense of control over the situation.

14. Written information reinforces teaching and serves as a resource at home.
15. This can help reassure the client that direct access for assistance is always available.

▲ **Documentation**

Discharge summary record
    Client and family teaching
    Outcome achievement or status

References/Bibliography

Bayless, W.A. (1988). The elements of permanent cardiac pacing. *Critical Care Nurse, 8*(7), 31–41.
Brenner, Z.R. (1988). Nursing diagnoses for rate-responsive pacemaker patients. *DCCN, 7*(5), 262–268.
Evans, N. (1985). Clinical assessment of pacemaker functions: The ICHD code. *DCCN, 4*(3), 140–145.

Hawthorne, J.W. (1986). How to choose a cardiac pacing system. *Cardiovascular Medicine, 35*(9), 10–11.

Huffman, M. (1988). Pacemaker battery change: An outpatient procedure. *AORN, 48*(4), 733–739.

LeBan, M.M., et al. (1988). Peripheral nerve conduction stimulation: Its effect on cardiac pacemakers. *Archives of Physical Medicine, 69*(9), 358–362.

Mickus, D., et al. (1986). Exciting external pacemakers. *American Journal of Nursing, 86*(4), 403–405.

Murdock, D. (1986). Pacemaker malfunction: Fact or artifact? *Heart & Lung, 15*(2), 150–154.

Owen, P.M. (1984). Defibrillating pacemaker patients. *American Journal of Nursing, 84*(9), 1129–1132.

Pietro, D.A. (1985). Recurrent dizziness and fatigue in a pacemaker patient. *Cardiovascular Medicine, 34*(6), 37–39.

Purcell, J.A., & Burrows, S.G. (1985). A pacemaker primer. *American Journal of Nursing, 85*(5), 553–568.

Tamarisk, N.K. (1988). Enhancing activity levels of patients with permanent cardiac pacemakers. *Heart & Lung, 17*(6), 698–707.

Percutaneous Transluminal Coronary Angioplasty

Percutaneous transluminal coronary angioplasty (PTCA) involves compression of atherosclerotic plaques by a catheter, which results in dilation of the stenosed coronary artery. After catheter insertion, a contrast medium is injected to visualize blood flow under fluoroscopy. Indications for PCTA include atherosclerotic disease affecting only one coronary artery and angina persisting for less than 1 year. Myocardial infarction (MI) is a serious risk associated with PCTA; if MI occurs during the procedure, surgical revascularization (coronary artery bypass surgery) is indicated.

Diagnostic Cluster

▲ Time Frame
Preprocedure and postprocedure

▲ Discharge Criteria
Before discharge, the client or family will:
1. Demonstrate insertion site care
2. Relate at-home activity restrictions and follow-up care
3. State signs and symptoms that must be reported to a health care professional

PREPROCEDURE PERIOD
Nursing Diagnoses

Anxiety/Fear (Individual, Family) related to the health status, angioplasty procedure, routines, outcome, and possible need for cardiac surgery

POSTPROCEDURE PERIOD
Collaborative Problems

Potential Complications:
Dysrhythmias
Acute Coronary Occlusion (Clot, Spasm, Collapse)
Myocardial Infarction
Arterial Dissection or Rupture
Hemorrhage/Hematoma at Angioplasty Site

Nursing Diagnoses

Impaired Physical Mobility related to prescribed bed rest and restricted movement of involved extremity
Potential Altered Health Maintenance related to insufficient knowledge of care of insertion site, discharge activities, diet, medications, signs and symptoms of complications, exercises, and follow-up care

Preprocedure: Nursing Diagnosis

▲ Outcome Criteria
The client and/or family will:
1. Verbalize concerns regarding the angioplasty procedure
2. Describe preangioplasty routines
3. Describe the procedure, the environment, and expected sensations
4. State the postprocedure routine and expected behaviors
5. Verbalize a decrease in anxiety and fear

Anxiety/Fear (Individual, Family) related to the health status, angioplasty procedure, routines, outcome, and possible need for cardiac surgery

Focus Assessment Criteria	Clinical Significance
1. Level of anxiety: mild, moderate, severe, or panic	1. High levels of anxiety interfere with learning.
2. Understanding of angioplasty procedure	2. Before angioplasty, the client's physician should explain:
	a. PTCA procedure
	b. Reason for and anticipated outcome of procedure

Focus Assessment Criteria

Clinical Significance

   c. Risks involved

   d. Possible need for emergency coronary artery bypass surgery

   e. Expectations regarding length of recovery and restrictions imposed during the recovery period.

      Preprocedure teaching provides information to help decrease fear of the unknown and to enhance the client's sense of control over the situation.

3. Past experiences with angioplasty or contact with others who have undergone the procedure

4. Concerns or fears regarding the angioplasty procedure

3. The client can be greatly influenced, either positively or negatively, by information from others.

4. The PTCA procedure can pose a threat to the client's body image and even life. Encouraging the client to share thoughts and feelings provides opportunities to clarify fears and provide realistic feedback.

Interventions

1. Attempt to reduce the level of anxiety and fear:
   a. Stay with the client and family as much as possible.
   b. Convey a sense of empathic understanding.
   c. Maintain a calm, quiet atmosphere; remove excessive stimuli from the client's room.
   d. Give the client and family time to verbalize feelings, fears, concerns regarding the PTCA procedure and health status.
2. Encourage participation of a social support system (e.g., family, friends, clergy, etc.).
3. Teach relaxation techniques, if needed (e.g., deep breathing, progressive muscle relaxation).
4. Reinforce the physician's explanation of the PTCA procedure. Notify the physician if additional explanations are indicated.

5. Provide instruction regarding pre-PTCA routines and care measures, covering:
   a. Nothing-by-mouth (NPO) status for 12 hours pre-PTCA, to reduce the nausea and vomiting that may occur with medication use
   b. Wearing a hospital gown for the procedure
   c. Removing nail polish
   d. May wear dentures
   e. Initiation of an intravenous (IV) line, to provide a site for medication administration if needed
   f. Shave and preparation
6. Provide instruction regarding the PTCA procedure, covering the following:
   a. Location (catheterization laboratory)
   b. Use of a mild sedative and local anesthetic so the client can be awake during the PTCA
   c. Cardiac monitoring

Rationale

1. Stress, anxiety, and fear can precipitate a sympathetic nervous system response that increases heart rate, blood pressure, and myocardial oxygen demand. Reducing these factors can reduce the demand placed on the already compromised heart.

2. Adequate support from others can help reduce and control anxiety.
3. These techniques decrease feelings of loss of control and enhance self-management of anxiety.
4. The physician is legally responsible for explaining the procedure to the client and family; the nurse, for evaluating if they require more information.
5–8. Specific explanations provide information to help reduce anxiety associated with the unknown and unexpected.

Interventions   *Rationale*

    d. Catheter insertion through femoral artery

    e. Catheter advancement to the diseased coronary artery

    f. Inflation of the catheter balloon to compress the plaque against the artery wall

    g. Physician's instructions to take deep breaths and cough during the procedure

    h. Catheter removal

    i. Application of pressure to the femoral artery site

7. Explain sensations the client may experience during the PTCA procedure.

    a. Visual
   - Monitoring equipment
   - Fluoroscope screen
   - Nurses and physicians with surgical scrubs and masks
   - Lights being turned on and off

    b. Auditory
   - Clicking of fluoroscopy camera
   - Questions and conversation from nurses and physicians
   - Audible alarms

    c. Tactile
   - Electrodes attached to body
   - Lying on a hard, cool surface
   - Burning on injection of local anesthetic at the groin
   - Pressure on PTCA catheter insertion into the femoral artery
   - Warm sensation on dye injection
   - Pressure on catheter removal
   - Chest pain on PTCA balloon inflation

8. Provide instruction regarding post-PTCA routines and care measures, covering the following:

    a. Frequent assessment of vital signs, groin site, and extremity

    b. Cardiac monitoring

    c. Bed rest for 24 hours

    d. Head of the bed elevated no more than 30 degrees for 24 hours

    e. Immobilizing the affected leg for 24 hours

    f. Applying hand pressure to the groin for 24 hours when coughing, sneezing, repositioning, or laughing

    g. The need to avoid straining (e.g., during turning, bowel movement, lifting head off pillow) for the first 24 hours post-PTCA

9. Present information or reinforce learning using written materials (e.g., booklets, instruction sheets) or audiovisual aids (e.g., slides and audio tapes, videotapes, heart models, diagrams, pictures).

9. Using multisensory strategies enhances learning.

10. Teach the client how to turn in bed while keeping the affected leg immobilized; request return demonstration.

10. Immobilizing the leg reduces the risk of bleeding.

11. Instruct the client to report promptly signs of altered tissue perfusion—numbness, tingling, decreased sensation, pain, or bleeding.

11. Early reporting enables prompt intervention to minimize the seriousness of complications.

▲ **Documentation**

Teaching record
    Client teaching
    Outcome achievement or status
Progress notes
    Emotional status
    Interventions
    Response to interventions
    Unusual emotional state

Postprocedure: Collaborative Problems

▲ *Nursing Goal*

The nurse will manage and minimize cardiac and vascular complications.

Potential Complication: Dysrhythmias
Potential Complication: Acute Coronary Occlusion (Clot, Spasm, Collapse)
Potential Complication: Myocardial Infarction
Potential Complication: Arterial Dissection or Rupture
Potential Complication: Hemorrhage/Hematoma at Angioplasty Insertion Site

Interventions

1. Monitor for signs and symptoms of acute coronary occlusion, myocardial infarction, or arterial dissection:
   a. Chest pain, pressure
   b. Increased heart rate
   c. Hypotension
   d. Tachypnea
   e. Abnormal heart sounds
   f. Restlessness
   g. Lethargy, confusion
   h. Weak pulses
   i. Moist, cool skin
   j. Decreased urine output
   k. Distended neck veins
   l. Nausea and vomiting
   m. Electrocardiographic (ECG) changes: ST segment elevation, abnormal Q waves
   n. Increased temperature
2. Monitor for signs and symptoms of dysrhythmias:
   a. Abnormal pulse rate, rhythm
   b. ST segment depression or elevation
   c. PR, QRS, or QT interval changes
   d. Palpitations
   e. Syncope
   f. Cardiac emergency (e.g., arrest, ventricular fibrillation)
3. Monitor for signs and symptoms of hemorrhage or hematoma:
   a. Bleeding on insertion site dressing
   b. Hematoma at site
   c. Ecchymoses at site
   d. Frank bleeding
   e. Increased heart rate, decreased blood pressure, increased respiratory rate
   f. Weak or absent peripheral pulses
   g. Inability to move the toes of the involved leg
   h. Numbness, tingling, burning, decreased sensations in the involved leg
   i. Cool, moist skin
   j. Pain or pressure at the insertion site
   k. Urine output < 30 mL/hr
   l. Restlessness, agitation, confusion
4. Instruct the client to report discomfort and changes in sensation.

Rationale

1. Cardiac pain results from decreased oxygenation of myocardial cells. The balloon dilatation causes coronary artery intimal injury; thrombi may develop at the site. Ischemia may be due to atherosclerosis, a thrombus, arterial spasm, or arterial dissection. The resulting symptoms are indicative of cardiac ischemia and hypoxia.

2. The balloon dilatation can cause myocardial ischemia. Ischemic muscle is electrically unstable, predisposing to dysrhythmias.

3. Hypovolemia results from fluid blood loss and decreased fluid intake. Bleeding at the PTCA catheter insertion site can result in shock. In a compensatory response to hypovolemia and hypoxia, the adrenal cortex releases catecholamines to constrict arterioles and venules in major organs (kidneys, liver, intestines), resulting in decreased urine output and peristalsis. In an attempt to increase blood oxygenation, respiratory and heart rates increase.

4. Reporting symptoms early enables prompt intervention to minimize the seriousness of complications.

▲ *Documentation*

Flow records
  Vital signs
  Intake and output
  Rhythm strips
  Dressing status
  Peripheral pulses, skin color

Related Physician-Prescribed Interventions

Medications
  Nitroglycerin
  Heparin
  Antiplatelets

Related Physician-Prescribed Interventions (Continued)

Intravenous Therapy
  IV line for direct venous access

Laboratory Studies
  Not indicated

Diagnostic Studies
  ECG

Therapies
  Activity restrictions   Site care

Postprocedure: Nursing Diagnoses

Impaired Physical Mobility related to prescribed bed rest and restricted movement of involved extremity

▲ Outcome Criteria

The client and family will:

1. State activity restrictions
2. Use the log-rolling technique when turning is necessary
3. Keep the involved leg immobilized at all times
4. Apply hand pressure to affected groin during coughing, sneezing, repositioning, laughing
5. Gradually increase activity when prescribed

Focus Assessment Criteria

1. Understanding of mobility restrictions

2. Presence of abnormal responses to activity:
   a. Dysrhythmias
   b. Greatly increased or decreased pulse rate; failure of the pulse rate to return to near resting rate 3 minutes after activity
   c. Excessively increased or decreased respiratory rate
   d. Progressive weakness
   e. Pallor or cyanosis
   f. Confusion
   g. Vertigo
   h. Uncoordination

Clinical Significance

1. Assessing the client's understanding of the need for mobility restrictions helps the nurse evaluate whether there is a need and what type of teaching he or she needs to help ensure compliance.
2. Abnormal physiological response to activity indicates the client's impaired ability to adapt to the increased need for oxygen, and necessitates further evaluation.

Interventions

1. Reinforce teaching regarding mobility restrictions:
   a. Bed rest for 24 hours
   b. Immobilization of involved leg
   c. Head of the bed elevated no more than 30 degrees for 24 hours
   d. Applying hand pressure to the groin during turning, bowel movements and lifting the head off the pillow for the first 24 hours
2. Use pillows to help maintain body alignment.
3. Assist with repositioning using the log-rolling technique.

4. Ensure that the call bell, water pitcher, tissues, and needed personal items are kept within the client's reach.
5. Promote progressive activity after 24 hours:
   a. Dangling legs over the side of the bed
   b. Sitting up in a chair
   c. Progressive ambulation
6. Progress self-care activities from partial to complete self-care as ability allows.

Rationale

1. While the arterial line and catheter sheath are in the femoral artery, the client must keep the involved leg immobilized to prevent dislodgment, line kinking, and bleeding at the site.

2,3. The involved leg must remain immobilized after removal so that a clot can form around the insertion site. Movement may increase pressure in the arterial system or cause the clot to dislodge.

4. Easy access to needed items can prevent unnecessary moving and reaching.

5,6. In the presence of cardiovascular disease, a gradual return to preprocedure activity level is needed to prevent hypoxia.

▲ Documentation

Flow records
  Vital signs
  Repositioning
  Ambulation

▲ Outcome Criteria

The outcome criteria for this diagnosis represent those associated with discharge planning. Refer to the discharge criteria.

Potential Altered Health Maintenance related to insufficient knowledge of care of insertion site, discharge activities, diet, medications, signs and symptoms of complications, and follow-up care

Focus Assessment Criteria	Clinical Significance
1. Readiness and ability to learn and retain information	1. A client or family failing to achieve learning goals requires a referral for assistance post-discharge.

Interventions

1. Explain and demonstrate care of an uncomplicated femoral artery PTCA insertion site:
   a. Wash with soap and water (bath and shower permitted).
   b. Wear loose clothing until the area is no longer tender.
   c. Place a bandage over the site if undergarments rub against it.
2. Provide instructions regarding discharge activities, covering the following:
   a. Progressive activity increase
   b. Rest periods as needed
   c. Restriction of driving for 1 week; may ride as a passenger (consult with the physician)
   d. Return to work (usually 1 week after uncomplicated PTCA; consult with the physician)
   e. Cardiac rehabilitation program approved by the physician
3. Provide instructions regarding cardiac diet, covering the following:
   a. Low-fat, low-cholesterol foods
   b. Possible sodium restriction (consult with the physician)
   c. Foods allowed
   d. Foods restricted
4. Teach the client and family to watch for and promptly report signs and symptoms of complications:
   a. Redness, drainage, warmth, increasing discomfort at the PTCA insertion site
   b. Chest pain
   c. Difficulty breathing
   d. Weakness, fatigue
   e. Pain, change in temperature of involved leg
5. Reinforce follow-up care prescribed by physician.
6. Present information or reinforce learning using written materials (e.g., pamphlets, instruction sheets) or audiovisual aids (e.g., slides and audio tapes, video tapes, diagrams, pictures).
7. Initiate referrals to a home health care agency or cardiac rehabilitation program, if needed.

Rationale

1. Precautions are needed to prevent infection and clot dislodgment.

2. Progressive activity and exercise gradually increases cardiac stroke volume, which increases the heart's efficiency without greatly altering heart rate. Return to independence in ADLs helps the client cope with necessary life style changes and promotes self-esteem.

3. Weight reduction reduces peripheral resistance and cardiac output. Excessive sodium intake causes water retention, leading to increased cardiac workload.

4. Early detection enables prompt intervention to prevent serious complications.
   a. These signs and symptoms point to infection.
   b. Chest pain results from myocardial hypoxia.
   c. Dyspnea may signal excessive fluid retention.
   d. Weakness and fatigue also may indicate hypoxia.
   e. Pain and temperature changes in the leg may indicate vascular or neurosensory impairment.
5. Reinforcing the need for follow-up can help promote compliance.
6. Printed and other instructional materials can provide a reference source for home use.

7. The client may need assistance with home management or cardiac rehabilitation.

▲ Documentation

Discharge summary record
    Client and family teaching
    Outcome achievement or status
    Referrals, if indicated

References/Bibliography

Bouman, C. (1984). Intracoronary thrombolysis and percutaneous transluminal coronary angioplasty. *Nursing Clinics of North America, 19*(2), 397–490.

Cimini, D., & Goldfarb, J. (1983). Standard of care for the patient with percutaneous transluminal coronary angioplasty. *Critical Care Nurse, 3*(6), 76–78.

Galan, K., Gruentzig, A., & Hollman, J. (1985). Significance of early chest pain after coronary angioplasty. *Heart & Lung, 14,* 105–109.

Guzzetta, C., & Dossey, B. (1984). *Cardiovascular nursing: Body-mind tapestry.* St. Louis: C.V. Mosby.

Lynn-McHale, D.J. (1986). Interventions for acute myocardial infarction: PTCA and CABGS. *Critical Care Nurse, 6*(2), 64–70.

McCarthy, C. (1982). Percutaneous transluminal coronary angioplasty: Therapeutic intervention in the cardiac catheterization laboratory. *Heart & Lung, 11,* 499–504.

Mullin, S. (1984). Percutaneous transluminal angioplasty. *Heart & Lung, 13,* 75–77.

Ott, B. (1982). Percutaneous transluminal coronary angioplasty and nursing implications. *Heart & Lung, 11,* 294–298.

Partridge, S. (1982). The nurse's role in percutaneous transluminal coronary angioplasty. *Heart & Lung, 11,* 505–511.

Purcell, J., & Giffin, P. (1981). Percutaneous transluminal coronary angioplasty. American Journal of Nursing, *81*(8), 1620–1626.

Shillinger, F. (1983). Percutaneous transluminal coronary angioplasty. *Heart & Lung, 12,* 45–51.

Underhill, S., Woods, S., Sivarajan, E., & Halpenny, C. (1982). *Cardiac nursing.* Philadelphia: J.B. Lippincott.

Willard, P. (1985a). *A patient's guide to PTCA.* Billerica, MA: C.R. Bard.

Willard, P. (1985b). Percutaneous transluminal angioplasty. *Point of View, 22,* 4–8.

Peritoneal Dialysis

Peritoneal dialysis—the repetitive instillation and drainage of dialysis solution into and from the peritoneal cavity—uses the process of osmosis to remove wastes, toxins, and fluid from the blood. The procedure is indicated for acute or chronic renal failure, severe fluid or electrolyte imbalances unresponsive to other treatments, and inadequate peritoneal blood flow.

Three modalities are available. *Manual* dialysis requires careful control of dialysate instillation (2 liters), dwell time (10 to 25 minutes), and outflow. *Continuous ambulatory* dialysis provides dialysate inflow with the disposable bag and tubing remaining connected, folded, and secured to the torso during dwell time (4 to 6 hours); four exchanges are completed daily. *Continuous cycled* dialysis comprises three to five exchanges performed automatically at night, with the abdomen left full during the day. The system alarms if inflow or outflow problems occur.

Diagnostic Cluster

▲ **Time Frame**

Pretherapy and intratherapy

▲ **Discharge Criteria**

Before discharge, the client and/or family will:

1. Be able to demonstrate home peritoneal dialysis procedures if appropriate
2. State signs and symptoms of infection
3. Discuss the expected impact of long-term dialysis on the client and family
4. State signs and symptoms that must be reported to a health care professional

Collaborative Problems

Potential Complications:
Hypovolemia/Hypervolemia
Electrolyte Imbalances
Uremia
Hemorrhage
Hyperglycemia
Bladder/Bowel Perforation
Inflow/Outflow Problems

Refer to:

Nursing Diagnoses

Potential for Infection related to access to peritoneal cavity, catheter exit site, and use of high dextrose concentration in dialysis solution

Potential Ineffective Breathing Pattern related to immobility, pressure, and pain

Altered Comfort related to catheter insertion, instillation of dialysis solution, outflow, suction, and chemical irritation of peritoneum

Potential Altered Health Maintenance related to insufficient knowledge of rationale of treatment, medications, home dialysis procedure, signs and symptoms of complications, community resources, and follow-up care

Potential Altered Family Processes related to the effects of interruptions of the treatment schedule on role responsibilities — Chronic Renal Failure

Powerlessness related to chronic illness and the need for continuous treatment — Chronic Renal Failure

Altered Nutrition: Less Than Body Requirements related to anorexia — Chronic Renal Failure

Collaborative Problems

▲ **Nursing Goal**

The nurse will manage and minimize complications of peritoneal dialysis.

Potential Complication: Hypovolemia or Hypervolemia
Potential Complication: Electrolyte Imbalances
Potential Complication: Uremia
Potential Complication: Hemorrhage
Potential Complication: Hyperglycemia
Potential Complication: Bladder or Bowel Perforation
Potential Complication: Inflow or Outflow Problems

Interventions

1. Monitor for signs and symptoms of hypervolemia:
   a. Edema
   b. Dyspnea, tachypnea
   c. Rales, frothy secretions
   d. Rapid, bounding pulse
   e. Hypertension
   f. Jugular vein distention
   g. S3 heart sounds

2. Monitor for signs and symptoms of hypovolemia:
   a. Dry skin and mucous membranes
   b. Poor skin turgor
   c. Thirst
   d. Rapid, weak pulse
   e. Tachypnea
   f. Hypotension with orthostatic changes
   g. Narrowed pulse pressure
   h. Altered level of consciousness
3. Monitor intake and output.
4. Enforce fluid restrictions, as ordered.

5. Weigh daily or before and after each dialysis treatment.
6. Monitor peritoneal dialysis inflow, dwell time, and outflow. *Inflow* (usually taking less than 15 minutes) is the infusion of dialysis solution by gravity into the peritoneal cavity. *Dwell time* (0 to 20 minutes) is the length of time that the dialysis solution remains in the peritoneal cavity, which determines the amount of diffusion and osmosis that occurs. *Outflow* (usually less than 20 minutes) is the emptying of the peritoneal cavity by gravity. A 1-hour cycle is usually used for intermittent peritoneal dialysis over 24 to 48 hours.
7. Monitor urine specific gravity.

8. Monitor for signs and symptoms of hypernatremia with fluid overload:
   a. Thirst
   b. Agitation
   c. Convulsions

Rationale

1. Hypervolemia may occur if dialysate does not drain freely or if excess intravenous (IV) or oral fluids have been infused or injected. Excess fluid greater than 5% of body weight is needed to produce edema. Fluid in lungs produces signs and symptoms of hypoxia. Hypertension results from fluid and sodium retention, increased peripheral resistance, increased rennin secretion, and decreased prostaglandins.

2. Hypovolemia may occur from excessive or too-rapid removal of dialysate fluid. Loss of tissue fluid reduces peripheral resistance, resulting in hypotension.

3. Urine output varies depending on renal status.
4. The physician may restrict fluid intake to insensible losses or the previous day's urine output.
5. Daily weights help evaluate fluid balance.

6. Catheter obstruction can prevent adequate inflow, reducing the effectiveness of treatment, or outflow, which can cause potentially dangerous dialysate retention.

7. Urine specific gravity less than 1.010 indicates fluid excess; more than 1.010 indicates hypovolemia. In renal failure, however, specific gravity may not change, because the kidneys cannot dilute urine.
8. The dialysate solution composition, rate of inflow, and rate of outflow can alter sodium levels.

Interventions

9. Monitor for signs and symptoms of hyponatremia:
    a. Lethargy, coma
    b. Weakness
    c. Abdominal pain
    d. Muscle twitching, convulsions
10. Monitor for signs and symptoms of hyperkalemia:
    a. Weakness, paralysis
    b. Muscle irritability
    c. Paresthesias
    d. Nausea, vomiting, abdominal cramping, diarrhea
    e. Irregular pulse
11. Monitor for signs and symptoms of hypokalemia:
    a. Weakness, paralysis
    b. Decreased or absent tendon reflexes
    c. Hypoventilation
    d. Polyuria
    e. Hypotension
    f. Paralytic ileus
12. Monitor for signs and symptoms of hypocalcemia:
    a. Hyperventilation
    b. Tetany
    c. Numbness and tingling
    d. Positive Trousseau's sign
    e. Positive Chvostek's sign
13. Monitor for signs and symptoms of hypermagnesemia:
    a. Weakness
    b. Hypoventilation
    c. Hypotension
    d. Flushing
    e. Behavioral changes
14. Monitor for signs and symptoms of hyperphosphatemia:
    a. Hyperventilation
    b. Tetany
    c. Numbness and tingling
    d. Positive Trousseau's sign
    e. Positive Chvostek's sign
15. Monitor for signs and symptoms of uremia:
    a. Skin and mucous membrane lesions
    b. Pericardial friction rub
    c. Pleural friction rub
    d. Gastrointestinal (GI) disturbances
    e. Peripheral neuropathy
    f. Vision changes
    g. Central nervous system (CNS) impairment
    h. Tachypnea
    i. Musculoskeletal changes
16. Monitor for vessel perforation and hemorrhage, marked by increasingly bloody dialysate return.
17. Explain the procedure and expected sensations, and provide support during temporary catheter insertion.

Rationale

9. Hyponatremia results from the dilutional effects of hypervolemia. Extracellular volume decrease lowers blood pressure and leads to hypoxia.

10. Prolonged dwell time can increase potassium fluctuations, which can affect neuromuscular transmission, reduce the action of GI smooth muscles, and impair electrical conduction of the heart.

11. Hypokalemia impairs neuromuscular transmission and reduces the action of respiratory muscles and GI smooth muscles. The kidneys become less sensitive to the effects of antidiuretic hormone and thus excrete large quantities of dilute urine.

12. Hypocalcemia can result as the citrate in transfused blood binds with circulating calcium. Respiratory alkalosis also binds calcium to protein, decreasing available calcium. Signs and symptoms reflect increased motor nerve excitability.

13. Possibly resulting from renal disease or excessive use of magnesium-based antacids, hypermagnesemia inhibits release of acetylcholine at the neuromuscular junction, causing decreased neuromuscular excitability and increased vasodilatation.

14. Respiratory alkalosis binds calcium to protein, decreasing available calcium and greatly increasing phosphorus absorption (80% to 90% of ingested phosphorus).

15. A multisystem syndrome, uremia is a manifestation of end-stage renal disease resulting from waste products of protein metabolism, including urea, creatinine, and uric acid.

16. Perforation of a blood vessel during catheter insertion can cause bloody dialysate, urine, or stool, or bleeding at the insertion site.

17. Explanations encourage the client to avoid sudden movement during catheter insertion.

Interventions

18. If bleeding persists, apply a pressure dressing and carefully monitor vital signs.
19. Monitor for signs and symptoms of hyperglycemia or hyperglycemia:
    a. Elevated or depressed blood glucose level
    b. Polyuria
    c. Polyphagia
    d. Polydipsia
    e. Abdominal pain
    f. Diaphoresis
20. Monitor for signs and symptoms of bladder or bowel perforation:
    a. Fecal material in dialysate
    b. Complaints of urgency
    c. Increased urine output with high glucose concentrations
    d. Complaints of pressure in the sensation to defecate
    e. Watery diarrhea
21. Have the client empty the bladder and bowel before insertion of the peritoneal dialysis catheter.
22. If inflow or outflow problems occur, do the following:
    a. Increase the height of the dialysate bag and lower the bed.
    b. Reposition the client and instruct him to cough.
    c. Remove the dressing to check for catheter obstruction.
    d. Check the dressing for wetness.

    e. Assess abdominal pain on outflow.

    f. Assess the amount of dialysate return.

    g. Ascertain whether heparin has been added to the dialysate.
23. Calculate inflow and outflow volume at the end of each dialysis cycle. Report discrepancies in accordance with hospital protocol.

Rationale

18. Pressure may stop the bleeding.

19. The amount of dextrose absorbed from the dialysate varies with duration of dialysis, dextrose concentration, and underlying client conditions. After dialysis is complete, hypoglycemia may occur because of increased insulin production during instillation of high dextrose concentrations.

20. Catheter insertion may perforate the bowel or bladder, allowing dialysate to infuse into the bowel or bladder.

21. Emptying the bladder and bowel decreases the risk of perforation during catheter insertion.

22. These measures can enhance the effectiveness of dialysis and prevent complications.
    a. Raising the bag and lowering the bed can help maximize gravity drainage.
    b. Repositioning and coughing may help clear a blocked or kinked catheter.
    c. The dressing can obscure an external obstruction or kink.
    d. A wet dressing can indicate leakage around the catheter.
    e. Abdominal pain may result from excessive suction on the abdominal viscera.
    f. Inadequate dialysate return (should be greater than or equal to inflow) necessitates further evaluation.
    g. Heparin can help prevent catheter blockage from fibrinous or proteinaceous material.
23. Accurate intake and output records help monitor flow and the safety and efficacy of treatment.

▲ **Documentation**

Flow records
    Vital signs
    Intake and output
    Weight (before and after dialysis)
    Dialysate color
    Abdominal girth
    Serum glucose (before and after dialysis)
    Urine specific gravity
    Other laboratory values (before and after dialysis)
Progress notes
    Changes in status
    Inflow or outflow problems
    Interventions

Related Physician-Prescribed Interventions
Medications
    Heparinized saline
Intravenous Therapy
    Not indicated
Laboratory Studies
    Refer to either the Acute or Chronic Renal Failure care plan
Diagnostic Studies
    Not indicated
Therapies
    Dialysate solution

Nursing Diagnoses

▲ *Outcome Criteria*

The client will be infection free.

Potential for Infection related to access to peritoneal cavity, catheter exit site, and use of high dextrose concentration in dialysis solution

Focus Assessment Criteria

1. Catheter site for redness, inflammation, purulent drainage, tenderness, warmth
2. Signs and symptoms of systemic infection:
   a. Fever
   b. Chills
   c. Diaphoresis
   d. Nausea and vomiting
   e. Abdominal pain and rebound tenderness
   f. Malaise
   g. Tachycardia
   h. Hypotension

Clinical Significance

1,2. Catheterization and instillation of dialysate entail an increased risk of local and systemic infection.

Interventions

1. If an automatic cycler is used, ensure use of sterile technique when setting up the equipment and performing dialysis.
2. Use sterile technique when assisting with catheter insertion or removal and when maintaining the system and insertion site.
3. Ensure complete skin preparation before catheter insertion.
4. When performing manual peritoneal dialysis, prevent contamination of spikes when changing dialysate bottles or bags; dry bottles and bags before spiking.
5. Monitor dialysate return for color and clarity.
6. Apply masks to all staff and the client during catheter insertion, catheter removal, and dressing changes.
7. Check all dialysate bottles and bags for clarity and broken seals before instilling.

8. Empty the dialysis warmer water every 36 hours.

Rationale

1–4. Aseptic technique reduces microorganisms and helps prevent their introduction into the system.

5. Cloudy return may indicate infection.
6. Masks help decrease the risk of contamination and infection transmission.

7. Cloudy dialysate may be contaminated. Poorly sealed containers are prone to microorganism growth.
8. Changing the water regularly can help minimize microorganism growth.

▲ *Documentation*

Progress notes
    Signs and symptoms of
        infection
Flow records
    Dressing changes

▲ *Outcome Criteria*

The client will demonstrate optimal respiratory function, as evidenced by bilateral breath sounds and arterial blood gases (ABGs) within normal limits.

Potential Ineffective Breathing Pattern related to immobility, pressure, and pain

Focus Assessment Criteria

1. Indicators of respiratory status:
   a. Respiratory rate and rhythm
   b. Abdominal girth
   c. Pain
   d. Dyspnea
   e. Cough
   f. Pleural friction rub
   g. Secretions

Clinical Significance

1. Hypoventilation may result from increased pressure on the diaphragm due to dialysate instillation. Pulmonary edema, pleuritis, infection, or uremic lung also may contribute to pulmonary malfunction.

Interventions

1. Encourage regular coughing and deep breathing exercises.

Rationale

1. These exercises promote lung expansion.

Interventions

2. Elevate the head of the bed during dialysis.

3. If the client experiences respiratory distress, immediately stop inflow or begin outflow.
4. Avoid the use of sedatives and narcotics.

Rationale

2. Head elevation facilitates ventilation while maintaining free flow of dialysate.
3. Stopping the flow reduces pressure on the diaphragm, possibly relieving distress.
4. These medications can further depress respiratory function.

▲ *Documentation*

Progress notes
   Abnormal respiratory status

▲ *Outcome Criteria*

The client will be as comfortable as possible during peritoneal dialysis and report any pressure or pain during the procedure.

Altered Comfort related to catheter insertion, instillation of dialysis solution, suction during outflow, and chemical irritation of peritoneum

Focus Assessment Criteria

1. Pain: Location, intensity, duration, quality, onset, precipitating factors

Clinical Significance

1. Constant abdominal distention and chemical irritation of the peritoneum contribute to abdominal pain during dialysis.

Interventions

1. Instruct the client to report excessive pain on catheter insertion or dialysate instillation. Have the client describe the pain's severity on a scale of 0 to 10 (0 = no pain; 10 = most severe pain).

2. Position the client to minimize pain while maintaining good air exchange and free-flowing dialysate.
3. If needed, administer lidocaine either in the dialysate, parenterally, or orally, as ordered.
4. As necessary, use nonpharmacological pain relief techniques, such as distraction, massage, guided imagery, and relaxation exercises.
5. Check the temperature of the dialysate before and during instillation.

6. If the client reports extreme pain during dialysis, decrease the inflow rate and consult with the physician to decrease temporarily the amount of dialysate instilled.
7. Investigate carefully any client reports of pain in the shoulder blades.

Rationale

1. Pain on catheter insertion calls for catheter repositioning; pain during dialysate instillation may result from various factors, including too-rapid inflow rate, cool dialysate temperature, and complications of treatment. A pain scale provides an objective methods of measuring the subjective pain experience.
2. Certain positions can reduce abdominal discomfort during instillation.

3. Lidocaine provides local anesthesia.

4. Nonpharmacological pain relief techniques can offer effective, safe alternatives to medication in some clients.
5. A too-cool dialysate temperature can cause abdominal cramps; too warm a temperature can cause tissue damage.
6. A slower instillation rate reduces intra-abdominal pressure and may decrease pain. A decrease in volume reduces the degree of abdominal distention, especially on initiation of dialysis.
7. Referred pain to the shoulders may indicate diaphragmatic irritation.

▲ *Documentation*

Progress notes
   Pain
   Relief measures instituted
   Client's response

▲ *Outcome Criteria*

The outcome criteria for this diagnosis represent those associated with discharge planning. Refer to the discharge criteria.

Potential Altered Health Maintenance related to insufficient knowledge of rationale of treatment, medications, home dialysis procedure, signs and symptoms of complications, community resources, and follow-up care

Focus Assessment Criteria

1. Readiness and ability to learn and retain information

Clinical Significance

1. A client or family failing to achieve learning goals requires a referral for assistance postdischarge.

Interventions

1. Reinforce the physician's explanations of renal disease and of the peritoneal dialysis procedure and its effects.

Rationale

1,2. The client's understanding can help increase compliance and tolerance of treatment.

Interventions

2. Discuss all prescribed medications, covering purpose, dosage, and side effects.
3. As appropriate, teach the client the following:
   a. Aseptic technique
   b. Catheter care and insertion
   c. Dialysate preparation
   d. Positioning during treatment
   e. Instilling additives to dialysate
   f. Inflow and outflow procedure
   Have the client perform return demonstrations so you can evaluate his or her ability to do the procedures safely and effectively.
4. Discuss how to manage inflow pain by ensuring proper temperature and flow rate of dialysate.
5. Teach the client to prevent constipation through adequate diet, fluid intake, and physical activity.
6. Teach the client to watch for and promptly report:

   a. Unresolved pain from inflow

   b. Outflow failure

   c. Low-grade fever, cloudy outflow, malaise
   d. Signs of fluid/electrolyte imbalance (see Collaborative Problems: Electrolyte Imbalances for specific signs and symptoms of various imbalances)
   e. Abdominal pain, stool changes, constipation
7. Provide information on where to purchase necessary supplies.
8. Teach the client to record the following:
   a. Vital signs and weight before and after dialysis
   b. Percent of dialysate and amount of inflow
   c. Amount of outflow
   d. Number of exchanges required
   e. Medications taken
   f. Problems
   g. Urine output and number and character of stools
9. Initiate referral to a home health agency for necessary follow-up.

10. Provide information on available community resources and self-help groups, e.g., National Kidney Foundation.

Rationale

3. Home peritoneal dialysis can be performed by many clients without assistance. Proper technique can help prevent infection and inflow and outflow problems.

4. Inflow pain can be caused by cold dialysate, too-rapid inflow, acid dialysate, and stretching of diaphragm.
5. Constipation or bowel distention impedes dialysate outflow.

6. Early detection of complications enables prompt intervention to minimize their seriousness.
   a. Unresolved inflow pain can indicate intraperitoneal infection.
   b. Outflow failure can be due to catheter obstruction, peritonitis, dislodged catheter, or a full colon.
   c. These signs can point to infection.
   d. Dialysis alters fluid and electrolyte levels, possibly resulting in imbalance.

   e. Bowel distention impedes outflow.

7. Knowledge of sources of supplies can prevent incorrect substitutions.
8. Accurate records aid in evaluating the effectiveness of the treatment.

9. The initial home care visit is needed to evaluate the client's suitability for home dialysis, taking into account factors such as physical condition, ability, environment, financial needs, and support system. Subsequent visits are indicated to assess the client for signs of infection, improper procedures, and complications (e.g., electrolyte, fluid, nutritional imbalances).

10. Access to resources and self-help groups may ease the difficulties of home dialysis and help minimize its impact on home life.

▲ *Documentation*

Discharge summary record
   Client and family teaching
   Outcome achievement or status
   Referrals, if indicated

References/Bibliography

Binkley, L.S. (1984). Keeping up with peritoneal dialysis. *American Journal of Nursing, 84,* 729–733.

Birdsall, C. (1986). How do you manage peritoneal dialysis? *American Journal of Nursing, 86,* 592–596.

Daly, B.J. (1985). *Intensive care nursing.* New York: Medical Examination Publishing.

Fleming, L.M., & Kane, J. (1984). Step-by-step guide to safe peritoneal dialysis. *RN, 47,* 44–47.

Millar, S. (1985). *AACN procedure manual for critical care.* Philadelphia: W.B. Saunders.

Moorhouse, M.F., Geissler, A.C., & Doenges, M.E. (1987). *Critical care plans.* Philadelphia: F.A. Davis.

Shelton, D. (1983). Procedure for chronic peritoneal dialysis. *Critical Care Nurse, 3*(3), 84–86.

Sorrels, A.J. (1981). Peritoneal dialysis: A rediscovery. *Nursing Clinics of North America, 16*(3), 515–529.

Stone, J.C. (1983). *Dialysis and the treatment of renal insufficiency.* New York: Grune & Stratton.

Tenckhoff, H. (1974). *Chronic peritoneal dialysis manual.* Seattle: University of Washington Press.

Walsh, J., Person, C., & Wieck, L. (1987). *Manual of home health care nursing.* Philadelphia: J.B. Lippincott.

Wieck, L., King, E., & Dyer, M. (1986). *Illustrated manual of nursing techniques.* Philadelphia: J.B. Lippincott.

Radiation Therapy

A local treatment used alone or in combination with surgery, chemotherapy, or immunotherapy, radiation therapy is indicated to cure or control cancer cell growth. It also can serve as palliative treatment to relieve pain, prevent fracture, or mobilize a client following a cord compression. When used in cancer treatment, radiation therapy aims to kill a maximum number of cancer cells while minimizing damage to normal tissue. Radiation effects occur at a cellular level and affect tissue, organs, and the entire body; they begin immediately on initiation of therapy and continue for a prolonged time. Specific cell reactions and side effects depend on the radiation dose, effect on deoxyribonucleic acid (DNA) and cell membrane, and the division rate of the cell.

Diagnostic Cluster

▲ **Time Frame**

Pretherapy and intratherapy

Collaborative Problems

Potential Complications:
Myelosuppression
Malabsorption
Pleural Effusion
Cerebral Edema
Inflammation
Renal Calculi
Fluid and Electrolyte Imbalance

Refer to:

Renal Failure

Nursing Diagnoses

Anxiety related to prescribed radiation therapy and insufficient knowledge of treatments and self-care measures

Potential Altered Oral Mucous Membrane related to dry mouth or inadequate oral hygiene

Impaired Skin Integrity related to effects of radiation on epithelial and basal cells and effects of diarrhea on perineal area

Potential Altered Sexuality Patterns related to fatigue, weakness, pain, self-concept changes, grief, impotence, and dyspareunia

Altered Comfort related to stimulation of the vomiting center and damage to the gastrointestinal mucosa cells secondary to radiation

Gastroenteritis

Fatigue related to systemic effects of radiation therapy

Inflammatory Joint Disease

Altered Comfort related to damage to sebaceous and sweat glands secondary to radiation

Cirrhosis

Altered Nutrition: Less Than Body Requirements related to decreased oral intake, reduced salivation, mouth discomfort, dysphasia, nausea/vomiting, and increased metabolic rate

Chemotherapy

Self-Concept Disturbance related to alopecia, skin changes, weight loss, sterility, and changes in role, relationships and life styles

Cancer (Initial Diagnosis)

Grieving related to changes in life style, role, finances, functional capacity, body image, and health losses

Cancer (Initial Diagnosis)

Altered Family Processes related to imposed changes in family roles, relationships, and responsibilities

Cancer (Initial Diagnosis)

▲ **Discharge Criteria**

Before discharge, the client and/or family will:

1. Relate skin care, oral care, and rest requirements
2. State an intent to discuss fears and concerns with a trusted friend
3. Relate signs and symptoms that must be reported to a health care professional

Collaborative Problems

▲ *Nursing Goal*

The nurse will manage and minimize complications of radiation therapy.

Potential Complication: **Myelosuppression**
Potential Complication: **Malabsorption**
Potential Complication: **Pleural Effusion**
Potential Complication: **Cerebral Edema**
Potential Complication: **Inflammation**
Potential Complication: **Renal Calculi**

Interventions

1. Monitor for signs of myelosuppression:
    a. Decreased white blood cell (WBC) and red blood cell (RBC) counts
    b. Decreased platelet count

2. Explain the risk of bleeding and infection. (Refer to the Corticosteroid Therapy care plan, page 542, for strategies to reduce the risk of infection.)

3. Monitor for signs and symptoms of malabsorption:
    a. Diarrhea
    b. Steatorrhea
    c. Abdominal pain
    d. Iron deficiency anemia
    e. Easy bleeding or bruising
    f. Paresthesias
    g. Skin and vision changes
    h. Fluid and electrolyte imbalances
    i. Weight loss
    j. Abnormal laboratory study results: vitamin B_{12}, folic acid, hemoglobin, hematocrit, electrolytes, prothrombin time

4. Monitor for signs and symptoms of pleural effusion:
    a. Dyspnea
    b. Cough
    c. Chest pain
    d. Tachycardia
    e. Tachypnea
    f. Bulging of intercostal spaces
    g. Decreased breath sounds
    h. Abnormal chest x-ray film

5. Monitor for signs and symptoms of cerebral edema:
    a. Restlessness, irritability, memory loss
    b. Somnolence
    c. Headache
    d. Vomiting
    e. Seizure activity
    f. Increased systolic blood pressure with widening pulse pressure

Rationale

1. The stem cell precursors of mature blood cells (WBCs, RBCs, and platelets) are highly radiosensitive. Irradiation of large areas of bone marrow results in decreased WBC and platelet cell production; RBCs are less affected because of their longer life span.

2. Decreased or nonfunctioning WBCs weaken the body's phagocytic defense against microorganisms. Platelets form a temporary plug to stop bleeding and activate clotting factors; decreased platelets can interfere with clotting.

3. Radiation damage to the small intestine results in shortening of intestinal villi and loss of absorptive surface. Radiation doses > 5,000 rads to the pelvis or abdomen can denude intestinal mucosa, impairing absorption of amino acids, carbohydrates, fats, fat-soluble vitamins (A, E, D, K), folic acid, vitamin B, and iron. Electrolyte imbalances also may occur.

4. High-dose radiation therapy to the lungs can cause lung inflammation (pneumonitis) and changes in membrane transfer capability, leading to fluid leakage into the interpleural space.

5. Radiation therapy administered to treat radiosensitive brain tumors such as medulloblastomas or metastatic brain tumors can cause cerebral edema. Effects mimic those of increased intracranial pressure.

Interventions   *Rationale*

    g. Bradycardia

    h. Depressed respirations

    i. Weakness

    j. Hemiparesis

    k. Vision changes

    l. Abnormal pupillary response to light

6. Monitor for signs and symptoms of mucositis:

    a. White patches on oral mucosa

    b. Reddened, swollen mucous membranes

    c. Ulcerated, bleeding lesions

6. Radiation therapy commonly causes tissue inflammation; higher doses generally produce more damage. Severe mucositis may necessitate interruption of radiation therapy.

7. Instruct the client to do the following:

    a. Perform diphenhydramine (Penadryl) mouth irrigations every 4 hours

    b. Take magnesium hydroxide (Maalox) to coat the oral mucosa

    c. Apply viscous lidocaine (Xylocaine) to the mucosa before meals

    d. Avoid alcohol, smoking, and spicy or acidic foods

    e. Avoid very hot or cold liquids and foods.

7. These agents can help reduce or ease the pain of local inflammation. Alcohol, smoking, spicy or acidic foods, and very hot or cold foods and liquids can irritate mucosa.

8. Monitor for signs and symptoms of pneumonitis:

    a. Shortness of breath (SOB)

    b. Hemoptysis

    c. Dry cough

8,9. Radiation to the chest or back can cause pneumonitis or esophagitis.

9. Monitor for signs and symptoms of esophagitis:

    a. Difficulty swallowing

    b. Sore throat

    c. Nausea and vomiting

10. Monitor for signs and symptoms of cystitis:

    a. Urinary urgency and frequency

    b. Hematuria

    c. Dysuria

    d. Negative urine cultures

10. Irradiation of the bladder can cause cystitis or urethritis. Symptoms mimic those of urinary tract or bladder infection, except with negative urine cultures.

11. Monitor for signs and symptoms of myelitis:

    a. Paresthesias in back or extremities

    b. Shocklike sensation on neck flexion

11,12. Radiation therapy to the head and neck can cause myelitis or parotitis. These problems usually are transient and not serious, and resolve spontaneously.

12. Monitor for signs and symptoms of parotitis:

    a. Painful, swollen parotid glands

13. Monitor for signs and symptoms of renal calculi:

    a. Flank pain

    b. Urinary urgency and frequency

    c. Renal colic

    d. Elevated uric acid level

    e. Hematuria

    f. Nausea and vomiting

13. Renal calculi are a potential complication of radiation therapy. They result from rapid lysis of tumor cells, which produces hyperuricemia, a predisposing condition to calculi formation.

▲ *Documentation*

Flow records
    Intake and output
    Abnormal laboratory values
    Assessments (skin, oral, respiratory, neurological)
    Stool for occult blood
    Daily weights

Related Physician-Prescribed Interventions

Dependent on cancer site, stage, and extent

Nursing Diagnoses

▲ **Outcome Criteria**

The client will:

1. Verbalize rationale for radiation treatment and treatment plan
2. Identify expected side effects and their management
3. Describe self-care measures to reduce fatigue, promote nutrition, manage skin problems, and prevent infection and bleeding

Anxiety related to prescribed radiation therapy and insufficient knowledge of treatments and self-care measures

Focus Assessment Criteria	Clinical Significance
1. Understanding of radiation principles	1–5. Many clients and their families poorly understand and fear radiation therapy; most often, their fears are based on assumptions about early types of radiation therapy, which often were crude and caused unfavorable outcomes. In contrast, current technology enables very precise and effective radiation treatment. Through careful assessment and thorough teaching, the nurse can help clear up misconceptions and thus reduce fear and anxiety.
2. Understanding of the treatment plan	
3. Understanding of the expected side effects of treatment	
4. Understanding of self-care measures to minimize side effects and promote health	
5. Misconceptions and concerns about radiation therapy	

Interventions

1. Encourage the client to share fears and beliefs regarding radiation. Delay teaching if the client is experiencing severe anxiety.
2. Review general principles of radiation therapy, as necessary. Provide written materials, such as a client education booklet from the National Cancer Institute.

3. Reinforce the physician's explanation of the treatment plan, covering the following items:
    a. The area to be irradiated
    b. Treatment schedule
    c. Dose to be administered
    d. Simulation to compute dose and delivery of radiation
    e. Markings and tattoos
    f. Shielding of vital organs
4. Review the general effects of radiation therapy:
    a. Fatigue
    b. Skin reactions
    c. Bone marrow depression
    d. Increased susceptibility to infection and bleeding
5. Explain site-specific radiation side effects:
    a. Neck
        • Mucositis
        • Dry mouth
        • Altered taste
        • Dental problems
        • Hoarseness
        • Dysphagia
    b. Head
        • Headache
        • Alopecia
        • Nausea and vomiting

Rationale

1. Sharing enables the nurse to identify sources of anxiety and correct misinformation. Severe anxiety prevents retention of learning.
2. A client undergoing radiation therapy is likely to have many questions about the treatment and its effects. Reinforcing information provided by the physician and radiologist and answering questions can help reduce the client's anxiety related to lack of knowledge.
3. This information can help reduce the client's anxiety associated with fear of the unknown and the unexpected.

4. Fatigue results from rapid cell lysis, increased metabolic rate, and bone marrow depression. Skin damage can occur as a direct local effect of radiation. Bone marrow depression increases the risk of infection, bleeding, and anemia.

5. Understanding what to expect can decrease anxiety related to fear of the unknown and the unexpected, and can help the client recognize and report adverse effects.

Interventions

    c. Chest and back
- Pneumonitis
- Esophagitis

    d. Abdomen and pelvis
- Nausea and vomiting
- Cystitis
- Tenesmus
- Diarrhea
- Abdominal cramps

6. Discuss measures to promote optimal nutrition:
    a. If beef and pork taste bad, try cheese, eggs, and chicken.
    b. Experiment with new seasonings to improve food taste.
    c. Moisten food to ease chewing and swallowing.
    d. If necessary, take antiemetics to control nausea.
    e. Increase intake of high-calorie and high-protein foods.
    f. Try protein supplements.
    g. Comply with prescribed vitamin therapy.

Rationale

6. Inadequate nutrition affects many clients receiving radiation therapy. Anorexia due to accumulation of waste products secondary to tissue destruction hinders adequate food intake. GI tract inflammation can cause nausea, vomiting, and diarrhea. Poor nutrition inhibits tissue repair and promotes anemia.

▲ Documentation

Progress notes
    Anxiety level
    Client teaching
    Outcome achievement or
        status

▲ Outcome Criteria

The client will:
1. Describe the possible effects of radiation on the oral cavity
2. Explain proper techniques for oral care

Potential Altered Oral Mucous Membrane related to dry mouth or inadequate oral hygiene

Focus Assessment Criteria

1. Understanding of possible effects of radiation on oral cavity:
    a. Mucositis
    b. Stomatitis
    c. Dental caries or tooth loss

2. Understanding of necessary oral hygiene measures
3. Oral cavity before treatment for any of the following:
    a. Loose teeth
    b. Dental caries
    c. Gingivitis
    d. Infection

Clinical Significance

1. Radiation therapy to the head and neck increases the acidity of saliva, which can lead to destruction of tooth enamel and increased risk of tooth decay. Radiation therapy also can damage the periodontal membrane, resulting in alveolar absorption of radiation and eventual tooth loss. Decreased WBC counts secondary to radiation therapy further increase the risk of mucositis and stomatitis.

2,3. Inadequate oral hygiene or preexisting dental problems increase the risk of infection and other complications.

Interventions

1. Explain the signs and symptoms of mucositis and stomatitis.

2. Stress the need to have caries filled and bad or loose teeth extracted before initiation of radiation therapy to the head and neck.
3. Emphasize the need for regular oral hygiene during and after therapy. Instruct the client to do the following:

Rationale

1. The client's understanding can help ensure early detection and prompt intervention to minimize problems.
2. Preexisting dental problems increase the risk of radiation-induced infection.

3. Proper oral hygiene eliminates microorganisms and reduces the risk of infection.

Interventions

    a. Brush with fluoridated toothpaste after meals

    b. Use a soft-bristle toothbrush

    c. Rinse the mouth with topical fluoride solution after each brushing

    d. Use a molded dental carrier and fluoride gel daily

4. If gingival tissue becomes inflamed, suggest a peroxide and water rinse.

5. Explain the need for dental examinations during and after the course of treatment.

Rationale

4. Rinsing removes debris and microorganisms without causing trauma to mucosal tissue.

5. The increased risk of dental caries and gum disease persists for months to years after completion of radiation therapy. Long-term follow-up dental care decreases the risk.

▲ **Documentation**

Flow records
    Mouth assessment
    Oral care
Teaching record
    Client teaching
    Outcome achievement or status

▲ **Outcome Criteria**

The client will relate strategies to reduce skin damage.

Impaired Skin Integrity related to effects of radiation on epithelial and basal cell damage and effects of diarrhea on perineal area

Focus Assessment Criteria	*Clinical Significance*
1. Skin in irradiated area(s)	1. Radiation therapy causes skin reactions ranging from mild erythema to weeping desquamation that leaves skin tissue (epidermal and basal layers) raw and irritated. The severity of reaction depends on the dose, depth, and area of irradiation. Moist areas, such as axillae, tend to develop more severe reactions. Healing usually occurs within a few weeks after completion of treatment. Some clients experience long-term fibrosclerotic changes in the subcutaneous layer, giving the affected area a taut, shiny appearance.
2. Nutritional status	2. Malnutrition and anemia commonly are associated with radiation therapy and can cause increased skin fragility. Combined with decreased mobility, this skin change can predispose the client to pressure ulcers.
3. Bowel patterns, perineal area	3. Radiation-induced diarrhea exposes the rectal and perineal areas to irritants that promote skin breakdown.

Interventions

1. Explain the effects of radiation on skin (e.g., redness, tanning, peeling, itching, hair loss, decreased perspiration), and monitor skin in the irradiated area(s).

2. Explain the need for optimal nutritional intake; provide instruction.

3. Teach precautions to protect skin integrity:

    a. If tattoos are used for skin markings, wash irradiated skin with a mild soap and tepid water; do not remove the markings.

Rationale

1. Radiation damages epithelial, sebaceous, and hair follicle cells, causing localized skin reactions. Understanding the reason for these effects can promote compliance with protective and preventive measures.

2. During radiation treatments, the body must build and repair tissue and protect itself from infection. This process requires increased intake of protein, carbohydrates, vitamins, and minerals (Constantian, 1980).

3. These measures can help maintain skin integrity.

    a. To reduce irritation, harsh soaps and hot water should be avoided. The tattoo must remain to guide evaluation and subsequent therapy, if it proves necessary.

Interventions

b. Avoid harsh soap, ointments, creams, cosmetics, and deodorants on treated skin unless approved by health care professionals.
c. Avoid exposure of radiated skin to sun, wind, and shaving.
d. Wear loose-fitting cotton clothing over treated skin.
e. Apply a water-soluble moisturizer, such as lanolin, for dry skin.
f. Apply cool air to the affected area; avoid heat lamps and warmth.

g. Use an electric razor only—no blades—to shave the irradiated area.
h. If moist desquamation is present, shower or irrigate the area frequently, and use a moist wound healing dressing.
4. Instruct the client to report any skin changes promptly.

5. Teach the client to keep the rectal and perineal area clean and to apply protective ointment after each cleaning.

Rationale

b. Harsh substances may increase the skin's vulnerability to damage.

c. This exposure can cause additional damage.

d. Loose-fitting cotton clothing can minimize irritation and injury to the epithelial surface.
e. Water-soluble moisturizers can prevent or treat dry skin.
f. Coldness reduces irritating sensory stimulation (e.g., pruritus) and prevents moist desquamation.
g. An electric razor can protect sensitive skin from razor cuts.
h. Showering or irrigation and moist wound dressings can help debride the area and aid healing.
4. Early detection of moist desquamation with shedding of surface epithelium enables prompt intervention to prevent severe skin damage and subsequent fibrosis.
5. Good hygiene and application of non–water-soluble ointments reduce the erosion of acidic excreta on the perineal area.

▲ **Documentation**

Flow records
   Skin assessments
Teaching record
   Client teaching
   Outcome achievement or status

▲ **Outcome Criteria**

The client will:

1. Relate possible effects of radiation on sexual patterns
2. Verbalize feelings regarding changes in sexual patterns

Potential Altered Sexuality Patterns related to fatigue, pain, self-concept changes, grief, and impotence or dyspareunia

Focus Assessment Criteria	*Clinical Significance*
1. Physical symptoms that may affect libido, e.g., fatigue, nausea and vomiting, diarrhea, anorexia, pain	1. Radiation therapy is associated with physical and psychosocial problems that may cause alterations in sexual patterns.
2. Radiation to the gonads, prostate, uterus, or cervix	2. Radiation to certain reproductive organs can result in changes in hormone levels, libido, and sexual function.
3. Fear, anxiety, depression, diminished self-concept	3. Fears, anxiety, grieving, and poor self-concept also inhibit libido.
4. Previous sexual activity patterns	4. Sexual expression is important to well-being and should be nurtured in all age groups. Assessment of pre-illness patterns helps guide the nurse in planning appropriate interventions.

Interventions

1. Promote open communication about sexual issues by bringing up the subject.

2. Discuss the possible effects of radiation on sexual function and libido:
   a. Hormonal changes
   b. Impotence
   c. Vaginal changes

Rationale

1. This conveys to the client your willingness to discuss sexual issues and concerns, which can promote sharing.
2. Understanding these possible effects and why they occur may help the client cope with the changes. Radiation to the gonads can cause hormonal changes that affect sexual desire. Radiation to the testes can cause permanent impotence due to destruction of Leydig's cells. Radiation of the cervix produces changes in vaginal size and lubrication, leading to dyspareunia and, eventually, to vaginal fibrosis and stenosis if regular vaginal dilatation is not done. Vaginal mucositis also may occur.

Interventions

3. Discuss the effects of fatigue, physical symptoms, and negative emotions and self-concept on libido.
4. Encourage the client to discuss sexual fears and concerns openly with his or her partner. Correct any misconceptions, e.g., that cancer is contagious or that radiation can harm a sexual partner.
5. If fatigue is a problem, suggest sexual activity in the morning or after naps.

6. Discuss management of dyspareunia:
   a. Water-soluble vaginal lubricant
   b. Sitz baths
   c. Avoiding intercourse when mucositis is present.
7. If the cervix was irradiated, discuss the need for regular vaginal dilatation (at least three times a week), either through intercourse or by using a manual obturator. (Refer to the Radical Vulvectomy care plan, page 478, for more information on vaginal dilatation.)
8. Teach the client and partner to identify and practice alternatives to intercourse that they can use for sexual expression, e.g., touching, body massage, masturbation.

Rationale

3. Fatigue, anxiety, fear, and depression can decrease libido and even cause temporary impotence.
4. Open communication helps strengthen a relationship and encourages positive coping.

5. In opposition to the prevailing cultural bias mandating spontaneity in sexual relations, the client may benefit from planning sexual encounters to coincide with times of peak energy.
6. Damage to vaginal mucosa produces decreased lubrication. Intercourse when mucositis is present can further damage cells and increase the risk of infection.

7. Regular dilatation helps prevent vaginal fibrosis and stenosis.

8. The client and partner should understand that sexual expression and gratification are not limited to intercourse, but that they encompass emotional closeness, communication, and other means of self-pleasure and giving pleasure to others.

▲ **Documentation**

Progress notes
  Dialogues
Teaching record
  Client teaching
  Outcome achievement or
    status

References/Bibliography

Constantian, M.B. (1980). *Pressure ulcers: Principles and Techniques of Management.* Boston: Little, Brown, and Co.

del Regato, J.A., & Spjut, H.J. (1984). *Cancer diagnosis, treatment, and prognosis.* St. Louis: C.V. Mosby.

Dudjak, L.A. (1988). Radiation therapy nursing care record: A tool for documentation. *Oncologic Nursing Forum, 15*(6), 763–777.

Dudjak, L.A. (1989). Mouth care for mucositis due to radiation therapy. *Cancer Nursing, 10*(3), 131–140.

Eilers, J., et al. (1988). Development, testing and application of the oral assessment guide for high-dose radiation and/or chemotherapy. *Oncologic Nursing Forum, 15*(3), 325–330.

Haylock, P.J. (1987). Radiation therapy. *American Journal of Nursing, 87*(11), 1441–1446.

Pape, L.H. (1988). Therapy-related acute leukemia: An overview. *Cancer Nursing, 11*(5), 295–302.

Strohl, R.A. (1988). The nursing role in radiation oncology: Symptom management of acute and chronic reactions. *Oncologic Nursing Forum, 15*(4), 429–434.

Total Parenteral Nutrition

Total parenteral nutrition (TPN) involves intravenous administration of an elemental diet (calories, vitamins, and minerals) in a hypertonic solution to a client who is unable to ingest or assimilate sufficient calories or who has increased metabolic needs that cannot be met by oral ingestion. Indications for TPN include cancer, chronic nausea and vomiting of any etiology, anorexia nervosa, massive burns, and gastrointestinal (GI) disorders such as inflammatory bowel disease and bowel obstruction.

Diagnostic Cluster

▲ Time Frame
Intratherapy

▲ Discharge Criteria
Before discharge, the client or family will:
1. Demonstrate proper catheter care and TPN administration at home
2. Discuss strategies for incorporating TPN management into activities of daily living (ADLs)
3. Verbalize precautions for medication use
4. Relate causes, prevention, and treatment of hypoglycemia and hyperglycemia
5. State signs and symptoms that must be reported to a health care professional

---

Collaborative Problems

Potential Complications:
Pneumothorax, Hemothorax, or Hydrothorax
Air Embolism
Sepsis
Hyperglycemia

Nursing Diagnoses

Potential for Infection related to catheter's direct access to bloodstream
Potential Self-Concept Disturbance related to inability to ingest food
Potential Activity Intolerance related to deconditioning
Potential Altered Health Maintenance related to insufficient knowledge of home care, signs and symptoms of complications, catheter care, and follow-up care (laboratory studies)

Collaborative Problems

▲ Nursing Goal
The nurse will manage and minimize complications of TPN.

Potential Complication: Pneumothorax, Hemothorax, or Hydrothorax
Potential Complication: Air Embolism
Potential Complication: Sepsis
Potential Complication: Hyperglycemia

Interventions
1. Monitor for signs and symptoms of pneumothorax, hemothorax, and hydrothorax:
   a. Acute chest pain
   b. Dyspnea

Rationale
1. The most common complication of subclavian catheter placement, pneumothorax can result from puncture or laceration of the pleura or lung. In most cases the air leak is self-limiting, and pneumothorax resolves spontaneously; some cases require aggressive intervention. The less common complications—hemothorax and hydrothorax—can occur from perforation of a great vessel during catheter insertion. It commonly is diagnosed when the physician cannot obtain a free flow of blood in the syringe.

Interventions

2. During the cannulation procedure, maintain the client in Trendelenburg's position with the head turned to the side.

3. Assist with radiography after cannula placement.

4. Monitor for signs and symptoms of air embolism during dressing and IV tubing changes and on accidental separation of IV connections:
   a. Acute, sharp chest pain
   b. Dyspnea
   c. Cyanosis
   d. Tachycardia
   e. Neck vein distention
   f. Hypotension

5. Secure the proximal catheter connection with a Luer-locking IV set, and tape all connections.

6. Instruct the client to perform Valsalva's maneuver during IV tubing disconnections.

7. Explain potential problems with tubing separation, and instruct the tubing to crimp the tubing near the entry site if it occurs.

8. Monitor for signs and symptoms of sepsis or catheter-related infection:
   a. Fever
   b. Chills
   c. Altered mental status
   d. Increased WBC count
   e. Sudden glucose intolerance
   f. Local signs of infection at the insertion site
   g. Positive blood cultures

9. Monitor for signs and symptoms of hyperglycemia:
   a. Kussmaul's respirations
   b. Polyuria
   c. Low urine specific gravity
   d. Glycosuria
   e. Mental status changes, e.g., lethargy, disorientation
   f. Elevated serum glucose
   g. Weight change

Rationale

2. Trendelenburg's position before and during subclavian catheter insertion provides maximum vein distention and minimizes the risk of complications.

3. A chest x-ray film confirms catheter placement and helps rule out complications.

4. Air embolism can occur with IV tubing changes, with accidental tubing situations, and during catheter insertion and disconnection. (For example, the client can aspirate as much as 200 cc of air from a deep breath during subclavian line disconnection.) Entry of air into the circulatory system can block blood flow and cause cardiac arrest.

5. These precautions can help prevent accidental disconnection.

6. Valsalva's maneuver with breath holding minimizes air aspiration and reduces the risk of embolism.

7. Immediate action can prevent air embolism.

8. The high glucose concentration of the TPN solution and frequent catheter manipulation put the client at high risk for infection.

9. Osmotic diuresis can result from inability to compensate for rapid instillation of high-glucose solution. The subsequent rise in serum glucose causes fluid shifts to the vascular compartment in an attempt to dilute the hyperosmolar glucose concentration. The increased fluid volume, along with the exogenous source, is lost rapidly in urine. If unrecognized and untreated, this condition can progress rapidly to nonketotic hyperglycemic coma.

▲ **Documentation**

Flow records
   Vital signs
   Intake and output
   Weight
   Serum glucose
   Urine specific gravity
   Catheter site
Progress notes
   Unusual complaints

Related Physician-Prescribed Interventions

Medications
   Not indicated

Intravenous Therapy
   Nutritional solution   Additives (e.g., insulin)

Laboratory Studies
   Serum albumin   Thyroxine-binding prealbumin
   Electrolytes   Complete blood count
   Serum transferrin   Amino acid profile
   24-hour creatinine excretion

Diagnostic Studies
   Chest x-ray film

Therapies
   Daily weights
   Catheter site care   Anthropometric measurements

Nursing Diagnoses

▲ Outcome Criteria

The client will:

1. Verbalize understanding of precautions for catheter care
2. Report any need for additional dressing changes

Potential for Infection related to the catheter's direct access to the bloodstream

Focus Assessment Criteria	*Clinical Significance*
1. Vital signs at least every shift	1. The TPN catheter provides a route for microorganism invasion of the bloodstream.
2. Local signs of infection at the catheter insertion site	2. Catheter irritation can lead to infection.
3. Serum WBC count	3. Elevated WBC count indicates active infection.

Interventions

1. Use aseptic technique and follow appropriate protocols when changing catheter dressings, IV tubing, and solutions.
2. Avoid administering other IV solutions piggyback into the TPN line unless otherwise ordered.

3. Discontinue lipid emulsions and change the infusion tubing immediately after infusion.

4. Secure proximal IV connections with a Luer-locking set, if possible.
5. Securely tape all IV connections.

6. Teach the client the following:
   a. The importance of proper catheter care
   b. The need to notify the nurse when the dressing becomes soiled or nonadherent
   c. How to crimp the tubing to stop flow should it become accidentally disconnected

Rationale

1. Aseptic technique can prevent contamination.

2. The risk of bacterial contamination increases with additional IV junctions, stopcocks, and ports. To minimize risk, the TPN line should be used exclusively for that purpose unless otherwise ordered.
3. Lipid emulsions and tubes hanging for more than 12 hours are prone to fungal contamination.
4. This precaution can help prevent disconnection and subsequent contamination.
5. Securing with tape helps prevent tissue trauma resulting from catheter manipulation.
6. The client's understanding of care and precautions can improve compliance and reduce the risk of complications.

▲ Documentation

Flow records
 Dressing and tubing changes
 Condition of IV insertion site

▲ Outcome Criteria

The client will:

1. Share feelings related to lack of oral ingestion
2. Verbalize the necessity of continued TPN therapy

Potential Self-Concept Disturbance related to inability to ingest food

Focus Assessment Criteria	*Clinical Significance*
1. Feelings and concerns related to the inability to ingest food orally.	1. Food and eating have many social and cultural implications besides nutritional intake. Prolonged or permanent NPO status can interfere with socialization and create isolation.

Interventions

1. Encourage the client to verbalize concerns related to lack of oral ingestion.

2. Explore possible alternatives to oral ingestion or substitute diversional activities.

3. Provide regular feedback on progress and positive reinforcement on appearance and weight gain.

Rationale

1. Sharing helps identify and clarify the client's concerns and problems, guiding the nurse in planning effective interventions.
2. Substituting activities for meals may help reduce the sense of loss related to lack of oral intake.
3. Feedback and reinforcement promote self-esteem and encourage continued compliance.

▲ **Documentation**

Progress notes
    Dialogues

▲ **Outcome Criteria**

The client will:

1. Verbalize the need for participation in progressive activity
2. Demonstrate correct performance of isometric and range-of-motion (ROM) exercises
3. Maintain current activity level and make progress toward improved conditioning

▲ **Documentation**

Progress notes
    Activity level
    Exercises performed

▲ **Outcome Criteria**

The outcome criteria for this diagnosis represent those associated with discharge planning. Refer to the discharge criteria.

Interventions

4. Arrange for visits from others on enteral nutrition, if feasible.
5. If permitted, allow the client to taste—but not swallow—desired foods.

Rationale

4. Sharing with others in the same situation allows mutual validation and support.
5. Placing food in the mouth without swallowing may help satisfy the need to taste and smell food.

Potential Activity Intolerance related to deconditioning

Focus Assessment Criteria	*Clinical Significance*
1. Muscle strength, ROM, gait, and balance before and throughout TPN therapy	1. TPN therapy without activity leads to inappropriate nutrient use and steady loss of muscle strength and joint ROM.

Interventions

1. Initiate an appropriate activity and exercise regimen, which may include the following:
   a. Active or passive ROM
   b. Isometric exercises
   c. Chair-setting
   d. Trapeze use
   e. Progressive ambulation
2. Advance activity according to improved tolerance.
3. Emphasize the importance of activity during TPN therapy, and discuss exercises that the client can perform without assistance, e.g., walking.

Rationale

1. Progressive activity or exercise promotes metabolism of TPN solution into muscle rather than fat and promotes muscle strengthening.

2. Excessive activity beyond limits of tolerance can cause activity intolerance and hypoxia.
3. The client's understanding can promote compliance with the activity and exercise program.

Potential Altered Health Maintenance related to insufficient knowledge of home care, signs and symptoms of complications, catheter care, and follow-up care (laboratory studies)

Focus Assessment Criteria	*Clinical Significance*
1. Understanding of the TPN procedure and reasons why it is indicated	1. Identifying learning needs guides the nurse in planning effective teaching strategies.
2. Available support persons to assist with TPN therapy at home, if applicable	2. The client may need assistance with home TPN management.
3. Readiness and ability to learn and retain information	3. A client or family failing to achieve learning goals requires a referral for assistance post-discharge.

Interventions

1. Reinforce teaching about TPN and the infusion and catheter insertion procedures.
2. Encourage the client and family to ask questions and express concerns about TPN therapy.
3. Explain the nutritional constituents of TPN solution and how it meets nutritional needs, using understandable terms.
4. Discuss reasons for the continued diagnostic tests: daily weights, urinalysis, and laboratory tests.
5. Teach and evaluate learning with return demonstration:
   a. Aseptic technique
   b. Preparation and storage of TPN solution

Rationale

1. The client's understanding can reduce misconceptions and encourage participation in care.
2. Sharing concerns and questions identifies learning needs and misconceptions, allowing the nurse to address problem areas.
3. Understanding the TPN constituents and their purpose can encourage compliance with therapy.
4. Ongoing monitoring is needed to evaluate therapy and nutritional status.

5. Home TPN can be performed by many clients and families without outside assistance. Proper technique is mandatory to prevent infection and air in the infusion line.

Interventions   *Rationale*

      c. Preparation of tubing for infusion
      d. Use of pump
      e. Discontinuation of infusion
      f. Heparinization of the catheter
      g. Catheter care
      h. Dressing changes

6. Teach about hyperglycemia:
      a. Signs and symptoms: nausea, weakness, thirst, headaches, elevated blood glucose level
      b. Prevention: maintain prescribed rate; avoid increasing the rate to "catch up"
      c. Treatment: consult with physician for possible insulin supplement

6. Because TPN solution contains high glucose concentrations, sudden changes in rate can increase blood glucose levels.

7. Teach about hypoglycemia:
      a. Signs and symptoms: sweating, pallor, palpitations, nausea, headache, shaking feeling, hunger, blurred vision
      b. Prevention: avoid stopping TPN too abruptly; slow TPN rate gradually to allow the body to decrease insulin production
      c. Treatment: glass of orange juice, teaspoon of honey

7. During TPN infusion, the body produces insulin in response to high glucose concentrations. Too much insulin in the TPN or too-rapid discontinuation of TPN can produce hypoglycemia.

8. Teach the client or family to report the following:
      a. Fever, malaise
      b. Redness or purulent drainage at catheter insertion site
      c. Unstable blood glucose level

8. Early detection of complications enables prompt intervention to minimize their seriousness.

9. Teach to keep records of these things:
      a. Daily weights
      b. Temperature
      c. Amount and infusion rate of TPN
      d. Serum glucose level (if advised to monitor)
      e. Any problems
      f. Oral intake

9. Accurate records aid in evaluating the safety and effectiveness of TPN therapy.

10. Refer to a home health agency for follow-up care.

10. The initial home care visit evaluates suitability for home TPN, considering client's ability, environment, financial needs; and support system. Subsequent visits are needed to assess the client's nutritional status, blood glucose levels, laboratory results, insertion site, and catheter patency.

▲ **Documentation**

Discharge summary record
    Client and family teaching
    Outcome achievement or
      status
    Referrals, if indicated

11. Provide a list of required equipment and supplies and of available sources.

11. Planning can prevent shortages and improper substitutions.

References/Bibliography

Crocker, K.S. (1988). AIDS-related GI dysfunction: Rationale for nutrition support. *Critical Care Nurse, 8*(3), 43–45.

DeMonaco, H.J. (1988). IV drug delivery: New technologies for consideration. *Journal of Intravenous Nursing, 11*(5), 316–320.

Grant, J.P. (1980). *Handbook of total parenteral nutrition.* Philadelphia: W.B. Saunders.

Irwin, M. (1988). Managing leaking gastrostomy sites. *American Journal of Nursing, 88*(3), 359–360.

McGee, L. (1987). Feeding gastrostomy: Nursing care, Part 2. *Journal of Enterostomy Therapy, 14*(5), 201–211.

Rombeau, J.L., & Caldwell, M.D. (1986). *Parenteral nutrition* (Vol. 2). Philadelphia: W.B. Saunders.

Souba, W.W., et al. (1989). Hyperalimentation in cancer. *CA, 39*(2), 105–114.

Tracheostomy

This procedure involves the creation of a temporary or permanent surgical opening into the trachea at the second, third, or fourth tracheal ring and insertion of an indwelling tube to permit ventilation and removal of secretions. Indications for tracheostomy include tracheal edema from trauma or allergic response, mechanical airway obstruction, inability to clear tracheobronchial secretions, prevention of aspiration in an unconscious client, and the need for mechanical ventilation.

Diagnostic Cluster

▲ Time Frame
Preprocedure and postprocedure

▲ Discharge Criteria
Before discharge, the client or family will:

1. Demonstrate the ability to perform coughing and deep breathing exercises
2. Demonstrate the ability to perform necessary pulmonary toileting procedures
3. State first aid measures for tracheal respiratory airway maintenance resuscitation
4. Demonstrate tracheostomy care measures
5. Verbalize precautions for drinking
6. State signs and symptoms that must be reported to a health care professional
7. Verbalize an intent to share feelings and concerns related to tracheostomy with significant other(s)
8. Identify available community resources and self-help groups

---

PREOPERATIVE PERIOD
Nursing Diagnoses

Anxiety related to lack of knowledge of impending surgery and implications of condition on life style (chronic)

POSTOPERATIVE PERIOD
Collaborative Problems

Potential Complications:
Hypoxia
Hemorrhage
Tracheal Edema

Nursing Diagnoses

Potential Ineffective Airway Clearance related to increased secretions secondary to tracheostomy, obstruction of inner cannula, or displacement of tracheostomy tube

Potential for Infection related to excessive pooling of secretions and bypassing of upper respiratory defenses

Impaired Verbal Communication related to inability to produce speech secondary to tracheostomy

Potential Altered Sexuality Patterns related to change in appearance or fear of rejection

Potential Altered Health Maintenance related to insufficient knowledge of tracheostomy care, precautions, signs and symptoms of complications, emergency care, and follow-up care

Preprocedure: Nursing Diagnosis

▲ Outcome Criteria
The client will:

1. State the reason for tracheostomy and the expected outcome
2. State anticipated limitations on speech and communication
3. Describe immediate postoperative care and self-care measures
4. Preoperatively, demonstrate the ability to communicate effectively using a method other than speech

Anxiety related to lack of knowledge of impending surgery and implications of condition on life style

Focus Assessment Criteria

1. Understanding of tracheostomy procedure, including previous experiences with surgery and anesthesia
2. Knowledge of the potential sequelae of tracheostomy, including these:
   a. Temporary or permanent status
   b. Changes in body function
   c. Change in appearance
   d. Limited speech
   e. Limited mobility

Clinical Significance

1,2. Assesssment of the client's knowledge guides the nurse in planning effective and appropriate teaching strategies. The nurse must determine if additional physician's explanations are needed for an informed consent.

Interventions

1. Reinforce the physician's explanations of the surgery and reason for it. As appropriate, explain that temporary tracheostomy is indicated in anticipated postoperative edema following biopsy, severe respiratory distress, and other disorders, and that permanent tracheostomy is an alternative to endotracheal or nasotracheal intubation.

2. Explain common terms and concepts; provide literature and actual equipment, if possible. Make sure the client is familiar with the following:
   a. Tracheostomy procedure
   b. Stoma
   c. Tracheostomy tube
   d. Suctioning and the suction catheter
   e. Tracheal humidity collar
   f. Tracheostomy ties
   g. Trachea bibs

3. Discuss potential sequelae of tracheostomy surgery, including the following:
   a. Change in body appearance
   b. Change in body functions, e.g., breathing, speaking, singing, coughing, and clearing secretions

4. Instruct the client on alternative means of communication, e.g., flip chart, picture board. Have the client use return demonstration to indicate mastery.

Rationale

1. Explaining what to expect may help reduce the client's anxiety related to fear of the unknown and unexpected.

2. Understanding of terminology improves comprehension and helps reduce anxiety.

3. Preparing the client for what to expect can reduce the anxiety of the unknown.

4. Having the client practice communication techniques before the procedure allows the nurse to detect and attempt to correct any serious flaws. Mastery of alternative communication can help decrease feelings of alienation and loneliness, enhance the client's sense of control, and reduce anxiety.

▲ **Documentation**

Progress notes
   Level of understanding
   Ability to use alternative
      communication method
   Client teaching

Postprocedure: Collaborative Problems

▲ **Nursing Goal**

The nurse will manage and minimize complications of a tracheostomy.

Potential Complication: Hypoxia
Potential Complication: Hemorrhage
Potential Complication: Tracheal Edema

Interventions

1. Monitor for signs and symptoms of respiratory distress:
   a. Restlessness, agitation, confusion
   b. Air hunger, inability to breathe
   c. Diminished or absent air exchange over the tracheostomy tube
   d. Use of accessory muscles of respiration, retraction of soft tissue around the tracheostomy
   e. Air crepitus around the stoma and in the neck and chest wall

2. Monitor for signs and symptoms of hemorrhage:
   a. Continuous oozing of blood, or bleeding around or inside the tracheostomy tube unrelated to suctioning
   b. Unusual edema around the stoma

Rationale

1. Respiratory distress can be caused by partial airway occlusion with a mucus plug or from a displaced tube. Unusual resistance encountered when advancing the tracheal suction catheter could indicate partial occlusion of the inner cannula. Subcutaneous air may indicate improper tracheostomy tube placement.

2. Hemorrhage can result from prolonged exposure of the carotid artery during surgery or radiation therapy, which dries and weakens the vessel wall and increases its susceptibility to injury.

Interventions

3. Elevate the head of the bed 30 to 40 degrees when the client is stable.

4. Provide supplemental tracheal humidification during the first 24 to 72 hours after tracheostomy surgery.

▲ *Documentation*

Flow records
  Vital signs
  Respiratory assessment
  Tracheostomy site

5. Keep a replacement cuffed tracheostomy tube and endotracheal tube at the client's bedside.

Related Physician-Prescribed Interventions
Medications
  Not indicated
Intravenous Therapy
  Not indicated
Laboratory Studies
  Arterial blood gas analysis
Diagnostic Studies
  Chest x-ray film
Therapies
  Supplemental humidification
  Oxygen therapy

Rationale

3. Tracheostomy tube placement stimulates increased secretions; elevating the head of the bed facilitates secretion drainage and helps decrease postoperative edema around the stoma.

4. Disruption of the normal mechanism for humidification of the tracheobronchial tree necessitates adding moisture to inspired air. Proper humidification helps liquify secretions and prevent encrustations and plug formation.

5. Displacement of the tracheostomy tube within the first 24 hours may necessitate emergency intubation until initiation of surgical intervention.

Nursing Diagnoses

▲ *Outcome Criteria*

The client will:
1. Maintain a patent tracheostomy tube
2. Cough effectively to clear the airway

Potential Ineffective Airway Clearance related to increased secretions secondary to tracheostomy, obstruction of inner cannula, or displacement of tracheostomy tube

Focus Assessment Criteria	*Clinical Significance*
1. Respiratory status	1. Baseline and ongoing assessment enables early detection of developing problems.
2. Cough	2. An effective cough effort is necessary to expel secretions.
3. Secretions	3. Assessing the amount and character of secretions helps detect infection and evaluate the risk of obstruction.

Interventions

1. Elevate the head of the bed 30 to 40 degrees.

2. Encourage the client to breathe deeply and cough regularly.
3. Provide adequate humidification of inspired air.

▲ *Documentation*

Flow records
  Intake and output
  Urine specific gravity
  Amount and character of
    secretions
  Humidification provided

4. Suction as necessary, maintaining sterile technique.
5. Regularly inspect and cleanse the tracheostomy tube.
6. Maintain optimal hydration status.

Rationale

1. This position facilitates optimal respiration by increasing drainage of secretions.
2. Deep breathing reduces pooling of secretions; coughing helps expel secretions.
3. Moisture is needed to replace the bypassed humidification normally provided by nasopharyngeal structures.
4. Suction removes secretions and prevents stasis.
5. Crusts of secretions can obstruct the airway or become a source of infection.
6. Hydration status affects the amount and character of secretions; a dehydrated client is at increased risk for mucus plug formation.

Potential for Infection related to excessive pooling of secretions and bypassing of upper respiratory defenses

Focus Assessment Criteria	*Clinical Significance*
1. Tracheostomy site: signs of infection	1. The tracheostomy site is at high risk for infection owing to its status as an open wound, possible tissue trauma from suctioning, and the culture medium provided by secretions.

Interventions	*Rationale*
1. Suction the tracheostomy tube every hour and as needed or as ordered, maintaining sterile technique and using a lubricated, appropriately sized (less than half the diameter of the tracheostomy tube) catheter. (Lubricate a nonsilicone tube catheter with water; a silicone catheter, with water-soluble, non–petroleum-based lubricant.) Decrease the frequency to suctioning as needed, as secretion formation decreases.	1. Regular suctioning removes pooled secretions, which provide a favorable medium for microorganism growth. Sterile technique provides additional infection protection. Too-large a catheter can obstruct the airway; a nonlubricated catheter can stick to the tracheostomy tube.
2. Assess stomal borders for unusual edema, signs of skin breakdown, drainage, bleeding, odor, erythema, lesions, and air crepitus.	2. Abnormal drainage can indicate infection (foul, purulent) or thoracic duct leakage (milky).
3. Change the tracheostomy dressing every shift and as needed.	3. Regular dressing changes help keep stomal borders dry and free of mucus.
4. Keep tracheostomy ties secure; use a square knot.	4. Continual movement of the tracheostomy tube can cause irritation, possibly leading to tissue erosion. An improperly tied tube also is prone to displacement by coughing or suctioning.
5. Avoid irritation of surrounding tissue by leaving one finger space between the ties and the neck.	5. The ties should be secure enough to prevent the tracheostomy tube from sliding up and down the trachea but not so tight as to compress the external jugular veins.
6. Cleanse around the stoma every 4 hours and as needed; use half-strength hydrogen peroxide and saline solution, and wipe with plain saline. Apply an antibacterial ointment if ordered. If the tracheostomy tube is sutured, clean around the stoma using a cotton swab.	6. Regular cleansing removes potential sources of contamination. The physician may elect to leave the stoma undressed during the immediate postoperative period to facilitate assessment and cleansing.

Impaired Verbal Communication related to inability to produce speech secondary to tracheostomy

Focus Assessment Criteria	*Clinical Significance*
1. Potential impediments to communication: a. Illiteracy or low reading level b. Hearing deficit c. Vision deficit d. Cognitive impairment e. Poor attention span or short-term memory f. Impaired hand–eye coordination or fine motor skills	1. Assessment of impediments before tracheostomy enables the nurse to plan appropriate teaching strategies and other interventions to maximize the client's communication ability postsurgery.
2. Understanding of tracheostomy and its effects on speech	2. The client's expectation of impaired speech encourages adaptation to alternative means of communication and prevents shock and fear at the inability to speak after surgery.

Interventions

1. Based on assessment findings, initiate appropriate consultations, e.g., speech pathologist, ophthalmologist, otorhinolaryngologist.
2. Before surgery, instruct the client on the expected effects of tracheostomy on speech. Explain the normal physiology of speech production and how tracheostomy disrupts this mechanism.

3. After identifying an appropriate alternative communication method, instruct the client to practice it preoperatively, if possible. Encourage staff and support persons to practice alternative communication also.
4. Keep a call light at the client's bedside, and post a note at the receiving desk reading "Client temporarily unable to speak."

5. Remove any extraneous barriers that can interfere with effective communication.
   a. Provide a calm, quiet environment.
   b. Decrease external stimuli, e.g., TV, radio, conversations of others.
   c. Face the client when communicating.
   d. Allow adequate time for the client to initiate, complete, and respond to communication.
   e. Avoid filling in gaps or completing sentences; allow the client to communicate as he or she wishes.
   f. Use restatement to ensure understanding.
   g. Use active listening skills.
   h. Provide emotional support, reassurance, and encouragement.

Rationale

1. The client may need intensive, specialized interventions to ensure effective communication.

2. The client's understanding that tracheostomy normally does not disrupt anatomical structures responsible for speech production, and that speech impairment is likely to be temporary, can help him cope with the impairment and may encourage use of alternative communication methods.
3. Using an alternative form of communication can help decrease anxiety and feelings of isolation and alienation, promote a sense of control over the situation, and enhance safety.

4. The client will be unable to use an intercom; the call light will help reduce feelings of isolation and provide reassurance that staff is available.
5. Effective communication techniques by the listener enhances understanding.

▲ **Documentation**

Progress notes
  Ability to communicate

▲ **Outcome Criteria**

The client will:
1. Discuss his or her feelings and concerns regarding the effect of tracheostomy on sexual functioning
2. Verbalize an intention to share with partner

Potential Altered Sexuality Patterns related to change in appearance, fear of rejection

Focus Assessment Criteria	*Clinical Significance*
1. Sexual history, including specific sexual needs or concerns of the client and partner	1. Obtaining a sexual history not only provides useful information but also validates that sexuality is an important component of health and well-being that warrants investigation.
2. Presence of any factors that could inhibit libido or sexual expression, e.g., pain, fatigue, limited mobility	2. This assessment helps determine whether the client's physical condition permits his or her usual form of sexual expression.

Interventions

1. Discuss the expected effects of tracheostomy on body functions (e.g., breathing, speaking, coughing, clearing secretions), appearance, and mobility.
2. Counsel the client about sexuality concerns, using the PLISSIT counseling model:
   a. *Permission.* Provide reassurance that shar-

Rationale

1. The client's understanding of the effects of surgery can help him or her accept and cope with the changes and maintain role relationships, self-esteem, and sexual identity.
2. The PLISSIT model allows the nurse to address the client's concerns in an organized, effective manner.

Interventions

      ing sexual feelings and concerns is healthy and that desiring sex and physical intimacy while ill is normal; encourage sharing with partner.

    b. *Limited information.* Provide only the information appropriate to the client's particular condition and concerns.

    c. *Specific instructions.* Provide detailed instructions and suggestions for dealing with a specific problem or concern.

    d. *Intensive therapy.* Initiate referrals to specialists for more intensive therapy, as necessary.

3. Reassure the client and partner that their concerns and fears are normal and expected.

4. Allow the partner to share his or her concerns in private, if possible. Areas of concern typically include the risk of hurting or even suffocating the client during sexual activity.

5. Encourage both the client and partner to look at the tracheostomy site.

6. Intervene to help clarify any misconceptions or to address specific areas of concern.

    a. Fear of suffocation: Explain that this is a remote possibility; encourage the client to wear a protective shield or stoma cover as an added precaution.

    b. Offensive odors and secretions: Encourage application of perfume or aftershave to mask odors, and wearing a stoma bib to hide secretions.

    c. Offensive appearance: Suggest covering the stoma bib with a scarf, high collar or turtleneck, or ascot; instruct a male client to wear shirts with a larger collar size to cover the stoma bib without binding.

    d. Fatigue: Encourage rest periods before engaging in sexual activity, and suggest positions that minimize the client's energy expenditure (e.g., client on bottom, both partners side-lying).

    e. Decreased libido: Explain that this is normal following surgery, owing to several factors including fatigue, concerns about appearance and odor, pain, and anxiety. Reassure the client that libido should return as these factors resolve.

7. Consult with a qualified sex therapist, if indicated.

Rationale

3. This reassurance can help reduce anxiety and facilitate positive coping.

4. Providing privacy may encourage the client's partner to share feelings and concerns, an important component in planning effective interventions.

5. Looking at the stoma can help the client and partner accept the reality of altered body function and appearance, which facilitates positive coping.

6. Addressing specific concerns and problems aids the client and partner in adapting to the changes.

7. The client and partner may benefit from the expertise of a specialist.

▲ *Documentation*

Progress notes
    Interactions
    Client teaching

▲ *Outcome Criteria*

The outcome criteria for this diagnosis represent those associated with discharge planning. Refer to the discharge criteria.

Potential Altered Health Maintenance related to insufficient knowledge of tracheostomy care, precautions, signs and symptoms of complications, emergency care, and follow-up care

Focus Assessment Criteria	Clinical Significance
1. Participation in self-care 2. Ability to perform self-tracheostomy care 3. Readiness and ability to learn and retain information	1,2. This assessment helps determine the client's suitability for home management of tracheostomy and identifies the need for any referrals. 3. A client or family failing to achieve learning goals requires a referral for assistance postdischarge.

Interventions

1. Teach tracheostomy home care measures:

   a. Skin care

   b. Suctioning

   c. Tube care

   d. Using a stoma cover or collar

   e. Obtaining necessary supplies (tracheostomy tubes, stoma adhesive or dressing pads, twill tape, saline solution, suctioning equipment)
2. Reinforce the importance of adequate humidity and of regular coughing and deep breathing exercises.
3. Explain the need for optimal oral hygiene.
4. Teach the client to protect the stoma from water when showering, shaving, washing hair, etc.
5. Instruct the client to avoid the following:
   a. Very hot or cold environments
   b. Exposure to gas fumes, dust, and aerosol sprays
6. Teach signs of infection to report, e.g., change of sputum to greenish-yellow.
7. Teach emergency management of tube displacement.

8. Explain why the client has a diminished sense of smell and taste; encourage adequate food intake despite altered taste.

9. Identify appropriate community resources and self-help groups, and encourage the client to contact them.

10. Initiate a referral to a home health agency.

Rationale

1. Proper tracheostomy care can help prevent infection and other complications.
   a. Skin must be protected from erosive secretions.
   b. Suctioning may be needed to provide airway patency.
   c. Proper tube care removes potential sources of infection and obstruction.
   d. A stoma bib protects the stoma, and filters out dust particles, and warms the air entering the trachea. It also increases the moisture concentration of inspired air, which eases breathing and helps liquefy secretions.
   e. Teaching where supplies can be obtained can reduce anxiety and shortages.

2. Adequate humidity decreases mucus crusting and facilitates expulsion of secretions.

3. Dysphagia may promote pooling of secretions.
4. A client with a tracheostomy is at risk for aspirating water through the stoma.

5. These factors and substances are irritating to mucus membranes and increase the risk of infection.

6. Early detection enables prompt treatment to prevent or minimize complications.
7. Understanding proper emergency management can prevent a panic response should displacement occur.

8. As a result of tracheostomy, inspired air bypasses the olfactory end organs, interfering with both smell and taste. Understanding this mechanism and its temporary nature can reduce anxiety.
9. The client may find it helpful to share experiences and concerns with others in a similar situation or may need assistance with aspects of home management.
10. A home visit is indicated to evaluate equipment and the client's ability to perform self-care.

▲ **Documentation**

Discharge summary record
   Client teaching
   Outcome achievement or
      status

References/Bibliography

Bell, C.W., et al. (1984). *Home care and rehabilitation in respiratory medicine.* Philadelphia: J.B. Lippincott.

Harris, R.B., et al. (1984). Clean vs. sterile tracheotomy care and level of pulmonary infection. *Nursing Research, 33*(2), 80–85.

Luce, J.M., Tyler, M., & Pierson, D.J. (1984). *Intensive respiratory care.* Philadelphia: W.B. Saunders.

Oerann, M.H., et al. (1983). Patient sensations following a tracheostomy: A discussion. *Critical Care Quarterly, 6*(2), 53–58.

Appendices

This care plan (Level I) presents nursing diagnoses and collaborative problems that commonly apply to clients (and their significant others) undergoing hospitalization for any medical disorder. Nursing diagnoses and collaborative problems specific to a disorder are presented in the care plan (Level II) for that disorder (see Unit II).

Diagnostic Cluster

Collaborative Problems

Potential Complications:
Cardiovascular
Respiratory

Nursing Diagnoses

Anxiety related to unfamiliar environment, routines, diagnostic tests, treatments, and loss of control

Potential for Injury related to unfamiliar environment and physical and mental limitations secondary to condition, medications, therapies, and diagnostic tests

Potential for Infection related to increased microorganisms in environment, the risk of person-to-person transmission, and invasive tests and therapies

(Specify) Self-Care Deficit related to sensory, cognitive, mobility, endurance, or motivation problems

Potential Altered Nutrition: Less Than Body Requirements related to decreased appetite secondary to treatments, fatigue, environment, and changes in usual diet; and to increased protein and vitamin requirements for healing

Potential Constipation related to change in fluid and food intake, routine, and activity level; effects of medications; and emotional stress

Sleep Pattern Disturbance related to unfamiliar, noisy environment, change in bedtime ritual, emotional stress, and change in circadian rhythm

Potential Spiritual Distress related to separation from religious support system, lack of privacy, or inability to practice spiritual rituals

Altered Family Process related to disruption of routines, change in role responsibilities, and fatigue associated with increased workload and visiting hour requirements

▲ Discharge Criteria

Specific discharge criteria vary depending on the client's condition; generally, all diagnoses in the above diagnostic cluster should be resolved before discharge.

Collaborative Problems

▲ *Nursing Goal*

The nurse will manage and minimize respiratory and cardiovascular complications.

Potential Complication: Cardiovascular
Potential Complication: Respiratory

Interventions

1. Monitor cardiovascular status:

    a. Radial pulse (rate and rhythm)

    b. Apical pulse (rate and rhythm)

    c. Blood pressure

    d. Skin (color, turgor, temperature, moisture)

2. Monitor respiratory status:
    a. Rate
    b. Rhythm
    c. Breath sounds

Rationale

1. Physiological mechanisms governing cardiovascular function are very sensitive to any changes in body function, making changes in cardiovascular status important clinical indicators.

    a. Pulse monitoring provides data to detect cardiac dysrhythmias, blood volume changes, and circulatory impairment.

    b. Apical pulse monitoring is indicated if the client's peripheral pulses are irregular, weak, or extremely rapid.

    c. Blood pressure represents the force exerted by blood against arterial walls. Hypertension (systolic pressure > 140 mm Hg, diastolic pressure > 85 mm Hg) may indicate increased peripheral resistance, increased cardiac output, or increased blood volume or viscosity. Hypotension can result from significant blood or fluid loss, decreased cardiac output, and certain medications.

    d. Skin assessment provides information for evaluating circulation, body temperature, and hydration status.

2. Respiratory assessment provides essential data for evaluating the effectiveness of breathing and detecting adventitious or abnormal breath sounds, which may indicate airway moisture, narrowing, or obstruction.

▲ *Documentation*

Flow records
    Pulse rate and rhythm
    Blood pressure
    Respiratory assessment
Progress notes
    Abnormal findings
    Interventions

Related Physician-Prescribed Interventions
Dependent on the underlying pathology

Nursing Diagnoses

▲ *Outcome Criteria*

The client will:

1. Communicate feelings regarding the condition and hospitalization
2. Verbalize, if asked, what to expect regarding routines and procedures

Anxiety related to unfamiliar environment and routines, insufficient knowledge of condition, diagnostic tests, and treatments, and loss of control

Focus Assessment Criteria

1. Physical condition

2. Sensory status:
    a. Vision
    b. Hearing
3. Intelligence and learning ability:
    a. Education
    b. Occupation
    c. Learning disabilities
    d. Language difficulties
4. Anxiety level: mild, moderate, severe, panic

Clinical Significance

1. Pain, fatigue, dyspnea, or other symptoms can increase a client's anxiety and hinder his motivation to learn, ability to concentrate, and retention of learning.

2,3. Impaired hearing, vision, cognition, or memory, a learning disability, or a language barrier can interfere with communication and learning. A client with any such problem needs alternative client teaching techniques.

4. Extreme anxiety impairs a client's learning and coping abilities.

Focus Assessment Criteria

5. Past experience with hospitalization

6. Specific stressors; nature of concerns

7. Support system: availability and quality

Clinical Significance

5. A client's expectations and perceptions of his hospital stay are influenced, both positively and negatively, by his past experience with hospitalization.

6. Every client experiences some emotional reaction to illness and hospitalization. The nature and degree of this reaction depend on how the client perceives his situation and its anticipated effects—physical, psychological, financial, social, occupational, spiritual.

7. Adequate support from family, friends, and other sources can provide comfort and help the client maintain self-esteem. Poor support can increase stress and impair the client's coping ability.

Interventions

1. Introduce yourself and other members of the health care team, and orient the client to the room (e.g., bed controls, call bell, bathroom).

2. Explain hospital policies and routines:
   a. Visiting hours
   b. Meal times and availability of snacks
   c. Vital sign monitoring
   d. Availability of newspapers
   e. Television rental and operation
   f. Storage of valuables
   g. Telephone use
   h. Smoking policy
   i. Policy for off-unit trips

3. Determine the client's knowledge of his condition, its prognosis, and treatment measures. Reinforce and supplement the physician's explanations as necessary.

4. Before any procedure requiring the client's informed consent, determine the client's ability to give this consent. He should understand the following:
   a. The specific nature of the procedure
   b. Possible alternative treatments or procedures
   c. Possible outcomes if procedure is not performed
   d. The potential for death or serious harm from the procedure
   e. Possible adverse effects during or after the procedure
   f. The client's right to refuse or to withdraw consent at any time after giving it
   Contact the physician if the client needs additional information or explanation.

5. Explain any scheduled diagnostic tests, covering the following:
   a. Description
   b. Purpose
   c. Pre-test routines

Rationale

1. A smooth, professional admission process and warm introduction can put a client at ease and set a positive tone for his hospital stay.

2,3. Providing accurate information can help decrease the client's anxiety associated with the unknown and unfamiliar.

4. The physician is legally responsible for providing a client with all relevant information before performing a procedure or providing a treatment. The nurse is responsible for evaluating the client's understanding of the physician's explanation, and for notifying the physician of the need for further explanation.

5-7. Teaching the client about tests and treatment measures can help decrease his fear and anxiety associated with the unknown, and improve his sense of control over the situation.

Interventions | *Rationale*

      d. Who will perform the procedure and where
      e. Expected sensations
      f. Post-test routines
      g. Availability of results
  6. Discuss all prescribed medications:
      a. Name and type
      b. Purpose
      c. Dosage
      d. Special precautions
      e. Side effects
  7. Explain any prescribed diet:
      a. Purpose
      b. Duration
      c. Allowed and prohibited foods

8. Provide the client with opportunities to make decisions about his care, whenever possible.

8. Participating in decision-making can help give a client a sense of control, which enhances his coping ability. Perception of loss of control can result in a sense of powerlessness, then hopelessness.

9. Explain and provide a copy of the hospital's or American Hospital Association's Patient Bill of Rights, which specifies the following rights:
    a. Respectful care
    b. Informed consent
    c. The right to refuse treatment
    d. Confidentiality of care and records

9. Knowledge of his rights and recourse as a hospitalized person may provide reassurance and help reduce the client's anxiety level.

10. Provide reassurance and comfort. Spend time with the client, encourage him to share feelings and concerns, listen attentively, and convey empathy and understanding.

10. Providing emotional support and encouraging sharing may help a client clarify and verbalize his fears, allowing the nurse to give realistic feedback and reassurance.

11. Correct any misconceptions and inaccurate information the client may express.

11. A common contributing factor to fear and anxiety is incomplete or inaccurate information; providing adequate, accurate information can help allay client fears.

▲ **Documentation**

Progress notes
   Unusual responses or situations

12. Allow the client's support persons to share their fears and concerns, and encourage them in providing meaningful and productive support.

12. Supporting the client's support persons can enhance their ability to help the client.

▲ **Outcome Criteria**

The client will:
1. Identify factors that increase his risk of injury
2. Describe appropriate safety measures

Potential for Injury related to unfamiliar environment and physical or mental limitations secondary to the condition, medications, therapies, and diagnostic tests

Focus Assessment Criteria	*Clinical Significance*
1. Vision and hearing 2. Mental status 3. Mobility	1–3. An unfamiliar environment and problems with vision, orientation, mobility, and fatigue can increase a client's risk of falling.

Interventions | *Rationale*

1. Orient the client to his environment (e.g., location of bathroom, bed controls, call bell). Leave a light on in the bathroom at night.

1. Orientation helps provide familiarity; a light at night helps the client find his way safely.

2. Instruct the client to wear slippers with nonskid soles and to avoid newly washed floors.

2. These precautions can help prevent foot injuries and falls from slipping.

3. Teach him to keep the bed in the low position, with side rails up at night.

3. The low position makes it easier for the client to get in and out of bed.

Interventions

4. Make sure that the telephone, eye glasses, and frequently used personal belongings are within easy reach.
5. Instruct the client to request assistance whenever he needs it.
6. As necessary, explain the unit's smoking policy and specify areas where smoking is permitted.
7. For an uncooperative, high-risk client, consult with the physician for a 24-hour sitter or restraints, as indicated.

Rationale

4. Keeping objects at hand helps prevent falls from overreaching and overextending.
5. Getting needed help with ambulation and other activities reduces a client's risk of injury.
6. A client smoking in a prohibited area may increase the risk of fire and injury.
7. In some cases, extra measures are necessary to ensure a client's safety and prevent injury to him and others.

▲ **Documentation**

Progress notes
    Client teaching
    Response to teaching

▲ **Outcome Criteria**

The client will describe or demonstrate appropriate precautions to prevent infection.

Potential for Infection related to increased microorganisms in the environment, risk of person-to-person transmission, and invasive tests or therapies

Focus Assessment Criteria	*Clinical Significance*
1. Personal hygiene	1. Poor personal hygiene encourages a microorganism population, increasing the risk of infection.
2. Nutritional status	2. Poor nutritional status increases a client's susceptibility to infection by impairing the phagocytic defense mechanism.
3. History of invasive tests or therapies (e.g., IV lines, indwelling urinary catheter)	3. Invasive tests or therapies can introduce microorganisms into the body.

Interventions

1. Teach the client to wash his hands regularly, especially before meals and after toileting.
2. Teach him to avoid coughing, sneezing, or breathing on others, and to use disposable tissues.
3. Follow institutional policies for IV and indwelling urinary catheter insertion and care.
4. Teach a client undergoing IV therapy not to bump or disturb the IV catheterization site.
5. Teach a client with an indwelling catheter in place to do the following:
   a. Avoid pressure on the catheter
   b. Wipe from front to back after a bowel movement
6. Instruct the client to watch for and report immediately any signs and symptoms of inflammation:
   a. Redness, pain at the catheter insertion site
   b. Bladder spasms and cloudy urine, for a client with an indwelling urinary catheter
   c. Feelings of warmth and malaise

Rationale

1. Proper handwashing deters the spread of microorganisms.
2. These techniques help prevent infection transmission through airborne droplets.
3. Proper insertion and care reduce the risk of inflammation and infection.
4. Movement of the device can cause tissue trauma and possible inflammation.
5. Catheter movement can cause tissue trauma, predisposing to inflammation. An indwelling catheter can be readily contaminated by feces.

6. Nosocomial infections occur in 5% to 6% of all hospitalized clients. Early detection enables prompt intervention to prevent serious complications and a prolonged hospital stay.

▲ **Documentation**

Flow records
    Catheter and insertion site
      care
Progress notes
    Abnormal findings

(Specify) Self-Care Deficit related to sensory, cognitive, mobility, endurance, or motivational problems

▲ **Outcome Criteria**

The client will:
1. Perform self-care activities (feeding, toileting, dressing, grooming, bathing), with assistance as needed
2. Demonstrate optimal hygiene after care is provided

Focus Assessment Criteria	*Clinical Significance*
1. Self-feeding ability	1–6. Assessing the client's abilities helps the nurse determine what assistance the client needs to achieve the greatest level of independence possible.
2. Self-bathing and grooming abilities	
3. Self-dressing ability	
4. Self-toileting ability	
5. Motivation for self-care	
6. Endurance	

Interventions

1. Promote the client's maximum involvement in self-feeding:
   a. Determine the client's favorite foods and provide them, when possible.
   b. As feasible, arrange for meals to be served in a pleasant, relaxed, familiar setting without too many distractions.
   c. Ensure good oral hygiene before and after meals.
   d. Encourage the client to wear his dentures and eye glasses when eating, as appropriate.
   e. Have the client sit upright in a chair at a table, if possible. If not, position him as close to upright as he can be.
   f. Provide some social contact during meals.
   g. Encourage a client who has trouble handling utensils to eat "finger foods" (e.g., bread, sandwiches, fruit, nuts).
   h. Provide needed adaptive devices for eating, e.g., plate guard, suction device under the plate or bowl, padded-handle utensils, wrist or hand splint with clamp, special drinking cup.
   i. Assist with meal set-up as needed—opening containers, napkins, and condiment packages; cutting meat; and buttering bread.
   j. Arrange foods so the client can eat them easily.

2. Promote the client's maximum involvement in bathing.
   a. Encourage and help set up a regular schedule for bathing.
   b. Keep the bathroom and bath water warm.
   c. Ensure privacy.
   d. Provide needed adaptive equipment, e.g., bath board, tub chair or stool, washing mitts, hand-held shower spray.
   e. Make sure the call bell is within easy reach of a client bathing alone.

3. Promote or provide assistance with grooming and dressing:
   a. Deodorant application
   b. Cosmetic application
   c. Hair care: shampooing and styling
   d. Shaving or beard care
   e. Nail and foot care

4. Promote the client's maximum involvement in toileting activities:
   a. Evaluate his ability to move to and use the toilet unassisted.
   b. Provide assistance and supervision only as needed.
   c. Provide needed adaptive devices, e.g., commode chair, spill-proof urinal, fracture bedpan, raised toilet seat, support rails.
   d. Whenever possible, encourage a regular elimination routine using the toilet and avoiding a bedpan or urinal.

Rationale

1–4. Enhancing a client's self-care abilities can increase his sense of control and independence, promoting overall well-being.

▲ *Documentation*

Flow records
  Assistance needed for self-care

▲ **Outcome Criteria**

The client will:

1. Ingest daily nutritional requirements in accordance with his activity level and metabolic needs
2. Relate the importance of good nutrition

Potential Altered Nutrition: Less Than Body Requirements related to decreased appetite secondary to treatments, fatigue, environment, and changes in usual diet; and to increased protein and vitamin requirements for healing

Focus Assessment Criteria

1. Usual dietary patterns (24-hour diet recall); caloric intake and types of foods

2. Height, daily weight

3. Presence of the following:
   a. Bowel sounds
   b. Nausea and vomiting
   c. Flatus

Clinical Significance

1. A 24-hour diet recall provides data to evaluate the quality of the client's diet and identify the need for modifications and teaching.
2. Daily weighing provides data to evaluate nitrogen balance; rapid weight gain can indicate edema.
3. Certain conditions and medications and prolonged immobility can disturb gastrointestinal (GI) function.

Interventions

1. Explain the need for adequate consumption of carbohydrates, fats, protein, vitamins, minerals, and fluids.
2. Consult with a nutritionist to establish appropriate daily caloric and food type requirements for the client.
3. Discuss with the client possible causes of his decreased appetite.

4. Encourage the client to rest before meals.

5. Offer frequent small meals instead of a few large ones.

6. Restrict liquids with meals and avoid fluids 1 hour before and after meals.
7. Encourage and help the client to maintain good oral hygiene.
8. Arrange to have high-calorie and high-protein foods served at the times that the client usually feels most like eating.
9. Take steps to promote appetite:
   a. Determine the client's food preferences and arrange to have these foods provided, as appropriate.
   b. Eliminate any offensive odors and sights from the eating area.
   c. Control any pain and nausea before meals.
   d. Encourage the client's support persons to bring allowed foods from home, if possible.
   e. Provide a relaxed atmosphere and some socialization during meals.
10. Give the client printed materials outlining a nutritious diet that includes the following:
    a. High intake of complex carbohydrates and fiber
    b. Decreased intake of sugar, salt, cholesterol, total fat, and saturated fats
    c. Alcohol use only in moderation
    d. Proper caloric intake to maintain ideal weight

Rationale

1. During illness, good nutrition can reduce the risk of complications and speed recovery (Salmond, 1980).
2. Consultation can help ensure a diet that provides optimal caloric and nutrient intake.

3. Factors such as pain, fatigue, analgesic use, and immobility can contribute to anorexia. Identifying a possible cause enables interventions to eliminate or minimize it.
4. Fatigue further reduces an anorexic client's desire and ability to eat.
5. Even distribution of total daily caloric intake throughout the day helps prevent gastric distention, possibly increasing appetite.
6. These fluid restrictions help prevent gastric distention.
7. Poor oral hygiene leads to bad odor and taste, which can diminish appetite.
8. This measure increases the likelihood of the client's consuming adequate calories and protein.
9. These measures can improve appetite and lead to increased intake.

10. Today, diet planning focuses on avoiding nutritional excesses (Taylor et al., 1989). Reducing fats, salt, and sugar can reduce the risk of heart disease, diabetes, certain cancers, and hypertension.

▲ **Documentation**

Flow records
　Dietary intake
　Daily weight

▲ *Outcome Criteria*

The client will maintain his pre-hospitalization bowel patterns.

Potential Constipation related to change in fluid or food intake, routine, or activity level; effects of medications; and emotional stress

Focus Assessment Criteria	*Clinical Significance*
1. Prehospitalization elimination patterns	1. These data help the nurse evaluate whether the client had any elimination problem before admission.
2. Laxative or enema use	2. Excessive use of these substances could cause constipation.
3. Character of bowel sounds, presence and degree of abdominal distention	3. Assessment helps the nurse monitor for the return of peristalsis, if absent.

Interventions

1. Auscultate bowel sounds.

2. Implement measures to promote a balanced diet that promotes regular elimination:
   a. Encourage increased intake of high-fiber foods, e.g., fresh fruit with skin, bran, nuts and seeds, whole-grain breads and cereals, cooked fruits and vegetables, fruit juices. (*Note:* If the client's diet is low in fiber, introduce fiber slowly to reduce irritation to the bowel.)
   b. Discuss the client's dietary preferences and plan diet modifications to accommodate them, whenever possible.
   c. Encourage the client to eat approximately 800 g of fruits and vegetables—the equivalent of about four pieces of fresh fruit and a large salad—daily to promote regular bowel movements.

3. Promote adequate daily fluid intake:
   a. Encourage intake of at least 2 liters (8 to 10 glasses) per day, unless contraindicated.
   b. Identify and accommodate fluid preferences, whenever possible.
   c. Set up a schedule for regular fluid intake.

4. Establish a regular routine for elimination:
   a. Identify the client's usual elimination pattern before the onset of constipation.
   b. Review the client's daily routine to find an optimal time for elimination, and schedule adequate time.
   c. Suggest that he attempt defecation about an hour following meals; instruct him to remain on the toilet for a sufficient length of time.

5. Attempt to stimulate the client's home environment for elimination:
   a. Have the client use the toilet rather than a bedpan or commode, if possible; offer a bedpan or commode only when necessary.
   b. Assist the client into proper position on the toilet, bedpan, or commode, as necessary.
   c. Provide privacy during elimination attempts—close the bathroom door or draw curtains around the bed, play the television or radio to mask sounds, use a room deodorizer.

Rationale

1. Bowel sounds indicate the nature of peristaltic activity.

2. A well-balanced diet high in fiber content stimulates peristalsis and regular elimination.

3. Adequate fluid intake helps maintain proper stool consistency in the bowel and aids regular elimination.

4. Devising a routine for elimination based on the body's natural circadian rhythms can help stimulate regular defecation.

5. A sense of normalcy and familiarity can help reduce embarrassment and promote relaxation, which may aid defecation.

Interventions

    d. Provide adequate comfort, reading material as a diversion, and a call bell for safety reasons.

  6. Teach the client to assume an optimal position on the toilet or commode (sitting upright, leaning forward slightly) or bedpan (head of bed elevated to put the client in high Fowler's position or at permitted elevation); assist him in assuming this position as necessary.

  7. Explain how physical activity affects daily elimination. Encourage and, as necessary, assist with regular ambulation, unless contraindicated.

Rationale

  6. Proper positioning takes full advantage of abdominal muscle action and the force of gravity to promote defecation.

  7. Regular physical activity aids elimination by improving abdominal muscle tone and stimulating appetite and peristalsis.

▲ **Documentation**

Flow records
  Bowel movements
  Bowel sounds

▲ **Outcome Criteria**

The client will report a satisfactory balance of rest and activity.

Sleep Pattern Disturbance related to an unfamiliar, noisy environment, a change in bedtime ritual, emotional stress, and a change in circadian rhythm

Focus Assessment Criteria	*Clinical Significance*
1. Usual sleep requirements	**1.** Sleep requirements vary among clients, depending on age, life style, activity level, stress, and other factors.
2. Usual bedtime routines, environment, position	**2.** Bedtime rituals may aid relaxation and promote sleep.
3. Quality of sleep	**3.** Only the client can subjectively evaluate the quality of sleep and his satisfaction or dissatisfaction with that quality.

Interventions

  1. Explain the sleep cycle:
    a. Stage I: Transitional stage between wakefulness and sleep (5% to 10% of total sleep)
    b. Stage II: Early sleep; the person is easily aroused (50% to 55% of total sleep)
    c. Stage III: Deeper sleep; arousal is more difficult (10% to 20% of total sleep)
    d. Stage IV: Deepest sleep; metabolism, brain waves slow (10% to 20% of total sleep).

  2. Discuss the reasons for differing individual sleep requirements, including age, life style, activity level, and other possible factors.

  3. Institute measures to promote relaxation:
    a. Maintaining a dark, quiet environment
    b. Allowing the client to choose pillows, linens, and covers, as appropriate
    c. Providing a regular bedtime ritual
    d. Ensuring good room ventilation
    e. Closing the door, if desired

  4. Schedule procedures to minimize the times you need to wake the client at night; as possible, plan for at least 2-hour periods of uninterrupted sleep.

Rationale

  1. A person typically goes through four or five complete sleep cycles each night. Awakening during a cycle may cause him to feel not well rested in the morning.

  2. Although many believe that a person needs 8 hours of sleep each night, no scientific evidence supports this belief. Individual sleep requirements vary greatly. Generally, a person who can relax and rest easily requires less sleep to feel refreshed. With age, total sleep time usually decreases—especially Stage IV sleep—and Stage I sleep increases.

  3. Sleep is difficult without relaxation. The unfamiliar hospital environment can hinder relaxation.

  4. In order to feel rested, a person usually must complete an entire sleep cycle (70 to 100 minutes) four or five times a night.

Interventions

5. Explain the need to avoid sedative and hypnotic drugs.

6. Assist with usual bedtime routine as necessary, e.g., personal hygiene, snack, music for relaxation.

7. Teach the client sleep-promoting measures:
   a. Eating a high-protein snack (e.g., cheese, milk) before bedtime
   b. Avoiding caffeine

   c. Attempting to sleep only when feeling sleepy

   d. Trying to maintain consistent nightly sleep habits

8. Explain the importance of regular exercise in promoting good sleep.

Rationale

5. These medications begin to lose their effectiveness after a week of use, requiring increasing dosages and leading to the risk of dependence.

6. A familiar bedtime ritual may promote relaxation and sleep.

7. These practices may help promote sleep.
   a. Digested protein produces tryptophan, which has a sedative effect.
   b. Caffeine stimulates metabolism and deters relaxation.
   c. Frustration may result if the client attempts to sleep when not sleepy or relaxed.
   d. Irregular sleeping patterns can disrupt normal circadian rhythms, possibly leading to sleep difficulties.

8. Regular exercise not only increases endurance and enhances the ability to tolerate psychological stress, but also promotes relaxation.

▲ **Documentation**

Progress notes
    Reports of unsatisfactory
    sleep

▲ **Outcome Criteria**

The client will maintain usual spiritual practices not detrimental to health.

Potential Spiritual Distress related to separation from religious support system, lack of privacy, or inability to practice spiritual rituals

Focus Assessment Criteria

1. Religious beliefs and ability to worship
2. Access to religious leader or group
3. Emotional response to inability to practice religious or spiritual rituals or separation from spiritual support system, e.g., calmness, anger, guilt, self-hatred, sadness

Clinical Significance

1,2. A client's religious beliefs and practices can be a source of comfort and strength.
3. Certain religious or spiritual beliefs and practices may conflict with prevalent health-care practices, and may be prohibited.

Interventions

1. Explore whether the client desires to engage in an allowable religious or spiritual practice or ritual; if so, provide opportunities for him to do so.
2. Express your understanding and acceptance of the importance of the client's religious or spiritual beliefs and practices.
3. Provide privacy and quiet for spiritual rituals, as the client desires and as practicable.
4. If you wish, offer to pray with the client or read from a religious text.

5. Offer to contact a religious leader or hospital clergy to arrange for a visit. Explain available services, e.g., hospital chapel, Bible.
6. Explore whether any usual hospital practices conflict with the client's beliefs, e.g., diet, hygiene, treatments. If so, try to accommodate the client's beliefs to the extent that policy and safety allow.

Rationale

1. For a client who places a high value on prayer or other spiritual practices, these practices can provide meaning and purpose and can be a source of comfort and strength.
2. Conveying a nonjudgmental attitude may help reduce the client's uneasiness about expressing his beliefs and practices.
3. Privacy and quiet provide an environment that enables reflection and contemplation.
4. The nurse—even one who does not subscribe to the same religious beliefs or values of the client—can still help him meet his spiritual needs.
5. These measures can help the client maintain spiritual ties and practice important rituals.
6. Many religions prohibit certain behaviors; complying with restrictions may be an important part of the client's worship.

▲ **Documentation**

Progress notes
    Spiritual concerns

▲ *Outcome Criteria*

The client and family members will:

1. Verbalize feelings regarding the diagnosis and hospitalization
2. Identify signs of family dysfunction
3. Identify appropriate resources to seek when needed

Altered Family Processes related to disruption of routines, change in role responsibilities, and fatigue secondary to stress, increased workload, and visiting requirements

Focus Assessment Criteria	*Clinical Significance*
1. Understanding of condition 2. Usual family coping patterns 3. Current response 4. Available resources	1–4. The family unit is a system based on interdependent members and patterns that provide structure and support. Hospitalization can disrupt these patterns, possibly leading to family dysfunction.

Interventions

1. Approach the family and attempt to create a private and supportive environment.
2. Provide accurate information, using simple terms.

3. Explore family members' perceptions of the situation.

4. Assess their current emotional response—e.g., guilt, anger, blame, grief—to the stresses of hospitalization.

5. Observe the dynamics of client–family interaction during visitations; evaluate the following:
   a. Apparent desire for visit
   b. Effects of visit
   c. Interactions
   d. Physical contact
6. Determine whether the family's current coping mechanism is effective.

7. Promote family strengths:
   a. Involve family members in caring for the client.
   b. Acknowledge their assistance.
   c. Encourage a sense of humor and perspective.
8. As appropriate, assist the family in reorganizing roles at home, resetting priorities, and reallocating responsibilities.
9. Warn family members to be prepared for signs of depression, anxiety, anger, and dependency in the client and other family members.

10. Encourage and help the family to call on their social network (e.g., friends, relatives, church members) for support.
11. Emphasize the need for family members to address their own physical and psychological needs. To provide time for this, suggest measures such as these:
    a. Taking a break and having someone else visit the client for a change
    b. Calling the unit for a status report rather than traveling to the hospital every day

Rationale

1. Approaching the family communicates a sense of caring and concern.
2. Moderate or high anxiety impairs the ability to process information; simple explanations impart useful information most effectively.
3. Evaluating family members' understanding can help identify any learning needs they may have.
4. A family member's response to another member's illness is influenced by the extent to which the illness interferes with his goal-directed activity, the significance of the goal interfered with, and the quality of the relationship.
5. These observations provide information regarding family roles and interrelationships and the quality of support family members provide for each other.

6. Illness of a family member may necessitate significant role changes, putting a family at high risk for maladaptation.
7. These measures may help maintain an existing family structure, allowing it to function as a supportive unit.

8. Reordering priorities may help reduce stress and maintain family integrity.

9. Anticipatory guidance can alert family members to impending problems, enabling intervention to prevent the problems from occurring.
10. Adequate support can eliminate or minimize family members' feelings that they must "go it alone."
11. A family member who ignores his own needs—e.g., sleep, relaxation, nutrition—and changes his usual health practices for the worst impairs his own effectiveness as a support person.

Interventions

12. If the family becomes overwhelmed, help them to prioritize their duties and problems and to act accordingly.
13. At the appropriate time, have family members list perceived problems and concerns. Then, develop a plan of action to address each item.
14. Encourage the family to continue their usual method of decision-making, including the client when appropriate.
15. As possible, adjust visiting hours to accommodate family schedules.
16. Identify any dysfunctional coping mechanisms:
    a. Substance abuse
    b. Continued denial
    c. Exploitation of one or more family members
    d. Separation or avoidance
    Refer for counseling, as necessary.
17. Direct the family to community agencies and other sources of emotional and financial assistance, as needed.
18. As appropriate, explore whether the client and family have discussed end-of-life decisions; if not, encourage them to do so.

19. When appropriate, instruct the client or family members to provide the following information:
    a. Person to contact in the event of emergency
    b. Person whom the client trusts with personal decisions
    c. Decision whether or not to maintain life support if the client were to become mentally incompetent
    d. Any preference for dying at home or in the hospital
    e. Desire to sign a living will
    f. Decision on organ donation
    g. Funeral arrangements; burial, cremation
    h. Any circumstances in which information should be withheld from the client (Carpenito, 1989)

Rationale

12. Prioritizing can help a family under stress focus on and problem-solve those situations requiring immediate attention.
13. Addressing each problem separately allows the family to identify resources and reduce feelings of being overwhelmed.
14. Joint decision-making reduces the client's feelings of dependency and reinforces that continued support is available.
15. This measure may help promote regular visitation, which can help maintain family integrity.
16. Families with a history of unsuccessful coping may need additional resources. Families with unresolved conflicts prior to a member's hospitalization are at high risk.

17. Additional resources may be needed to help with management at home.

18. Intense stress is experienced when families and health care providers are faced with decisions regarding either initiation or discontinuation of life-support systems or other medical interventions that prolong life—e.g., nasogastric tube feeding (Johnson & Justin, 1988). If the client's wishes are unknown, additional conflicts arise—especially if the family disagrees with decisions made by the health care providers, or vice versa.
19. During an episode of acute illness, these discussions may not be appropriate. Clients and families should be encouraged to discuss their directions to be used to guide future clinical decisions, and their decisions should be documented. One copy should be given to the person designated as the decision-maker in the event the client becomes incapacitated or incompetent, with the other copy retained in a safe deposit box.

▲ **Documentation**

Progress notes
  Interactions with family
  Assessment of family functioning
  End-of-life decisions, if known

References/Bibliography

Carpenito, L.J. (1989). *Nursing diagnosis: Application to clinical practice* (3rd ed.). Philadelphia: J.B. Lippincott.

Johnson, R.A., & Justin, R. (1988). Documenting patients' end-of-life decisions. *Nurse Practitioner, 13*(6), 41.

Salmond, S. (1980). How to assess the nutritional status of acutely ill patients. *American Journal of Nursing, 80*(3), 922.

Taylor, C., Lillis, C., & LaMone, P. (1989). *Fundamentals of nursing.* Philadelphia: J.B. Lippincott.

This care plan (Level I) presents nursing diagnoses and collaborative problems that commonly apply to clients (and their significant others) experiencing all types of surgery. Nursing diagnoses and collaborative problems specific to a surgical procedure are presented in the care plan (Level II) for that procedure (see Unit II).

Diagnostic Cluster

▲ **Time Frame**

Preoperative and postoperative periods

PREOPERATIVE
Nursing Diagnosis

Anxiety/Fear related to surgical experience, loss of control, unpredictable outcome, and insufficient knowledge of preoperative routines, postoperative exercises and activities, and postoperative changes and sensations

POSTOPERATIVE
Collaborative Problems

Potential Complications:
Hemorrhage
Hypovolemia/Shock
Evisceration
Dehiscence
Infection (Peritonitis)
Urinary Retention
Thrombophlebitis
Paralytic Ileus

Nursing Diagnoses

Potential Altered Respiratory Function related to immobility secondary to postanesthesia state and pain

Potential for Infection related to increased susceptibility to bacteria secondary to wound

Impaired Physical Mobility related to surgical interruption of body structures, flatus, and immobility

Potential Altered Nutrition: Less Than Body Requirements related to increased protein and vitamin requirements for wound healing and decreased intake secondary to pain, nausea, vomiting, and diet restrictions

Potential Colonic Constipation related to decreased peristalsis secondary to immobility and the effects of anesthesia and narcotics

Activity Intolerance related to pain and weakness secondary to anesthesia, tissue hypoxia, and insufficient fluid and nutrient intake

Potential Altered Health Maintenance related to insufficient knowledge of care of operative site, restrictions (diet, activity), medications, signs and symptoms of complications, and follow-up care

▲ **Discharge Criteria**

Before discharge, the client and/or family will:

1. Describe any at-home activity restrictions
2. Describe at-home wound and pain management
3. Discuss fluid and nutritional requirements for proper wound healing
4. List the signs and symptoms that must be reported to a health care professional
5. Describe necessary follow-up care

Preoperative: Nursing Diagnosis

▲ Outcome Criteria

The client will:

1. Communicate feelings regarding the surgical experience
2. Verbalize, if asked, what to expect regarding routines, environment, and sensations
3. Demonstrate postoperative exercises, splinting, and respiratory regimen

Anxiety/Fear related to surgical experience, loss of control, unpredictable outcome, and insufficient knowledge of preoperative routines, postoperative exercises and activities, and postoperative changes and sensations

Focus Assessment Criteria	*Clinical Significance*
1. Specific stressors and nature of concerns	1. Every client experiences some emotional reaction to surgery; the nature and degree of this reaction depend on how the client perceives the surgery and its anticipated effects—physical, psychological, financial, social, occupational, spiritual.
2. Past experiences or knowledge regarding surgery 3. Understanding of the planned surgical procedure	2,3. Accurate knowledge of the planned procedure and care routines can help reduce anxiety and fear related to the unknown.
4. Available support system	4. Adequate support from family, friends, and other sources can help the client cope with surgery and recovery.

5. Anxiety level:
  a. Mild (alert and aware of the situation, learning and coping abilities intact)
  b. Moderate (physical signs present—e.g., increased pulse rate, muscle tremors; concentration difficult)
  c. Severe (more overt signs present—e.g., hyperventilation, tachycardia; perception altered greatly; learning and coping severely impaired)
  d. Panic (hyperactivity and other overt physical signs present, perception completely distorted, learning and coping impossible)
	5. Extreme anxiety impairs the client's learning and coping abilities.

6. Readiness and ability to learn and retain information	6. A client or family failing to achieve learning goals requires a referral for assistance post-discharge.

Interventions

1. Provide reassurance and comfort; stay with the client, encourage him to share his feelings and concerns, listen attentively, and convey a sense of empathy and understanding.
2. Correct any misconceptions and inaccurate information the client has about the procedure.

3. Determine whether the client desires spiritual support, e.g., visit from clergy or other spiritual leader, religious article, or ritual. Arrange for this support if necessary.
4. Allow and encourage family members and significant others to share their fears and concerns. Enlist their support for the client, but only if it is meaningful and productive.

Rationale

1. Providing emotional support and encouraging the client to share allows him to clarify his fears and provides opportunities for the nurse to provide realistic feedback and reassurance.
2. Modifiable contributing factors to anxiety include incomplete and inaccurate information. Providing accurate information and correcting misconceptions may help eliminate fears and reduce anxiety.
3. Many clients need spiritual support to enhance coping ability.

4. Effective support from family members, other relatives, and friends can help the client cope with the surgery and recovery.

Interventions

5. Notify the physician if the client exhibits severe or panic anxiety.

6. Notify the physician if the client needs any further explanations about the procedure; beforehand, the physician should explain the following:
   a. Nature of the surgery
   b. Reason for and expected outcome of surgery
   c. Any risks involved
   d. Type of anesthetic that is to be used
   e. Expected length of recovery and any postoperative restrictions and instructions

7. Involve family members or significant others in client teaching, whenever possible.

8. Provide instruction (bedside or group) on general information pertaining to the need for active participation, preoperative routines, environment, personnel, and postoperative exercises.

9. Present information or reinforce learning using written materials (e.g., books, pamphlets, instruction sheets) or audiovisual aids (e.g., videotapes, slides, posters).

10. Explain the importance and purpose of all preoperative procedures:

    a. Enemas

    b. Nothing-by-mouth (NPO) status

    c. Skin preparation

    d. Laboratory studies

    e. Preoperative medications

11. Discuss expected intraoperative procedures and sensations:
    a. Appearance of the operating room and equipment
    b. Presence of surgical staff
    c. Administration of anesthesia
    d. Appearance of the postanesthesia recovery room
    e. Recovery from anesthesia

12. Explain all expected postoperative routines and sensations:

Rationale

5. Immediate notification enables prompt assessment and possible pharmacological intervention.

6. The physician is responsible for explaining the surgery to the client and family; the nurse, for determining their level of understanding and then notifying the physician of the need to provide more information.

7. Knowledgeable family members or significant others can serve as "coaches" to remind the client of postoperative instructions and restrictions.

8. Preoperative teaching provides the client with information, which can help decrease anxiety and fear associated with the unknown and enhance his sense of control over the situation.

9. Simultaneous stimulation of multiple senses augments the learning process. Written materials can be retained and used as a reference after discharge. These materials may be especially useful for caregivers who did not participate in client teaching sessions.

10. This information can help relieve anxiety and fear associated with lack of knowledge of necessary preoperative activities and routines.
    a. Enemas are sometimes given to empty the bowel of fecal material, which can help reduce the risk of postoperative bowel obstruction as peristalsis resumes.
    b. Eliminating oral fluids preoperatively reduces the risk of aspiration postoperatively.
    c. Tests and studies establish baseline values and help detect any abnormalities before surgery.
    d. Preoperative sedatives reduce anxiety and promote relaxation, which increases the effectiveness of anesthesia and decreases secretions in response to intubation.

11. Again, the client's understanding of expected procedures and sensations can help ameliorate fears.

12. Explaining what the client can expect, why the procedures are done, and why certain sensations may occur can help reduce fears associated with the unknown and unexpected.

	Interventions		*Rationale*
a.	Parenteral fluid administration	**a.**	Parenteral fluids replace fluids lost from NPO state and blood loss.
b.	Vital sign monitoring	**b.**	Careful monitoring is needed to determine status and track any changes.
c.	Dressing checks and changes	**c.**	Until wound edges heal, the wound must be protected from contaminants.
d.	Nasogastric (NG) tube insertion and care	**d.**	An NG tube promotes drainage and reduces abdominal distention and tension on the suture line.
e.	Indwelling (Foley) catheter insertion and care	**e.**	A Foley catheter drains the bladder until muscle tone returns as anesthesia is excreted.
f.	Other devices, such as intravenous (IV) lines, pumps, and drains	**f.**	Nausea and vomiting are common side effects of preoperative medications and anesthesia; other contributing factors include certain types of surgery, obesity, electrolyte imbalance, rapid position changes, and psychological and environmental factors. Pain commonly occurs as medications lose their effectiveness.

g. Symptoms including nausea, vomiting, and pain

h. The availability of analgesics and antiemetics, if needed

13. As applicable, teach the client (using return demonstration to ensure understanding and ability), how to do the following:
    a. Turn, cough, and deep-breathe
    b. Support the incision site while coughing
    c. Change position in bed every 1 to 2 hours
    d. Sit up, get out of bed, and ambulate as soon as possible after surgery (prolonged sitting should be avoided)

14. Explain the importance of progressive activities postoperatively, including early ambulation and self-care as soon as the client is able.

15. Explain important hospital policies to family members or significant others, e.g., visiting hours, number of visitors allowed at one time, location of waiting rooms, how the physician will contact them after surgery.

16. Evaluate the client's and family's or significant others' ability to achieve preset, mutually planned learning goals.

13. Again, the client's understanding of postoperative care measures can help reduce anxiety associated with the unknown, and it can promote compliance. Teaching the client about postoperative routines before surgery ensures that his understanding is not impaired by the continuing effects of sedation postoperatively.

14. Activity improves circulation and helps prevent pooling of respiratory secretions. Self-care promotes self-esteem and can help enhance recovery.

15. Providing family members and significant others with this information can help reduce their anxiety and allow them to support the client better.

16. This assessment identifies the need for any additional teaching and support.

▲ **Documentation**

Flow records
   Client teaching
   Progress notes
   Unusual interactions

Postoperative: Collaborative Problems

▲ **Nursing Goal**

The nurse will manage and minimize complications post-surgery.

Potential Complication: **Hemorrhage**
Potential Complication: **Hypovolemia/Shock**
Potential Complication: **Evisceration**
Potential Complication: **Dehiscence**
Potential Complication: **Infection (Peritonitis)**
Potential Complication: **Urinary Retention**
Potential Complication: **Thrombophlebitis**
Potential Complication: **Paralytic Ileus**

Interventions

1. Monitor for signs and symptoms of hemor-rhage/shock:
   a. Increased pulse rate with normal or slightly decreased blood pressure
   b. Urine output < 30 mL/hr
   c. Restlessness, agitation, decreased menta-tion
   d. Increased respiratory rate
   e. Diminished peripheral pulses
   f. Cool, pale, or cyanotic skin
   g. Thirst
2. Monitor fluid status; evaluate the following:
   a. Intake (parenteral and oral)
   b. Output and other losses (urine, drainage, and vomiting)
3. Monitor the surgical site for bleeding, dehis-cence, and evisceration.
4. Teach the client to splint the surgical wound with a pillow when coughing, sneezing, or vomiting.
5. If dehiscence or evisceration occur do the fol-lowing:
   a. Place the client in low Fowler's position

   b. Instruct the client to lie still and quiet

   c. Cover protruding viscera with a warm ster-ile dressing
6. Do not initiate fluids until bowel sounds are present; begin with small amounts. Monitor the client's response to resumption of fluids and foods, and note the nature and amount of any emesis.
7. Monitor for signs of paralytic ileus:
   a. Absent bowel sounds
   b. Flatus
   c. Abdominal distention
8. Monitor for signs and symptoms of infection/ sepsis (refer also to the nursing diagnosis Po-tential for Infection, page 647 of this Appen-dix):
   a. Increased temperature
   b. Chills
   c. Malaise
   d. Elevated white blood cell (WBC) count
   e. Increasing abdominal tenderness
   f. Wound tenderness, redness, or edema
9. Monitor for signs of urinary retention:
   a. Bladder distention
   b. Urine overflow (30–60 mL of urine every 15 to 30 minutes)

10. Instruct the client to report bladder discomfort or inability to void.
11. If the client does not void within 8 to 10 hours after surgery or complains of bladder discomfort, do the following:

Rationale

1. The compensatory response to decreased cir-culatory volume aims to increase blood oxy-gen through increased heart and respiratory rates and decreased peripheral circulation (manifested by diminished peripheral pulses and cool skin). Decreased oxygen to the brain results in altered mentation.

2. Fluid loss during surgery and as a result of NPO status can disrupt fluid balance in a high-risk client. Stress can cause sodium and water retention.
3. Careful monitoring enables early detection of complications.
4. Splinting reduces stress on the suture line by equalizing pressure across the wound.

5. Rapid interventions can reduce the severity of complications.
   a. Low Fowler's position uses gravity to mini-mize further tissue protrusion.
   b. Lying still and quiet also minimizes tissue protrusion.
   c. A warm sterile dressing helps maintain tis-sue viability.
6,7. Intraoperative manipulation of abdominal or-gans and the depressive effects of narcotics and anesthetics on peristalsis can cause para-lytic ileus, usually between the third and fifth postoperative day. Pain typically is localized, sharp, and intermittent.

8. Microorganisms can be introduced into the body during surgery or through the incision. Circulating pathogens trigger the body's de-fense mechanisms: WBCs are released to de-stroy some pathogens, and the hypothalamus raises the body temperature to kill others. Wound redness, tenderness, and edema result from lymphocyte migration to the area.

9. Anesthesia produces muscle relaxation, af-fecting the bladder. As muscle tone returns, spasms of the bladder sphincter prevent urine outflow, causing bladder distention. When urine retention increases the intravesical pres-sure, the sphincter releases urine and control of flow is regained.
10. Bladder discomfort and failure to void may be early signs of urinary retention.
11. These measures may help promote relaxation of the urinary sphincter and facilitate voiding.

Interventions

 a. Warm the bedpan.
 b. Encourage the client to get out of bed to use the bathroom, if possible.
 c. Instruct a male client to stand when urinating, if possible.
 d. Run water in the sink as the client attempts to void.
 e. Pour warm water over the client's perineum.

12. If the client still cannot void, follow protocols for straight catheterization, as ordered.

13. Monitor for signs and symptoms of thrombophlebitis:
 a. Positive Homans' sign (pain on dorsiflexion of the foot, due to insufficient circulation)
 b. Calf tenderness, unusual warmth, or redness

14. Encourage the client to perform leg exercises. Discourage placing pillows under the knees, use of a knee gatch, crossing the legs, and prolonged sitting.

Rationale

12. Straight catheterization is preferable to indwelling catheterization because it carries less risk of urinary tract infection from ascending pathogens.

13. Vasoconstriction due to hypothermia decreases peripheral circulation. Anesthesia and immobility reduce vasomotor tone, resulting in decreased venous return with peripheral blood pooling. In combination, these factors increase the risk of thrombophlebitis.

14. These measure help increase venous return and prevent venous stasis.

▲ Documentation

Flow records
 Vital signs (pulses, respirations, blood pressure, temperature)
 Circulation (color, peripheral pulses)
 Intake (oral, parenteral)
 Output (urinary, tubes, specific gravity)
 Bowel function (bowel sounds, defecation, distention)
 Wound (color, drainage)
Progress notes
 Unusual complaints or assessment findings
 Interventions

Related Physician-Prescribed Interventions

Medications
Preoperative
 Sedatives
 Narcotic analgesics
 Anticholinergics

Postoperative
 Narcotic analgesics
 Antiemetics

Intravenous Therapy
Fluid and electrolyte replacement

Laboratory Studies
Complete blood count   Urinalysis
Chemistry profile

Diagnostic Studies
Chest x-ray film
Electrocardiography

Therapies
Indwelling catheterization   Incentive spirometry
Wound care   Liquid diet progressed to full diet as tolerated
Preoperative NPO status   Antiembolic hose

Postoperative: Nursing Diagnoses

▲ Outcome Criteria

The client will exhibit clear lung fields.

Potential Altered Respiratory Function related to immobility secondary to postanesthesia state and pain

Focus Assessment Criteria	*Clinical Significance*
1. Respiratory status: **a.** Rate and rhythm **b.** Breath and lung sounds **c.** Effectiveness of coughing effort	**1.** In the immediate postoperative period, hypoventilation and decreased sensorium, resulting from CNS depression by narcotics and anesthesia, increase the risk of aspiration.

Focus Assessment Criteria

2. Risk factors for postoperative respiratory problems:
   a. Smoking
   b. Obesity
   c. Chronic respiratory disease
   d. Liver dysfunction
   e. Prolonged immobility
   f. Surgical incision near the diaphragm
   g. Debilitation
   h. Malnutrition or dehydration

Clinical Significance

2. Even after recovery from anesthesia, respiratory effort is reduced owing to fatigue, pain, and immobility. These effects—particularly in combination with one or more of the listed risk factors—increase a client's risk of postoperative respiratory problems.

Interventions

1. Auscultate the lung fields for diminished and abnormal breath sounds.

2. Take measures to prevent aspiration:
   a. Position the client on his side with pillows supporting the back and the knees slightly flexed.
   b. Keep the bed flat.
3. Reinforce preoperative client teaching on the importance of turning, coughing, and deep breathing and leg exercises every 1 to 2 hours.
4. Promote the following:
   a. Breathing exercises
   b. Splinting the incision site
   c. Frequent turning
   d. Leg exercises
   e. Incentive spirometry, if indicated
5. Encourage adequate oral fluid intake, as indicated.

Rationale

1. Presence of rales indicates retained secretions. Diminished breath sounds may indicate atelectasis.
2. In the postoperative period, decreased sensorium and hypoventilation contribute to increased risk of aspiration.

3. Postoperative pain may discourage compliance; reinforcing the importance of these measures may improve compliance.
4. Exercises and movement promote lung expansion and mobilization of secretions. Incentive spirometry promotes deep breathing by providing a visual indicator of the effectiveness of the breathing effort.

5. Adequate hydration liquefies secretions, enabling easier expectoration, and prevents stasis of secretions, which provide a medium for microorganism growth. It also helps decrease blood viscosity, which reduces the risk of clot formation.

▲ **Documentation**

Flow record
    Temperature
    Respiratory rate and rhythm
    Breath sounds
    Respiratory treatments and client's response
Progress notes
    Unsatisfactory response to respiratory treatments

▲ **Outcome Criteria**

The client will demonstrate healing with evidence of intact, approximated wound edges or granulation tissue.

Potential for Infection related to increased susceptibility to bacteria secondary to wound

Focus Assessment Criteria

1. Surgical site and drains
2. Type and progression of wound healing
3. Signs of infection or delayed healing

Clinical Significance

1–3. Surgical interruption of skin integrity disrupts the body's first line of defense against infection and allows direct entry of microorganisms. In most cases, a surgical wound should close within 24 hours by primary intention.

Interventions

1. Monitor for signs and symptoms of wound infection:
   a. Increased swelling and redness
   b. Wound separation
   c. Increased or purulent drainage
   d. Prolonged subnormal temperature or significantly elevated temperature

Rationale

1. Tissue responds to pathogen infiltration with increased blood and lymph flow (manifested by edema, redness, and increased drainage) and reduced epithelialization (marked by wound separation). Circulating pathogens trigger the hypothalamus to elevate the body temperature; certain pathogens cannot survive at higher temperatures.

Interventions

2. Monitor wound healing by noting the following:
   a. Evidence of intact, approximated wound edges (primary intention)
   b. Evidence of granulation tissue (secondary and tertiary intention)

3. Teach the client about factors that can delay wound healing:
   a. Dehydrated wound tissue

   b. Wound infection

   c. Inadequate nutrition and hydration

   d. Compromised blood supply

   e. Increased stress or excessive activity

4. Take steps to prevent infection:
   a. Wash hands before and after dressing changes.
   b. Wear gloves until the wound is sealed.
   c. Thoroughly clean the area around drainage tubes.
   d. Keep tubing away from the incision.
   e. Discard unused irrigation solutions after 24 hours.

5. Explain when a dressing is indicated for wounds healing by primary intention and by secondary intention.

6. Minimize skin irritation by the following means:
   a. Using the least amount of tape possible or using Montgomery straps, if indicated
   b. Changing saturated dressings often

7. Protect the wound and surrounding skin from drainage by these methods:
   a. Using a collection pouch, if indicated
   b. Applying a skin barrier

8. Teach and assist the client in the following:
   a. Supporting the surgical site when moving
   b. Splinting the area when coughing, sneezing, or vomiting
   c. Reducing flatus accumulation

9. Consult with an enterostomal or a clinical nurse specialist for specific skin care measures.

Rationale

2. A surgical wound with edges approximated by sutures usually heals by primary intention. Granulation tissue is not visible and scar formation is minimal. In contrast, a surgical wound with a drain or an abscess heals by secondary intention or granulation, with more distinct scar formation. A restructured wound heals by third intention and results in a wider and deeper scar.

3.
   a. Studies report that epithelial migration is impeded under dry crust; movement is three times faster over moist tissue.
   b. The exudate in infected wounds impairs epithelialization and wound closure.
   c. To repair tissue, the body needs increased protein and carbohydrate intake and adequate hydration for vascular transport of oxygen and wastes.
   d. Blood supply to injured tissue must be adequate to transport leukocytes and remove wastes.
   e. Increased stress and activity result in higher levels of chalone, a mitotic inhibitor that depresses epidermal regeneration.

4. These measures help prevent introduction of microorganisms into the wound, and they also reduce the risk of transmitting infection to others.

5. A wound healing by primary intention requires a dressing to protect it from contamination until the edges seal (usually 24 hours). A wound healing by secondary intention requires a dressing to maintain adequate hydration; the dressing is not needed after wound edges seal.

6. Preventing skin irritation eliminates a potential source of microorganism entry.

7. Protecting the skin can help minimize excoriation by acid drainage. A semipermeable skin barrier provides a moist environment for healing and prevents entry of bacteria.

8. A wound typically requires 3 weeks for strong scar formation. Stress on the suture line before this occurs can cause disruption.

9. Management of a complex wound or impaired healing requires expert nursing consultation.

▲ *Documentation*

Flow record
   Wound care
      Evidence of healing
Progress notes
   Abnormal wound condition
      (e.g., signs of infection, drainage)

▲ *Outcome Criterion*

The client will report progressive reduction of pain and an increase in activity.

Impaired Physical Mobility related to surgical interruption of body structures, flatus, and immobility

Focus Assessment Criteria

1. Source of the pain, such as:
   a. Surgical site
   b. Chest tube site
   c. Invasive line
   d. Generalized discomfort
   e. Angina
   f. Flatus
2. Severity of pain, based on a scale of 0 to 10 (0 = no pain; 10 = the most severe pain), rated as follows:
   a. At its best
   b. At its worst
   c. After each pain relief measure
3. Physical signs of pain, e.g., increased heart and respiratory rates, elevated blood pressure, restlessness, facial grimacing, guarding)

4. Factors that influence pain tolerance:
   a. Knowledge of pain and its cause
   b. Meaning of pain
   c. Ability to control pain
   d. Energy level
   e. Stress level
   f. Cultural background
   g. Response of others

Clinical Significance

1. Postoperative surgical site pain results from destruction of nerves and tissue during surgery. When assessing a client's pain, you must try to differentiate between postoperative incision pain and the discomfort stemming from flatus or immobility, in order to intervene appropriately.
2. Such a rating scale provides an objective means of evaluating the subjective experience of pain.

3. Clients experience and express pain in different ways; some are reluctant to verbalize pain or request pain medications. Objective signs may alert the nurse to such a client's pain.
4. Pain tolerance refers to the duration and the intensity of pain that a client is willing to endure. Pain tolerance differs greatly among clients and also may vary in an individual client in different situations.

Interventions

1. Collaborate with the client to determine effective pain relief interventions.

2. Express your acceptance of the client's pain. Acknowledge the pain's presence, listen attentively to his complaints, and convey that you are assessing the pain because you want to understand it better, not because you are trying to determine whether it really exists.
3. Reduce the client's fear and clear up any misinformation by doing the following:
   a. Teaching what to expect; describing the sensation as precisely as possible, including how long it should last
   b. Explaining pain relief methods, such as distraction, heat application, and progressive relaxation
4. Explain the difference between involuntary physiological responses and voluntary behavioral responses regarding drug use.
   a. Involuntary physiological responses:
      • Drug tolerance is a physiological phenomenon in which, after repeated doses, the prescribed dose begins to lose its effectiveness.

Rationale

1. A client experiencing pain may feel a loss of control over his body and his life. Collaboration can help minimize this feeling.
2. A client who feels the need to convince health care providers that he actually is experiencing pain is likely to have increased anxiety, which can lead to increased pain.

3. A client who is prepared for a painful procedure with a detailed explanation of the sensations that he will feel usually experiences less stress and pain than a client who receives vague or no explanations.

4. Many clients and families are misinformed regarding the nature and risks of drug addiction and consequently may be reluctant to request pain medication.

Interventions   *Rationale*

- Physical dependence is a physiological state that results from repeated administration of a drug. Withdrawal is experienced if the drug is abruptly discontinued. Tapering down the drug dosage helps manage withdrawal symptoms.

b. Voluntary behavioral responses:
- Drug abuse is the use of a drug in any manner that deviates from culturally acceptable medical and social uses (McCafferty, 1979). Addiction is a behavioral pattern of drug use characterized by overwhelming involvement with the use of the drug and the securing of its supply, and the high tendency to relapse after withdrawal (Jaffe, 1975).

5. Provide the client with privacy for his or her pain experience; e.g., close curtains and room door, ask others to leave the room.

5. Privacy allows the client to express pain in his or her own manner, which can help reduce anxiety and ease pain.

6. Provide optimal pain relief with prescribed analgesics:

6.

   a. Determine the preferred administration route—by mouth, intramuscular, intravenous, or rectal. Consult with the physician.

   a. The proper administration route optimizes the efficacy of pain medications. The oral route is preferred in most cases; for some drugs, the liquid dosage form may be given to a client who has difficulty swallowing. If frequent injections are necessary, the intravenous (IV) route is preferred to minimize pain and maximize absorption; however, IV administration may produce more profound side effects than other routes.

   b. Assess vital signs—especially respiratory rate—before and after administering any narcotic agent.

   b. Narcotics can depress the respiratory center of the brain.

   c. Consult with a pharmacist regarding possible adverse interactions between the prescribed drug and other medications the patient is taking, e.g., muscle relaxants, tranquilizers.

   c. Some medications potentiate the effects of narcotics; identifying such medications before administration can prevent excessive sedation.

   d. Take a preventive approach to pain medication; i.e., administer medication before activity (e.g., ambulation) to enhance participation (but be sure to evaluate the hazards of sedation); instruct the client to request pain medication as needed before the pain becomes severe.

   d. The preventive approach may reduce the total 24-hour dose as compared to the p.r.n. approach; it also provides a more constant blood drug level, reduces the client's craving for the drug, and eliminates the anxiety associated with having to ask for and wait for p.r.n. relief.

   e. After administering pain medication, return in ½ hour to evaluate its effectiveness.

   e. Each client responds differently to pain medication; careful monitoring is needed to assess individual response. For example, too often every surgical client is expected to respond to 50 mg of meperidine (Demerol) every 3 to 4 hr regardless of body size, type of surgery, or previous experiences.

7. Explain and assist with noninvasive and nonpharmacological pain relief measures:
   a. Splinting the incision site
   b. Proper positioning
   c. Distraction
   d. Breathing exercises

7. These measures can help reduce pain by substituting another stimulus to prevent painful stimuli from reaching higher brain centers. In addition, relaxation reduces muscle tension and may help increase the client's sense of control over the pain.

Interventions

    e. Massage

    f. Heat and cold application

    g. Relaxation techniques

8. Progress the client to ambulating without assistance if possible:

    a. Assist to sitting position with legs dangling.

    b. Assess ability to walk and need for assistance (one or two persons, walker, cane).

    c. Explain the projected distance to be ambulated.

    d. Instruct to report weakness or vertigo and to take deep breaths during activity.

    e. Progress from out of bed to a chair at bedside, to walking to chair across room, to walking in hall with assistance.

9. Teach the client to expel flatus by the following measures:

    a. Walking as soon as possible after surgery

    b. Changing positions regularly, as possible, e.g., lying prone, assuming the knee–chest position.

Rationale

8. Walking will increase venous return, prevent venous stasis, expand lung tissue and reduce the incidence of atelectasis.

9. Postoperatively, sluggish peristalsis results in accumulation of nonabsorbable gas. Pain occurs when unaffected bowel segments contract in an attempt to expel gas. Activity speeds the return of peristalsis and the expulsion of flatus; proper positioning helps gas rise for expulsion.

▲ Documentation

Medication administration record
  Type, route, and dosage schedule of all prescribed medications
Progress notes
  Unsatisfactory relief from pain-relief measures

▲ Outcome Criteria

The client will resume ingestion of the daily nutritional requirements, which include the following:

1. Selections from the four basic food groups
2. 2000 to 3000 mL of fluids
3. Adequate fiber, vitamins, and minerals

Potential Altered Nutrition: Less than Body Requirements, related to increased protein and vitamin requirements for wound healing and decreased intake secondary to pain, nausea, vomiting, and diet restrictions

Focus Assessment Criteria	*Clinical Significance*
1. Nutritional status (intake, weight)	1. Wound healing requires sufficient intake of protein, carbohydrates, vitamins, and minerals for fibroblast formation and granulation tissue and collagen production.

2. Presence of the following:
  a. Bowel sounds
  b. Nausea
  c. Vomiting
  d. Flatus
	2. Gastrointestinal (GI) function is impaired by many surgeries, anesthesia, oral intake restrictions, and immobility. The more rapidly a client resumes his normal diet postoperatively, the more quickly normal GI function will return.

Interventions

1. Explain the need for an optimal daily nutritional intake, including these items:

    a. Increased protein and carbohydrate intake

    b. Increased intake of vitamins A, B, B_2, B_6, B_{12}, C, D, and E and niacin

    c. Adequate intake of minerals (zinc, magnesium, calcium, copper)

2. Take measures to reduce pain:

    a. Plan care so that painful or unpleasant procedures are not scheduled before mealtimes.

    b. Administer pain medication ½ hour before meals, as ordered.

3. Explain the possible causes of the client's nausea and vomiting:

    a. Side effects of preoperative medications and anesthesia

Rationale

1. Understanding the importance of optimal nutrition may encourage the client to comply with the dietary regimen.

2. Pain causes fatigue, which can reduce appetite.

3. The client's understanding of the source and normalcy of nausea and vomiting can reduce anxiety, which may help reduce symptoms.

Interventions

    b. Surgical procedure
    c. Obesity
    d. Electrolyte imbalance
    e. Gastric distention
    f. Too-rapid or strenuous movement
Reassure the client that these symptoms are normal.

4. Take steps to reduce nausea and vomiting:
    a. Restrict fluids before meals and large amounts of fluids at any time; instead, encourage the client to ingest small amounts of ice chips or cool clear liquids (e.g., dilute tea, Jell-o water, flat ginger ale or cola) frequently, unless vomiting persists.
    b. Teach the client to move slowly.

    c. Reduce or eliminate unpleasant sights and odors.
    d. Provide good mouth care after the client vomits.
    e. Teach deep breathing techniques.

    f. Instruct the client to avoid lying down flat for at least 2 hours after eating. (A client who must rest should sit or recline with his head at least 4 inches higher than his feet.)
    g. Ensure patency of any nasogastric (NG) tube.
    h. Teach the client to practice relaxation exercises during episodes of nausea.

5. Maintain good oral hygiene at all times.

6. Administer an antiemetic agent before meals, if indicated.

Rationale

4.
    a. Gastric distention from fluid ingestion can trigger the vagal visceral afferent pathways that stimulate the medulla oblongata (vomiting center).

    b. Rapid movements stimulate the vomiting center by triggering vestibulocerebellar afferents.
    c. Noxious odors and sights can stimulate the vomiting center.
    d. Good oral care reduces the noxious taste.

    e. Deep breaths can help excrete the anesthetic agent.
    f. Pressure on the stomach can trigger vagal visceral afferent stimulation of the vomiting center in the brain.

    g. A malfunctioning NG tube can cause gastric distention.
    h. Concentrating on relaxation activities may help block stimulation of the vomiting center.

5. A clean, refreshed mouth can stimulate appetite.

6. Antiemetics prevent nausea and vomiting.

▲ **Documentation**

Flow record
    Intake (amount, type, time)
    Vomiting (amount, description)

▲ **Outcome Criteria**

The client will resume effective preoperative bowel function.

Potential Colonic Constipation related to decreased peristalsis secondary to immobility and effects of anesthesia and narcotics

Focus Assessment Criteria	*Clinical Significance*

1. Preoperative and postoperative elimination patterns
2. Abdominal status:
    a. Distention
    b. Bowel sounds
	1,2. Postoperatively, decreased GI motility can result from disruption of autonomic innervation due to stress, surgical manipulation of the intestine, immobility, and the effects of medications. Preoperative elimination patterns and postoperative abdominal status serve as criteria for assessing bowel function.

Interventions

1. Assess bowel sounds to determine when to introduce liquids. Allow the client to progress to solid food when liquids are tolerated.

Rationale

1. Presence of bowel sounds indicates return of peristalsis.

Interventions

2. Explain the effects of daily activity on elimination. Assist with ambulation when possible.

3. Promote factors that contribute to optimal elimination.
   a. Balanced diet:
      • Review a list of foods high in bulk, e.g., fresh fruits with skins, bran, nuts and seeds, whole grain breads and cereals, cooked fruits and vegetables, and fruit juices.
      • Discuss dietary preferences.
      • Encourage intake of approximately 800 g of fruits and vegetables (about four pieces of fresh fruit and a large salad) for normal daily bowel movement.
   b. Adequate fluid intake:
      • Encourage intake of at least 8 to 10 glasses (about 2000 mL) daily, unless contraindicated.
      • Discuss fluid preferences.
      • Set up a regular schedule for fluid intake.
   c. Regular time for defecation:
      • Identify the normal defecation pattern before the onset of constipation.
      • Review daily routine.
      • Include time for defecation as part of the regular daily routine.
      • Discuss a suitable time, based on responsibilities, availability of facilities, and so on.
      • Suggest that the client attempt defecation about 1 hour following a meal and remain in the bathroom a suitable length of time.
   d. Simulation of the home environment:
      • Have the client use the bathroom instead of a bedpan, if possible; offer a bedpan or a bedside commode if the client cannot use the bathroom.
      • Assist into position on the toilet, commode, or bedpan if necessary.
      • Provide privacy; e.g., close the door, draw curtains around the bed, play a TV or radio to mask sounds, make room deodorizer available.
      • Provide for comfort (e.g., provide reading materials as a diversion) and safety (e.g., make a call bell readily available).
   e. Proper positioning:
      • Assist the client to a normal semi-squatting position on the toilet or commode, if possible.
      • Assist onto a bedpan if necessary, elevating the head of the bed to high Fowler's position or to the elevation permitted.
      • Stress the need to avoid straining during defecation efforts.

4. Notify the physician if bowel sounds do not return within 6 to 10 hours or if elimination does not return within 2 to 3 days postoperatively.

Rationale

2. Activity influences bowel elimination by improving abdominal muscle tone and stimulating appetite and peristalsis.

3.
   a. A well-balanced diet high in fiber content stimulates peristalsis.

   b. Sufficient fluid intake is necessary to maintain bowel patterns and promote proper stool consistency.

   c. Taking advantage of circadian rhythms may aid in establishing a regular defecation schedule.

   d. Privacy and a sense of normalcy can promote relaxation, which can enhance defecation.

   e. Proper positioning uses the abdominal muscles and the force of gravity to aid defecation. Straining can activate Valsalva's response, which may lead to reduced cardiac output.

4. Absence of bowel sounds may indicate paralytic ileus; absence of bowel movements may indicate obstruction.

▲ **Documentation**

Flow record
   Bowel movements
   Bowel sounds

▲ *Outcome Criteria*

The client will increase tolerance to activities of daily living (ADLs), as evidenced by the following:

1. Progressive ambulation
2. Ability to perform ADLs

Activity Intolerance related to limited mobility and weakness secondary to anesthesia, tissue hypoxia, and insufficient fluids and nutrients

Focus Assessment Criteria	*Clinical Significance*
1. Degree of activity progression	1,2. Surgery, NPO status, and pain can compromise a client's energy and ability to participate in ADLs. The client should demonstrate steady activity progression.
2. Response to activity	

Interventions

1. Encourage progress in the client's activity level each shift, as indicated:

   a. Allow the client's legs to dangle first; support him from the side.
   b. Place the bed in high position and raise the head of the bed.
   c. Increase the client's time out of bed by 15 minutes each time. Allow him to set a comfortable rate of ambulation, and agree on a distance goal for each shift.
   d. Encourage the client to increase activity when pain is at a minimum or after pain relief measures take effect.

2. Increase the client's self-care activities from partial to complete self-care, as indicated.

3. If the client is not progressing at the expected or desired rate, do the following:
   a. Take vital signs prior to activity
   b. Repeat vital sign assessment after activity
   c. Repeat again after the client has rested for 3 minutes.
   d. Assess for abnormal responses to increased activity:
      • Decreased pulse rate
      • Decreased or unchanged systolic blood pressure
      • Excessively increased or decreased respiratory rate
      • Failure of pulse to return to near the resting rate within 3 minutes after discontinuing activity
      • Complaints of confusion or vertigo
      • Uncoordinated movements

▲ *Documentation*

Flow record
    Vital signs
    Ambulation (time, amount)
Progress notes
    Abnormal or unexpected response to increased activity

4. Plan regular rest periods according to the client's daily schedule.
5. Identify and encourage the client's progress. Keep a record of progress, particularly for a client who is progressing slowly.

Rationale

1. A gradual increase in activity allows the client's cardiopulmonary system to return to its preoperative state without excessive strain.
   a. Dangling the legs helps minimize orthostatic hypotension.
   b. Raising the head of the bed helps reduce stress on suture lines.
   c. Gradual increases toward mutually established, realistic goals can promote compliance and prevent overexertion.

2. The client's participation in self-care improves his physiological functioning and reduces fatigue from inactivity, and also improves his sense of self-esteem and well-being.

3. Activity tolerance depends on the client's ability to adapt to the physiological requirements of increased activity. The expected immediate physiological responses to activity are increased pulse rate and amplitude, increased systolic blood pressure, and increased respiratory rate and depth. After 3 minutes, pulse rate should decrease to within 10 beats/minute of the client's usual resting rate. Abnormal findings represent the body's inability to meet the increased oxygen demands imposed by activity.

4. Regular rest periods allow the body to conserve and restore energy.
5. Encouragement and realization of progress can give the client an incentive for continued progression.

▲ *Outcome Criteria*

The outcome criteria for this diagnosis represent those associated with discharge planning. Refer to the discharge criteria.

Potential Altered Health Maintenance related to insufficient knowledge of care of operative site, restrictions (diet, activity), medications, signs and symptoms of complications, and follow-up care

Focus Assessment Criteria	*Clinical Significance*
1. Readiness and ability to learn and retain information	1. A client or family failing to achieve learning goals requires a referral for assistance post-discharge.

Interventions

1. As appropriate, explain and demonstrate care of an uncomplicated surgical wound:
   a. Washing with soap and water
   b. Dressing changes using clean technique

2. As appropriate, explain and demonstrate care of a complicated surgical wound:
   a. Aseptic technique
   b. Handwashing before and after dressing changes
   c. Avoiding touching the inner surface of the soiled dressing and discarding it in a sealed plastic bag
   d. The use of sterile hemostats, if indicated
   e. Wound assessment—condition and drainage
   f. Wound cleaning
   g. T-tube care, if indicated
   h. Dressing reapplication

3. Reinforce activity restrictions, as indicated, e.g., bending, lifting.

4. Explain the importance of the following:
   a. Avoiding ill persons and crowds
   b. Drinking 8 to 10 glasses of fluid daily
   c. Maintaining a balanced diet

5. Review with the client and family the purpose, dosage, administration, and side effects of all prescribed medications.

6. Teach the client and family to watch for and report signs and symptoms of possible complications:
   a. Persistent temperature elevation
   b. Difficulty breathing, chest pain
   c. Change in sputum characteristics
   d. Increasing weakness, fatigue, pain, or abdominal distention
   e. Wound changes, e.g., separation, unusual or increased drainage, increased redness or swelling
   f. Voiding difficulties, burning on urination, urinary frequency, or cloudy, foul-smelling urine
   g. Pain, swelling, and warmth in the calf
   h. Other signs and symptoms of complications specific to the surgical procedure performed

7. Whenever possible, provide written instructions.

8. Evaluate the client's and family's understanding of the information provided.

Rationale

1. Uncomplicated wounds have sealed edges after 24 hours and therefore do not require aseptic technique or a dressing; however, a dressing may be applied if the wound is at risk for injury.

2. Aseptic technique is necessary to prevent wound contamination during dressing changes. Handwashing helps prevent contamination of the wound and the spread of infection. Proper handling and disposal of contaminated dressings helps prevent infection transmission. Daily assessment is necessary to evaluate healing and detect complications.

3. Avoiding certain activities decreases the risk of wound dehiscence before scar formation occurs (usually after 3 weeks).

4. Wound healing requires optimal nutrition, hydration, and rest, as well as avoiding potential sources of infection.

5. Complete understanding can help prevent drug administration errors.

6. Early detection and reporting of danger signs and symptoms enable prompt intervention to minimize the severity of complications.

7. Written instructions provide an information resource for use at home.

8. Knowledge gaps may indicate the need for a referral for assistance at home.

▲ *Documentation*

Flow records
    Discharge instructions
    Follow-up instructions
Discharge summary record
    Status at discharge (pain, activity, wound healing)
    Achievement of goals (individual or family)

References/Bibliography

Association of Operating Room Nurses. (1986). *AORN standards and recommended practices for perioperative nursing.* Denver: AORN.

Cassidy, V.R., & Oddi, L.F. (1986). Legal and ethical aspects of informed consent: A nursing research perspective. *Journal of Professional Nursing, 2*(6), 343–349.

Douglas, S., & Larson, E. (1986). There's more to informed consent than information. *Focus on Critical Care, 13*(2), 43–47.

Hathaway, D. (1985). Effect of preoperative teaching on postoperative pain: A replication and explanation. *International Journal of Nursing Studies, 22*(3), 267–280.

Jaffe, J.H. (1975). Drug addiction and drug abuse. In L.S. Goodman & A. Gilman (Eds.). *Goodman and Gilman's pharmacological basis of therapeutics* (5th ed.). New York: Macmillan.

McCafferty, M. (1979). *Nursing management.* Philadelphia: J.B. Lippincott.

Schecter, N. (1987). Pain: Acknowledging it, assessing it, treating it. *Contemporary Pediatrics, 4*(7), 16–46.

Vaughn, J.B., & Nemcek, M.A. (1986). Postoperative flatulence: Causes and remedies. *Today's OR Nurse, 8*(10), 19–23.

Ziemer, M.M. (1983). Effects of information on postsurgical coping. *Nursing Research, 32*(5), 282–287.

This diagnostic cluster represents the standard of care applying to all clients and families undergoing outpatient surgery. (*Note:* The postoperative nursing diagnoses listed in the following diagnostic cluster, as well as their applicable interventions and rationales, are the same as those in Appendix II, Generic Care Plan for Surgical Clients. Please refer to Appendix II for more information.)

Diagnostic Cluster

▲ **Discharge Criteria**

Before discharge, the client or family will:

1. Describe any at-home activity restrictions
2. Describe at-home wound and pain management
3. Discuss fluid and nutritional requirements for proper wound healing
4. List the signs and symptoms that must be reported to a health care professional
5. Describe necessary follow-up care

PREOPERATIVE
Nursing Diagnosis

Fear related to scheduled outpatient surgery and insufficient knowledge of preparation, routines, and postoperative condition

POSTOPERATIVE
Collaborative Problems

Potential Complications:
Hemorrhage
Hypovolemia/Shock

Nursing Diagnoses

Potential Altered Respiratory Function related to immobility secondary to postanesthesia state and pain

Potential for Infection related to increased bacteria secondary to wound

Impaired Physical Mobility related to surgical interruption of body structures, flatus, and immobility

Potential Altered Health Maintenance related to insufficient knowledge of operative site care, diet and activity restrictions, medications, signs and symptoms of complications, and follow-up care

Preoperative: Nursing Diagnosis

▲ **Outcome Criteria**

The client will:

1. Discuss preadmission requirements
2. Relate what he can expect before and after surgery

Fear related to scheduled outpatient surgery and insufficient knowledge of preparation, routines, and postoperative condition

Focus Assessment Criteria

1. Specific stressors and nature of concerns

2. Past experiences or knowledge regarding surgery
3. Understanding of the planned surgical procedure
4. Available support system

5. Anxiety level:
   a. Mild (alert and aware of the situation, learning and coping abilities intact)
   b. Moderate (physical signs present—e.g., increased pulse rate, muscle tremors; concentration difficult)
   c. Severe (more overt signs present—hyperventilation, tachycardia, etc.; perception greatly altered; learning and coping severely impaired)
   d. Panic (hyperactivity and other overt physical signs present, perception completely distorted, learning and coping impossible)
6. Readiness and ability to learn and retain information

Clinical Significance

1. Every client experiences some emotional reaction to surgery; the nature and degree of this reaction depend on how the client perceives the surgery and its anticipated effects—physical, psychological, financial, social, occupational, spiritual.
2,3. Accurate knowledge of the planned procedure and care routines can help reduce anxiety and fear related to the unknown.

4. Adequate support from family, friends, and other sources can help the client cope with surgery.
5. Extreme anxiety impairs client's learning and coping abilities.

6. A client or family failing to achieve learning goals requires a referral for assistance postdischarge.

Interventions

1. Provide reassurance and comfort; stay with the client, encourage him to share his feelings and concerns, listen attentively, and convey a sense of empathy and understanding.
2. Correct any misconceptions and inaccurate information the client has about the procedure.

3. Notify the physician if the client needs any further explanations about the procedure; beforehand, the physician should explain the following:
   a. Nature of the surgery
   b. Reason for and expected outcome of surgery
   c. Any risks involved
   d. Type of anesthetis that is to be used
   e. Expected length of recovery and any postoperative restrictions and instructions

Rationale

1. Providing emotional support and encouraging sharing may help the client clarify and verbalize his fears, allowing the nurse to provide realistic feedback and reassurance.
2. Modifiable contributing factors to anxiety include incomplete and inaccurate information. Providing accurate information and correcting misconceptions may help eliminate fears and reduce anxiety.
3. The physician is responsible for explaining the surgery to the client and family; the nurse, for determining their level of understanding and then notifying the physician of the need to provide more information.

Interventions

4. Contact the physician if the client exhibits severe or panic anxiety.

5. Provide the client and family with the following information:
   a. Time to report for surgery
   b. Nothing-by-mouth (NPO) requirements
   c. Expected preadmission testing, health history, and physical assessment
   d. The need to bring any test results to the unit on the day of surgery
   e. The need to be accompanied by a responsible adult
   f. The importance of leaving valuables at home

6. Explain preoperative routines:
   a. Vital sign measurement
   b. Removal of eye glasses, contact lenses, jewelry, and dentures
   c. Administration of preoperative medications

7. Explain expected postoperative routines and sensations, including the following, as applicable:

   a. Parenteral fluid administration

   b. Vital sign monitoring

   c. Dressing checks and changes

   d. Nasogastric (NG) tube insertion and care

   e. Indwelling (Foley) catheter insertion and care

   f. Symptoms including nausea, vomiting, and pain, and the availability of analgesics and antiemetics

8. As applicable, teach the client (using return demonstration to ensure understanding and ability) how to do the following:
   a. Turn, cough, and deep-breathe
   b. Support the incision site while coughing
   c. Change position in bed every 1 to 2 hours
   d. Sit up, get out of bed, and ambulate as soon as possible after surgery (prolonged sitting should be avoided)

9. Involve family members or significant others in all client teaching, as appropriate.

10. Explain important hospital policies to family members or significant others, e.g., visiting

Rationale

4. Immediate notification enables prompt assessment and possible pharmacological intervention.

5,6. This information can help relieve anxiety and fear associated with lack of knowledge of necessary preoperative activities and routines.

7. Explaining what the client can expect, why the procedures are done, and why certain sensations may occur can help reduce fears associated with the unknown and unexpected.
   a. Parenteral fluids replace fluids lost from NPO state and blood loss.
   b. Careful monitoring is needed to determine status and track any changes.
   c. Until wound edges heal, the wound must be protected from contaminants.
   d. An NG tube promotes drainage and reduces abdominal distention and tension on the suture line.
   e. A Foley catheter drains the bladder until muscle tone returns as anesthesia is excreted.
   f. Nausea and vomiting are common side effects of preoperative medications and anesthesia; other contributing factors include certain types of surgery, obesity, electrolyte imbalance, rapid position changes, and psychological and environmental factors. Pain commonly occurs as medications lose their effectiveness.

8. Again, the client's understanding of care measures can help reduce anxiety associated with the unknown. Teaching the client about postoperative routines before surgery ensures that his understanding is not impaired by the continuing effects of sedation postoperatively.

9. Knowledgeable family members and significant others can serve as "coaches" to remind the client of postoperative instructions and restrictions.

10. Providing family members and significant others with this information can help reduce

Interventions

hours, number of visitors allowed at one time, location of waiting rooms, how the physician will contact them after surgery.

11. Explain the factors evaluated to determine a client's readiness for discharge:
    a. Physiological stability (vital signs, hydration status, and respiratory function)
    b. Level of orientation
    c. Drainage at operative site
    d. Degree of pain
    e. Degree of nausea and vomiting
    f. Ability to ambulate
    g. Ability to void

12. If indicated, explain the possibility that the client may require an overnight stay.

13. If appropriate, suggest that the client's young children stay with relatives or friends for the first 1 or 2 days after the client's discharge to home.

Rationale

their anxiety and allow them to support the client better.

11. This information can help reassure the client and support persons that discharge is to be delayed until the client's physiological status indicates readiness.

12. If the client needs more time to recover from anesthesia and return to his preoperative level of functioning, discharge is postponed until the next day. Explaining this possibility can offer reassurance.

13. The client is likely to need plenty of rest for the first few days after discharge. A client with young children may benefit from having them stay elsewhere during this period.

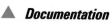 **Documentation**

Progress notes
  Unusual interactions
Discharge summary record
  Client teaching
  Achievement or status of
    outcome criteria

Clinical Situations

Abdominal aortic aneurysm resection, 351–353
Acquired immunodeficiency syndrome, 312–320
Acute renal failure, 180–184
Amputation, 355–362
Anticoagulant therapy, 507–509
Arterial bypass grafting in the lower extremity, 364–367
Arteriography, 510–513
Atherosclerosis, 78–83

Cancer (end-stage), 330–341
Cancer (initial diagnosis), 322–329
Cardiac catheterization, 514–517
Carotid endarterectomy, 369–372
Casts, 518–523
Cataract extraction, 373–379
Cerebrovascular accident, 202–211
Cesium implant, 524–531
Chemotherapy, 532–541
Chronic obstructive pulmonary disease, 96
Chronic renal failure, 185–194
Cirrhosis, 110–115
Colostomy, 380–390
Congestive heart failure, 57–59
Corneal transplant, 461–466
Coronary artery bypass grafting, 392–401
Corticosteroid therapy, 542–546
Cranial surgery, 402–407

Deep venous thrombosis, 70–73
Diabetes mellitus, 116–133

End-stage cancer, 330–341
Enteral nutrition, 548–553
Enucleation, 408–417
External arteriovenous shunting, 555–558
Extracorporeal renal surgery, 484–486

Fractured hip and femur, 418–423
Fractures, 288–290

Gastroenteritis, 158–160
Glaucoma, 260–264

Hemodialysis, 559–564
Hemodynamic monitoring, 565–570
Hepatitis (viral), 134–136
Hypertension, 74–77
Hypothyroidism, 137–141
Hysterectomy, 424–428

Ileostomy, 429–440
Immobility, 243–249
Infectious arthritis, 296–305
Inflammatory bowel disease, 161–172
Inflammatory joint disease, 296–305

Laminectomy, 441–444
Laryngectomy, 445–446
Leukemia, 342–347
Long-term venous access devices, 572–576

Mastectomy, 447–451
Mechanical ventilation, 577–581
Multiple sclerosis, 213–218
Myocardial infarction, 60–69

Nephrectomy, 484–486
Nephrostomy, 484–486
Neurogenic bladder, 250–258

Obesity, 142–148
Ophthalmic surgery, 452–459
Osteoporosis, 291–295

Pacemaker insertion, 582–588
Pancreatitis, 149–155
Parkinson's disease, 219–222
Penetrating keratoplasty, 461–466
Peptic ulcer disease, 173–177
Percutaneous transluminal coronary angioplasty, 590–595
Peripheral arterial disease, 78–83
Peritoneal dialysis, 597–603
Pneumonia, 104–108
Pressure ulcers, 266–272
Prostatectomy, 467–471

Radiation therapy, 605–612
Radical neck dissection, 472–477
Radical vulvectomy, 478–483
Raynaud's syndrome, 85–88
Renal calculi, 195–199
Renal surgery, 484–486
Rheumatoid arthritis, 296–305

Seizure disorders, 223–227
Spinal cord injury, 227–241
Stroke, 202–211
Systemic lupus erythematosus, 308–311

Thermal injuries, 274–285
Thoracic surgery, 487–491
Total joint replacement (hip, knee), 492–495
Total parenteral nutrition, 613–617
Tracheostomy, 618–624

Unconsciousness, 243–249
Ureteral stents, 484–486
Urolithiasis, 195–199
Urostomy, 496–503

Venous stasis ulcers, 89–92

Nursing Diagnoses

Collaborative Problems*

* The prefix Potential Complications (PC) has been omitted for easier use of the index only.

* The prefix Potential Complications (PC) has been omitted for easier use of the index only.

* The prefix Potential Complications (PC) has been omitted for easier use of the index only.

* The prefix Potential Complications (PC) has been omitted for easier use of the index only.

* The prefix Potential Complications (PC) has been omitted for easier use of the index only.

Index

Page numbers in *italics* indicate figures; those followed by *t* indicate tabular material.